Advances in Intelligent Systems and Computing

Volume 1431

The series "Advances in Intelligent Systems and Computing" contains publications on theory, applications, and design methods of Intelligent Systems and Intelligent Computing. Virtually all disciplines such as engineering, natural sciences, computer and information science, ICT, economics, business, e-commerce, environment, healthcare, life science are covered. The list of topics spans all the areas of modern intelligent systems and computing such as: computational intelligence, soft computing including neural networks, fuzzy systems, evolutionary computing and the fusion of these paradigms, social intelligence, ambient intelligence, computational neuroscience, artificial life, virtual worlds and society, cognitive science and systems, Perception and Vision, DNA and immune based systems, self-organizing and adaptive systems, e-Learning and teaching, human-centered and human-centric computing, recommender systems, intelligent control, robotics and mechatronics including human-machine teaming, knowledge-based paradigms, learning paradigms, machine ethics, intelligent data analysis, knowledge management, intelligent agents, intelligent decision making and support, intelligent network security, trust management, interactive entertainment, Web intelligence and multimedia.

The publications within "Advances in Intelligent Systems and Computing" are primarily proceedings of important conferences, symposia and congresses. They cover significant recent developments in the field, both of a foundational and applicable character. An important characteristic feature of the series is the short publication time and world-wide distribution. This permits a rapid and broad dissemination of research results.

Indexed by DBLP, INSPEC, WTI Frankfurt eG, zbMATH, Japanese Science and Technology Agency (JST).

All books published in the series are submitted for consideration in Web of Science.

For proposals from Asia please contact Aninda Bose (aninda.bose@springer.com).

More information about this series at https://link.springer.com/bookseries/11156

Kevin Daimi · Abeer Al Sadoon
Editors

Proceedings of the ICR'22 International Conference on Innovations in Computing Research

Springer

Editors
Kevin Daimi
University of Detroit Mercy
Detroit, MI, USA

Abeer Al Sadoon
Kent Institute Australia
Sydney, NSW, Australia

ISSN 2194-5357 ISSN 2194-5365 (electronic)
Advances in Intelligent Systems and Computing
ISBN 978-3-031-14053-2 ISBN 978-3-031-14054-9 (eBook)
https://doi.org/10.1007/978-3-031-14054-9

This Springer imprint is published by the registered company Springer Nature Switzerland AG
The registered company address is: Gewerbestrasse 11, 6330 Cham, Switzerland

Preface

ICR 2022, the First International Conference on Innovations in Computing Research, was held in Athens, Greece, from August 29 to 31, 2022, at the Novotel Hotel. ICR'22 was sponsored by the Spanish National Research Council (CSIC), Spain; Australian Computer Society (ACS), Australia; Polytechnic Institute of Porto, Portugal; University of Detroit Mercy, USA; Features Analytics, Belgium; and Flexens Ltd, Finland.

ICR'22 encompasses six tracks: Data science, computer and network security, Internet of things, health informatics and biomedical imaging, smart cities and smart energy, and computer science and engineering education

The conference received many submissions. Only 45 papers were selected by the program committee for presentation at the conference. There were two presentation modes: online (virtual) and on-site at Novotel hotel. 15 papers were presented online, and 30 papers were presented on-site. These proceedings contain the revised versions of the papers that took the comments of the reviewers into consideration. Only the program committee members were used as reviewers, and no secondary reviewers were allowed. The revisions were not re-reviewed. The authors assume full responsibility for the contents of their final papers. All papers were checked for plagiarism using the Turnitin App.

It gave us great pleasure to experience the great dedication of the advisory committee, organization committee, and program committee. This dedication greatly contributed to the success of ICR'22. Without the excellent papers that were accepted by the program committee, this conference would have not existed. Therefore, we are delighted to thank all the authors for their hard work to come up with excellent original papers and for their productive cooperation with us to incorporate the comments of the reviewers that participated in improving their papers and submitting their camera-ready papers on time.

We are grateful to the editorial director in charge of the Springer book series: Advances in Intelligent Systems and Computing: Dr. Thomas Ditzinger. We greatly appreciate his valuable help and support. We would also like to thank Gowrishankar Ayyasamy, the project coordinator of ICR'22 proceedings book project.

August 2022

Kevin Daimi
Abeer Al Sadoon

Organization

ICR 2022

The 1st International Conference on Innovations in Computing Research (ICR'22)
Athens, Greece
August 29–31, 2022

Advisory Committee

Luis Hernandez Encinas	Spanish National Research Council (CSIC), Spain
Guilermo Francia III	University of West Florida, USA
Solange Ghernaouti	Swiss Cybersecurity Advisory and Research Group., Switzerland
Åsa Hedman	Flexens Ltd, Finland
Hiroaki Kikuchi	Meiji University, Japan
Stefan Pickl	University of the Federal Armed Forces Munich, Germany
Peter Schartner	Alpen-Adria-Universität Klagenfurt, Austria
Cristina Soviany	Features Analytics SA, Belgium

Organization Committee

Conference Chair

Hiroaki Kikuchi	Meiji University, Japan

Program Chairs

Abeer Alsadoon	Charles Sturt University, Australia
Kevin Daimi	University of Detroit Mercy, USA

Posters Chairs

Mary Ann Hoppa	Norfolk State University, USA
Flaminia Luccio	Ca' Foscari University of Venice, Italy
Esmiralda Moradian	Stockholm University, Sweden

Sessions/Workshops Chairs

Luis Coelho	Polytechnic Institute of Porto, Portugal
Ioanna Dionysiou	University of Nicosia, Cyprus
Cathryn Peoples	Ulster University, UK

Publicity Chairs

Anna Allen	IICSER, Australia
Carl Wilson	ZRD Technology, USA

Web Chair

Teresa Martinez	Kent Institute Australia, Australia

Program Committee

Smart Cities and Smart Energy

Mohammed Akour	Yarmouk University, Jordan
Nourhène Ben Rabah	ESIEE-IT, France
Lasse Berntzen	University of South-Eastern Norway, Norway
Manuel I. Capel	Universidad de Granada, Spain
Adrian Castillero Franco	IE Business School, UAE
María del Mar Gómez	Universidad Rey Juan Carlos, Spain
Diala Abi Haidar	Dar Al Hekma University, Saudi Arabia
Karina Kervin	IBM, USA
Pinar Kirci	Bursa Uludag University, Turkey
Sergio Ilarri	University of Zaragoza, Spain
Yi-Jing Li	King's College London, UK
Natarajan Meghanathan	Jackson State University, USA
Dmitry Namiot	Lomonosov Moscow State University, Russia
Fatma Newagy	Ain Shams University, Egypt
Mais Nijim	Texas A&M University—Kingsville, USA
Jun-Seok Oh	Western Michigan University, USA
Kenza Oufaska	International University of Rabat, Morocco

Cathryn Peoples	Ulster University, UK
Alessandro Ruggiero	University of Salerno, Italy
Monica Siroux	INSA Strasbourg, France
Vivian Sultan	California State University—Los Angeles, USA
Fakhrul Hazman Yusoff	Universiti Teknologi MARA, Malaysia
Hailu Xu	California State University, USA
Sotirios Ziavras	New Jersey Institute of Technology, USA

Internet of Things

Iness Ahriz	CEDRIC Lab Conservatoire National des Arts et Métiers, France
Ali Alwan Al-Juboori	Ramapo College of New Jersey, USA
Nourhène Ben Rabah	ESIEE-IT, France
Khalil Challita	Notre Dame University-Louaize, Lebanon
Adrian Castillero Franco	IE Business School, UAE
Jide Edu	King's College London, UK
Hicham H. Hallal	American University of Sharjah, UAE
Marie Khair	Notre Dame University, Lebanon
Irene Kopaliani	Princeton University, USA
Nour El Madhoun	EPITA Engineering School, France
Maggie Mashaly	German University in Cairo, Egypt
Mais Nijim	Texas A&M University—Kingsville, USA
Slobodan Petrovic	Norwegian University of Science and Technology (NTNU), Norway
Cathryn Peoples	Ulster University, UK
Sunny Raj	Oakland University, USA
Alessandro Ruggiero	University of Salerno, Italy
Amparo Fuster Sabater	Spanish National Research Council (CSIC), Spain
Sorin Soviany	National Institute for Research and Development in Informatics, Romania
Hailu Xu	California State University, USA
Suhad Yousif	Al-Nahrain University, Iraq

Health Informatics and Biomedical Imaging

Iman Abdel Aal	Alexandria University, Egypt
Nidhal Abdulaziz	University of Wollongong in Dubai, UAE
Abdullah Alamoodi	Sultan Idris Educational University (UPSI), Malaysia
Thair Al-Dala'in	Western Sydney University, Australia
Hasan AlMarzouqi	Khalifa University, UAE
Violeta Bulbenkiene	Klaipeda University, Lithuania
John Chelsom	Fordham University, UK

Nectarios Costadopoulos	Charles Sturt University, Australia
Dillon Chrimes	University of Victoria, Canada
Luis Coelho	Polytechnic Institute of Porto, Portugal
Sammy Danso	The University of Edinburgh Medical School, UK
Ahmed Dawoud	Western Sydney University (WSU), Australia
António Dourado	University of Coimbra, Portugal
Christopher Druzgalski	California State University, USA
Selena Firmin	Federation University Australia, Australia
José Manuel Fonseca	NOVA University of Lisbon, Portugal
George Gregoriou	University of Nicosia, Cyprus
Ahmad Kayed	Sohar University, Oman
Karina Kervin	IBM, USA
Marie Khair	Notre Dame University, Lebanon
William Klement	Dalhousie University, Canada
Irene Kopaliani	Princeton University, USA
Liwan Liyanage	Western Sydney University (WSU), Australia
Panicos Masouras	Cyprus University of Technology, Cyprus
Junfeng Qu	Clayton State University, USA
Tarik A. Rashid	University of Kurdistan Hewler, Iraq
Sara Seabra dos Reis	Instituto Superior de Engenharia do Porto, Portugal
Alessandro Ruggiero	University of Salerno, Italy
Cristina Soviany	Features Analytics SA, Belgium
Karl A. Stroetmann	University of Victoria, Canada
Suhad Yousif	Al-Nahrain University, Iraq

Computer Science and Computer Engineering Education

Laila Ahddar	VP CISO, Global R&D, IDEMIA, France
Bilal Al-Ahmad	The University of Jordan, Jordan
Karim Baïna	Mohammed V University in Rabat, Morocco
Rita DiLeo	University of Scranton, USA
Violeta Bulbenkiene	Klaipeda University, Lithuania
Raafat Elfouly	Rhode Island College, USA
Vladimir Estivill-Castro	Universitat Pompeu Fabra, Spain
Selena Firmin	Federation University Australia, Australia
José Manuel Fonseca	NOVA University of Lisbon, Portugal
Hadi Khalilia	University of Trento, Italy
Feng Cheng	Hasso-Plattner-Institute, University of Potsdam, Germany
George Dimitoglou	Hood College, USA
Ioanna Dionysiou	University of Nicosia, Cyprus
Luis Hernández Encinas	Spanish National Research Council (CSIC), Spain

Stevens Fox	State of Washington Office of Cybersecurity, USA
Hicham H. Hallal	American University of Sharjah, United Arab Emirates
Iman M. A. Helal	Cairo University, Egypt
Imane Aly Saroit Ismail	Cairo University, Egypt
Chadi El Kari	University of the Pacific, USA
Ievgeniia Kuzminykh	King's College London, UK
Wadha Khalid Labda	Qatar University, Qatar
Edison Loza-Aguirre	Escuela Politécnica Nacional, Ecuador
J. Todd McDonald	University of South Alabama, USA
Suzanne Mello-Stark	Rhode Island College, USA
Hoda M. O. Mokhtar	Egypt University of Informatics (EUI), Egypt
Nader Nassar	IBM, USA
Nkaepe Olaniyi	Kaplan Open Learning, UK
Srujal Patel	Kent Institute Australia, Australia
Robert Polding	IE Business School, Spain
Razwan Mohmed Salah	The University of Duhok, Iraq
Maher Salem	King's College London, UK
Andreas Savva	University of Nicosia, Cyprus
Karpoor Shashidhar	Sam Houston State University, USA
Nicolas Sklavos	University of Patras, Greece
Vasso Stylianou	University of Nicosia, Cyprus

Computer and Network Security

Fawaz Alazemi	Kuwait University, Kuwait
Roberto Omar Andrade	Escuela Politécnica Nacional, Ecuador
Samia Bouzefrane	Conservatoire National des Arts et Métiers, Paris, France
Oli Buckley	University of East Anglia, UK
Khalil Challita	Notre Dame University-Louaize, Lebanon
Sammy Danso	The University of Edinburgh Medical School, UK
Feng Cheng	Hasso-Plattner-Institute, University of Potsdam, Germany
Ahmed Dawoud	Western Sydney University, Australia
George Dimitoglou	Hood College, USA
Ioanna Dionysiou	University of Nicosia, Cyprus
Levent Ertaul	California State University East Bay, USA
Diala Abi Haidar	Dar Al Hekma University, Saudi Arabia
Luis Hernández Encinas	Spanish National Research Council (CSIC), Spain
Hicham H. Hallal	American University of Sharjah, United Arab Emirates

Contents

Health Informatics and Biomedical Imaging

Detection of Unconsciousness in Falls Using Thermal Vision Sensors

Marcos Lupión[1](✉), Vicente González-Ruiz[1], Juan F. Sanjuan[1], Javier Medina-Quero[2], and Pilar M. Ortigosa[1]

[1] Department of Informatics, University of Almería, CeiA3, Almería, Spain
{marcoslupion,vruiz,jsanjuan,ortigosa}@ual.es
[2] Department of Computer Science, University of Jaen, Jaen, Spain
jmquero@ujaen.es

Abstract. Unattended falls, where the injured person may be unconscious, are among the most frequent causes of death worldwide among the elderly population. Several fall detection methods using devices, such as wearable sensors and cameras, have been deployed in Smart Homes to detect and minimize the response time against these types of accidents. Some related works have proposed to trigger an alarm when a fall is detected. However, there is a lack of considering the state in which the person has been left after the fall. This work proposes a fall detection system using low-resolution thermal cameras that detects falls and classifies the falls depending on the state of conscience of the user. Thus, once detected in a risky state, a voice assistant routine starts to measure the degree of conscience of the person and make an emergency call only when necessary. The system is deployed in the Smart Home of the University of Almeria and validated with one user, triggering the alarm in all falls that lead to an unconscious state.

Keywords: Fall detection · Thermal sensors · Recurrent neural network · Fall classification · Alert system

1 Introduction

Age reduces people's psychomotor skills and reflexes, increasing the number of falls over the years due to demographic change. The effects of falls are the second leading cause of death worldwide among people over 60 years of age [18]. In this situation, it is essential to act promptly in order to avoid difficult situations for health [15, 17].

In most cases, the environments in which older people live are not fully adapted to their physical conditions. This is one of the reasons why they frequently resided in long-stay centers. So, in the event of a fall, they need to request the attention of health professionals or family members as soon as possible.

Thanks to the Internet of Things (IoT), smart environments are being created in which fall detection is conducted by systems with sensors located in the environments. These systems have a high accuracy in detecting falls and allow people to live alone and send some alerts in case of emergency [6]. In this case, emergency services are connected to the system and can act at the earliest to assist a person.

K. Daimi and A. Al Sadoon (Eds.): ICR 2022, AISC 1431, pp. 3–12, 2022.
https://doi.org/10.1007/978-3-031-14054-9_1

In some cases, when using visible cameras, their privacy concern, which intimidates people living at home, avoids their deployment in real environments. For this reason, low-resolution thermal vision sensors are proposed [12]. These sensors maintain the user's privacy and provide images with enough information to detect falls in the environment. Other goals, such as activity recognition, person identification, and intrusion detection, have also been achieved using these sensors. In addition, these tasks can also be performed in dark situations.

In the context described above, we propose an automatic fall detection system that uses thermal cameras to recognize if the user has been able to get up or otherwise remains motionless on the ground.

The remainder of this manuscript is organized as follows: in Sect. 2, related works are discussed, Sect. 3 describes the proposed system, Sect. 4 the evaluation of the system performed, and Sect. 5 provides the conclusions of the work and future improvements.

2 Related Works

In the related literature, several works tackle the problem of fall detection. Indeed, these solutions use different sensors, devices, and algorithms to carry out this task.

The early works used binary sensors [16] to detect falls. However, although they were allowed to classify several Activities of Daily Living (ADLs), the detection accuracy was low because they did not provide the required information. Thus, as a solution, wearable devices were proposed to gather data (accelerometer and gyroscope) that describe the movement, orientation, and acceleration in body parts such as arms or legs. Using these devices, falls systems having high accuracy were developed [2, 10]. The main problem with these devices lies in their high battery consumption, as high-bit-rate data have to be processed on the device or using a central device, transmitting the information periodically. Users always have to wear these devices for the fall detection system to work, but sometimes the fall can happen when the user is not wearing the device, and therefore the system fails in detecting this fall. Several solutions use smartphones to detect falls [1], as they incorporate similar sensors as the wearable ones, and they also fail if the user is not wearing the smartphone when falling.

As a solution, these environments incorporate cameras, and mainly deep learning approaches have been developed to detect falls achieving state-of-the-art performance [5]. Nevertheless, a constant recording of the inhabitant's behavior is reported to be intrusive [12]. To tackle this problem, in this work, we have incorporated thermal vision cameras, and similar performance [8] has been obtained while preserving privacy. Other works face the problem of multi-occupancy, being able to detect falls when there is more than one user in the scene [20]. Thermal images, in most cases, are processed using deep learning algorithms, more precisely, convolutional and recurrent neural networks (CNN and RNN, respectively), which enable the systems to learn patterns from the images and also the temporal relationship between them [7]. Applying CNN to raw thermal images could produce large networks. Therefore, several works use the pose of the user instead of a raw thermal image to detect falls [13, 19]; in this case, a pose-estimation pre-processing has to be performed before classifying data.

In brief, fall detection systems using different sensing devices have arrived to obtain a high degree of accuracy in fall detection [11]. However, in several works, the alarm system is not developed, which is fundamental to deploy the system in natural environments [3]. Several works, when detecting a fall, send a notification to medical staff or family [4, 14], but do not take into account the state of the person who falls.

In this work, a novel fall detection system based on thermal vision sensors is proposed to solve the limitations of current works. The contributions are the following:

- A lightweight fall detection CNN-LSTM artificial neural network (ANN) is proposed, executed in an IoT device placed in a Smart Home.
- A new method to detect the unconscious state of the fallen person is developed.
- A voice-controlled system that triggers an alert in case of not answering the system's questions or answering incorrectly.

3 Methodology

The current work aims to detect falls in a Smart Home using thermal vision sensors. Figure 1 shows the whole system deployed in the Smart Home. First, an IoT device that records data using thermal cameras and processes them using an ANN implementation is deployed in the Smart Home. The ANN classifies data in two states: normal behavior and fall. When detecting a fall, if the person does not recover, a voice assistant is started and makes sure the user is not conscious. It asks some questions to the user, and triggers an alarm if the person does not answer or answers incorrectly. With this verification method provided by the voice assistant, false positives emergency calls do not occur.

In this section, the details of the different parts of the systems are developed.

3.1 IoT Device

We have designed an IoT device (Fig. 2) to record images and run the fall detection algorithm concurrently as a fall detection system. It is composed of three main devices:

- Raspberry Pi Model 4. It is a well-known single-board computer incorporated into many IoT projects.

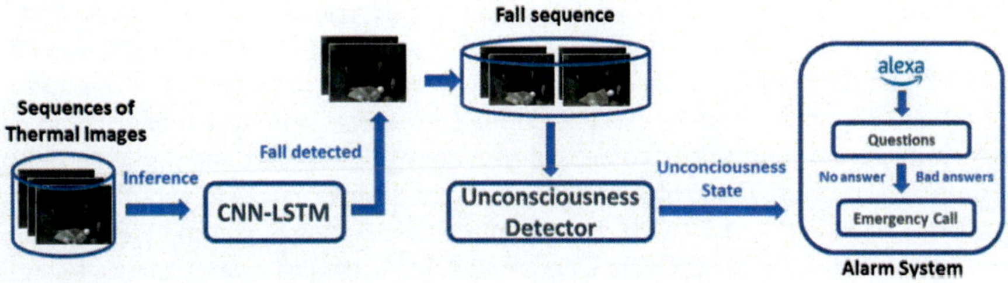

Fig. 1. IoT fall detection system

- FLIR Lepton 3.5. It is a thermal vision sensor used to capture thermal images.
- PureThermal 2 Smart I/O Module. This device lets the communication between the thermal vision sensor and Raspberry Pi.

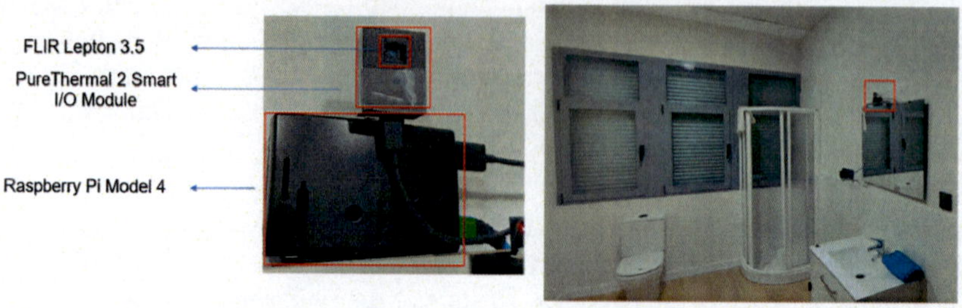

Fig. 2. On the left, the device and its components. On the right, the location of the device.

3.2 Neural Network Architecture

An artificial neural network (ANN) [9] is an algorithm based on the behavior of the human brain and lets us solve several tasks in the field of artificial intelligence, such as data classification, anomaly detection, or artificial vision.

In this work, thermal images are the input model obtained from a thermal vision sensor. These images have to be classified in a binary label as *normal* or *fall*. In deep learning, images are processed using convolutional layers, which perform the convolution operation on images and output feature maps having patterns found in the images from the dataset.

Thus, to classify the convolutional layers' output, multi-layer perceptrons are usually incorporated. These layers are usually called "fully connected layers". They are modelled with a different number of units and depth and let the system map the visual features extracted in the convolutional layers to the system's output. In general, ANNs that process images are developed using convolutional and fully connected layers.

In the ANNs mentioned above, the classification of an image in one or several classes is performed without considering other temporal components. In this case, before a user falls, the state is always *normal*. In addition, in most cases, after a fall, the user stands up, and the state is *normal*. As can be appreciated, the temporal component of a sequence of images has to be considered to classify the user's state. We have incorporated recurrent layers into neural networks to tackle this sequential dependence. These layers can act as a memory in the neural network and classify current data, considering previously classified data. The most popular long-memory layers are LSTM.

An LSTM has three main steps: convolutional, recurrent, and fully connected. In the first step, there are four blocks composed of a convolutional (C), max-pooling (MP), and dropout (D) layer. These blocks include several dropout layers to avoid overfitting the network. Second, an LSTM layer containing 32 neurons is incorporated. Finally, three fully connected layers (FC) are incorporated, being the last layer (Output), a single neuron layer having sigmoid as an activation function, therefore, outputs values between 0 (normal) and 1 (fall). Therefore, a total of three different layers are used to build the proposed ANN (Fig. 3).

The proposed ANN has a total of 158,097 parameters to learn.

In this case, the thermal vision sensor records images at 9 FPS. Thus, the input of the ANN is a sequence containing 9 images (1 s). Therefore, each second, the ANN outputs a state (normal or fall) instead of classifying each image in the sequence. This

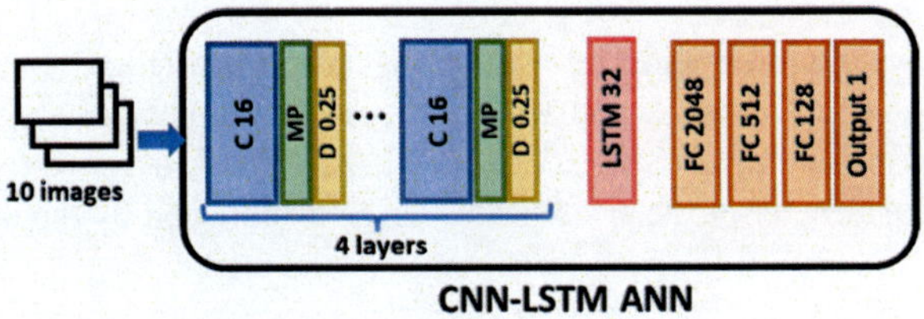

Fig. 3. Proposed neural network

approach lets the ANN consider the user's movement to predict the state instead of simply classifying the raw static image.

3.3 Unconsciousness Detection

The detection of unconsciousness is based on the expected reduction of the overall motion magnitude in the captured images after detecting a fall when this undesired situation happens. For this, we estimate the amount of motion in the scene by computing the energy of the differences $\Sigma i, j(Aij - Bij)^2$ found between two consecutive images (**A** and **B**) that does not represent moving objects and consider this value as a minimum threshold below of that the camera is capturing no motion. Thus, the unconsciousness alarm is activated when this threshold is reached several times in consecutive frames after detecting a fall.

3.4 Alert System

In case of noticing a state of "unconsciousness", the alarm system is triggered.

First, after processing a batch of images labeled as fallen, the IoT device detects unconsciousness. After the detection, it communicates with the Alexa device deployed in the Smart Home through an API. At this moment, an Alexa skill starts and tries to communicate with the person who has fallen. Alexa asks several questions to check that the person is conscious of this communication. These questions are basic ones: "tell me the name of a person who lives here." If the person does not answer or the answers are incorrect, the alert system immediately calls the emergency service; nevertheless, the system logs in and stores all the fall sequence images if the person answers correctly.

4 Experimental Results

4.1 Dataset and Training Configuration

In this work, a new dataset is recorded, taking into account the *unconsciousness* state of several falls. The dataset contains 4,070 images having dimensions 160x120. A total of 11 falls (3 represent the unconsciousness state) were simulated in a controlled way. In this case, all the images are from the same person in the same location of the Smart Home.

Figure 4 shows the three states into which the system classifies the individual. Normal) when the user is not fallen; Fall) when the user falls but he/she is also moving; Unconsciousness) when the user has fallen, and he/she does not move for more than 10 s. This time is a parameter of the system and can be established by the user.

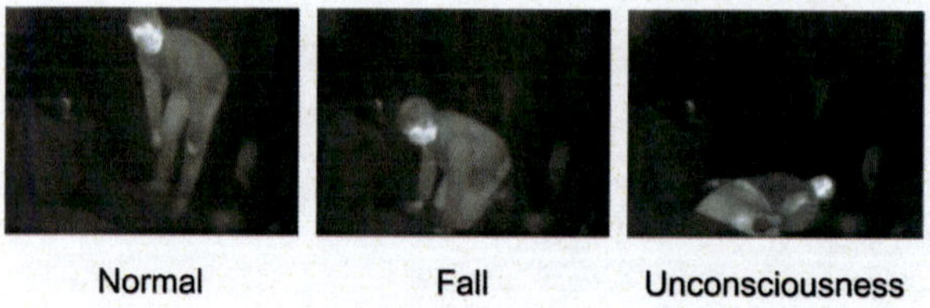

Fig. 4. States of the user

An early stopping method has been incorporated for training configurations because the initial number of epochs is set to 1,000. In this stopping method, the training is finished when the number of epochs the ANN executes without improving the indicated loss equals a given value. In this case, the given value was set to 30, and the loss used to stop training is the binary cross-entropy value on the validation dataset.

4.2 Results

In this section, the evaluation of the proposed method is discussed.

In this case, the batch size is set to 1, as the window size of each data is 10 images. Figure 5 shows the evolution in training and evaluation loss. The network avoids overfitting thanks to the dropout layers incorporated. The total number of epochs to train the model is 22.

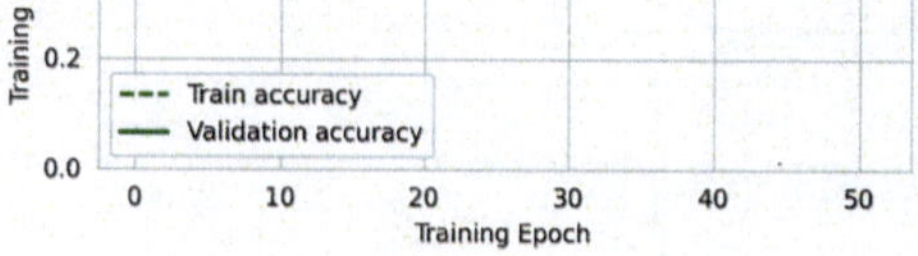

Fig. 5. Train and evaluation loss

Once trained, the ANN was used to predict the labels of the validation dataset. These results are shown in a confusion matrix (Fig. 6). It can be appreciated that there are only 3 cases where the ANN failed to predict the input data class. In this case, 2 sequences were classified as a normal state, despite being a fall state. Only once a normal state sequence has been classified as a fall. In this case, the dataset is unbalanced, so the class with more data tends to be the predominant one.

In addition to the confusion matrix, several metrics are calculated to evaluate the performance of the model. These metrics are: precision (Eq. 1), recall (Eq. 2) and F1-Score (Eq. 3). In these equations, *TP* is the number of True Positives, *FP* is the number of False Positives and *FN* is the number of false negatives.

$$Precision = \frac{TP}{TP + FP} \tag{1}$$

$$Recall = \frac{TP}{TP + FN} \tag{2}$$

$$F1 = \frac{2 * TP}{2 * TP + FP + FN} \tag{3}$$

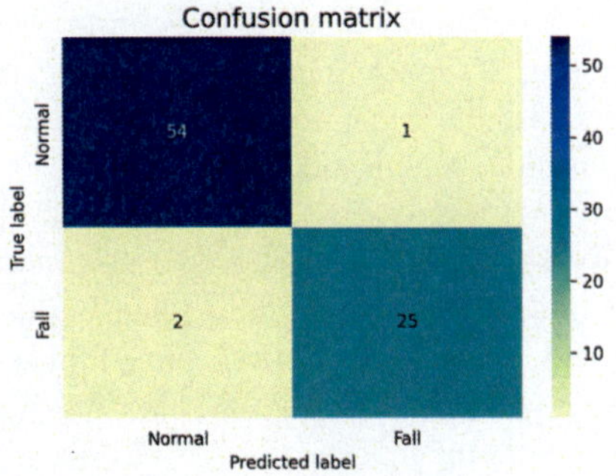

Fig. 6. Confusion matrix

Table 1 shows the previous metrics calculated on the ANN defined in this work.

In this case, precision in fall class is the most important metric, as it describes the ability of the algorithm to detect a fall when it happens. In this case, its value is 92.59%. Note that this value is only taking into account the classification of the different windows in the dataset. As falls last for over some seconds, sometimes the system will not detect every window of images as a fall, but the alarm will be triggered because some windows will be detected as falls in 92.59% of the registers.

As for the recall value on falls, it shows that the fall detection system will produce only a few cases of false positives. These few cases are not a problem as the system has to detect a fall in consecutive time windows to trigger the alarm.

Therefore, the fall detection neural network has no accuracy of 100%, but the post-processing allows the system to trigger the alarm only when needed.

A critical factor in the system is when the fall is produced and triggered by the alarm. The system analyses the images in real-time, obtaining a label every 9 frames indicating whether a fall has been detected or not. If a fall is detected in more than 2 sequences in a row (1.8 s), the unconsciousness detection system is activated, checking whether the fall

Table 1. Evaluation metrics

Metric	Normal	Fall
Precision	98.18	92.59
Recall	96.42	96.15
F1	97.29	94.33

has caused the user to become unconscious. Given the results, this system takes 7.5 s on average to detect the state of unconsciousness when the fall begins. This delay is because the user is in motion in the first few seconds of the fall. Once unconsciousness is detected, the skill that asks the user questions is initiated. If not correctly recorded, the alarm to the emergency service is triggered within 30 s of the detection of unconsciousness.

5 Conclusions and Future Works

The ANN was trained during 22 epochs and achieved a precision of 92.59 in the fall class. Despite the imbalanced and tiny dataset, this precision value ensures fall detection in more than 90% cases. In addition, this model minimizes the number of false positives (96.15% of recall).

Furthermore, in this work, when a fall is detected in several consecutive images, they are processed in parallel to detect an unconscious state. In this case, the energy of the pixel-wise difference (residue) between two consecutive frames is calculated, triggering an alarm when no movement is detected.

Regarding the alarm system, the introduction of the voice assistant interaction when detecting a fall improves the detection of urgent falls and avoids false alarms due to a non-important fall, which implies a better use of the emergency resources that have to go to the house.

In future works, we will extend the system to those cases where some other no human movement is not readily appreciated, such as, for example, a pet that is close to the fallen user. This kind of movement can make the current system fail when detecting the unconscious state of the user. We are also planning to use better motion estimations, such as the optical flow. Finally, a larger dataset with different inhabitants, locations, and camera orientations will be collected to develop a robust model for heterogeneous contexts.

Acknowledgements. This research was funded by the Spanish Ministry of Economy and Competitiveness grant number RTI2018-095993-B-I00; by the Junta de Andalucía grant number P18-RT-1193 and by the University of Almería grant number UAL18-TIC-A020-B. Marcos Lupión Lorente is a fellow of the Spanish 'Formación del Profesorado Universitario' program (FPU19/02756).

References

1. Aguiar, B., Rocha, T., Silva, J., Sousa, I.: Accelerometer-based fall detection for smartphones. In: 2014 IEEE International Symposium on Medical Measurements and Applications (MeMeA), pp. 1–6 (2014)
2. Chen, X., Jiang, S., Lo, B.: Subject-independent slow fall detection with wearable sensors via deep learning. In: 2020 IEEE SENSORS, pp. 1–4 (2020)
3. Gharti, P.: A study of fall detection monitoring system for elderly people through IoT and mobile based application devices in indoor environment. In: 2020 5th International Conference on Innovative Technologies in Intelligent Systems and Industrial Applications (CITISIA), pp. 1–9 (2020)
4. Gupta, A., Srivastava, R., Gupta, H., Kumar, B.: IoT based fall detection monitoring and alarm system for elderly. In: 2020 IEEE 7th Uttar Pradesh Section International Conference on Electrical, Electronics and Computer Engineering (UPCON), pp. 1–5 (2020)
5. Gutiérrez, J., Rodríguez, V., Martin, S.: Comprehensive review of vision-based fall detection systems. Sensors **21**(3) (2021). https://www.mdpi.com/1424-8220/21/3/ 947
6. Hu, C.L., et al.: Using camera array to detect elderly falling and distribute alerting media for smart home care. In: 2019 8th International Conference on Innovation, Communication and Engineering (ICICE), pp. 98–101 (2019)
7. Jeong, S., Kang, S., Chun, I.: Human-skeleton based fall-detection method using LSTM for manufacturing industries. In: 2019 34th International Technical Conference on Circuits/Systems, Computers and Communications (ITC-CSCC), pp. 1–4 (2019)
8. Kido, S., Miyasaka, T., Tanaka, T., Shimizu, T., Saga, T.: Fall detection in toilet rooms using thermal imaging sensors. In: 2009 IEEE/SICE International Symposium on System Integration (SII), pp. 83–88 (2009)
9. Kriegeskorte, N., Golan, T.: Neural network models and deep learning. Curr. Biol. **29**(7), R231–R236 (2019)
10. Lu, N., Wu, Y., Feng, L., Song, J.: Deep learning for fall detection: three-dimensional CNN combined with LSTM on video kinematic data. IEEE J. Biomed. Health Inform. **23**(1), 314–323 (2019)
11. Quero, J.M., Burns, M., Razzaq, M.A., Nugent, C., Espinilla, M.: Detection of falls from non-invasive thermal vision sensors using convolutional neural networks. Proceedings **2**(19) (2018). https://www.mdpi.com/2504-3900/2/19/1236
12. Rafferty, J., Synnott, J., Nugent, C.: A hybrid rule and machine learning based generic alerting platform for smart environments. In: 2016 38th Annual International Conference of the IEEE Engineering in Medicine and Biology Society (EMBC), pp. 5405–5408 (2016)
13. Ramirez, H., Velastin, S.A., Meza, I., Fabregas, E., Makris, D., Farias, G.: Fall detection and activity recognition using human skeleton features. IEEE Access **9**, 33532–33542 (2021)
14. Rathi, N., Kakani, M., El-Sharkawy, M., Rizkalla, M.: Wearable low power pre-fall detection system with IoT and bluetooth capabilities. In: 2017 IEEE National Aerospace and Electronics Conference (NAECON), pp. 241–244 (2017)
15. Rubenstein, L.Z.: Falls in older people: epidemiology, risk factors and strategies for prevention. Age Ageing **35**(Suppl 2), ii37–ii41 (2006)
16. Tan, T.H., Badarch, L., Zeng, W.X., Gochoo, M., Alnajjar, F.S., Hsieh, J.W.: Binary sensors-based privacy-preserved activity recognition of elderly living alone using an RNN. Sensors (Basel, Switz.) **21**(16), 5371 (Aug 2021). https://www.ncbi.nlm.nih.gov/pmc/articles/PMC8398125/
17. Terroso, M., Rosa, N., Torres Marques, A., Simoes, R.: Physical consequences of falls in the elderly: a literature review from 1995 to 2010. Eur. Rev. Aging Phys. Act. **11**(1), 51–59 (2014). https://eurapa.biomedcentral.com/articles/10.1007/s11556-013-0134-8

18. World Health Organization: falls, 21 April 2021. https://www.who.int/news-room/fact-sheets/detail/falls. Accessed 07 Mar 2022
19. Wu, J., Wang, K., Cheng, B., Li, R., Chen, C., Zhou, T.: Skeleton based fall detection with convolutional neural network. In: 2019 Chinese Control and Decision Conference (CCDC), pp. 5266–5271 (2019)
20. Zhong, C., Ng, W.W.Y., Zhang, S., Nugent, C.D., Shewell, C., Medina-Quero, J.: Multi-occupancy fall detection using non-invasive thermal vision sensor. IEEE Sens. J. **21**(4), 5377–5388 (2021)

Work Disability Risk Prediction Using Machine Learning, Comparison of Two Methods

Katja Saarela[1](✉), Vili Huhta-Koivisto[2], and Jukka K. Nurminen[1]

[1] University of Helsinki, Helsinki, Finland
{katja.saarela,jukka.k.numinen}@helsinki.fi
[2] Aalto University, Espoo, Finland
vili.huhta-koivisto@cgi.com

Abstract. The risk of work disability can be predicted with machine learning and using various data sources. In this study, we compare two methods that use different data sources, occupational health care data and pension decision register data. The first method, medical report data classification for two classes (M_{Health}), reached an accuracy of 72% by using neural networks. This tool is used in occupational health care to help in the screening process of the patients. The second method, pension data prediction ($M_{Pension}$), achieved an accuracy of 69–78% depending on the algorithm used. Using pension decision register data, disability was best predicted by old age, high use of sickness benefits and rehabilitation allowance in previous years, and low or no earnings in previous years. Based on the experiments, machine learning techniques appear to be a potential tool to support expert work and decision-making.

Keywords: Machine learning · Neural networks · NLP · ULMFit

1 Introduction

Virtually all OECD countries share the problem of too many employees leaving the labor market permanently due to disability or health problems [1]. It is in the common interest of society, the employer, the employee, and the pension fund administration to keep the employees healthy and able to work. The risk factors for the disability should be identified promptly, as early intervention is known to be cost-effective, and more effective than later treatments. Thus, it is important to identify people who are at high risk of ending up in disability pension as early as possible. Many statistical dependencies between factors predicting disability, like duration of sickness absence, diagnosis, socioeconomic status, and disability, are known from previous cohort or multicohort studies (for example in Finland Airaksinen *et al.* [2] and Salonen *et al.* [3], in Sweden Salonen *et al.* [4] and in Germany Bethge *et al.* [5]. Airaksinen *et al.* [2] found eight factors that lead to disability pension: age, self-rated health, no. of sick absences during the previous year, socioeconomic position, chronic illness, trouble falling asleep, Body Mass Index (BMI), and smoking. ML (Machine Learning) methods are widely developed to predict certain disability types (for example musculoskeletal diseases [6], fatigue [7], and lung function

K. Daimi and A. Al Sadoon (Eds.): ICR 2022, AISC 1431, pp. 13–21, 2022.
https://doi.org/10.1007/978-3-031-14054-9_2

[8]), whereas Reho [9] inspects the relation between occupational health care visits and disability risk. However, there are only a few proposed methods for the work disability risk prediction on a general level. The most closely related work comes from disease prediction, where diseases have been predicted from medical reports using NLP (Natural Language Processing) tools (for example Pham *et al.* [10]). We aim to predict whether the person has a high risk to get a disability for work for any reason, for example, diseases or a combination of them. In this study, we will compare two methods, our method [11], work disability risk prediction using occupational health care data and NLP (M_{Health}), and prediction using pension decision register's structural data ($M_{Pension}$) [12, 13]. First, we will introduce M_{Health} and $M_{Pension}$, and next, we will compare the data and the results of these two methods. Finally, we will discuss our future research and have a conclusion on the results.

2 M_{Health}: Work Disability Prediction with Occupational Health Care Data

In the first method, we use occupational health care data and predict work disability using medical report data [11]. By finding high-risk patients early, we can help them more efficiently and more cost-efficiently compared to later detection and treatment. Data used for the research is anonymized medical reports from occupational health care. More specifically, the data is a collection of medical reports describing patients' visits to occupational health doctors. Each patient has three separate texts, the first one describing the situation before the visit; the second containing observations made during the visit, and the last one containing the treatment plan. These three texts are combined into a single text that is then used for the prediction.

After the visits, medical professionals have labeled these patients to have either no risk or risk of disability. Doctors perform the labeling based on their expertise and guidelines created by the health care company providing the data. In this case, we do not know whether the persons started their disability pension, labeling was just the doctor's opinion on the risk. 59% of the cases were labeled as having a risk so classes were a bit imbalanced. We have 17 000 recorded patient visits. However, patients with some information missing or combined medical records shorter than 100 characters are removed to achieve more consistent results. After the removal of incomplete, unlabeled, and too short records, there are 9 000 recorded visits left. No other information was used for predictions. There are not many machine-learning approaches capable of working with Finnish texts, while the data source is this small. The limited size of training data was the main reason why only models capable of transfer learning were considered for this case. A low number of training examples makes transfer learning an important tool as this significantly lowers requirements for data and computational power. In practice, this means that base of the language model is pre-trained with a generic corpus and then fine-tuned with specific examples. In the end, modeling was done with Fastai's ULMFiT (Universal Language Model Fine-tuning for Text Classification) tools for Python [14]. Other possible tools that were considered were Bidirectional Encoder Representation from Transformers (Bert) [15] and Transformer-XL [16]. ULMFit is a neural net architecture that is based on ASGD (Average-Stochastic Gradient Descent) weight-dropped long short term memory network (AWD-LSTM). Ultimately, Finnish ULMFit, a pre-trained ULMFit language model for the Finnish language, was used as a starting point for the language model. The model was trained on Azure's virtual machine containing GPUs for better training performance. Preprocessing of data consisted of two separate tasks. First, retrieving and cleaning data to suit the environment's requirements. Secondly, transforming data so that a neural network could utilize it. Texts were cleaned and data was split into training and validation sets. 30% of labeled examples were used as a validation set and the rest were used for the model training. The final model consists of two parts, the language model that is responsible for language understanding and the classifier. Where training classifiers require labels, the language model can be trained with just texts. Therefore, the language model could be trained with every available medical record, not just ones that were labeled. Therefore, the volume of data used in the language model training was greater than in the classifier training. Results were evaluated by comparing target labels to the ones predicted by the model. The confusion matrix and associated measures were used as an easy way to get an overview of the performance, and individual predictions were inspected against their respective text to find possible problems.

3 $M_{Pension}$: Work Disability Prediction with Pension Decision Register

In the second method, Varis [12, 13] used pension decision register data and predicted work disability using structural data. Finnish Center for Pensions has access to an extensive database covering almost all Finnish employees and pensioners. The data includes income data and pension decisions. Varis predicted given disability pensions after two years they have submitted their first disability pension application. The teaching material consisted of the anonymized data on socioeconomic, incomes, and social benefits of 240000 persons. Varis used data from the period 2–10 years before they started their disability pension. In this first group, all the persons started their disability pension. 240000 randomly selected persons who had not received a disability pension during the reference period were used as controls. Varis strived to include as accurately as possible in the teaching material people who could potentially retire on a disability pension. Thus, people who were already retired were removed. The project tool was the Python programming language and its open-source machine learning add-ons, especially Scikit-learn. Varis divided the material into teaching data (60% of the data) and test data (40% of the data). Data was processed typically, such as normalizations of floating-point numbers, transformations of categorical variables into dummy variables, and processing of missing values.

Varis experimented with a few different classifier algorithms that yielded very similar prediction accuracy results: Random forest, 77.8%, XGBoost (advanced decision tree), 77.3, Logistic regression with L1 regularization, 77.0%, Decision tree, 69%, and Simple 1–4 hidden layer NLP neural networks, 78% prediction accuracy. During the experiment, no actual time series models were used, but annual time series of the variables were used. As the result of the experiment, it became clear that socio-economic, earnings, and benefits data can be used to predict the starting of a disability pension with some accuracy. About 78% of the pensions starting after two years could be correctly predicted, leaving about 22% undetected by the algorithm. All machine learning algorithms gave similar results. Correspondingly, high levels of education, high earnings, and marriage reduced the likelihood of starting a disability pension. Unemployment benefits increased the probability of receiving a disability pension, but earnings-related unemployment benefits reduced the probability. The analysis with the pension decision register data showed that disability pensions for musculoskeletal and respiratory diseases were the best predictors. It was more difficult to predict disability pensions for mental health reasons. Many of these statistical dependencies are known from previous multi-cohort or cohort studies [2–5]. Varis got similar results using pure machine learning methods. Disability was best predicted by old age, high use of sickness benefits and rehabilitation allowance in previous years, and low or no earned income in previous years. Low levels of education, unemployment, and singlehood also predicted the ending up in disability pension. Based on the experiment, ML techniques appear to be potential tools to support expert work.

4 Comparison of Data Sources in M_{Health} and $M_{Pension}$

Next we will compare the two separate data sources used in M_{Health} and $M_{Pension}$. The data sources are shown in Fig. 1. Both methods use anonymized data.

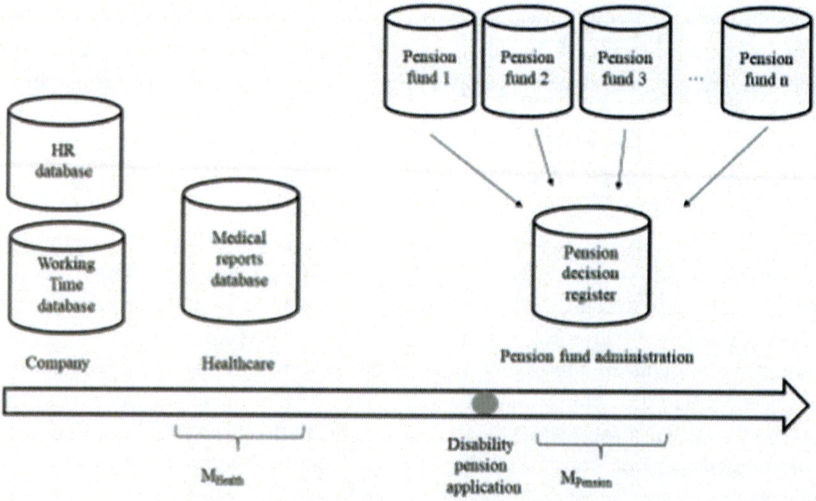

Fig. 1. Data sources for M_{Health} and $M_{Pension}$.

When a person is in working life, her information can be found in the company's HR system and working time system as well as in occupational health care company's information systems. The employer knows her sick leave information and the occupational health care company has more detailed information about the reason for the absence, such as medical reports written by a doctor. It would be useful for the prediction if this information could be combined to get the most comprehensive picture possible but there are legal issues that restrict this. For example, pension funds cannot get information on the insured before he has submitted his pension application. When a person becomes ill, he or she first goes on sick leave. In Finland, after a year of sick leave, a person has the opportunity to apply for a rehabilitation allowance, a fixed-term disability pension. After one year of rehabilitation support, a person can apply for a permanent disability pension. The pension fund administration receives information about the person at the stage when the first disability pension application arrives for them. At this point, a person's health is already quite poor and often problems have accumulated.

The biggest difference in the methods is that the M_{Health} compares results to the expert's opinions. We do not know if the person gets the disability pension or not, but it is not our purpose because we want to avoid disability pensions by screening potential risk cases and using interventions. Our AI model aims to replicate the estimations of experts. On the other hand, in the $M_{Pension}$ we know if the person has gotten the disability pension. This increases the reliability of the data and results as they are based on actual events.

5 Comparison of Results of M_{Health} and $M_{Pension}$

Figures 2 and 3 present the models' ROC curves. Figures 4 and 5 present the confusion matrixes of the models. Matrixes have been drawn from the points of ROC curves that give the best overall accuracy.

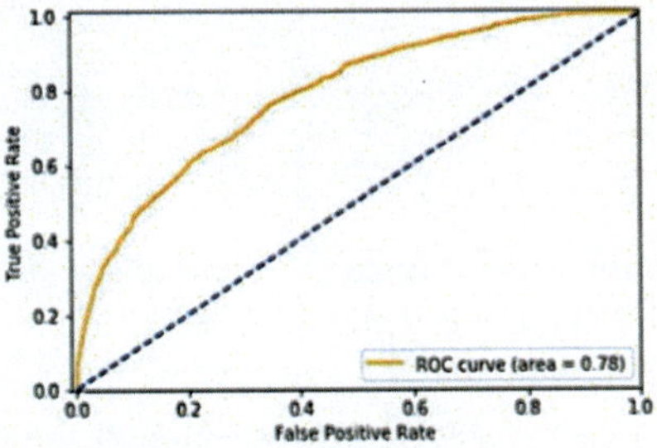

Fig. 2. M_{Health} ROC curve.

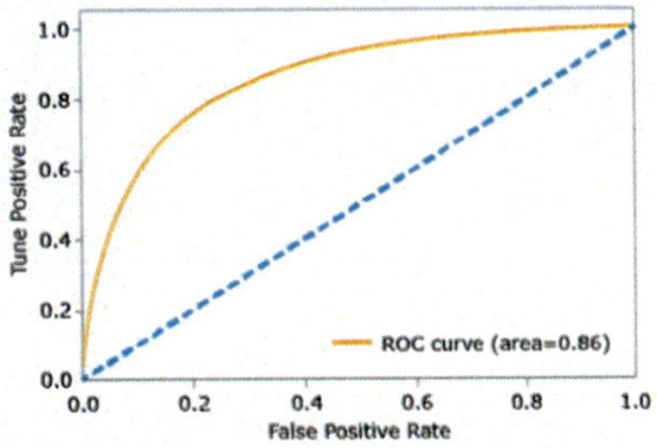

Fig. 3. $M_{Pension}$ ROC curve.

The comparison of the results of M_{Health} and $M_{Pension}$ can be found in Table 1.

If the model gives a **false positive prediction**, it means in the health care company case, that the doctor goes through the situation with the patient shortly but further help is not needed. The situation is similar in the pension fund administration case. A person responsible for rehabilitation can contact the insured and discuss his or her situation. If the model gives many false positives, it is laborious for personnel, and the advantages of using AI are missed. From the employee's or insured's view false early intervention can cause effects in both positive and negative manner. The topic is important and we will discuss it more in future research. On the other hand, if the model gives a **false negative prediction**, it means that the real risk case is ignored. In the occupational health care company case, it affects too late intervention, which is less cost-efficient and efficient.

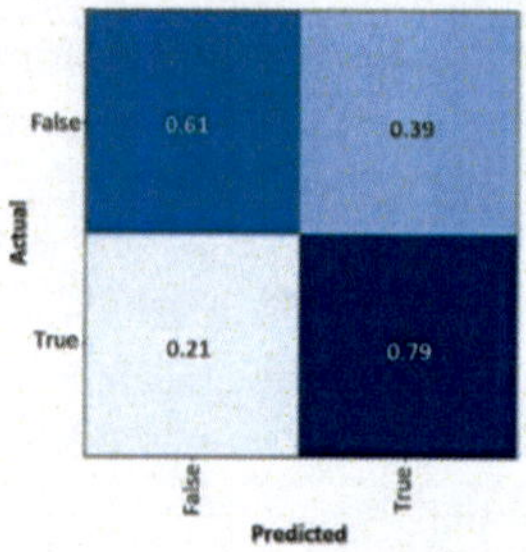

Fig. 4. M_{Health} confusion matrix.

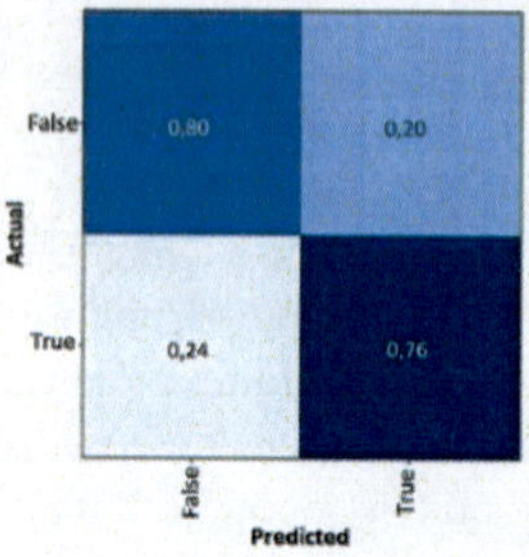

Fig. 5. $M_{Pension}$ confusion matrix.

Table 1. Comparison of the results of M_{Health} and $M_{Pension}$.

Result	M_{Health}	$M_{Pension}$	Result	M_{Health}	$M_{Pension}$
Positives	1800	96000	**False negatives**	378 (61%)	23040 (80%)
Negatives	1200	96000	**Accuracy** = $\frac{TP+TN}{TP+TN+FP+FN}$	72%	78%
True positives	1422 (79%)	72960 (76%)	**Sensitivity** = $\frac{TP}{TP+FN}$	79%	76%
True negatives	732 (39%)	76800 (20%)	**Specificity** = $\frac{TN}{TN+FP}$	61%	80%
False positives	468 (21%)	19200 (24%)			

The situation is similar to a pension case – rehabilitation is started too late when problems have typically accumulated. On the other hand, there are many other ways to predict disability risk than the AI. Experts do the estimation regularly when meeting the patient in the appointments and as mentioned earlier, different multi-cohort studies are done to find the factors, which are increasing the disability risk.

Both data sets gave certainly good results for the **accuracy** of the prediction. M_{Health} reached an accuracy of 72% by using neural networks. $M_{Pension}$ achieved an accuracy of 78% when neural networks were used. That means, that the AI algorithm can predict reasonably well whether the person has a high risk to get on the disability pension. AI can support the experts, but it is not accurate enough to work independently. When comparing our results with other studies, we must observe that they are typically done using a certain disease. For example, Bergström et al. [17] got 67–93% prediction accuracy for the patients with back pain, while the most accurate results were for disability pension cases.

Sensitivity refers to the probability of a positive test, conditioned on truly having the condition. In the M_{Health} sensitivity means, how well patients with work disability risk are identified from the data compared to health care expert's classification. In the $M_{Pension}$ sensitivity means, how well work disability pension is predicted compared to real disability pension decision. Sensitivity scores were on a similar level in both methods. In the M_{Health} sensitivity was 79% and $M_{Pension}$ 76%. It is important to find risk cases from both health care and pension data, so the sensitivity must be as high as possible in both methods.

Specificity refers to the probability of a negative test, provided one does not have the condition. In the M_{Health} specifity means, how well patients without work disability risk are identified from the data compared to health care expert's classifications. In the $M_{Pension}$ specifity means, how well cases where a disability pension is not granted can be predicted compared to real disability pension decisions. The methods differ more in the specificity. In the M_{Health} the specificity was pretty low, 61%, whereas the specificity in the $M_{Pension}$ was much better, 80%. When using this kind of algorithm in screening the risk individuals, it is not so critical for the patient if we falsely classify him as a risk case and discuss the topic of disability risk with him even if the patient is not at risk. In practice, an expert will go through these positive classifications before the customer appointment and thus these discussions are not held. This naturally causes some extra work, but the efficiency is improved as all the negatively classified cases can be disregarded. Thus, the rather low specificity in the M_{Health} is not so problematic. On the other hand, if we are using that kind of algorithm in support of pension decisions, which is the situation when using the $M_{Pension}$, specificity must be quite high to avoid false pension decisions.

6 Discussion

The final model of research with occupational health companies shows that the model can probably be used as a tool that helps reduce work in the screening process. However, the error rate is still so high that it should not be trusted blindly, and humans should inspect the results. Increased forecasting accuracy or easy transferability from context to context would greatly increase the usefulness of the model. When thinking about proactive help for a patient, a discussion with the doctor and patient can be held and it is not a big problem if we get false positives. When dealing with disability pension decisions, both false positives and negatives have a great impact. We cannot give a permanent pension decision for the wrong reasons and we also must find those people who need it. Some decisions in the insurance business can be done without a human in the decision-making, but the disability pension process should make the right decisions in almost 100% of cases, which is at least today impossible. But, on the other hand, also humans make errors, and decisions are typically done using documents only without meeting the patient, which makes AI possible to use in the decision-making as the machine is more precise and can go through all the documents more carefully than a human.

The forecasting accuracy should be significantly improved by further development of the forecasting model and the introduction of data from new sources, for example, combining health and pension data and adding more social data. Once it gets easier to combine more extensive datasets and form health care ecosystems to get over legal restrictions, AI will offer improved tools to help identify risk groups and plan preventive methods. We will investigate later the possible ecosystem models used in work disability prediction. We must also take into consideration the legal restrictions of data sharing between different organizations. We will also study consent management and trust creation in digital environments. If we could use both methods together, we could get better results. Pension companies could use M_{Health}, the NLP algorithm, for medical certificates, which are an appendix for disability pension applications. This could improve results for the pension register case, $M_{Pension}$. On the other hand, occupational health care companies could use more structural data, such as self-rated health, trouble falling asleep, BMI, and smoking, which could be received from surveys during the visits to the doctor. There are legal restrictions for that – pension fund administration cannot have data from the pension applicant before the application is submitted.

With using machine learning in disability risk prediction, we want to provide proactive health and rehabilitation services to employees as early as possible to keep people healthy and capable to work. On the other hand, this kind of use of AI could lead to a society where people can be discriminated against when applying for work or insurance with their disability risk, this is not the society we are aiming for and thus ethics of AI is so important.

7 Conclusions

It is important to find ML methods for work disability prediction to screen efficiently potential risk individuals to provide preventive help and thus avoid disability pensions. We compared two ML methods for that purpose. The method M_{Health} is an NLP model that predicts work disability risk based on medical records. There are two classification groups: no disability risk and disability risk. The model is created based on Fastai's ULMFiT using 6000 labeled Finnish medical records as training data and 3000 labeled texts for validation. Medical experts labeled texts to the risk and non-risk cases and the algorithm tried to learn the classification. The method $M_{Pension}$, on the other hand, tried different algorithms and utilizes structural data. Data consists of pension decision register data of 240 000 persons retired on a work disability pension and same size data set of randomly selected persons not retired on a disability pension. In this method, we knew the real disability pension decisions and the algorithm tried to predict a given decision. Results are quite similar in both methods, work disability risk can be predicted with accuracy of 70–80%. M_{Health} and $M_{Pension}$ had quite similar results on sensitivity (79% and 76%, respectively), but methods differ on specificity (61% and 80%, respectively). This is enough to use these methods to support expert work but the decision-maker must still be a human and the responsibility for the decision cannot be on AI but on the expert.

References

1. OECD. Sickness, Disability and Work: Breaking the Barriers. OECD Publishing, Paris, (2010)
2. Airaksinen, J., et al.: Development and validation of a risk prediction model for work disability: multicohort study. Sci. Rep. **7**(13578), 1–12 (2017)
3. Salonen, L., Blomgren, J., Laaksonen, M.: From long-term sickness absence to disability retirement: diagnostic and occupational class differences within the working-age Finnish population. BMC Public Health **20**(1), 1–11 (2020)

4. Salonen, L., Alexanderson, K., Rugulies, R., et al.: Combinations of Job demands and job control and future trajectories of sickness absence and disability pension an 11-year follow-up of two million employees in Sweden. J. Occup. Environ. Med. **62**(10), 795–802 (2020)
5. Bethge, M., Spanier, K., Köhn, S., et al.: Self-reported work ability predicts health-related exit and absence from work, work participation, and death: longitudinal findings from a sample of German employees. Int. Arch. Occup. Environ. Health **94**(4), 591–599 (2020). https://doi.org/10.1007/s00420-020-01608-4
6. Shiri, R., et al.: A screening tool for the risk of disability retirement due to musculoskeletal disoders. Scand. J. Work Environ. Health **44**(1), 37–46 (2018)
7. van Amelsvoort, L.G.P.M., Kant, I.J., Beurskens, A.J.H.M., Schröer, C.A.P., Swaen, G.M.H.: Fatigue as a predictor of work disability. Occup. Environ. Med. **59**(10), 712–713 (2002)
8. Reho, T.: Frequent attenders of occupational health primary care and work disability. Tampere University Dissertations 225 (2020)
9. Lindström, I., Pallasaho, P., Remes, J., et al.: Does lung function predict the risk of disability pension? An 11-year register-based follow-up study. BMC Public Health **20**(165), 1–11 (2020)
10. Pham, A.D., et al.: Natural language processing of radiology reports for the detection of thromboembolic diseases and clinically relevant incidental findings. BMC Bioinform. **15**(1), 266 (2014)
11. Huhta-Koivisto, T.: Work disability risk prediction with machine learning. Master thesis. Aalto University, School of Electrical Engineering, Espoo, 56 p. (2020)
12. Varis, J.: Eläketurvakeskuksen koneoppimiskokeilu – näin se tehtiin! Finnish Centre for Pensions, blog post. https://www.etk.fi/blogit/elaketurvakeskuksen-koneoppimiskokeilu-nain-se-tehtiin/. Accesed 17 Apr 2018
13. European Pensions: Finnish AI testing successfully identifies future retirees facing disability pension. https://www.europeanpensions.net/ep/Finnish-AI-successfully-identifies-future-retirees-facing-disability-pension.php. Accesed 17 Apr 2018
14. Howard, J., Ruder, S.: Universal language model fine-tuning for text classification, In: Proceedings of the 56th Annual Meeting of the Association for Computational Linguistics, vol. 1 (2018)
15. Devlin, J., Ming-Wei, C., Lee, K., Toutanova, K.: BERT: pre-training of deep bidirectional transformers for language understanding (2019). arXiv:1810.04805v2
16. Vaswani, A., et al.: Attention is all you need. In: Advances in Neural Information Processing Systems, pp. 5998–6008 (2017)
17. Bergström, G., Hagberg, J., Busch, H., Jensen, I., Björklund, C.: Prediction of sickness absenteeism, disability pension and sickness presenteeism among employees with back pain. J Occup. Rehabil. **24**(2), 278–286 (2014)

Breast Tumor Segmentation in Ultrasound Images Based on U-NET Model

Epimack Michael, He Ma(✉), and Shouliang Qi

Northeastern University, Shenyang, China
{mahe,qisl}@bmie.neu.edu.cn

Abstract. Breast cancer is the second leading cause of cancer death among women in the United States. If detected and diagnosed in the early stages, it increases survival rates and lowers treatment costs. Emerging deep learning methods have enabled researchers to achieve remarkable results in the classification and segmentation of natural images and computer vision tasks. However, medical images continue to face challenges due to a lack of ground truth for segmentation tasks. As a result, this study proposed and developed automatic methods for segmenting breast lesions from ultrasound images with few label images. The proposed U-NET model employs GELU activation function and has been tested on a total of 620 breast ultrasound images, which includes 310 benign and 310 malignant cases. The quantitative analysis includes accuracy, loss function, dice similarity coefficient, and precision. The qualitative analysis compares original images, masks, image predicted, and the output result, which is mask predicted binary image. The proposed U-NET model outperformed previous methods, achieving a DSC of 99.62%, a loss of 3.01%, an accuracy of 98.15%, and a precision of 91.82%. In addition, we have identified some of the innovations made to the original U-NET model.

Keywords: Ultrasound image · Deep learning · Images segmentation · U-NET segmentation · GELU activation

1 Introduction

Among women in the United States, breast cancer ranks second among cancer-related deaths. According to the American Cancer Society predicts that in 2021, 49,290 new cases of female breast ductal carcinoma and 101,280 cases of melanoma have diagnosed in the United States [1]. WHO statistics indicate that in 2020, 2.3 million women were diagnosed with breast cancer, resulting in 685,000 deaths [2]. Breast cancer detected in the early stages increases survival and decreases mortality by 40.0% in both men and women [3–5]. A breast ultrasound (BUS) is one of the most widely used imaging methods for detecting breast cancer. It's common because it is non-invasive and less expensive than other image modalities and also is capable of seeing internal organs in the body in real time compared to other imaging modalities [6, 7] and [8]. Since 2015, the U-NET model has grown in popularity, and many academics have experimented with new approaches

K. Daimi and A. Al Sadoon (Eds.): ICR 2022, AISC 1431, pp. 22–31, 2022.
https://doi.org/10.1007/978-3-031-14054-9_3

to make the original U-NET model more powerful. To the best of our knowledge, no research has been done to evaluate the improvements made to the original U-UNET model for breast cancer segmentation using 2D ultrasound images. Furthermore, the majority of previous start-of-art works used the RELU activation function. The proposed work employs the Gaussian Error Linear Unit (GELU) activation function instead of the rectified linear (RELU) activation function. Some recent studies are shown below:

Vakanski et al. [9] suggested a new method for integrating a visual salience map into an in-deep learning model for tumor segmentation in breast ultrasound images (BUS). The proposed model included attention blocks in the form of a U-Net model. The method makes use of 510 BUS images gathered from three hospitals. The method achieved a dice similarity coefficient (DSC) of 90.5%, an intersection over union (IOU) of 83.8%, an accuracy (ACC) of 98.0%, and an area under the ROC Curve (AUC-ROC) of 95.7%.

Bra et al. [10] proposed a new form of the U-NET model based on a selective kernel (SK) U-Net convolutional neural network for mass segmentation of ultrasound images (CNN). A total of 882 mass breast ultrasound images was used to assess the model. The SK-U-NET model achieved a mean DSC of 82.6%, an ACC of 97.9%, and an area under the curve (AUC) of 95.8% after benign and malignant tumors were combined by adjusting receptive fields.

Singh et al. [11] proposed an effective automated way to segment tumors in breast ultrasound images based on a contextual information-aware conditional generative adversarial learning framework. The proposed method uses atrous convolution, which captures spatial and scale contexts that can handle different sizes and shapes of the tumor. The proposed method used 350 breast ultrasound images, of which 150 were malignant tumor images and 100 were benign tumor images. The method achieved a DSC of 93.76%, an accuracy of 99.26%, IOU of 88.82%, a sensitivity of 90.11%, and a specificity of 99.73%.

Han et al. [12] suggested semi-supervised segmentation of lesions. The proposed method used for segment breast ultrasound images based on attentional generative adversarial network. The proposed method was trained and tested using two datasets which comprised of 2D BUS images of female patients. The training dataset contained 2000 ultrasound images of which 100 were annotated images and 1900 were annotated images. The method was tested 963 ultrasound images. The method achieved a DSC of 87.12%, Jaccard index (JI) of 77.62%, and precision of 86.38%.

Ramadan et al. [13] proposed automatic detection and segmentation of breast ultrasound images based on saliency guided. The proposed method uses 163 lesion images, of which 53 were cancer images and 110 were benign lesions. The method achieved a DSC of 84.00%, Jaccard index of 73.09%, true positive rate (TPR) of 76.81%, and a BF of 98.15%.

Qu et al. [14] proposed a global attention up sample combined with deep supervision based on a full-resolution residual network. The proposed method was tested on two data sets. The first dataset consisted of 163 breast ultrasounds images, of which 53 were malignant and 110 were benign tumor images. In addition, the second data set consisted of 980 breast ultrasound images, of which 595 were malignant and 385 were benign tumor images. The proposed method achieved a DSC of 84.3%, a Jaccard index of 75.2%, and an F1 score of 84.3%. Pan et al. [15] proposed a bidirectional LSTM neural network and an attention mechanism to automatically segment entire breast ultrasound images. The proposed model used 124 patients based on 170 volumes, of which 3636 slices were labelled as 2D. The model achieved a DSC of 81.78%, recall of 80.67%, precision of 82.92%, and a Hausdorff distance (HD) of 11.1367%.

Amiri et al. [16] proposed two-stage breast ultrasound image segmentation by employing the U-NET model based on the augmentation of images. The performance of the proposed method was tested using 163 B-mode US images, of which 110 were benign and 53 were malignant lesions. The proposed method achieved a DSC of 86.5%.

Yang et al. [17] proposed tumor detection from breast ultrasound images using mammary gland attentive U-NET. The proposed model is based on a deep learning model which incorporates anatomical knowledge of the human breast. The method was tested using 971 BUS images from four different sources with a pixel size of 500 × 500. The method achieved an accuracy of 92.7%.

Guo et al. [18] proposed an expanded U-NET model for segmentation and recognition of breast ultrasound images. The proposed method was tested using 192 BUS, of which 177 were benign and 23 were malignant tumor images. The method achieved a Dice coefficient of 90.5% and an IOU coefficient of 82.7% based on the expanded training method.

Alzahrani et al. [19] proposed breast ultrasound image segmentation based on the deep learning method. The original U-NET architecture was modified by including pre-trained inception residual blocks to segment (BUS) images. The method was tested using two datasets that include UDIAT with 4800 BUS images and BUSI with 4992 BUS images. The method achieved a DSC of 94.8%, IOU of 90.3%, a recall of 94.6%, a precision of 95.2% and an accuracy of 99.5%.

Tong et al. [20] proposed a lesion segmentation of breast ultrasound images based on an improved U-NET MALF model. The proposed improvement to the U-NET model was based on a mixed attention loss function. The method was evaluated using 316 BUS images, of which 145 were malignant and 171 were benign tumors. The method achieved a precision of 90.6%, a recall of 83.2%, an accuracy of 95.7% and a DSC of 91.1%.

Zhuang et al. [21] proposed a residual dilated attention gate U-NET to segment the tumors in BUS images. The plain neural units were replaced with residual units to enhance the edge information that overcomes the network performance degradation problem caused by deep networks. The model increases the receptive field and acquires more characteristic information. Dilated convolutions use the feature maps obtained from the encoder. The performance of the proposed method was tested on 1062 BUS images and produced mean intersection over union which provided performances above 80.0%. The following are the contributions made by this paper:

- It identifies some improvements made to the original U-NET Model.
- It generates group truth, which is then fed into the U-NET model.
- It summarizes deep learning segmentation based on breast ultrasound images.
- It proposes a U-NET model based using GELU activation function.

The rest of this article is organized as follows: Sect. 2 introduces the materials and methods used in this research. The experimental findings are presented in Sect. 3. The paper is concluded in Sect. 4.

2 Materials and Methods

We present here a method for segmenting breast ultrasound images based on U-NET. The proposed model consists of two parts: a contracting path (encoding) and an expansive path (decoding). The U-NET model was initially designed to segment microscopy images and was developed by Ranneberger as an improvement to fully convolutional networks (FCN) [22]. The study showed that the U-NET model has been successful in medical image segmentation compared with other deep learning models in terms of pixel detection and architecture segmentation, and it also does not require thousands of annotated medical images.

2.1 Data Acquisition

The medical dataset collected from the hospital can be in 2D or 3D images. The 2D breast ultrasound image dataset used in this study was acquired from the imaging department of a local Chinese hospital. The 2D images were selected over the 3D dataset because the 2D dataset requires less memory usage and 2D models are more lightweight due to a number of learned parameters. As a result, 2D models can accurately detect and accurately segment breast lesion boundaries. The data set consisted of 620 breast ultrasound images at a resolution of 500 $\times$ 500 pixels, including 310 benign and 310 malignant lesions. According to the pathology report, the breast images were confirmed as benign or malignant breast tumors. An example of an ultrasound image with a benign and malignant breast tumor are shown in Fig. 1 and Fig. 2. In addition, based on a mark drawn by radiologists, we developed a binarization-based segmentation algorithm to obtain the ROI.

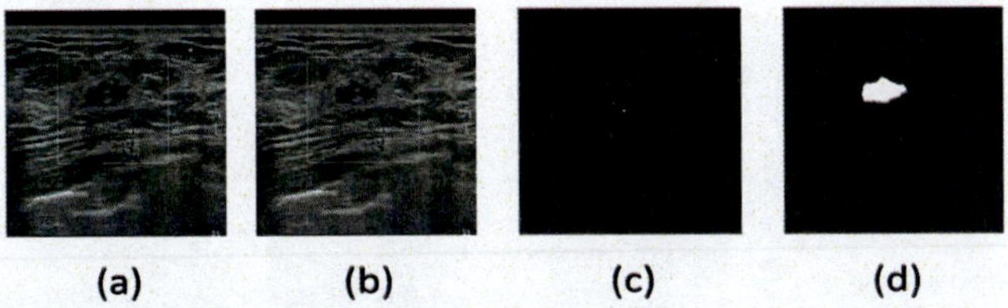

Fig. 1. An example of an ultrasound image with a benign breast tumor: (a) Original image, (b) Mask image (c) Outline detection (d) Ground truth image.

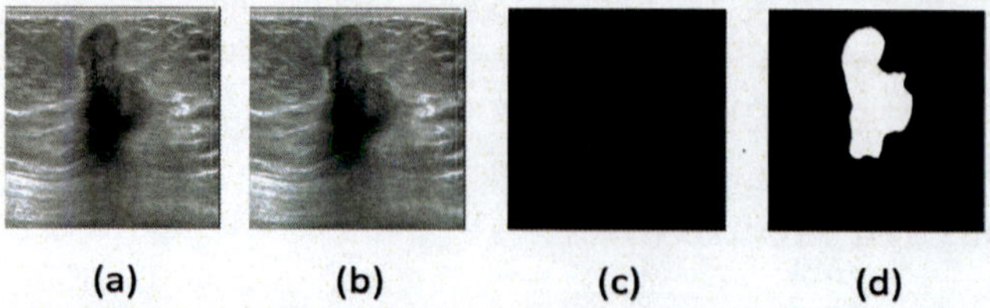

Fig. 2. An example of an ultrasound image with a malignant breast tumor: (a) Original image, (b) Mask image (c) Outline detection (d) Groundtruth image.

2.2 U-Net Topology

The suggested U-NET model was created in Python with the TensorFlow and Keras packages, and trained and tested with Google Colab, a free cloud GPU. Figure 3 show the proposed U-NET topology. In the encoding path, the input images are RGB with 16 channels and have a convolution of 5×5 followed by 4 max pooling. In the decoder path, we use transposed convolution. The method employs GELU instead of RELU's activation function. The dimensions of input images were maintained to be the same as output images by using padding in each max pooling. In addition, the overfit of the model was avoided by employing dropout in each convolution block.

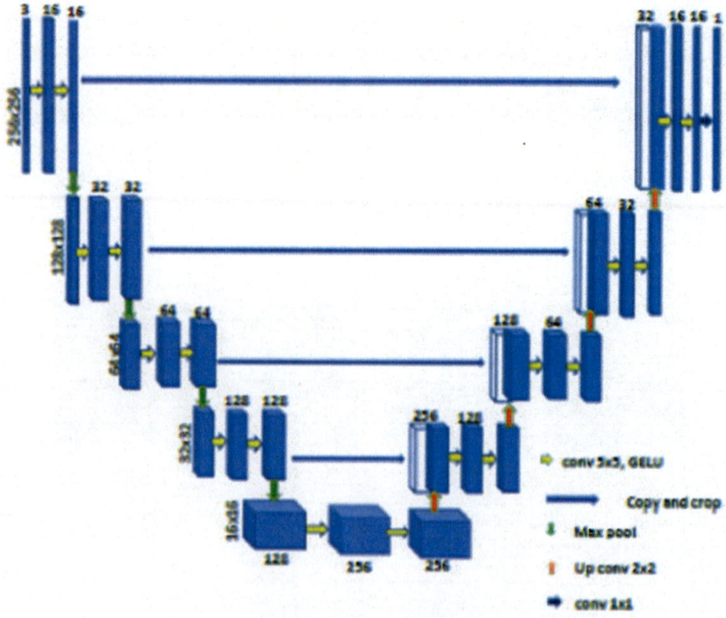

Fig. 3. U-Net topology.

2.3 Training Procedure

The dataset was split into training (80%) and testing (20%) images. The breast ultrasound images, and ground truths were used to train the proposed U-NET model. The datasets were normalized with 0 and 1, a binary cross-entropy loss function was used, and the network was optimized using the Adam optimizer. The dropout used was 0.005, the learning rate was 0.00000001, the batch size was 16, and the epochs were 500, but the early stop was 22. In addition, no image augmentation was done.

2.4 Evaluation

The performance of the segmentation model is evaluated using three quantitative indicators, namely; loss function, accuracy (ACC), and dice similarity coefficient (DSC) [23] and precision. Dice is the commonest segmentation evaluation metric for medical image task [24] and is used to compare the ground truth and the automatic segmentation results.

$$\text{Dice} = \frac{2 \times \text{True positive}}{2 \times \text{True positive} + \text{False negative} + \text{False positive}} \tag{1}$$

$$\text{Accuracy} = \frac{\text{Number of True Positives} + \text{True Negatives}}{\text{Total Observations}} \tag{2}$$

$$\text{Precision} = \frac{\text{Number of True Positives}}{\text{Number of Predicted Positives}} \tag{3}$$

3 Results

In this section, we compared previous state-of-the-art deep learning models, including U-NET, Residual dilated attention gate, PPU-NET, FCN, Semi-supervised segmentation, Multi-U-NET, LSTM, and CNN. We compared the results with ground truth ROIs that were manually annotated by expert radiologists and also results produced by the U-NET model. The obtained results were compared with the previous method as shown in Table 1. In addition, Table 1 shows some of the innovations made to the original U-NET model, which include: integrating visual saliency into a DL model, selective kernel (SK) U-NET CNN, U-NET model incorporating VGG16, Expanded U-NET, Inception encoder embedded into U-NET, Improved U-NET MALF, and plain neural units are replaced with residual units. Also, Fig. 4 shows quantitative analysis such as (a) 3.01% loss, (b) 98.15% accuracy, (c) a dice coefficient of 99.62%, and (d) precision of 91.82%. In addition, Fig. 5 indicates qualitative analysis, which shows a (visuality) comparison between the original images, mask, image predicted and the output result of the proposed method, which is mask predicted binary. Based on the presented results, based on quantitative analysis. The proposed U-NET model determines the suitability for segmentation of breast ultrasound images as it outperforms previous deep learning models.

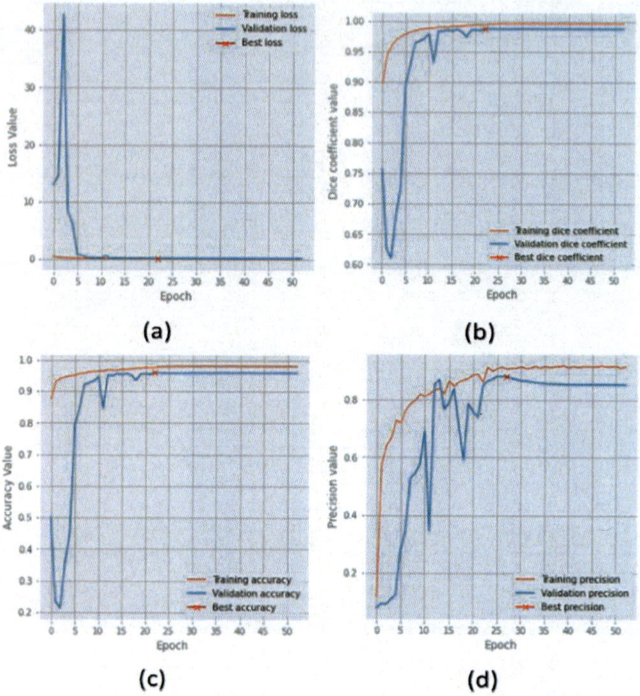

Fig. 4. The comparison of the proposed U-NET model: (a) Loss, (b) Dice coefficient (c) Accuracy and, (d) Precision.

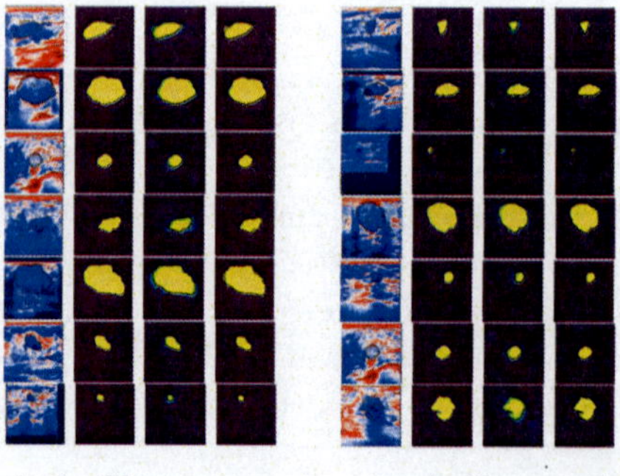

Fig. 5. The qualitative analysis of the segmented results: the first row (image), second row (mask), third row (image predicted), and four row (mask predicted binary)

Table 1. Performance evaluation in comparison to previous related state-of-the-art works

Refer	Method	No of Image	Metrics	Innovation
[9]	U-NET	510	Dice coefficient of 90.5%, IOU of 83.8%, Accuracy of 98.0% and AUC-ROC of 95.7%	Integrate visual saliency into a DL model
[10]	U-NET	882	Dice coefficient of 82.6%, Accuracy of 97.9% and AUC of 95.82%	Selective kernel (SK) U-NET CNN
[11]	Conditional generative adversarial	350	Dice coefficient of 93.76%, Accuracy of 99.20%, IOU of 88.82%, Sensitivity of 90.11%, and Specificity of 99.73%	Contextual-information-aware GAN
[12]	BUS-GAN	2800	Dice coefficient of 87.12%, Jaccard Index of 77.62%, and Precision of 86.38%	Uses of unannotated BUS images to improve segment performance
[13]	Saliency-guided au- detection and segmentation	163	Dice coefficient of 84.0%, Jaccard. In supervised of 73.09% TPR of 76.81% and BF of 98.15%	new saliency guided method
[14]	Attention-supervised full-resolution residual network	980	Dice coefficient of 84.0%, Jaccard In- of 75.26%, and F1 of 84.3%	Combined FRRN, attention mechanism, & deep supervised
[15]	BLSTM	3636	DSC of 80.67%, HD of 11.1367, and Pre- precision of 82.9%	Incorporating BLSTM & SC-attention module into FCN.
[16]	U-NET	163	DSC of 86.5%	Double U-NET techniques
[17]	U-NET & VGG16	971	Accuracy of 86.5%	DL model incorporated VGG16
[18]	U-NET	192	DSC of 90.5% and IOU coefficient of 82.7%	Expanded U-NET
[19]	U-NET	9792	DSC of 94.8%, IOU of 90.3%, recall of 94.6%, precision of 95.2% and Accuracy of 99.5%	Inception encoder embedded into U-NET
[20]	U-NET	316	Precision of 90.6%, recall of 83.2%, accuracy of 95.7% and DSC of 91.1%	Improved U-NET MALF
[21]	Residual Dilated At- Gate U-NET	1062	IOU 80.0%	Plain neural units are replaced with residual units
Proposed	U-NET	620	DSC of 99.62%, loss of 3.01%, accuracy of 98.15%, and precision of 91.82%	GELU

4 Conclusions

In this paper, we propose breast ultrasound image segmentation based on the U-NET model. The proposed method is based on the U-NET algorithm to segment 2D breast ultrasound images in real-time, and it outperformed previous deep leaning models. In addition, we have identified some innovations that have been made to the original U-NET model. Some of these innovations include, integrating visual saliency into a DL model, selective kernel (SK) U-Net CNN, U-NET model incorporating VGG16, Expanded U-NET, Inception encoder embedded into U-NET, Improved U-net MALF, and plain neural units are replaced with residual units. The proposed U-NET model employs GELU activation function and has been tested on a total of 620 breast ultrasound images, which includes 310 benign and 310 malignant cases. In our future work, the model is going to be tested on different data sets to test its generalizability. The method will be divided into three experiments, based on benign, malignant, and benign combined with malignant tumors. In addition, the same hyper-parameters will be used during training in three experiments to ensure the fairness of the model.

References

1. Siegel, R.L., Miller, K.D., Fuchs, H.E., Jemal, A.: Cancer statistics, 2021. CA: Cancer J. Clin. **71**(1), 7–33 (2021)
2. World Health Organization: Global health observatory. World Health Organization, American Cancer Society, Geneva, Atlanta (2018)
3. Coleman, C.: Early detection and screening for breast cancer. Semin. Oncol. Nurs. **33**(2), 141–155 (2017)
4. Loud, J.T., Murphy, J.: Cancer screening and early detection in the 21st century. Semin. Oncol. Nurs. **33**(2), 121–128 (2017)
5. Smith, N.B., Webb, A.: Introduction to Medical Imaging: Physics Engineering and Clinical Applications. Cambridge University Press, Cambridge (2010)
6. Kim, W.H., et al.: Ultrasonographic assessment of breast density. Breast Cancer Res. Treat. **138**(3), 851–859 (2013)
7. Huang, Y.-L., Chen, D.-R., Liu, Y.-K.: Breast cancer diagnosis using image retrieval for different ultrasonic systems. In: 2004 International Conference on Image Processing, ICIP 2004, vol. 5, pp. 2957–2960. IEEE (2004)
8. Sennoga, C.A.: Ultrasound imaging, bioengineering innovative solutions for cancer, pp. 123–161 (2020)
9. Vakanski, A., Xian, M., Freer, P.E.: Attention-enriched deep learning model for breast tumor segmentation in ultrasound images. Ultrasound Med. Biol. **46**(10), 2819–2833 (2020)
10. Byra, M., et al.: Breast mass segmentation in ultrasound with selective kernel U-net convolutional neural network. Biomed. Signal Process. Control **61**, 102027 (2020)
11. Singh, V.K., et al.: Breast tumor segmentation in ultrasound images using contextual-information-aware deep adversarial learning framework. Expert Syst. Appl. **162**, 113870 (2020)
12. Han, L., et al.: Semi-supervised segmentation of lesion from breast ultrasound images with attentional generative adversarial network. Comput. Methods Program. Biomed. **189**, 105275 (2020)
13. Ramadan, H., Lachqar, C., Tairi, H.: Saliency-guided automatic detection and segmentation of tumor in breast ultrasound images. Biomed. Signal Process. Control **60**, 101945 (2020)

14. Qu, X., Shi, Y., Hou, Y., Jiang, J.: An attention-supervised fullresolution residual network for the segmentation of breast ultrasound images. Med. Phys. **47**, 5702–5714 (2020)
15. Pan, P., Chen, H., Li, Y., Cai, N., Cheng, L., Wang, S.: Tumor segmentation in automated whole breast ultrasound using bidirectional LSTM neural network and attention mechanism. Ultrasonics **110**, 106271 (2020)
16. Amiri, M., Brooks, R., Behboodi, B., Rivaz, H.: Two-stage ultrasound image segmentation using U-net and test time augmentation. Int. J. Comput. Assist. Radiol. Surg. **15**, 981–988 (2020)
17. Yang, K., Suzuki, A., Ye, J., Nosato, H., Izumori, A., Sakanashi, H.: Tumor detection from breast ultrasound images using mammary gland attentive U-NET. In: International Forum on Medical Imaging in Asia 2021, vol. 11792, p. 1179202. International Society for Optics and Photonics (2021)
18. Guo, Y., Duan, X., Wang, C., Guo, H.: Segmentation and recognition of breast ultrasound images based on an expanded U-NET. PLoS One **16**(6), e0253202 (2021)
19. Alzahrani, Y., Boufama, B.: Deep learning approach for breast ultrasound image segmentation. In: 2021 4th International Conference on Artificial Intelligence and Big Data (ICAIBD), pp. 437–442. IEEE (2021)
20. Tong, Y., Liu, Y., Zhao, M., Meng, L., Zhang, J.: Improved U-NET malf model for lesion segmentation in breast ultrasound images. Biomed. Signal Process. Control **68**, 102721 (2021)
21. Zhuang, Z., Li, N., Joseph Raj, A.N., Mahesh, V.G., Qiu, S.: An RDAU-NET model for lesion segmentation in breast ultrasound images. PLoS One **14**, e0221535 (2019)
22. Ronneberger, O., Fischer, P., Brox, T.: U-NET: convolutional networks for biomedical image segmentation. In: Navab, N., Hornegger, J., Wells, W., Frangi, A. (eds.) MICCAI 2015. LNCS, vol. 9351, pp. 234–241. Springer, Cham (2015). https://doi.org/10.1007/978-3-319-24574-4_28
23. Adegun, A.A. Viriri, S. Ogundokun, R.O.: Deep learning approach for medical image analysis. Comput. Intell. Neurosci. **2021** (2021)
24. Dice, L.R.: Measures of the amount of ecologic association between species. Ecology **26**(3), 297–302 (1945)

Heart Attack Classification System Using Neural Network Trained with Particle Swarm Optimization

Askandar H. Amin[1](✉), Botan K. Ahmed[2], Bestan B. Maaroof[3,4], and Tarik A. Rashid[5]

[1] Technical College of Informatics, Sulaimani Polytechnic University, Sulaimani, KRG, Iraq
askandar.hamid@spu.edu.iq

[2] Administration and Economics, University of Sulaimani, Sulaimani, KRG, Iraq
botan.ahmed@univsul.edu.iq

[3] IT Department, College of Commerce, University of Sulaimani, Sulaimani, KRG, Iraq
bestan.maaroof@univsul.edu.iq

[4] School of Information Technology, Fanshawe College, London, Canada

[5] Computer Science and Engineering Department, University of Kurdistan Hewler, Erbil, KRG, Iraq
tarik.ahmed@ukh.edu.krd

Abstract. The prior detection of a heart attack could lead to the saving of one's life. Putting specific criteria into a system that provides an early warning of an imminent attack will be advantageous to a better prevention plan for an upcoming heart attack. Some studies have been conducted for this purpose, but yet the goal has not been reached to prevent a patient from getting such a disease. In this paper, Neural Network trained with Particle Swarm Optimization (PSONN) is used to analyze the input criteria and enhance heart attack anticipation. A real and novel dataset that has been recorded on the disease is used. After preprocessing the data, the features are fed into the system. As a result, the outcomes from PSONN have been evaluated against those from other algorithms. Decision Tree, Random Forest, Neural network trained with Backpropagation (BPNN), and Naive Bayes were among those employed. Then the results of 100%, 99.2424%, 99.2323%, 81.3131%, and 66.4141% are produced concerning the mentioned algorithms, which show that PSONN has recorded the highest accuracy rate among all other tested algorithms.

Keywords: Heart attack · Particle swarm optimization · Neural network · Backpropagation · Swarm intelligence

1 Introduction

Each year, around twelve million people die due to heart attacks around the globe. The disease affects poor and rich people, both men and women. There are great means specialists set to follow, and the good news is that the disease can be prevented through

K. Daimi and A. Al Sadoon (Eds.): ICR 2022, AISC 1431, pp. 32–41, 2022.
https://doi.org/10.1007/978-3-031-14054-9_4

some steps to help [1]. The main purpose of conducting this research is to showcase where people suffer heart attacks based on some criteria using a recent dataset collected from actual patients who either had a heart attack or not [2].

To contribute, the way this study covers is to enter into the field of Artificial Intelligence for extra accuracy and to save time in assessing such a case in the future application of the model generated by this case study. Furthermore, the result has a higher level of accuracy since the dataset collected from actual cases of the mentioned disease, is based on some features that all people have in common that have a major impact on this type of disease; heart attack. This is a long-lasting disease, it has a long history, and so much research has been done to identify and understand it. The American College of Cardiology (ACC) states that the earliest example of coronary artery disease was discovered in an Egyptian princess, who died of a heart attack near the end of her illness in her forties living between the years 1580 and 1550 B.C. [3].

No final therapy or direct prevention has indeed been released to date to stop heart attacks, and this is an urgent issue when the person affected should be treated at the very early stage of it as quickly as possible. Consequently, more investigation needs to be taken into account to better understand the reasons why one gets a heart attack and to find a quick and effective solution to it for a specific patient, either to monitor the body's activities during old age or in hospitals using artificial intelligence microsystems placed on the patient's body for any of our elderly people. To cope with the disease and/or to specify if one is about to get a heart attack, it is necessary to update the datasets time by time that is used to let the systems that are working concerning that disease be aware of the changes happening in the human body and to treat the algorithms more accurately to prevent someone from dying.

The system testing the dataset that has been used is very user-friendly and has an upgraded hybrid algorithm, combining two great algorithms into one, better to work on datasets for a realistic outcome. So in the upcoming sections, it will be discussed how the algorithms, which have been combined into one piece, are used in a prepared system to train and test such new or any datasets to collect results. In our case, is the patient close to getting a heart attack or not. After that, the methodology for using the system and the grabbed results will be presented in a discussion.

The rest of the paper is divided into the following sections: Literature Review is explained in Sect. 2, Methodology is described in Sect. 3. Section 4, displays the results, and finally, the main points are concluded in Sect. 5.

2 Literature Review

As mentioned earlier in this paper, heart attack early detection has continuously gained the attention of researchers, especially those in the artificial intelligence field. Various studies and research have been conducted for this purpose, as early detection of a heart attack is a huge step toward saving many people's lives. Research conducted by Feshki and Shijani [4] presented the Particle Swarm Optimization system (PSO) and feed-forward neural network for feature ranking on affected factors. The proposed system had the impact of the reduction of thirteen effective cardiovascular factors to eight optimized features. As a result of the assessment of the selected features, the system showed a high accuracy rate of 91.94%.

Shanthi proposed an adaptive neuro-fuzzy inference system [5]. The proposed system relied on some features based on the lifestyle of the patient taken as input to the system and then neuro-fuzzy inference predicts the probability of cardiovascular disease. Ali et al. [6] proposed an automated diagnostic system based on deep neural networks (DNN) for making predictions for heart disease. Then X^2 statistical model was conducted for feature refinement. The Cleveland dataset was used for testing and training. The results claimed better performance compared to the previously presented neural networks.

Very recent work has been done by Wang et al. [7] to predict heart attack in stroke patients. They used an undersampling, clustering-oversampling algorithm (UCO) for imbalanced data processing as well as feature extraction. The output from UCO120 was fed into five different classifiers, and the test results showed that the random forest had gained an accuracy of 70.29%, which was the best performance among the other classifiers. Another study conducted by Ali et al. [8] used two support vector machines (SVM). The first linear SVM was used for feature selection as well as the removal of extraneous features. The second SVM was used for prediction.

Javeed et al. [9] proposed an intelligent hybridized random search algorithm (RSA) with random forest (RF) as an intelligent learning system for heart failure detection. In the proposed RSA-RF system, RSA was used for feature selection and RF was used for prediction based on the selected features from RSA. Another recent piece of research work has been done by Maghdid et al. [2]. The same dataset was used as we used in this current work. They used three techniques; BPNN was one of them, but in the current work, a PSONN [10] is proposed as well. They used two more techniques, the Fuzzy Inference System (FIS) and Adaptive Neuro-Fuzzy System (ANFIS) as predictors for heart attack. The experimental results showed ANFIS to be the most efficient model compared with the other two techniques.

3 Methodology

For this research, the dataset collected by Maghdid et al. [2] is used to detect heart attack systems which are suggested based on the particle swarm optimization neural network (PSONN). This process falls into two steps; firstly, the neural network with two hidden layers is structured to receive the data set [2]. The neural network's weights and biases will be optimized using particle swarm optimization (PSO). Secondly, the PSONN is tested with the dataset to see how well it has been trained [10].

3.1 Dataset

The dataset used for this paper is the same one that was collected from the Surgical Specialty Cardiac Centre's "Directorate of Health-Erbil" Kurdistan Regional Government Iraq, 2018. The size of the provided dataset is 1319 with 8 attributes as shown in Table 1; age, gender, pulse, blood pressure systolic, blood pressure diastolic, glucose, CK-MB, and troponin with only one output; either indicates the existence of a heart attack (positive) or not (negative). The actual data set can be obtained here [11].

According to the provided information, the medical dataset is to classify whether it is a heart attack or not. The data has been encoded in an excel sheet as follows: the male

Table 1. Data attributes & their descriptions

Attributes	Descriptions
Age	Age of the patient in the year
Gender	Gender of the patient (male or female)
Heart rate	Maximum heart rate achieved 10 to 160–180
Systolic blood pressure	Resting systolic blood pressure (in mm Hg on admission to the hospital) (70–190)
Diastolic blood pressure	Resting diastolic blood pressure (in mm Hg on admission to the hospital) (40–100)
Blood sugar	(Blood sugar >120 mg/dl) (1–900 mg/dl)
CK-MB	Enzyme CK-MB (male upto-6.22 female upto-4.88) It is Creatine Kinase Enzymes
Troponin	Enzyme Troponin (0.0–0.014)

is set to 1 and the female to 0. The glucose column is set to 1 if it is >120, otherwise 0. As for the output, positive is set to 1 and negative to 0 (see Fig. 1).

	A	B	C	D	E	F	G	H	I	J
1	Age	Gender	Pulse	Pressure high	Pressure low	Glucose	CK-MB	Troponin	Target	Target
2	64	1	66	160	83	1	1.8	0.012	0	negative
3	21	1	94	98	46	1	6.75	1.06	1	positive
4	55	1	64	160	77	1	1.99	0.003	0	negative
5	64	1	70	120	55	1	13.87	0.122	1	positive
6	55	1	64	112	65	1	1.08	0.003	0	negative
7	58	0	61	112	58	0	1.83	0.004	0	negative
8	32	0	40	179	68	0	0.71	0.003	0	negative
9	63	1	60	214	82	0	300	2.37	1	positive
10	44	0	60	154	81	1	2.35	0.004	0	negative
11	67	1	61	160	95	0	2.84	0.011	0	negative
12	44	0	60	166	90	0	2.39	0.006	0	negative
13	63	0	60	150	83	1	2.39	0.013	0	negative
14	64	1	60	199	99	0	3.43	5.37	1	positive
15	54	0	94	122	67	0	1.42	0.012	0	negative
16	47	1	76	120	70	1	2.57	0.003	0	negative
17	61	1	81	118	66	1	1.49	0.017	1	positive
18	86	0	73	114	68	0	1.11	0.776	1	positive
19	45	0	70	100	68	0	0.606	0.004	0	negative
20	37	0	72	107	86	1	2.89	0.003	0	negative

Fig. 1. A snapshot of the medical dataset in excel (20 out of 1319)

3.2 Neural Network Trained with Particle Swarm Optimization

An elaborated and inherited network based on particle swarm optimization and neural network (PSONN). The proposed PSONN was developed from a neural network (NN) model trained by particle swarm optimization (PSO) for optimizing the weights and biases of the neural network. PSO is used to obtain the optimum weights, and then the optimized weights are fed into the neural network for decision making in the testing

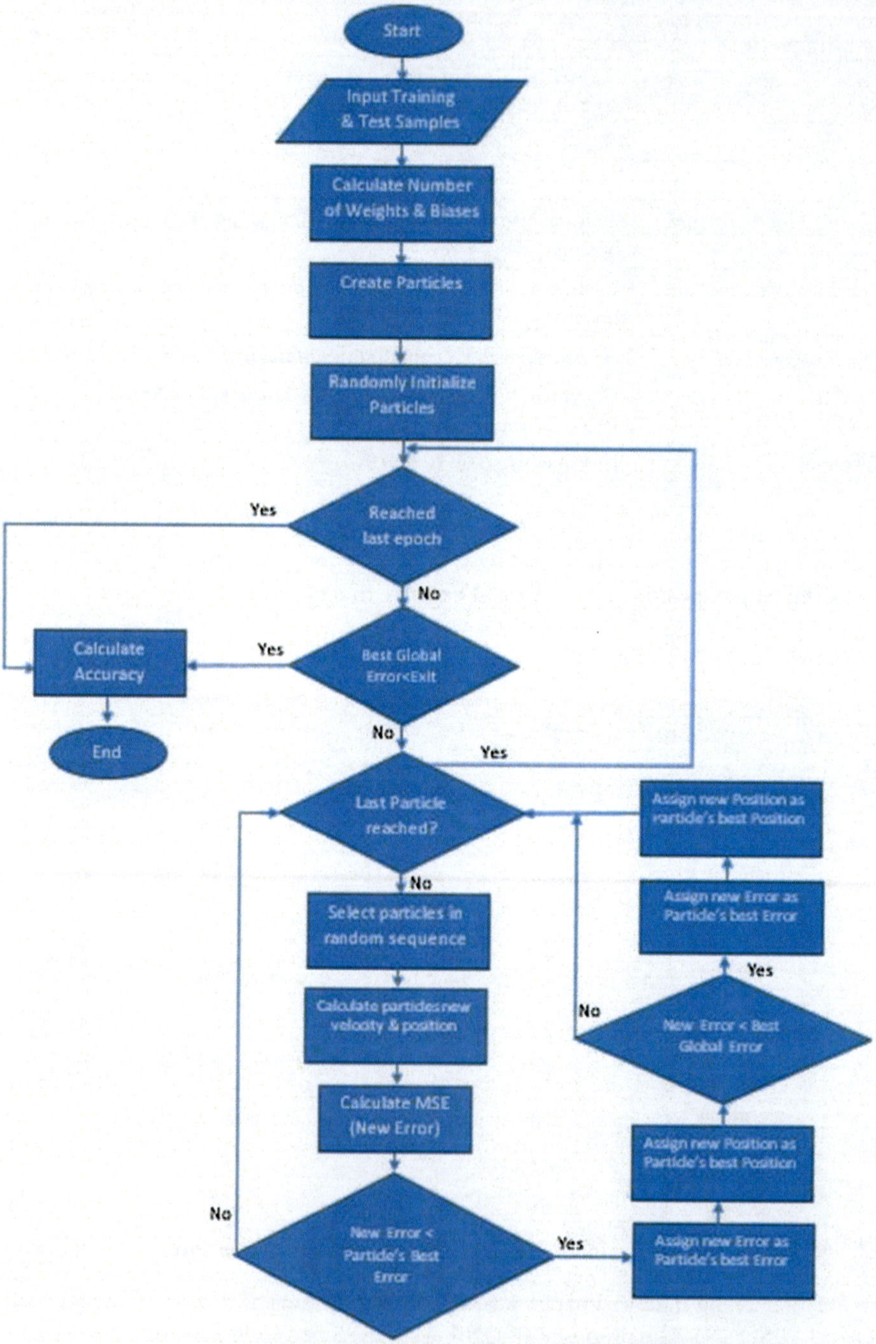

Fig. 2. Flow chart for PSONN algorithm [10].

phase. Then, afterward, these weights are fed into the NN to test the system (PSONN). The flow chart for PSONN algorithms is shown below (Fig. 2).

4 Results and Discussions

The results obtained by the algorithm are as follows for the PSONN model described in the methodology section. Table 2 displays the results of the PSONN model having different epochs applied.

Table 2. Results of the PSONN model for different epochs.

ID	# of epochs	# of features	# of observations	# of hidden layers	MAE	RMSE	Training accuracy
	Train phase						
1	200	8	1055	2	0	0	100.00%
2	500	8	1055	2	0	0	100.00%
3	700	8	1055	2	0	0	100.00%
	Test phase						
1	200	8	264	2	0	0	100.00%
2	500	8	264	2	0	0	100.00%
3	700	8	264	2	0	0	100.00%

Table 2 indicates the accuracy of PSONN with having different epochs it achieved 100% accuracy during the training and testing phases.

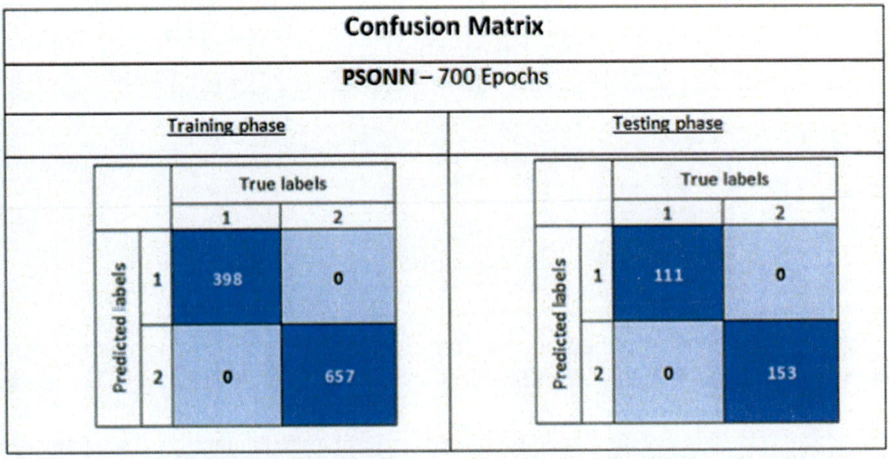

Fig. 3. Confusion matrix for 700 epochs for PSONN model.

Figure 3 demonstrates the accuracy of PSONN during the training and testing phases. The above outcomes were collected when PSONN was configured to run for 700 epochs. The result is that increasing the number of epochs will significantly improve the performance of the PSONN. However, it increases the time and computational power when generating the model. PSONN was tested when there were 700 epochs. It was capable of correctly classifying all the observations during the training and testing phases without any errors. Even after 10,000 epochs of the heart attack dataset, the PSONN algorithm achieves 100% accuracy. Consequently, some other techniques are applied to the same data to achieve a proper result that satisfies researchers.

The Weka tool has been used as a machine learning tool and techniques have been developed using some approaches on how to best fit the data in the tool [12–14]. After loading the data into the tool, it is normalized for better comparison between the features of the dataset. Then four techniques are applied by dividing the dataset into 70% for training and 30% for testing. The results vary; first, the Decision Tree algorithm includes two hidden layers, each having five nodes, and for 500 epochs, the accuracy is the highest compared to the other three algorithms, which average 99.2424%. Second, with slightly lower accuracy, is the Random Forest technique, with 99.2323%. Third, the Backpropagation Neural Network received 81.3131% of the accuracy, and Naive Bayes came in last with 66.4141% of the accuracy. All the results are shown in the below figures along with their confusion matrixes included in them.

```
=== Summary ===

Correctly Classified Instances         393               99.2424 %
Incorrectly Classified Instances         3                0.7576 %
Kappa statistic                          0.9839
Mean absolute error                      0.0129
Root mean squared error                  0.0871
Relative absolute error                  2.7335 %
Root relative squared error             17.9625 %
Total Number of Instances              396

=== Detailed Accuracy By Class ===

                 TP Rate  FP Rate  Precision  Recall   F-Measure  MCC      ROC Area  PRC Area  Class
                 0.988    0.000    1.000      0.988    0.994      0.984    0.990     0.995     positive
                 1.000    0.012    0.980      1.000    0.990      0.984    0.990     0.970     negative
Weighted Avg.    0.992    0.005    0.993      0.992    0.992      0.984    0.990     0.986

=== Confusion Matrix ===

   a   b   <-- classified as
 244   3 |   a = positive
   0 149 |   b = negative
```

Fig. 4. Accuracy of weka decision tree on the heart attack dataset.

Figure 4 illustrates that the Decision Tree algorithm gives the best accuracy for the heart attack dataset which is 99.2424% that correctly classified 393 out of 396 in the testing phase; to mention, all the negative cases of 149 cases were correctly categorized.

Figure 5 clarifies that the Random Forest algorithm gives another great accuracy for the heart attack dataset which is 99.2323%. It categorized 148 out of 149 for negative cases and missed only 6 cases out of 247 positive circumstances.

```
=== Summary ===

Correctly Classified Instances         389               98.2323 %
Incorrectly Classified Instances         7                1.7677 %
Kappa statistic                          0.9626
Mean absolute error                      0.03
Root mean squared error                  0.1051
Relative absolute error                  6.3392 %
Root relative squared error             21.6845 %
Total Number of Instances              396

=== Detailed Accuracy By Class ===

                 TP Rate  FP Rate  Precision  Recall   F-Measure  MCC      ROC Area  PRC Area  Class
                 0.976    0.007    0.996      0.976    0.986      0.963    0.997     0.998     positive
                 0.993    0.024    0.961      0.993    0.977      0.963    0.997     0.988     negative
Weighted Avg.    0.982    0.013    0.983      0.982    0.982      0.963    0.997     0.994

=== Confusion Matrix ===

   a   b   <-- classified as
 241   6 |   a = positive
   1 148 |   b = negative
```

Fig. 5. Accuracy of Weka Random Forest on the heart attack dataset.

```
=== Summary ===

Correctly Classified Instances         322               81.3131 %
Incorrectly Classified Instances        74               18.6869 %
Kappa statistic                          0.6071
Mean absolute error                      0.2562
Root mean squared error                  0.3544
Relative absolute error                 54.1912 %
Root relative squared error             73.1281 %
Total Number of Instances              396

=== Detailed Accuracy By Class ===

                 TP Rate  FP Rate  Precision  Recall   F-Measure  MCC      ROC Area  PRC Area  Class
                 0.830    0.215    0.865      0.830    0.847      0.608    0.896     0.945     positive
                 0.785    0.170    0.736      0.785    0.760      0.608    0.896     0.785     negative
Weighted Avg.    0.813    0.198    0.816      0.813    0.814      0.608    0.896     0.885

=== Confusion Matrix ===

   a   b   <-- classified as
 205  42 |   a = positive
  32 117 |   b = negative
```

Fig. 6. Accuracy of Weka Backpropagation Neural Network on the heart attack dataset.

Figure 6 proves that the Backpropagation Neural Network algorithm gives the accuracy of 81.3131% for the heart attack dataset with two hidden layers of five nodes each. It incorrectly classified 42 positives and 32 negatives out of 396 cases in total for the testing phase.

Figure 7 shows that the Naive Bayes algorithm gives the lowest accuracy for the heart attack dataset which is 66.4141%. Surprisingly, it covered all the 149 negative cases but missed 133 of the positive cases out of 247 positive circumstances.

```
=== Summary ===

Correctly Classified Instances         263               66.4141 %
Incorrectly Classified Instances       133               33.5859 %
Kappa statistic                          0.3921
Mean absolute error                      0.3343
Root mean squared error                  0.5481
Relative absolute error                 70.7018 %
Root relative squared error            113.0935 %
Total Number of Instances              396

=== Detailed Accuracy By Class ===

                 TP Rate  FP Rate  Precision  Recall   F-Measure  MCC      ROC Area  PRC Area  Class
                 0.462    0.000    1.000      0.462    0.632      0.494    0.840     0.914     positive
                 1.000    0.538    0.528      1.000    0.691      0.494    0.840     0.681     negative
Weighted Avg.    0.664    0.203    0.823      0.664    0.654      0.494    0.840     0.826

=== Confusion Matrix ===

   a   b   <-- classified as
 114 133 |   a = positive
   0 149 |   b = negative
```

Fig. 7. Accuracy of Weka Naive Bayes on the heart attack dataset.

5 Conclusion

In this paper, PSONN was used to classify heart attacks. A relatively big dataset was used for classification purposes. PSONN outperformed other competitive algorithms, such as Decision Tree, Random forest, BPNN, and Naive Bayes. Thus, the PSONN model can be relied on by hospitals to predict patients' states according to the experimental results that we obtained. For future work, this algorithm could be tested with different datasets to ensure and verify its performance.

References

1. WHO | Avoiding heart attacks and strokes, WHO (2016). http://www.who.int/cardiovascular_diseases/publications/avoid_heart_attack_report/en/. Accessed 06 May 2021
2. Maghdid, S., Rashid, T., Ahmed, S., Zaman, K., Rabbani, M.: Analysis and prediction of heart attacks based on design of intelligent systems. J. Mech. Contin. Math. Sci. **14**(4), 628–645 (2019). https://doi.org/10.26782/jmcms.2019.08.00051
3. Earliest case of coronary artery disease found in Egyptian princess - American College of Cardiology. https://www.acc.org/about-acc/press-releases/2011/04/05/16/22/mummies. Accessed 06 May 2021
4. Feshki, M., Shijani, O.: Improving the heart disease diagnosis by evolutionary algorithm of PSO and feed forward neural network. In: 2016 Artificial Intelligence and Robotics (IRANOPEN) 2016, pp. 48–53, August 2016. https://doi.org/10.1109/RIOS.2016.7529489
5. Shanthi, S.: Cutomized prediction of heart disease with adaptive neuro fuzzy inference system. Int. J. Adv. Res. Comput. Commun. Eng. **6**(2), 14–18 (2017). https://doi.org/10.17148/IJARCCE.2017.6204
6. Ali, L., Rahman, A., Khan, A., Zhou, M., Javeed, A., Khan, J.A.: an automated diagnostic system for heart disease prediction based on χ^2 statistical model and optimally configured deep neural network, vol. 7, pp. 34938–34945 (2019). https://doi.org/10.1109/ACCESS.2019.2904800

7. Wang, M., Yao, X., Chen, Y.: "An imbalanced-data processing algorithm for the prediction of heart attack in stroke patients. IEEE Access **9**, 25394–25404 (2021). https://doi.org/10.1109/ACCESS.2021.3057693
8. Ali, L., et al.: an optimized stacked support vector machines based expert system for the effective prediction of heart failure. IEEE Access **7**, 54007–54014 (2019). https://doi.org/10.1109/ACCESS.2019.2909969
9. Javeed, A., Zhou, S., Yongjian, L., Qasim, I., Noor, A., Nour, R.: An intelligent learning system based on random search algorithm and optimized random forest model for improved heart disease detection. IEEE Access **7**, 180235–180243 (2019). https://doi.org/10.1109/ACCESS.2019.2952107
10. Rashid, T., Ahmad, H.: Lecturer performance system using neural network with Particle Swarm Optimization. Comput. Appl. Eng. Educ. **24**(4), 629–638 (2016). https://doi.org/10.1002/cae.21737
11. Maghdid, S., Rashid, T.: An extensive dataset for the heart disease classification system. Mendeley data **2** (2022). https://doi.org/10.17632/65gxgy2nmg.2
12. Witten, I., Frank, E., Hall, M.: The WEKA workbench. In: Online Appendix for Data mining: Practical Machine Learning Tools and Techniques, 4th edn. Morgan Kaufmann, Burlington (2016)
13. How to Build Regression Models (Weka Tutorial #1). https://www.youtube.com/watch?v=t5mylGHE2Fg. Accessed 30 July 2022
14. Ahmad, H., Rashid, T.: Lecturer performance analysis using multiple classifiers. J. Comput. Sci. **12**(5), 255–264 (2016). https://doi.org/10.3844/jcssp.2016.255.264

Electroencephalography Image Classification Using Convolutional Neural Networks

Mohammad Gouse Galety[1(✉)], Firas Al-Mukhtar[1], Fanar Rofoo[1], A. V. Sriharsha[2], and Rebaz Maaroof[1]

[1] Catholic University in Erbil, Erbil, Kurdistan Region, Iraq
{m.galety,f.almukhtar,fanar.rofoo,rebaz.maaroof}@cue.edu.krd
[2] Sree Vidyanikethan Engineering College, Tirupathi, India

Abstract. A phenomenal, neurological, and disordered expression of emotions is released as eccentric bio-signals with varied electrical voltages in the brain. An involuntary state of being seized reflects the brain generates electroencephalonsignals read through encephalography and analyzed for many purposes in science and technology. The signal data sets can be commonly applied for classification tasks using DCNN; generally, inaccurate results are posted. However, the datasets are pre-classified during preservation and making up a repository; a class is likely to possess features of other classes, leading to classification uncertainty, which is more particular in EEG datasets. Imbalanced classification prevails due to uncertainty, and heterogeneous entropies influence features in data sets independently, wherefore a multi-label classification employs to anatomize the data containing multiple categorical features. EEG signal image datasets are converted into scaled and normalized image patch forms, smoothened with pooling using Geometric Parameterized ReLU. Multi-label classification is achieved on source EEG signal image data sets using classical DCNN and variations with GPReLU on sets of image patches. ROC assesses the quality of the framework chosen for multi-label classification.

Keywords: Electro-encephalography · Deep convolutional neural network · GPReLu · Bio-signals · Multi-label classification · Epilectical · Entropy

1 Introduction

From the perspective of science or mythology, a significant number of literature demands the prevalence of epileptical seizures. In contrast, the central nervous system's underpowering and overpowering brain electrical stations influence physical acts, irrespective of age and gender. A neuronal discharge is a physical emanation of chemical charges, usually a chemical blip in isolation, while brain motor functions, the interaction of neurons for the successes or failures during the formation of thoughts, unpredictable and unwarned leading to loss of attention of physical body. Many miscommunications rise in the brain internally and externally through the peripheral and constituent parts of the body. This syndrome is not common to all the subjects of patients; the only non-invasive

K. Daimi and A. Al Sadoon (Eds.): ICR 2022, AISC 1431, pp. 42–52, 2022.
https://doi.org/10.1007/978-3-031-14054-9_5

method to read the electrical status of the brain is EEG, which generates multichannel readings. Classifiers are applied to determine the absolute impression of seizure while detection [6]. The chance of building a multi-label classification model persists for most applications due to uncertainty, voluminosity, and multiple classes.

2 Literature

A CNN can correspond to past and future data analyses, mitigating with certainty and state of the data, a high-level cognitive accomplishment, drawing a phenomenal model of studies of the human brain. As recent research demands quick learning and the disposition of conclusions, machine learning and deep learning methods [7] hold anessential position over usual signal processing methods. Optimization and Optimal Search heuristics [24, 25] also contribute to the discovery of peculirar characteristics of the signal data. In [8], the application of machine learning for seizure detection using the CHB-MIT Scalp database of EEG has been treated, and sublime performance factors are yielded. In [9, 21], Qin. et al. proposed a framework for bi-clustering and extreme learning methods, which can almost binary classification of seizure and non-seizure on EEG data. Though not of enough importance, analogue methods are applied [10, 22] for new variants of the time-frequency domain using local mean decomposition blended with support vector machines for the classification based on EEG features. The EEG signal recordings are decomposed for an empirical study [11, 23], and a wavelet-based transform analysis with least squares is executed on focal and non-focal classes.

As opined by Krizhevsky et al. [12], almost eight learned layers and three fully connected layers with five convolutional layers accomplishes the classification of images. The equation to get the output $\boldsymbol{f}$ from the standard model of neuron $\boldsymbol{f}\ (\boldsymbol{x}) = \tan\mathbf{h}\boldsymbol{x}$ or as equivalent to $f(x) = (1 + \mathrm{e}^{-\mathrm{x}})^{-1}$. The saturating nonlinearities are very slow than that of non-saturating concerning time factors. The proposed architecture has promised 78.1% of accuracy in the classification.

As Sharma et al. [13, 20] proposed, the various classifiers take features as inputs from EEG signals; the performance is empirically proven with respective frequencies and structures in the readings. A single-channelled EEG signals database with several epochs with iterative filtering and decomposition, non-stationary signal decomposition methods are employed (Table 1).

The EEG signals are collected and classified, as usual, preictal, ictal and seizure classes. Acharya et al. [14] propounded that EEG signals are classified automatically with a deep CNN model; the basic model of CNN models aremature enough to achieve the goal of classification. Still, the proposed model [14] has improved convergence upto 88.67% evenly upon iterations of applications on samples. Yimin Hou et al. appliedto decode the EEG signals and identified four-class motor imagery using weighted minimum norm estimation. A global classifier is incrementally built to accomplish the perfection of classification using deep convolutional neural networks, with an accuracy of approximately 93.30% from the computed mean of results. W-L Mao et al. in [15] introduced the simple CNN architecture for the classification of EEG signal data, aiming to identify different characteristics that influence epilepsy using electroencephalography. Ciaran Cooney et al. [17, 19] proposed the conceptual inferences drawn from the encephalography data,

Table 1. Applications of DCNN on EEG signal image datasets in varied applications.

S. no.	Authors	CNN and methods	Epileptical status	Accuracy
1	Rajendra Acharya et al.	13 layer DCNN	Normal, preictal and seizure classes	88.67%
2	Yimin Hou et al.	Weight minimum norm estimation, CNN for motor imagery	Summarized to be as Ictal, Preictal	93.30%
3	W-L Mao et al.	CNN with complete wavelet transform methods	Normal epileptic seizures	72.49%
4	Ciaran Cooney et al.	CNN in BCI, transfer learning	Tuning BCI using TL	35.68%
5	Lan Ma et al.	CNN based joint-biometric system	EEG-based 10-class classification	88.00%

Brain-Computer Interfaces. The work in [16] also compares other TL methods. Finding the state of the human mind is yet another challenge versed in [18]; using the electrical signals, a set of biometric drawings determine the state of mind, where brainwave patterns are introduced to code the biometrics.

3 Related Work

The electrical signals are non-uniform and boundless, as uncertainty and entropy aspects influence the datasets at intervening temporal points; the seizure detection and brainwave pattern detection through classification has much importance in the research.

3.1 Entropy in EEG

Entropy measures the uncertainty in data, which almost represents the quantitative output of some predictable configuration. Entropy is used to measure the disorder in a system in general. The concept of entropy is applied to electroencephalography to measure the signals' uncertainty or random patterns. The application of entropy measure on signals is challenging, such that the experiment is a priori; therefore, the meaning to be derived out of randomness is not known. Based on the signal-noise ratio, the entropy measure is influenced bythe time-domain and frequency-domain of the signals. Thus, it is assumed that the input for the experimentation for finding the epileptic seizures have already been treated with entropy measures and corrected with suitability meaningfully. The application of classification deserves good consistency apart from high accuracy. The characteristics of a patient with epilepsy are traced in the recordings as four periods: interictal, pre-ictal, seizure and post-ictal.

3.2 CNN's and EEG

The challenging element in the diagnosis of epilepsy is classification. An epileptic signal classification was proposed by Yunyuan et al. [1] transforms epileptic signals into power spectrum density energy diagrams. Further, a Deep CNN is employed for variety based on the features selected from the four categorical epileptic states interictal, pre-ictal, seizure and post-ictal. Case studies from CHB-MIT epileptic EEG data were instrumental in the proofs of the experiments. The classification model has been proven to be an excellent performance compared to other LSTM based DCNN algorithms. J.X.Chen et al. [2] has proposed a CNN model for classifying epileptic disorder data, which employs end-to-end learning of signals and states of epilepsy with spatial and temporal dimensions. A Bayesian model is proposed in the framework, which does emotional binary classification. A verified DEAP dataset with 32 subjects is used in the framework. RahibAbiyev et al. [3] has proposed yet another CNN model for epileptic EEG data classification, stating that epilepsy is a chronic neurological disorder and yields different types of EEG data and needs an ensemble of methods in CNN for classification. Tengfei Song et al. [4] has proposed that DGCNN, deep graph convolutional neural networks have a profound influence in CNN's classification models, so far employed. Cheng Lian Liu et al. [5] worked on different montage points of the EEG data sets and tested on multi-view convolutional neural networks.

3.3 EEG Signals to EEG Images

There are five exciting sub-bands of frequencies for EEG, viz., alpha, beta, theta, delta, and gamma, which usually span the 0 Hz to 64 Hz range; almost all the frequencies are prone to noise. The frequency of all possible power shots of EEG is 1763.61 Hz, which is considered sampling frequency. Conditionally the maximum frequency for extracting EEG with the slightest noise is 86.81 Hz or evenly half in the sampling frequency is considered. Some wavelet transformation does not allow the extraction of specific signals; the 0 Hz to 64 Hz range is regarded as the ideal frequency. An example is delegated with all five possible frequencies of an interictal EEG signal.

The generic Structure of a converted EEG data file consists of the readings collected at each pass of scanning at specific frequencies of a subject (Table 2).

Numbers of trials are executed on various sensor positions of unipolar setup, with a considerable number of samples about each subject. Time, matching conditions and channels are observed and recorded as shown above. The sensor values readings are registered for the issues with different positions are between −48.33 and 31.057. At which FP1: between −6.48 and 23.794, at FP2: between −7.406 and 20.915, at FC1: between −4.405 and 8.779 at FC2: between −2.625 and 7.629 at FC3: between −5.493 and 9.644 at FC4: between −6.002 and 8.158 at FC5: between −16.541 and 17.151 at FC6: between −8.667 and 9.888.

4 Experimental Setup

One of the essential categories and frequently used in multi-label classification is the transformation method. A multi-label classification problem employs a technique to convert either into a single-label classification or regression.

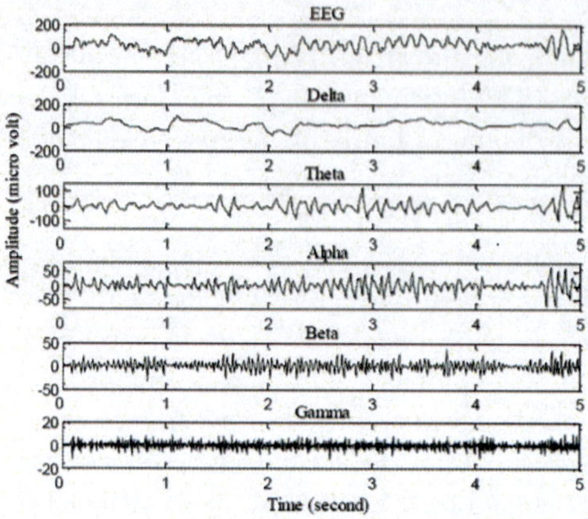

Fig. 1. A sample image of EEG Interictal signals after decomposition of band-limited into five sub-bands

Table 2. Generic Structure of the EEG interictal signals

Unnamed: 0	Trail number	Sensor position	Sample num	Sensor value	Subject identifier	Matching condition	Channel	Name	Time
2	7	30	FP1	2	−5.503	a	S1 obj	Co2a000364	0.007812
3	8	30	FP1	3	−3.550	a	S1 obj	Co2a000364	0.011719
4	9	30	FP1	4	−0.621	a	S1 obj	Co2a000364	0.015625
5	10	30	FP1	5	1.821	a	S1 obj	Co2a000364	0.019531
6	11	30	FP1	6	2.309	a	S1 obj	Co2a000364	0.0.23438

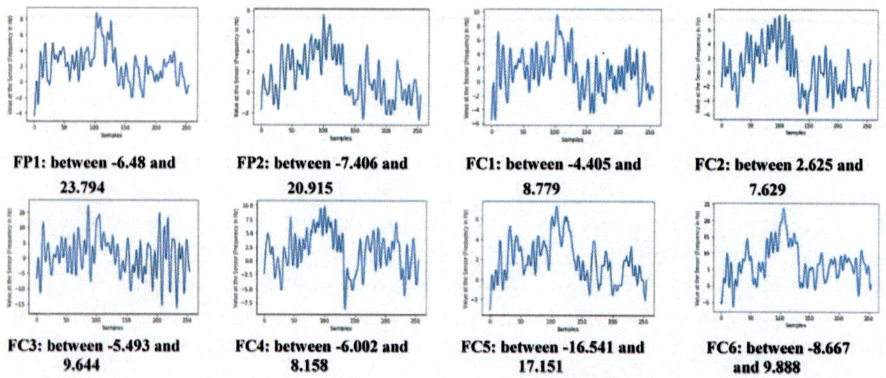

Fig. 2. The sensor value readings on selected subjects at positions of FP1, FP2, FC1, FC2, FC3, FC4, FC5, FC6.

The class frequency is based on the data set's data frequencies. Based on the frequency of the class, the merge process of the class into another is based on the entities and the entropies of the class, which also yields to the predictive method of adapting

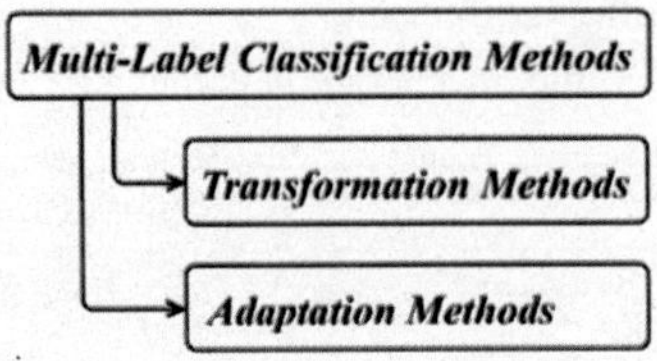

Fig. 3. Types of multi-label classification methods.

into multi-label classification. At the core, the problem transformation is employed and then to overcome the ambiguity of sharing the class labels, an adaptation mechanism is introduced based on the frequencies and entropies. A set of labels |L| is noted to compare all the other classes whether or not they belong to the set, but for some applications number of labels that have to be compared is too large, and for some, it is tiny. The two factors called label cardinality and label density is thus introduced to address the issues. The following definitions clarify the computation of the two factors.

$$LabelCadinality(D) = \frac{1}{|D|}\sum\nolimits_{i=1}^{|D|}|Y_i| \tag{1}$$

The cardinality D is represented as the average number of labels for the examples of D.

$$LabelCadinality(D) = \frac{1}{|D|}\sum\nolimits_{i=1}^{|D|}\frac{|Y_i|}{|L|} \tag{2}$$

The cardinality D is represented as the average number of labels for the examples of D concerning L. In the present work, the features of each label are ascertained for the merging of the classes and comparing with the said L. The features of the EEG signal data are observed in different texture forms and represented as a template to refer to the similarity among the classes. Therefore, first, the identification and declaration of class labelling are introduced in the simple CNN based on the EEG signals' similarity features about different instances of different subjects.

5 Network Setup

The convolutional layers of the network consisting of ReLU and parametric ReLU (pReLU) are the vital components of the sequential model of the proposed CNN. The parametric ReLU (pReLU) parameter is derived from computing the Geometric Mean of two positive values.

5.1 Parametric ReLU (pReLU)

The proposed DCNN has elementary four convolution layers with eight feature maps. A usual kernel size of 3 × 3 pixels is set up with ReLU to prevent intermediate saturations in each layer. Generally, a series of sampled and tested positive integers are determined for the parameter coefficients and tested in the ReLU, where all the values converge in

Table 3. Validation parameters

Parameter	Computation
Accuracy	$\frac{TP+TN}{TP+TN+FP+FN}$
Error Rate	$\frac{FP+FN}{TP+TN+FP+FN}$
Positive Predict Value (PPV)	$\frac{TP}{TP+FP}$
Sensitivity	$\frac{TP}{TP+FN}$
Specificity	$\frac{TN}{TN+FP}$

pooling. Instead of a series of values, a geometric mean of the select values is considered a parameter for the variable in the ReLU function to improve the efficiency.

As the initial step of the operations of DCNN, the size of feature maps is reduced even to 2×2 using Max-Pooling, further appended with normalization layers to enable quicker convergence after each max-pooling layer. The max-pool layer generates eight features, which are further input to the fully connected layer. The fully connected layer consists of 256 neurons.

Features of the EEG image data are collected into a select category of image patches with EEGF = 50, and the size of EEGF × EEGF segments are prepared. During the experiment, in the augmented dataset, patches are asserted as non-overlapping, tested by flipping horizontally and vertically; about 19,269 patches result as seizures and 36,635 were negative, which can be matched with pathological observations.

Table 4. Setup of Image Patches for Experiment

No. of images (patches) with seizures	
Training	9669
Testing	4800
Validation	4800
Total number	19269

The experiment is conducted by testing the model with 0 to 150 epochs. It is observed that during iterations between and around 66th and 70th epoch, accuracies are measured 96% approximately. Table 3 shows that for the training (50%), validation (25%) and testing (25%) of the total number of patches are considered.

6 Results

The overall experiment is executed around 150 iterations; a patch-based method is employed in the model during the investigation. Further, it is derived that pathological symptoms of seizures the accuracy, sensitivity, specificity of 0.967, 0.958 and 0.948 respectively exists and for no-sign of taking as 0.987, 0.974 and 0.958 respectively (Tables 5 and 6).

Table 5. Number of images patches per class of validation obtained

Positive class		Negative class	
Positive prediction	Negative prediction	Positive prediction	Negative prediction
True positive	False negative	False positive	True negative
46	6	43	38
52	7	37	33
55	7	34	30
62	8	27	24
68	9	21	19
74	9	15	14
76	10	13	12
80	10	9	8
86	12	5	6

Table 6. Validation parameters obtained from the experiment

	Seizure	No-sign
Accuracy	0.967	0.987
Sensitivity	0.958	0.974
Specificity	0.948	0.958

The number of image patches per class during validation considered to enable predictions in experimentation is shown in Table 4 (Fig. 4).

With selected image patches and their relevance of classification into normal and seizure, the above graphs comply with the model described for the DCNN.

Thus, the model has achieved 74% of higher accuracy where each of the EEG signal image entities in the dataset can be classified with two labels, 'typical' and 'seizure', with the relevant percentage of their existence in the source image data sets. The following table shows the labelling percentages for the few selected signal images (Fig. 5).

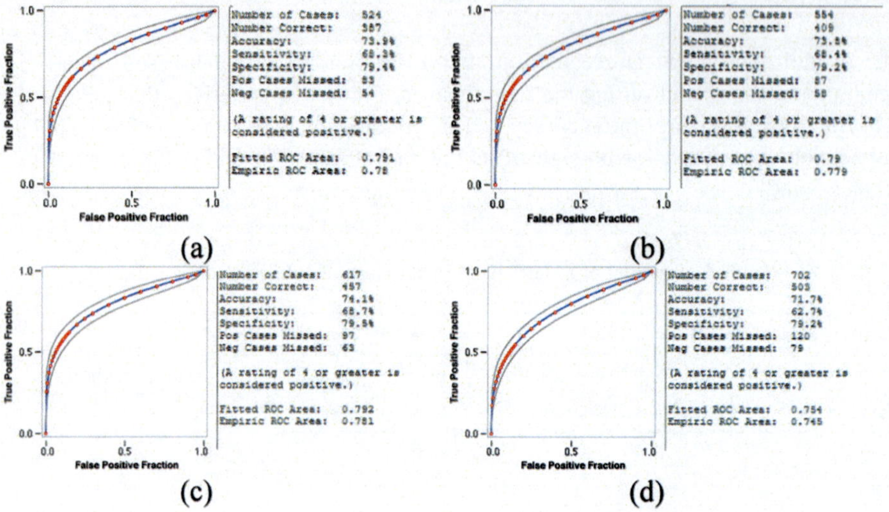

Fig. 4. Repeater operating characteristic curve, representing the relevance of classification in the proposed DCNN

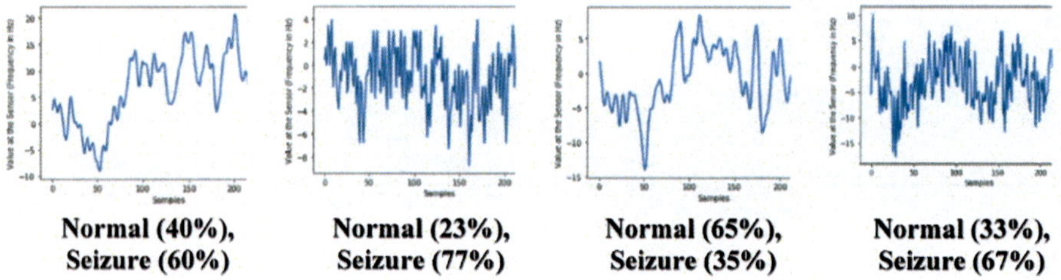

Fig. 5. EEG signal image entities classified with multiple labels

7 Conclusion

EEG data of a subject with seizures and without seizures have been used in the proposed work. The collected EEG signals are converted into images using pyimage. The proposed model is tested on the dataset. Algorithmically, the signal is converted into data set in the form of a CSV file for each subject and for each time the signals are recorded. The dataset represented for illustrations Fig. 1, 2, 3, in this article, collected from Children's Hospital Boston (CHB) and the Massachusetts Institute of Technology (MIT), contains long-term EEG records from 24 pediatric patients. The proposed model for multi-label classification has shown the results with a specific percentage of labelling that each EEG signal image entity belongs to. The performance of the model is achieved upto 74% accurate. Several experiments on EEG signal data sets have been conducted in the erstwhile research. Based on the application, they achieve different levels of accuracy and performance metrics are found to be appropriate for specific models. Practically, the complete image of the graph cannot be input into the model, so patches of the images in the EEG signal image datasets are considered for training, testing and validations. The model proposed they proved with geometric values of the parameters supplied to the ReLU and has achieved a significant level of learning to define the labels of the source image entities.

References

1. Gao, Y., Gao, B., Chen, Q., Liu, J., Zhang, Y.: Deep convolutional neural network-based epileptic electroencephalogram (EEG) signal classification. Front. Neurol. **11**, 375 (2020)
2. Chen, J.X., Zhang, P.W., Mao, Z.J., Huang, Y.F., Jiang, D.M., Zhang, Y.N.: Accurate EEG-based emotion recognition on combined features using deep convolutional neural networks. IEEE Access **7**, 44317–44328 (2019)
3. Abiyev, R., Arslan, M., Idoko, J.B., Sekeroglu, B., Ilhan, A.: Identification of epileptic EEG signals using convolutional neural networks. Appl. Sci. **10**(12), 4089 (2020)
4. Song, T., Zheng, W., Song, P., Cui, Z.: EEG emotion recognition using dynamical graph convolutional neural networks. IEEE Trans. Affect. Comput. **11**(3), 532–541 (2018)
5. Liu, C., Xiao, B., Hsaio, W.-H., Tseng, V.S.: Epileptic seizure prediction with multi-view convolutional neural networks. IEEE Access **7**, 170352–170361 (2019)
6. Usman, S.M., Usman, M., Fong, S.: Epileptic seizures prediction using machine learning methods. Comput. Math. Methods Med. **2017**, 10 (2017)
7. Li, G., Lee, C.H., Jung, J.J., Youn, Y.C., Camacho, D.: Deep learning for EEG data analytics: a survey. Concurr. Comput.: Pract. Exp. **32**(18), e5199 (2020)
8. Shoeb, A., Guttag, J.: Application of machine learning to epileptic seizure onset detection. In: 27th International Conference on Machine Learning (ICML), 21–24 June 2010, Haifa, Israel (2010)
9. Lin, Q., Ye, S., Wu, C., Gu, W., Xue, Y.: A novel framework based on bi-clustering for automatic epileptic seizure detection. Int. J. Mach. Learn. Cybernet. **10**, 1–13 (2017)
10. Zhang, T., Chen, W.Z.: LMD Based features for the automatic seizure detection of EEG signals using SVM. IEEE Trans. Neural Syst. Rehab. Eng. **25**(8), 1100–1108 (2017)
11. Bhattacharyya, A., Sharma, M., Pachori, R.B., Sircar, P., Acharya, U.R.: A novel approach for automated detection of focal EEG signals using empirical wavelet transform. Neural Comput. Appl. **29**(8), 47–57 (2016). https://doi.org/10.1007/s00521-016-2646-4
12. Krizhevsky, A., Sutskever, I., Hinton, G.E.: ImageNet classification with deep convolutional neural networks. Adv. Neural. Inf. Process. Syst. **25**, 1097–1105 (2012)
13. Sharma, R., Pachori, R.B., Upadhyay, A.: Automatic sleep stages classification based on iterative filtering of electroencephalogram signals. Neural Comput. Appl. **28**(10), 2959–2978 (2017). https://doi.org/10.1007/s00521-017-2919-6
14. Acharya, U.R., Oh, S.L., Hagiwara, Y., Tan, J.H., Adeli, H.: Deep convolutional neural network for the automated detection and diagnosis of seizure using EEG signals. Comput. Biol. Med. **100**, 270–278 (2018)
15. Emami, A., Kunii, N., Matsuo, T., Shinozaki, T., Kawai, K., Takahashi, H.: Seizure detection by convolutional neural network-based analysis of scalp electroencephalography plot images. NeuroImage Clin. **22**, 101684 (2019)
16. Mao, W.L., Fathurrahman, H.I.K., Lee, Y., Chang, T.W.: EEG dataset classification using CNN method. J. Phys. Conf. Ser. **1456**(1), 012017 (2020)
17. Cooney, C., Folli, R., Coyle, D.: Optimizing layers improve CNN generalization and transfer learning for imagined speech decoding from EEG. In: 2019 IEEE International Conference on Systems, Man and Cybernetics (SMC), pp. 1311–1316. IEEE (2019)

18. Ma, L., Minett, J.W., Blu, T., Wang, W.S.Y.: Resting-state EEG-based biometrics for individual identification using convolutional neural networks. In: 2015 37th Annual International Conference of the IEEE Engineering in Medicine and Biology Society (EMBC), pp. 2848–2851. IEEE (2015)
19. Cooney, C., Folli, R., Coyle, D.: Optimizing layers improve CNN generalization and transfer learning for imagined speech decoding from EEG. In: 2019 IEEE International Conference on Systems, Man, and Cybernetics (SMC). IEEE (2019)
20. Mohammad, G.G., et al.: An empirical study on COVID-19 for social contact tracing on classification perspective. Int. J. Comput. Appl. Technol. **66**(3–4), 303–308 (2021). https://doi.org/10.1504/IJCAT.2021.120455
21. Galety, M., Al Mukthar, F.H., Maaroof, R.J., Rofoo, F.: Deep neural network concepts for classification using convolutional neural network: a systematic review and evaluation. Technium Roman. J. Appl. Sci. Technol. **3**(8), 58–70 (2021). https://doi.org/10.47577/technium.v3i8.4554
22. Sahu, B., et al.: MMFA-SVM: new bio-marker gene discovery algorithms for cancer gene expression. Mater. Today: Proc. (2021). https://doi.org/10.1016/j.matpr.2020.11.617
23. Reshma, G., et al.: Deep learning-based skin lesion diagnosis model using dermoscopic images. Intell. Autom. Soft Comput. **31**, 621–634 (2022)
24. Sriharsha, A.V., et al.: Improvisation of k-NN classifier on semantically secure encrypted relational data. Int. J. Comput. Eng. Technol. (IJCET) **8**(3), 1–10 (2017)
25. Sriharsha, A.V., et al.: Music inspired HS algorithm for determining software design patterns. Issues **1**, 230–238 (2014)

BeCaked$^+$: An Explainable AI Model to Forecast Delta-Spreading Covid-19 Situations for Ho Chi Minh City

Cuong Nguyen[1,2], Minh Nguyen[1,2], Duc Nguyen[1,2], Duc Nguyen[4], Thinh Nguyen[1,2], Khuong Nguyen-An[1,2], Chon Le[1,2,3], and Tho Quan[1,2](✉)

[1] Ho Chi Minh City University of Technology (HCMUT), Ho Chi Minh City, Vietnam
{cuong.nguyen1605,minh.nguyenhuynh.2257,duc.nguyenquang,ntthinh, nakhuong,ltchon,qttho}@hcmut.edu.vn, chonlt@hcmunre.edu.vn
[2] Vietnam National University Ho Chi Minh City, Linh Trung Ward, Thu Duc District, Ho Chi Minh City, Vietnam
[3] Ho Chi Minh City University of Natural Resources and Environment (HCMUNRE), Ho Chi Minh City, Vietnam
[4] Hanoi University of Science and Technology (HUST), Hanoi, Vietnam
duc.nq204876@sis.hust.edu.vn

Abstract. Covid-19 is a global disaster that needs computing power to analyze, predict and interpret. So far, there have been several models doing the job. With a huge amount of daily data, deep learning models can be trained to achieve highly accurate forecasts but their mechanism lacks explainability. Epidemiological models, e.g. SIR, on the other hand, can provide insightful analyses, but they require appropriate parameter values, which might be complicated in certain locations.

The fourth wave of the pandemic in *Ho Chi Minh City* (HCMC), Vietnam in 2021, brought valuable lessons along with accurate and specific data. Hence, we introduce an explainable AI model, known as BeCaked$^+$, to predict and analyze the pandemic situation efficiently from the collected data. BeCaked$^+$ combined deep learning and epidemiological models enhanced by specific parameters related to the policies endorsed by the government. Such a combination makes BeCaked$^+$ so accurate and a tool that provides information for policymakers to respond appropriately. One take a try BeCaked$^+$ at http://www.cse.hcmut.edu.vn/BeCaked.

Keywords: BeCaked$^+$ · Covid-19 · Ho Chi Minh City · Delta-variant · Explainable AI · Epidemic model · Time-series forecasting

1 Introduction

SARS-Cov-2 has spread rapidly through most the countries in the world and has caused an infamous global pandemic (Covid-19 pandemic). In Vietnam, the spread of the *Delta* since the fourth Covid-19 wave in May 2021 has caused significant damages and losses, especially in Ho Chi Minh City (HCMC). Though the government has made every effort, such as quarantine (like previous waves) and vaccination, the city still experienced

K. Daimi and A. Al Sadoon (Eds.): ICR 2022, AISC 1431, pp. 53–64, 2022.
https://doi.org/10.1007/978-3-031-14054-9_6

significant deceased cases. Currently, as the situation in HCMC has been under control, a model needs to be developed to forecast and interpret data from the past to prevent similar sufferings in the future.

Typically, there are two major approaches for pandemic forecasting including *compartmental* and *time forecasting* models. While the latter enjoys good accuracy, the former has the advantage of *explainability*. Hence, in 2020 we introduced a prediction model, which combined the *Susceptible-Infectious-Recovered-Deceased* (SIRD) [1] and deep learning, known as *BeCaked* [2]. BeCaked includes two sub-models, a compartmental model in epidemiology, and a deep learning system. When a new outbreak occurred in HCMC in May 2021, we upgraded BeCaked with a new version named BeCaked$^+$, which offers the following contributions: (1) we propose a new model combining compartmental and learning techniques for Covid-19 forecast interpretation; (2) we introduce a set of specific parameters to address the situation in HCMC during the fourth wave; and (3) we implement the model as a Web application where everyone can visit daily at http://www.cse.hcmut.edu.vn/BeCaked.

2 Background Compartmental Models in Epidemiology

SIR model [3] is a classical model in epidemiology. It assumes that the fixed population N is divided into three *compartments* that can vary over time as below:

- S (susceptible): individuals who have not been infected with the disease,
- I (infectious): individuals who are currently infected,
- R (recovered): individuals who have recovered from the disease and have immunity to it.

Initially, most people are susceptible (S), and the others are in the I state. Each person in S interacts with the infectious population and becomes contagious with the effective contact rate of the disease (β). Each infectious individual has the rate of μ of being recovered. These interactions are expressed in Fig. 1(a), assuming that the recovered people cannot be reinfected with the disease (i.e. not get reinfected and not infect others)

$$\begin{cases} \frac{dS}{dt} = -\frac{\beta}{N}SI \\ \frac{dI}{dt} = \frac{\beta}{N}SI - \gamma I \\ \frac{dR}{dt} = \gamma I. \end{cases} \quad (a) \qquad \begin{cases} \frac{dS}{dt} = -\frac{\beta}{N}SI \\ \frac{dI}{dt} = \frac{\beta}{N}SI - \gamma I - \mu I \\ \frac{dR}{dt} = \gamma I \\ \frac{dD}{dt} = \mu I. \end{cases} \quad (b) \qquad (1)$$

In addition, SIRD is an extension of SIR. Compared to SIR model, SIRD has four states, namely S (susceptible), I (infectious), R (recovered) and D (deceased). The meanings of S, I, and R are the same as those in the SIR model while the D state represents deaths due to the disease. At any given time, t, $S(t)$, $I(t)$, $R(t)$, $D(t)$ denote the number of the individuals in each corresponding compartment, and they satisfy $S(t) + I(t) + R(t) + D(t) = N$. SIRD model is described by the system of equations (1b). Similar to the SIR model, there are relations in this model, which are depicted in Fig. 1(b).

3 Related Works

Pure Time Series Forecasting. In 2020, Hernandez et al. proposed a method [4] that estimated the parameters of *Autoregressive Integrated Moving Average* (ARIMA) [5] to predict the number of infected cases for many countries. Another work by A. Ghany et al. proposed a simple *Multi-layer Perceptron* (MLP) network [6] to forecast the time series data of the epidemic. This method tries to fit the data to the regression models directly without the basis of epidemiological theory. The model returns a beautiful curve fitting with the actual data, but the process is unexplainable. Thus, this direction is a black box, which results in a lack of reliability.

Compartmental Model. Chatterjee et al. [7] improved the SIRD model by reducing the infection rate β over time to reflect the effect of lockdown policies, then they tuned parameters to simulate and analyze the actual situation. Berger et al. [8] proposed a more complex model based on *Susceptible-Exposed-Infectious-Recovered* (SEIR) by considering symptomatic, testing, and vaccination factors. Using models in epidemiology is more explainable since they are built based on epidemiological theory, but the accuracy of this direction does not reach the deep learning models' accuracy as it is less adaptable to new data.

The BeCaked Model. As mentioned in Sect. 1, this work is an improvement of BeCaked that was proposed in 2020. The BeCaked is a model based on Encoder-Decoder architecture. The Encoder is an LSTM network to extract features of epidemic time-series data (i.e number of susceptible cases, infected cases, recovered cases, deceased cases) and return a set of parameters for the SIRD model, then the Decoder takes these parameters and the input to predict the epidemic data in the future. Compared to BeCaked, BeCaked$^+$ upgrades the epidemic model inside Decoder to a more complex model, the Encoder is also integrated with a new network with higher performance. Besides, the method to solve the differential system in Decoder is different, and a new objective function is introduced. The next section will describe the BeCaked$^+$ model in more detail.

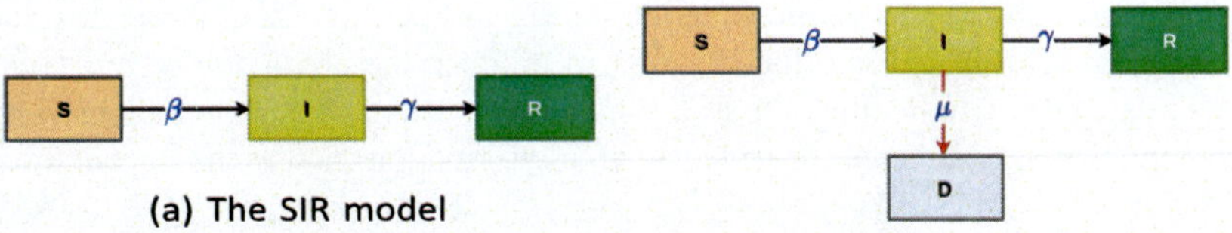

(a) The SIR model (b) The SIRD model

Fig. 1. Standard SIR and SIRD model

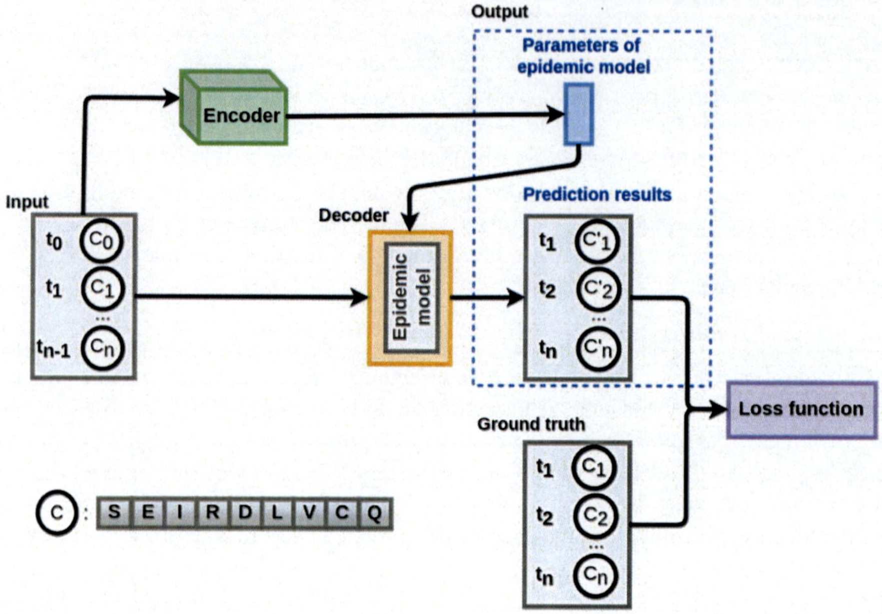

Fig. 2. The overall structure of our method. We use an Encoder block to encode Covid-19 time series data into a set of parameters. This set and the input are then fed to the Decoder block to predict the situations of the next days. These components will be discussed more deeply in later sections.

4 The BeCaked$^+$ Model

4.1 The Overview of BeCaked$^+$

An overview of BeCaked$^+$ is depicted in Fig. 2. Our method comprises an encoder and a decoder, which try to minimize the reconstruction error between ground truth and output from the encoding-decoding process. First, the input data from t_0 day to t_{n-1} day goes through the Encoder to produce the parameters of the epidemic model. The obtained parameters describe the pandemic situation during this period. Then, these parameters and the input data are fed into the Decoder to produce the prediction results from t_1 day to t_n day. Furthermore, the output of Encoder can be analyzed comprehensively by the epidemiologist, which will provide valuable information such as the impact level of each factor.

4.2 BeCaked$^+$ Compartmental Model

This work improves and extends the SIRD model to create a more suitable model that describes the epidemic evolution in HCMC. In addition to the original SIRD model, we also consider other factors such as the effects of restriction, vaccination, quarantine, and critical population. Each individual in the population is assigned to only one of the nine compartments which are S (*Susceptible*), E (*Exposed*), I (*Infected*), R (*Recovered*), D (*Deceased*), L (*Locked*), V (*Vaccinated*), C (*Critical*), and Q (*Quarantined*).

As a compartmental epidemic model, relations between compartments are indispensable, which are depicted in Fig. 3. The dynamics of the pandemic and the constraints between parameters of the model are given in Eq. 2.

$$\begin{cases} M = S + V + E + R \\ \frac{dS}{dt} = -\frac{\beta SE}{M} - \tau S - \rho S + \hat{\rho} L - \varphi S + \hat{\varphi} Q \\ \frac{dE}{dt} = \frac{(\beta S + \zeta V)E}{M} - \eta E - \psi E \\ \frac{dI}{dt} = \eta E - \gamma_1 I - \theta I + \delta L + \omega Q \\ \frac{dR}{dt} = \gamma_1 I + \gamma_2 C \\ \frac{dD}{dt} = \mu C \\ \frac{dL}{dt} = \rho S - (\delta + \hat{\rho}) L \\ \frac{dV}{dt} = -\frac{\zeta VE}{M} + \tau S \\ \frac{dC}{dt} = \theta I - \gamma_2 C - \mu C \\ \frac{dQ}{dt} = \varphi S + \psi E - (\omega + \hat{\varphi}) Q. \end{cases} \quad (a) \qquad \begin{cases} \gamma_2 + \mu < 1 \\ \gamma_1 + \theta < 1 \\ \delta + \hat{\rho} < 1 \\ \eta + \psi < 1 \\ \omega + \hat{\varphi} < 1 \\ \zeta < \beta. \end{cases} \quad (b) \qquad (2)$$

In short, let $\boldsymbol{x}_t = [S(t), E(t), I(t), R(t), D(t), L(t), V(t), C(t), Q(t)]$, and $\boldsymbol{p}$ be parameters of the epidemic model, we can rewrite the system of Eq. 2 as $\frac{d\boldsymbol{x}_t}{dt} = f(\boldsymbol{x}_t, \boldsymbol{p})$.

Almost all people are in S, E, or I state at first. M denotes the current number of people that can make interaction in the community. The people in S can be vaccinated, quarantined, or moved to restricted areas; in other words, they are transferred into V, Q, or L with the probability of τ, φ, ρ, respectively (corresponding to τS, φS, ρS in Eq. 2a reflecting population changes). It should be noticed that minus marks indicate decreases and plus signs show increases. Besides, the corresponding probability that a restrictcted area comes back to normal is $\hat{\rho}$ (given in terms of $\hat{\rho} L$). The vaccinated population (V) and susceptible population (S) interacting with the exposed (E) becomes exposed with the rate of ζ and β (corresponding to $\frac{\zeta VE}{}$ and $\frac{\beta SE}{}$ where $\frac{E}{}$ denotes the probability that one interaction between a person in E with another, ζ and β are the probability that a person is exposed after interacting with exposed people). We assume that ζ is lower than β because of the vaccine effectiveness. If ζ is zero, the vaccine offers immunizable protection against the disease. Each exposed person has a rate of ψ of staying in quarantine zones, while the quarantined ones have the rate of $\hat{\varphi}$ that they finish the quarantine period without being positive for Covid-19 (given in terms of ψE and $\hat{\varphi} Q$). The probability that the exposed, locked, and quarantined populations are confirmed to have Covid-19 are η, δ, and ω, respectively (corresponding to ηE, δL and ωQ). Each currently infected case (I) has a rate of $\vartheta\theta$ of getting serious (C) (the term ϑI). The recovery of an infected person and a critical patient is determined by the γ_1 and γ_2 rate, respectively (corresponding to $\gamma_1 I$ and $\gamma_2 C$). The population of critical patients (C) has a death rate of μ and then moves to the D state (the term μC).

4.3 Encoder

We design the Encoder based on *Temporal Convolutional Network* (TCN) [9] to capture the features of all input data (i.e epidemic data of 10 days in the past, which 9 elements per day corresponding to 9 compartments of the compartmental model that will be described in the Sect. 4.2. The way to preprocess the raw data in the real life to obtain this input

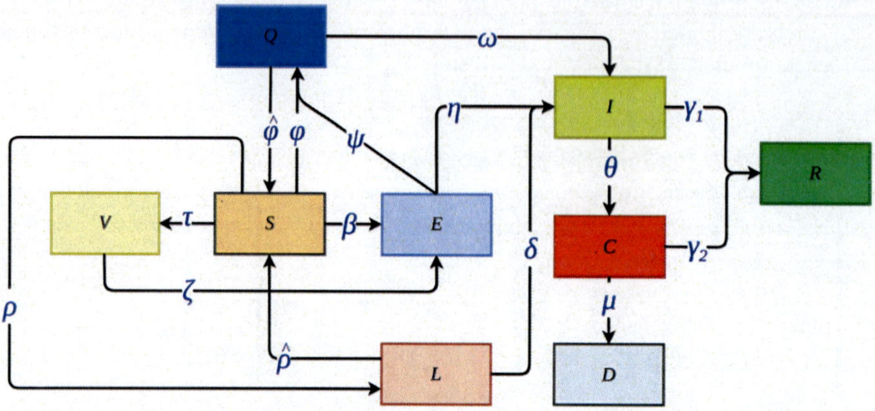

Fig. 3. The relations between the compartments

will be described in Sect. 5.1). TCN applies the *Causal convolution* rather than the usual convolution. Causal convolution is normally used for temporal data to ensure that the prediction at any time step does not depend on the future time steps. Since the input and output of TCN have the same shape, an average-pooling layer is used to reduce the size of the window. Besides, we also need a flattened layer and a fully-connected layer to get the desired output from the Encoder. We propose to use some well-known techniques to improve the performance, which are residual connections and attention mechanisms. Moreover, a regularization, concretely Dropout is applied to prevent overfitting. The output of the Encoder is a set of parameters per day mentioned in Sect. 4.2. Formally, with the input

$$X = \begin{bmatrix} S_0\ E_0\ I_0\ R_0\ D_0\ L_0\ V_0\ C_0\ Q_0 \\ S_1\ E_1\ I_1\ R_1\ D_1\ L_1\ V_1\ C_1\ Q_1 \\ \vdots \\ S_9\ E_9\ I_9\ R_9\ D_9\ L_9\ V_9\ C_9\ Q_9 \end{bmatrix},$$

the Encoder will generate the output

$$P = \begin{bmatrix} \beta_0\ \tau_0\ \rho_0\ \hat{\rho}_0\ \varphi_0\ \hat{\varphi}_0\ \zeta_0\ \eta_0\ \psi_0\ \eta_0\ \gamma_{1_0}\ \gamma_{2_0}\ \theta_0\ \delta_0\ \omega_0\ \mu_0\ \theta_0 \\ \beta_1\ \tau_1\ \rho_1\ \hat{\rho}_1\ \varphi_1\ \hat{\varphi}_1\ \zeta_1\ \eta_1\ \psi_1\ \eta_1\ \gamma_{1_1}\ \gamma_{2_1}\ \theta_1\ \delta_1\ \omega_1\ \mu_1\ \theta_1 \\ \vdots \\ \beta_9\ \tau_9\ \rho_9\ \hat{\rho}_9\ \varphi_9\ \hat{\varphi}_9\ \zeta_9\ \eta_9\ \psi_9\ \eta_9\ \gamma_{9_9}\ \gamma_{2_9}\ \theta_9\ \delta_9\ \omega_9\ \mu_9\ \theta_9 \end{bmatrix}$$

The overall Encoder architecture is shown in Fig. 4.

ResNeXt. To improve the performance of TCN, we suggest using ResNeXt blocks [10] in hidden layers. The main idea of ResNeXt blocks is to perform a set of transformations with the input, and then the intermediate outputs are summed. Each transformation is a different path from the input to the output. Thus, many routes will extract various features, helping the model learn better.

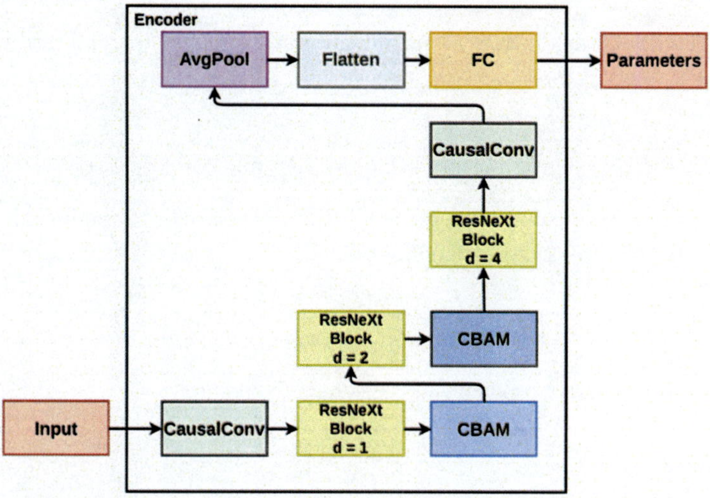

Fig. 4. The overview of the Encoder. In the beginning, we used a Causal Convolution Block to process the input. This block ensures that the output only depends on the previous input (i.e., the number of infectious in the following days can not affect the number of current infections). Next, a ResNeXt Block is used to extract features, and then we apply CBAM to focus on both temporal and channel dimensions. We repeat this process three times with dilation of 1, 2, and 4, respectively, to capture all of the 10-day input based on TCN architecture.

Convolutional Block Attention Module (CBAM). CBAM was proposed by Woo et al. in 2018 [11]; they apply CBAM to improve CNN architectures by inferring attention maps along two separate dimensions, channel and spatial, sequentially. To apply this idea to our model, we use 1D filters instead of 2D ones, and simultaneously two dimensions correspond to channel and temporal. This way, we can concentrate on the prominent features in both dimensions. We briefly summarize this idea as below.

Let F be an intermediate feature map, $F \in \mathrm{R}^{C\times L}$. Our modified CBAM first calculates a channel attention map $M \in \mathrm{R}^{C\times 1}$, then a temporal attention map $M_t \in \mathrm{R}^{1\times L}$.

In the channel attention module, it receives the input F, then squeezes temporal dimension by using both global max-pooling and global average-pooling parallelly. Each branch continues to go through a shared MLP. An addition operation aggregates the outputs of two branches. We receive the channel attention map after the gained output is forwarded to the sigmoid function. Formally, the channel attention operation can be written as

$$\begin{aligned} M_c(F) &= \sigma(MLP(MaxPooling(F)) + MLP(AvgPooling(F))) \\ &= \sigma(MLP(MaxPooling(F) + AvgPooling(F))). \end{aligned}$$

In the temporal attention module, to prepare the input, the feature map F is multiplied by M_c element by element. We also use both global max-pooling and average-pooling operations to aggregate across the channel dimension, then concatenate them to produce temporal descriptors. We apply a causal convolutional layer and sigmoid activation to temporal descriptors to generate a final attention map. The temporal attention can be written as

$$F' = M_c(F) \odot F$$
$$M_t(F') = \sigma\left(Conv\left(\left[MaxPooling\left(F'\right); AvgPooling\left(F'\right)\right]\right)\right).$$

where σ is the sigmoid activation and *Conv* is a 1D causal convolutional layer. For brevity, the overall process is equivalent to

$$F' = M_c(F) \odot F,$$
$$F'' = M_t\left(F'\right) \odot F', \tag{3}$$

where $\odot$ is Hadamard product and F'' is the refined output.

4.4 Decoder

The Decoder receives the input data in the interval from t_0 day to t_{n-1} day (X) as well as the output of the Encoder (P) to produce the prediction results from t_1 day to t_n day ($\hat{Y}$). The nature of the Decoder is to solve ordinary differential equations, which is done by the semi-implicit Euler [12] method to avoid the stiffness of the system.

4.5 Parameter Estimation

We use *Weighted Mean Square Error* to compute the gap between the predicted output and the actual data, each compartment has a different weight

$$\mathcal{L}_1 = \frac{1}{n}\sum_{t=1}^{n} w\left(x_t - \hat{x}_t\right)^2,$$

with $\boldsymbol{w}$ is a vector including weights for each compartment while $\boldsymbol{x}_t, \hat{\boldsymbol{x}}_t$ are vectors from actual data and predicted output respectively:

$$\boldsymbol{x}_t = [S(t), E(t), I(t), R(t), D(t), L(t), V(t), C(t), Q(t)],$$
$$\hat{\boldsymbol{x}}_t = [\hat{S}(t), \hat{E}(t), \hat{I}(t), \hat{R}(t), \hat{D}(t), \hat{L}(t), \hat{V}(t), \hat{C}(t), \hat{Q}(t)].$$

However, $_1$ only considers the relation between the input data and the predicted result according to the system of equations (2a). We adopt another loss based on the idea of *Physics-informed neural networks* [13] to constrain the relation between prediction at time-step t and one at time-step $t + 1$ tightly according to the system (2a).

$$\mathcal{L}_2 = \frac{1}{n-1}\sum_{t=1}^{n-1} w\left(\frac{dx_t}{dt} - f(x_t, p)\right)^2.$$

Besides, to satisfy the conditions (2b), we consider an L2 regularization loss L_3 to penalize whenever these constraints are violated. In summary, the final loss is

$$L = L_1 + \lambda_1 L_2 + \lambda_2 L_3,$$

where λ_1 and λ_2 are adjustable weights.

5 Empirical Evaluation

5.1 Dataset, Metrics, and Setting

We use the actual data provided by Ho Chi Minh Center for Disease Control (HCDC). The raw data includes daily reports about the epidemic in HCMC in particular, and we then process them to match the model's input format. In more detail,

- $R(t)$, $D(t)$, $V(t)$ are the total recovered cases, total deceased cases, total vaccinated human at the time t, respectively. They are calculated by accumulating the daily data.
- $I(t)$ is the current infected cases, calculated by the total number of infections, excluding the total number of recovered cases and the number of deceased.
- $L(t)$, $Q(t)$, $C(t)$ are the current number of people living inside lockdown regions, number of people living inside quarantine zones, and emergency cases, respectively. They are reported clearly and do not need to be preprocessed.
- $E(t)$ is the current number of people in latent time (exposed) and is estimated to be four times $I(t)$, based on the result [14] revealing the exposure time of the Delta variant approximate four days.

From our dataset, we split it into training and testing sets by the rates of 80_20, respectively, and the testing set consists of the actual data over four consecutive weeks. We use Mean Squared Error (MSE) and Mean Absolute Percentage Error (MAPE) as metrics to evaluate on four indices, namely I, R, D and C. Our source code is implemented in PyTorch. To train the model, we use Adam optimizer [15] with a cosine annealing scheduler [16]. The initial learning rate is 0.0001, and the minimum one is 0.0000001.

5.2 Baseline Models

The typical ARIMA model is used to compare with our method. ARIMA is a well-known model for time-series forecasting. Nevertheless, ARIMA is a univariate model that can only receive and predict one variable, so we build a different ARIMA model for each index. In addition, we also adopt an RNN-based baseline that is a two-layer LSTM and a multivariate single-step model (named Pure-LSTM, which is similar to the method of A Ghany mentioned in the Sect. 3). It forecasts all four indices simultaneously. To measure the effectiveness of the Encoder based on TCN, we also consider *L-BeCaked*, a model that is quite similar to BeCaked+, but its encoder is based on LSTM.

5.3 Quantitative Results

Both MSE and MAPE indicate that the higher an error, the further the distance between the prediction and the actual data. As shown in Table 1, our method performs better than the others. Though Pure-LSTM is more complex than ARIMA, it is less effective. Nevertheless, there is a considerable gap between ARIMA and our method. Especially when HCMC has attempted to reduce severe cases per day, predicting the number of critical cases is essential, for which our approach is well qualified.

5.4 Model Analysis

To better understand the advantages of our method, it should be noted again that BeCaked$^+$ is explainable as further discussed.

Table 1. Performance of BeCaked$^+$ is consistently better than other baselines.

Model	MAE				MAPE			
	I	*R*	*D*	*C*	*I*	*R*	*D*	*C*
ARIMA	9707.786	12519.643	458.571	704.036	0.062	0.050	0.027	0.615
Pure-LSTM	10239.042	21853.690	431.653	765.448	0.066	0.088	0.026	0.661
L-BeCaked	9103.990	**2320.005**	1852.554	954.378	0.058	**0.009**	0.111	0.822
BeCaked$^+$	**3663.312**	6481.097	**309.719**	**122.656**	**0.023**	0.026	**0.019**	**0.104**

Explainability of BeCaked$^+$. BeCaked$^+$ can serve not only as a regression system with good fit curves for compartments of the epidemic model (i.e Infected, Exposed, etc.) but also as an analytical system to generate the parameters of the epidemic model with an explanation of the regressed value at the same time. Therefore, the parameters of the epidemic model can be used by epidemiologists to comprehensively analyze the factors influencing the evolution of the pandemic. For instance, if the number of infected people becomes alarming at present, we can study and figure out the major reasons causing such a situation. Hence, we have solid bases to alleviate the pandemic.

As mentioned above, one key reason why our approach can be explainable is thanks to the parameters of the epidemic model. Given the input data, the Encoder not only generates the parameters reflecting the pandemic situation but also makes sure these parameters are highly accurate and reliable. The Encoder captures the relationships between days in the input data, e.g, increases or decreases in states, and encodes them in terms of the parameters of the epidemic model.

To explore the parameters, we can apply a method, called sensitivity analysis. It is usually used to figure out how changes in input variables affect target variables. In this work, we use the LHS-PRCC method to estimate the sensitivity of the model's parameters. In particular, a high sensitivity value indicates that the corresponding parameter has a significant impact on figures of the pandemic. Thus, we focus more on solutions that can mitigate the effects of the parameters which are making the pandemic worse. The obtained results are shown in Fig. 5.

Our work shows that the number of infected cases mostly depends on quarantine (corresponding to $\omega, \varphi, \hat{\varphi}$), vaccination (corresponding to τ), and lockdown (corresponding to ρ). The significant sensitivities of ω and φ with the number of infected cases indicate that most people in quarantine areas are more likely to be infected. Significantly, the contact rates (corresponding to β and ζ) do not significantly affect the number of infected cases. This can be explained by the city enforcing a curfew during the period

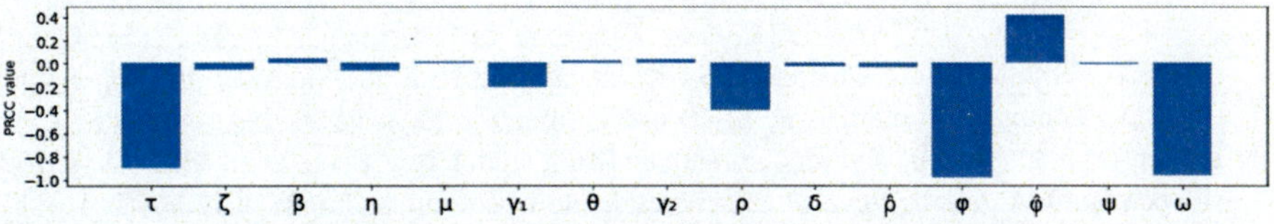

Fig. 5. PRCC scores of parameters with *I* compartment. The closer the absolute value of this point is to one, the more sensitive the corresponding parameter is to the model.

we apply the model, people having fewer interactions with each other, or the vaccination has probably reduced the risk of infection by contact.

Looking at this result, we can suggest to policymakers that our city can release the lockdown carefully and slowly while also improving the quarantine strategy.

6 Conclusion

We proposed BeCaked$^+$, an extended model of the SIRD integrated with Deep Learning to estimate the parameters describing the evolution of the pandemic. The results provided by our method are more accurate and liable than other baselines. Another advantage of BeCaked$^+$ is the explainability, which is illustrated to explain the situation of HCMC during the fourth wave starting from May 2021. Furthermore, BeCaked$^+$ can give results displayed visually for end-users and can be used by epidemiologists to analyze the evolution of the pandemic.

Acknowledgement. This research is funded by the Ho Chi Minh City University of Technology (HCMUT), VNU-HCM, under grant number **SVKSTN-2021-KH&KTMT-41**. We acknowledge the support of time and facilities from HCMUT, VNU-HCM for this study. We also would like to express our sincerest gratitude to Mr. Hong Son Bui, Prof. Hung Son Nguyen, Dr. Truong-Minh Vu, Dr. Thu Anh Nguyen, Dr. Viet-Cuong Nguyen, and Mr. Minh Canh Khuu for giving us the useful and valuable actual data, servers, and advice.

References

1. Bailey, N.T., et al.: The Mathematical Theory of Infectious Diseases and Its Applications, 2nd edn., Charles Griffin & Company Ltd., High Wycombe (1975)
2. Nguyen, D., et al.: BeCaked: an explainable artificial intelligence model for COVID-19 forecasting. Sci. Rep. (2022). https://doi.org/10.21203/rs.3.rs-454474/v1
3. Kermack, W.O., McKendrick, A.G.: A contribution to the mathematical theory of epidemics. Proc. R. Soc. London. Ser. A, Contain. Pap. Math. Phys. Character **115**(772), 700–721 (1927)
4. Hernandez-Matamoros, A., et al.: Forecasting of COVID-19 per regions using ARIMA models and polynomial functions. Appl. Soft Comput. **96**, 106610 (2020)
5. Saboia, J.L.M.: Autoregressive integrated moving average (ARIMA) models for birth forecasting. J. Am. Stat. Assoc. **72**(358), 264–270 (1977)
6. Ghany, K.K.A., et al.: COVID-19 prediction using LSTM algorithm: GCC case study. Inform. Med. Unlocked **23**, 100566 (2021)

7. Chatterjee, S., Sarkar, A., Chatterjee, S., Karmakar, M., Paul, R.: Studying the progress of COVID-19 outbreak in India using SIRD model. Indian J. Phys. **95**(9), 1941–1957 (2020)
8. Berger, D., et al.: Testing and reopening in an SEIR model. Rev. Econ. Dyn. **43**, 1–21 (2020)
9. van den Oord, A., et al.: WaveNet: a generative model for raw audio. SSW **125**, 2 (2016)
10. Xie, S., et al.: Aggregated residual transformations for deep neural networks. In: 2017 IEEE Conference on Computer Vision and Pattern Recognition (CVPR), pp. 5987–5995 (2017)
11. Woo, S., Park, J., Lee, J.-Y., Kweon, I.S.: CBAM: convolutional block attention module. In: Ferrari, V., Hebert, M., Sminchisescu, C., Weiss, Y. (eds.) ECCV 2018. LNCS, vol. 11211, pp. 3–19. Springer, Cham (2018). https://doi.org/10.1007/978-3-030-01234-2_1
12. Hu, Y.: Semi-implicit Euler-Maruyama scheme for stiff stochastic equations. In: Körezlioğlu, H., Øksendal, B., Üstünel, A.S. (eds) Stochastic Analysis and Related Topics V. Progress in Probability, vol. 38, pp. 183–202. Birkhäuser Boston, Boston (1996). https://doi.org/10.1007/978-1-4612-2450-1_9
13. Raissi, M., Perdikaris, P., Karniadakis, G.: Physics-informed neural networks: a deep learning framework for solving forward and inverse problems involving non- linear partial differential equations. J. Comput. Phys. **378**, 686–707 (2019)
14. Li, B., et al.: Viral infection and transmission in a large, well-traced outbreak caused by the SARS-CoV-2 Delta variant. medRxiv (2021)
15. Kingma, D.P., Ba, J.: Adam: a method for stochastic optimization. In: 3rd International Conference on Learning Representations, ICLR 2015, San Diego, CA, USA, 7–9 May 2015, Conference Track Proceedings (2015)
16. Loshchilov, I., Hutter, F.: SGDR: stochastic gradient descent with warm restarts. Learning, vol. 10, p. 3

SpringNet: A Novel Deep Neural Network Architecture for Histopathological Image Analysis

Matej Halinkovic(✉) and Wanda Benesova

Faculty of Informatics and Information Technologies, Slovak University of Technology in Bratislava, Bratislava, Slovakia
{xhalinkovicm,vanda_benesova}@stuba.sk

Abstract. Reliable and capable tools are needed for segmentation and classification of nuclei in histopathology images to improve the workflow of histopathologists and lessen the burden of diagnosis. Analyzing histopathology images can be challenging for deep learning models due to the various sources of noise. We propose a pipeline for segmenting and classifying nuclei, trained on a combination of datasets to ensure robustness. This makes our pipeline capable of generalizing on image tiles with varying Hematoxylin & Eosin concentrations. For nuclei classification, we present a novel convolutional neural network classifier that demonstrate state-of-the-art classification performance on the Lizard dataset.

Keywords: Deep learning · Convolutional neural networks · Computational pathology · Nuclei segmentation · Nuclei classification · Medical imaging

1 Introduction

Medical imaging is an important tool for diagnosing a variety of diseases. It is an expansive field that can be divided into many categories based on the source of the image and its purpose. Computer vision is uniquely suited to improve this tool, helping pathologists make a more accurate diagnosis and reducing the costs and therefore increasing the availability of potentially life-saving procedures.

Computer vision can be applied to medical imaging effectively in the form of computer-aided diagnosis. Deep learning computer vision models have been successfully applied to problems such as the diagnosis of skin lesions [1], the comparison of suspected tumors in X-ray scans [2], the prediction of the status of HER2 [3], and many more.

During microscopic imaging, pathologists analyze tissue slides at varying magnification levels. Magnifying tissues lets us observe nuclei, cells, glands, etc. Such detailed visualization can be used to detect abnormal cell structures, analyze blood components, or track disease growth [4]. Microscopic imaging plays an important role in several clinical applications, including cancer diagnosis. Microscopic images are more complicated than those produced by radiology, making them more challenging for computer vision methods [4].

K. Daimi and A. Al Sadoon (Eds.): ICR 2022, AISC 1431, pp. 65–75, 2022.
https://doi.org/10.1007/978-3-031-14054-9_7

Although successful models for nucleus segmentation and predicting cellular composition exist, they often struggle to maintain their performance when presented with a different dataset. Our goal is to create a solution validated on varied data to help prove its usefulness in real-world applications.

We focus on applying computer vision to histopathological images of colon tissue stained with Hematoxylin and Eosin with the goal of segmenting and classifying nuclei. Segmentation and classification is done in separate steps to allow for a greater degree of control and the usage of the classification model as a potential refinement agent for segmentation. The data we analyze contains a wide variety of samples representing normal, inflammatory and cancerous conditions of colon tissue [5]. This wide collection of data allowed us to create a robust pipeline capable of generalizing its workflow to different conditions, thus making the pipeline more usable in real-world applications.

In this paper, we introduce our contributions as follows:

- We propose a method for stabilizing and improving the performance of U-Net [6] binary segmentation on a histological dataset with highly varied data.
- We propose a novel convolutional neural network architecture for the effective classification of nuclei from 15×15 pixel image patches. We called this model *SpringNet*, due to the utilization of *Spring blocks* which we designed as a method of building deep models for images with low spatial dimensionality.

2 Related Work

Histopathology is proving to be one of the most difficult challenges when it comes to computer vision in medical imaging. It relies on whole slide images (WSIs) that can reach a resolution of up to 150000×150000 pixels [3]. The size of WSIs makes it difficult to train a model on entire images, and splitting them into patches can be problematic due to the fact that most histopathological tasks require visual context.

As a result of the complexity of the field, current state-of-the-art methods propose various deep learning approaches [7] for tackling the challenges of nucleus segmentation and classification.

The segmentation baseline in histopathology has been established by the U-Net architecture [6]. Many more recent models, such as Hover-Net [8] and HookNet [9], build on the concepts introduced by U-Net, such as the use of convolutional blocks and skip connections, to create models capable of semantic segmentation for simultaneous segmentation and classification of nuclei.

Building separate convolutional neural networks (CNNs) has also been explored as a way of annotating specific patches of WSIs. Human annotation of nuclei requires expert knowledge and is time consuming. Annotations must be precise for them to be useful to histopathologists, which means that the performance of semantic segmentation models is often insufficient. The Lizard dataset [5] which relies on Hover-Net for segmenting its images also utilizes a separate CNN model for improving the categorization of inflammatory nuclei. Deep active learning has been explored [10] as a way for training a reliable nuclei annotator without the need for a large amount of expertly labeled data.

Topological features play an important role in the analysis of WSIs. However, learning topological features from entire WSIs requires dense computation and the optimal topological representation is ambiguous [11]. Graph Neural Networks (GNNs) are uniquely suited for analyzing data with complex topological dependencies. For this reason Graph Convolutional Networks (a combination of CNN and GNN) have also been successful in the field.

DeepGraphSurv [11] proposes a method for annotating regions of interest in WSIs using the VGG-16 architecture [12] as a tool to create vertices that can be used as input for its GNN. First, the VGG-16 model extracts feature vectors, which are then reduced by using principal component analysis to extract the most important local features used as vertices. A graph created from this process is then used in the proposed DeepGraphSurv model.

A common feature among the current state-of-the-art solutions is the need to post-process the output of models to varying degrees. While semantic segmentation models have proven to be successful, they still require post-processing to produce annotations of sufficient quality. The analysis of histopathological images might benefit from separating the segmentation and classification steps for better optimization and increased potential for interpretability.

2.1 Lizard Dataset

We chose the Lizard dataset [5][1] as a source of data for training our models. This dataset is in fact a combination of 5 other datasets, containing histological image regions of colon tissue at a 20× objective magnification. The dataset includes segmentation masks and class labels for epithelial cells, connective tissue cells, lymphocytes, plasma cells,

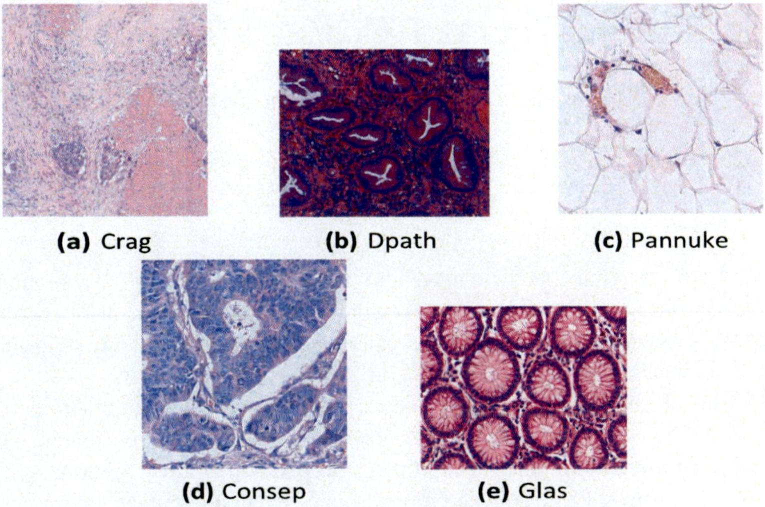

Fig. 1. Examples of datasets compiled in the Lizard dataset [5]

[1] Available from: https://warwick.ac.uk/fac/cross_fac/tia/data/lizard/.

neutrophils and eosinophils [5]. Overall, the lizard dataset contains 238 histopathological images of colon tissue with 495,179 annotations.

The Lizard dataset was created using an iterative process where each image was segmented using Hover-Net, the segmentation was refined using NuClick [13], nucleus sub-types were refined using a separate CNN classifier, and the output was validated by histopathologists.

We decided to use the large and robust Lizard dataset to train and validate our model with the goal of creating a method for segmenting and classifying nuclei that is capable of generalizing even when presented with previously unseen data. The diversity of the dataset ensures that our solution is resilient to variations in histopathological images that often cause models to struggle to maintain their performance (Fig. 1).

3 Our Solution

In our approach (see Fig. 2), we decided to separate the segmentation and classification tasks. This lets us optimize each process separately, with a greater degree of control and it lets our classification model act as a refinement agent for segmentation. Separate classification will also lend itself better for increasing interpretability in the future.

First, we extract and normalise the patches, then the normalised patches are segmented using the U-Net [6] model, the output of this segmentation is processed to create image patches centred on each segmented nucleus, and finally they are classified using our novel model, SpringNet (see Sect. 3.3).

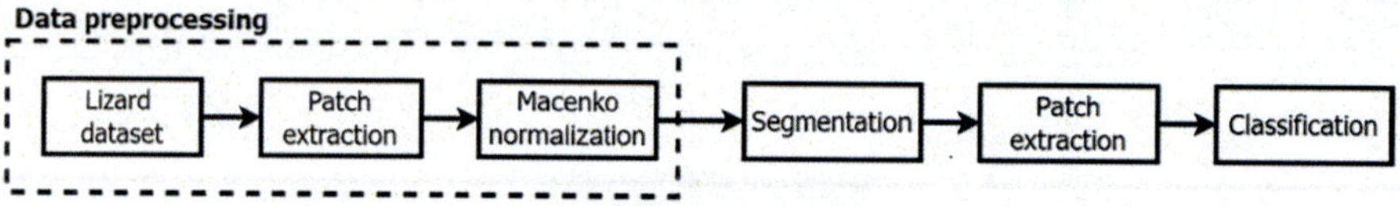

Fig. 2. The pipeline of our solution

3.1 Data Pre-processing

The lack of accurately labelled data needed to train complex models for computational histopathology presents a considerable bottleneck to the advancement of research in the field. We took steps during dataset selection and data pre-processing to ensure our solution is as robust and as capable of generalization as possible.

The Lizard dataset provides data from a variety of sources, which lets us build a robust solution capable of generalization. However, since the original sources contain images with varying resolutions (from 500×500 pixels to 4500×4500 pixels), and varying Hematoxylin & Eosin concentrations, we needed to implement a pre-processing pipeline to standardize the source images for our models.

In Fig. 3 we demonstrate the data preprocessing steps we took before training. First, we extracted patches with the size of 256×256 pixels using a sliding window with a step of 128×128 pixels and mirror padding. This ensures a uniform size for all images when used by our models and increases the amount of usable data for training due to the 50% overlap.

Second, we applied the Macenko method [14] for normalizing histology slides to counteract differences in staining between images. This method of normalization uses optical density values to calculate stain vectors and saturations to improve the ability to quantitatively analyze slides stained using Hematoxylin & Eosin.

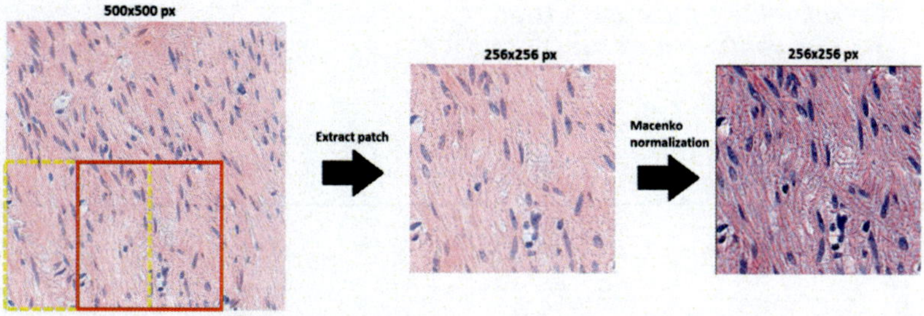

Fig. 3. Image preprocessing pipeline

3.2 Segmentation

The U-Net model was chosen as our segmentation model due to its proven [15] success in the field of biomedical image segmentation. We utilized a U-Net model with a depth of 4 and input image dimensions of 256 × 256 pixels. During training, we employed a custom distance loss function in addition to pixel-wise cross-entropy and Dice loss. The distance loss function (see Algorithm 1) penalized False Positive predictions based on their Euclidean distance from the nearest True Positive.

From the visual analysis of the U-Net's output in Fig. 4, we can see that segmentation has several weaknesses. The model struggles with edge definition in almost every nucleus, which could be improved by using one of the improved U-Net variants [16]. Further issues appear to be more fundamentally related to the source data. In some cases, the model segments the nucleus correctly, but the annotation contains the rest of the cell as well. In other cases, the model fails to distinguish visual artifacts and marks them as nuclei. However, it is possible that at least some of the False Positive predictions are caused by incorrect annotations and not incorrect segmentation.

Algorithm 1: Custom distance loss

```
Data: true_mask, predicted_mask
differences ← XOR(true_mask, predicted_mask)
pos_differences ← AND(true_mask, differences)
dst_map ← EUCLIDEAN_DST_TRANSFORM(pos_differences)
max_dst ← MAX(dst_map)
for each pixel in dst_map do
    if pixel.value > max_dst/3 then
        pixel.value ← max_dst
    end
end
avg_loss ← AVG(dst_map)
Result: Average distance loss
```

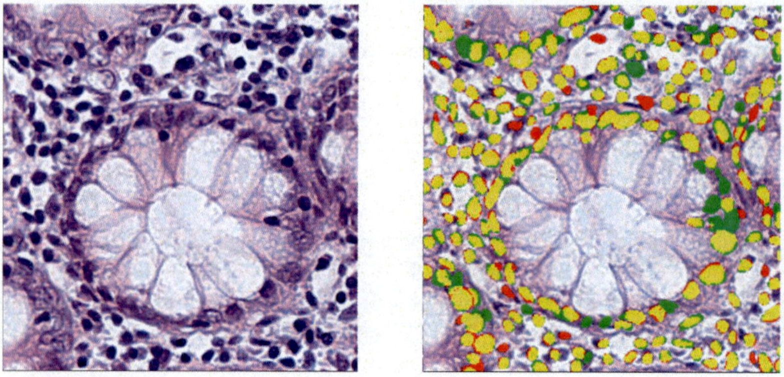

(a) Segmentation patch example **(b)** Segmentation output example

Fig. 4. U-Net segmentation output. Green - False Negative; Red - False Positive; Yellow - True Positive

The output mask of the segmentation model was used as a basis for creating a dataset for our classifier. Using contour analysis, we located the centroids of the nuclei in the mask and extracted a 15×15 pixels area around it. The resulting patch was labeled based on per-pixel class labels contained in the original dataset. Example outputs from this extraction can be seen in Fig. 5. The most common value was chosen as the overall label of the patch, with the 'Background' label only being assigned if the selected region contained no other class labels.

(a) Lymphocyte **(b)** Background **(c)** Lymphocyte **(d)** Epithelial

Fig. 5. Example patches with extracted class labels

3.3 SpringNet: Proposed Novel Model for Nucleus Classification

In this section, we propose SpringNet (see Fig. 7), a novel convolutional neural network for nuclei classification. SpringNet uses sequential Spring blocks (see Fig. 6) that we designed as a method of building deep models for images with low spatial dimensionality to extract complex features by utilizing channel-wise pooling.

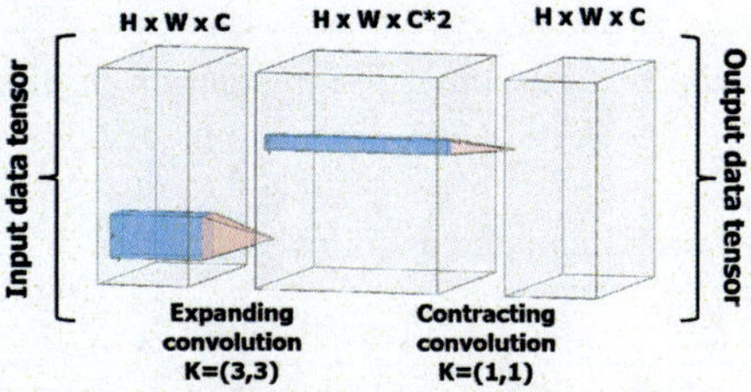

Fig. 6. Spring block

Relying on channel-wise pooling lets us propagate salient features throughout the network without increasing the number of feature maps. This allows us to build a deep network while minimizing the need to use pooling layers for spatial dimensionality reduction, which is beneficial due to the small size of the input patches.

A stride convolution is included between the Spring blocks to increase channel-wise dimensionality while decreasing spatial dimensionality. The final Spring block is followed by three fully connected layers for final classification.

Summation skip connections are implemented to reduce the impact of vanishing gradients due to the depth of our network.

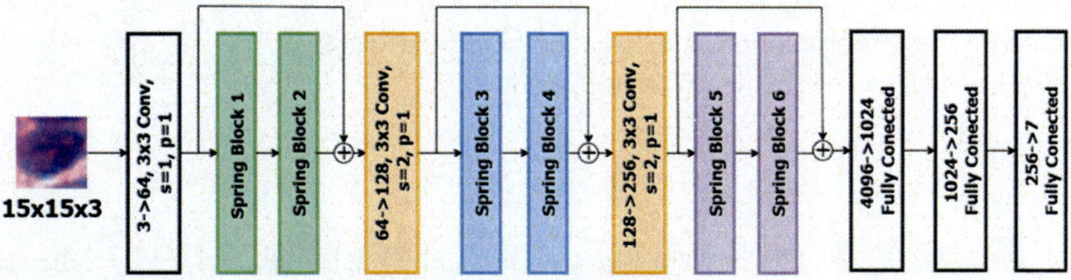

Fig. 7. SpringNet architecture

3.4 Results

In segmentation, we were able to achieve a Dice coefficient [17] of **0.81** on our test subset of data using the U-Net architecture described in Sect. 3.2. This result outperforms the U-Net baseline on the Lizard dataset, which achieved a Dice coefficient of **0.74** during validation and **0.61** during testing.

We attribute this improvement in U-Net performance to our usage of Macenko's normalization method which helped minimize the variation between the various sources of data, thus improving our model's generalization capabilities. The authors of the mentioned baseline did not use any form of normalization, and did not provide information about the representatives of the test data. This makes it likely that during their experiments, the U-Net model overfitted to a certain subset of the dataset, reducing its capability to generalize.

It is comparable to the baseline binary segmentation results of Hover-Net, which achieved a Dice coefficient of **0.80** on test data, and thus appears to be less susceptible to variations in data.

The Dice coefficient was calculated as follows [17]:

$$\mathbf{dc} = \frac{2 * \text{True Positives}}{2 * \text{True Positives} + \text{False Positives} + \text{False Negatives}} \tag{1}$$

SpringNet performs well when it comes to classification on the Lizard dataset. It was trained on 308,754 nuclei patches and tested on 17,153 nuclei patches. The proposed architecture with Spring blocks and residual connections that allowed us to build a deep model achieved an accuracy of **76.3%** and Cohen's kappa of **0.681** on test data when excluding the *Background* class, to make a more accurate comparison. In contrast, Hover-Net achieved an average classification accuracy of **70.3%** and an average Cohen's kappa of **0.651** when evaluated by histopathologists [5].

When also considering classification with the *Background class* included, our approach achieved an accuracy of **71%** and Cohen's kappa of **0.637**. This approach could also be used for further refinement of the segmentation output, by removing nuclei classified as *Background* from the predicted segmentation mask based on their coordinates stored during patch extraction.

The complete confusion matrix of test predictions can be seen in Fig. 8, and a summary of test information is available in Table 1 and Table 2.

Cohen's kappa was calculated as follows [18]:

$$\mathbf{k} = \frac{\mathbf{p_0} - \mathbf{p_e}}{1 - \mathbf{p_e}} \tag{2}$$

where p_0 is the relative observed agreement among raters and p_e is the hypothetical probability of chance agreement.

Table 1. Size of data used for testing

	Binary segmentation: test subset size	Classification: test subset size
HoverNet	N/A	1800 nuclei
Our approach	2289 patches	17153 nuclei

Table 2. Comparison of results between our approach and the Hover-Net baseline

	Binary segmentation: dice coefficient	Classification: accuracy	Classification: Cohen's kappa
HoverNet	0.80	70.3%	0.651
Our approach	**0.81**	**76.3%**	**0.681**

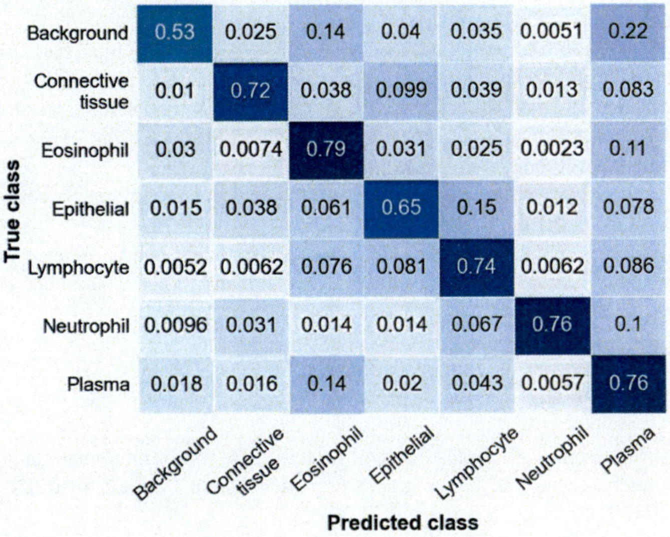

Fig. 8. Normalized confusion matrix of nuclei classification on test data

4 Conclusions

Our proposed solution for nuclei segmentation and classification using a two-step approach with a U-Net binary segmentation model and a custom SpringNet classifier achieved competitive results on the Lizard dataset when compared to the Hover-Net baseline. The focus on data preprocessing using Macenko's normalization and the implementation of a custom loss function allowed us to slightly outperform Hover-Net with a binary segmentation Dice score of **0.81** versus Hover-Net's baseline of **0.80**. SpringNet nucleus classification also outperforms the classification baseline, with an accuracy of **76.3%** and Cohen's kappa of 0.681 on test data versus Hover-Net's accuracy of **70.3%** and Cohen's kappa of **0.651**.

Further improvements could be achieved by implementing a more complex segmentation model to reduce the amount of model-induced error in the pipeline. The SpringNet architecture needs to be further refined by optimizing model depth and data dimensionality. A transition to concatenation based DenseNet-like [19] skip connections also need to be explored.

Due to the nature of histopathology and the need for explainable decisions in computer aided diagnosis, further research on model interpretability should also be conducted.

References

1. Chen, Z., Bei, Y., Rudin, C.: Concept whitening for interpretable image recognition. Nat. Mach. Intell. **2**(12), 772–782 (2020)
2. Chen, C., Li, O., Tao, C., Barnett, A.J., Su, J., Rudin, C.: This Looks like That: Deep Learning for Interpretable Image Recognition. Curran Associates Inc., Red Hook (2019)
3. Lu, W., Graham, S., Bilal, M., Rajpoot, N., Minhas, F.: Capturing cellular topology in multi-gigapixel pathology images. In: Proceedings of the IEEE/CVF Conference on Computer Vision and Pattern Recognition Workshops, pp. 260–261 (2020)
4. Dey, N., Ashour, A., Ashour, A., Singh, A.: Digital analysis of microscopic images in medicine. J. Adv. Microsc. Res. **10**(1), 1–13 (2015)
5. Graham, S., et al.: Lizard: a large-scale dataset for colonic nuclear instance segmentation and classification. In: Proceedings of the IEEE/CVF International Conference on Computer Vision, pp. 684–693 (2021)
6. Ronneberger, O., Fischer, P., Brox, T.: U-Net: convolutional networks for biomedical image segmentation. In: Navab, N., Hornegger, J., Wells, W., Frangi, A. (eds.) MICCAI 2015. LNCS, vol. 9351, pp. 234–241. Springer, Cham (2015). https://doi.org/10.1007/978-3-319-24574-4_28
7. Krithiga, R., Geetha, P.: Breast cancer detection, segmentation and classification on histopathology images analysis: a systematic review. Arch. Comput. Methods Eng. **28**(4), 2607–2619 (2021)
8. Graham, S., et al.: Hover-net: simultaneous segmentation and classification of nuclei in multi-tissue histology images. Med. Image Anal. **58**, 101563 (2019)
9. Van Rijthoven, M., Balkenhol, M., Siliņa, K., Van Der Laak, J., Ciompi, F.: Hooknet: multi-resolution convolutional neural networks for semantic segmentation in histopathology whole-slide images. Med. Image Anal. **68**, 101890 (2021)
10. Shao, W., Sun, L., Zhang, D.: Deep active learning for nucleus classification in pathology images. In: 2018 IEEE 15th International Symposium on Biomedical Imaging (ISBI 2018), pp. 199–202 (2018)
11. Li, R., Yao, J., Zhu, X., Li, Y., Huang, J.: Graph CNN for survival analysis on whole slide pathological images. In: Frangi, A., Schnabel, J., Davatzikos, C., Alberola-López, C., Fichtinger, G. (eds.) MICCAI 2018. LNCS, vol. 11071, pp. 174–182. Springer, Cham (2018). https://doi.org/10.1007/978-3-030-00934-2_20
12. Simonyan, K., Zisserman, A.: Very deep convolutional networks for large-scale image recognition. arXiv preprint arXiv:1409.1556 (2014)
13. Koohbanani, N.A., Jahanifar, M., Tajadin, N.Z., Rajpoot, N.: Nuclick: a deep learning framework for interactive segmentation of microscopic images. Med. Image Anal. **65**, 101771 (2020)
14. Macenko, M., et al.: A method for normalizing histology slides for quantitative analysis. In: 2009 IEEE International Symposium on Biomedical Imaging: From Nano to Macro, pp. 1107–1110. IEEE (2009)
15. Litjens, G., et al.: A survey on deep learning in medical image analysis. Med. Image Anal. **42**, 60–88 (2017)
16. Siddique, N., Paheding, S., Elkin, C.P., Devabhaktuni, V.: U-net and its variants for medical image segmentation: a review of theory and applications. IEEE Access **9**, 82031–82057 (2021)

17. Dice, L.R.: Measures of the amount of ecologic association between species. Ecology **26**(3), 297–302 (1945)
18. Cohen, J.: A coefficient of agreement for nominal scales. Educ. Psychol. Meas. **20**(1), 37–46 (1960)
19. Iandola, F., Moskewicz, M., Karayev, S., Girshick, R., Darrell, T., Keutzer, K.:Densenet: implementing efficient convNet descriptor pyramids. arXiv preprint arXiv:1404.1869 (2014)

Automated Tracking and Navigation of Spine Surgery with the Aid of Augmented and Virtual Reality: A Review and Taxonomy

Odimegwu C. Joseph[1], Nawzat Sadiq Ahmed[2], Somkiat Kitjongthawonkul[4], Nada AlSallami[5](✉), Syed Altaf[4], and Shahad Ahmed[3]

[1] Study Group Australia, Darlinghurst, Australia
[2] Duhok Polytechnic University, Duhok, KRG, Iraq
nawzat.ahmed@dpu.edu.krd
[3] The University of Duhok, Duhok, KRG, Iraq
[4] Kent Institute Australia, Melbourne, Australia
{somkiat.kitjongthawonkul,syed.altaf}@kent.edu.au
[5] Worcester State University, Worcester, MA, USA
nada.alsallami@yahoo.com

Abstract. Background and Aim: The application of augmented reality (AR) navigation & tracking in spine and orthopaedic have been very limited during spinal surgeries because the component of AR has not been subjected to objective evaluation and validation. This study aimed to evaluate and validate the application of AR in tracking and navigation of spine surgery to be sure that they can guarantee intraoperative accuracy and precision by reviewing journals on the focused subject. Methodology: We introduce the augmented reality surgical navigation (ARSN) which consists of the Data acquisition, automated tracking and navigation, and navigation feedback (DANF) workflow that we consider the necessary factors for seamless, accurate, precise, and flexible operation during spinal surgery. We propose that these system components should become a yardstick for evaluating and validating the applicability, and appropriateness of any navigation and tracking systems that have existed or that will exist. Result: DANF is evaluated based on its fitness for purpose. A comparison of this system was carried out with the models presented in existing pieces of literature. Findings reveal that AR is feasible and provides high precision and can deploy in surgery.

Keywords: Surgical navigation · Precision · Accuracy · Augmented reality · Automatic tracking · Pedicle screw

1 Introduction

In the context of surgery, AR is a technological tool that superimposes a computer-generated image on a surgeon's view of the surgical field. The use of AR in spine surgery is to enhance accurate tracking and navigation around intricate and minute structures of the spine, as well as to facilitate flexibility for the surgeon to ensure accuracy of data

K. Daimi and A. Al Sadoon (Eds.): ICR 2022, AISC 1431, pp. 76–83, 2022.
https://doi.org/10.1007/978-3-031-14054-9_8

during the surgery. As far as the subspeciality of spine surgery is concerned, AR-based navigation is currently commercially available majorly for simulation and training. Also, the use of a wireless tablet computer AR for neuro navigation system in the surgical planning and surgery of a couple of cases in China by [3] remains one of the few documented use of AR-system during surgery. However, despite the promises that it holds, AR use for neuro navigation in actual spinal surgeries remains limited due to lack of conviction on its accuracy, precision and flexibility [4] and because its use in final surgery is not yet approved by the FDA [5]. As a result of these, the incorporation of AR into automated navigation and tracking is still in its infancy age in spinal surgery [6]. The objective of this paper is to evaluate the existing model of augmented reality navigation and tracking techniques used in spine surgery and compare them on the component that we proposed which is based on the quality of data acquired, image calibration & registration, verification and navigation feedback that the system presents to the spine surgeons who are the end-users. Intra-operatively acquired images are integrated into the guidance environment to give accurate and precise target identification and on-target instrument navigation and tracking based on real-time feedback. Despite the promises that it holds, AR use for neuro-navigational in actual spinal surgeries remains limited due to lack of conviction on its accuracy, precision and flexibility and because the FDA does not yet approve its use in final surgery. As a result, the incorporation of AR into automated navigation and tracking is still in its infancy age in spinal surgery [1]. The objective of this paper is to evaluate the existing model of AR navigation and tracking techniques used in spine surgery and compare them on the component that we proposed which is based on the quality of data acquired, image calibration & registration, verification and navigation feedback that the system presents to the spine surgeons who are the end-users. We presented DANF algorithm. Moreover, we described the methods and process of every model of AR navigation and automated tracking systems that are worth using and evaluating for use in spinal surgery. The rest of the work is organized as follows. In Sect. 2, the selected previous works on navigation and automated tracking systems are discussed by categorizing them based on technology and techniques. In Sect. 3, the proposed taxonomy components are developed and discussed based on their subcomponents and instances. Section 4 includes the validation and evaluation of proposed taxonomy components. The discussion is given in Sect. 5. At last, the conclusion of the study and the future work are given in Sect. 6.

2 Literature Review

Elmi-Terander et al. [2] published the outcome of a clinical trial that they performed to assess the accuracy and feasibility of the same model on spinal tracking and navigation on cadaveric subjects. According to their reports, mean navigation time was 90 ± 53 s with an accuracy of 2.2 ± 1.3 mm. Carl et al. [3] used the operating microscope heads-up display for establishing and that could be easily integrated in the normal surgical procedure. In conjunction, the microscope video was superimposed on the segmented 3-D constructions that were semi-transparently visualized along with different display modes of picture information. Elmi-Terander et al. [4] used AR Surgical Navigation with Intra-operative 3D imaging system to place pedicle screws in the thoracic and lumbosacral spine of 20 patients. They further prove the accuracy of pedicle screw placement using augmented reality surgical navigation (ARSN) in a clinical trial. This solution proves the accuracy of 94.1% in using AR for navigation in a larger sample. Pietruskia et al. [5] experimented on two different intraoperative navigation systems based on simple (sAR) and navigated (nAR) AR technology, with the view of finding better options. This work fused the data obtain from computed tomography image after performing 126 osteotomies with preoperative CT scans and objectively compare the outcomes. Ma et al. [1] experiment demonstrated that AR surgical navigation system based on ultrasound-assisted registration for pedicle screw placement has an acceptable clinically desired targeting accuracy and reduces radiation exposure. Ma et al. [1] offered a solution by conducting eight K-wire insertion experiment. Ultrasound probes were used to acquire images of the vertebrae; it used the agar phantom to evaluate the targeting accuracy of AR-guided insertion. Hajek et al. [6] demonstrated a surgical procedure of closing the calibration loop between patients, C-arm and the surgeon with AR using a technique called marker-less and dynamic tracking concept. Hajek et al. [6] developed their solution by using an inside out SLAM-based tracking of the C-arm with respect to the exact same map of the environment, via means of an additional tracker rigidly attached to the C-shaped gantry. Wu et al. [7] compared three different approaches in lumbar spondylolisthesis surgery to determine the best approach that guaranteed patient satisfaction, shorter hospital stay and low processing time. This research offered a solution to the dilemma of the choice of method for better surgery. Wu et al. [7] proposed a system that they named the Augmented Reality Computer Assisted Spine Surgery (ARCASS). It consists of four successive stages that are pre-operative, 3-D modelling and calibration of the camera-projector system, image alignment, marker detection and tracking. Of all the works reviewed, that of Burström et al. [8] was the most impressive. This research assessed the possibility and accuracy of pedicle cannulation using AR in surgical navigation and automated tracking of spine surgery. They used a hybrid OR with a robotic C-arm along with optical cameras to track and measure the accuracy of pedicle screw insertions in spine surgery. This was proven to have an accuracy of 97.4%–100%.

3 System Components

The proposed system ARSN is based on reviewing eight works on both augmented and virtual reality in hard tissue surgery. The search was conducted on both CSU and Macquarie's journal database and returned 1452 research, 48 of these publications met our inclusive criteria. To obtain quality research work, we limited our journal to a highly ranked journal. Also, for the purpose of getting relevant information and latest innovations in our domain, we reduce our search to 2017, 2018 and 2019 only. We discard any paper that works on soft tissue with the same technique and technology, as our search were focus on hard tissue only. We look out for papers that explain in detail the proposed technique and its applications. For wider view of our study, we looked at different applications of augmented and virtual reality which include training and education purpose, but it wasn't considered in the table below. Out of the 48 journals, we reviewed based on our inclusive criteria, 8 of them were selected to be best solutions as summarized in Table 1. below. We consider each component and discuss the solutions that were given in

Table 1. Classification of AR and VR aided tracking and navigation of spine surgery.

RREF	TTYPE OF SURGER	DATA		NAVIGATION PROCESSING	FEEDBACK		
		RAW	VISUALLY PROCESSED		PL	DISP	INTERACTION TOOLS
(Burstrom et al.,2019), [8]	Spine surgery	CBCT X-Ray optical input from four cameras	A: Accuracy of the tracked needle D:3D CBCT of the region of interest PK: N/S	A hybrid Operating room (hybrid OR), robotic C-arm with optical camera Automatic spine segmentation and pedicle identification algorithm.	AC	M	Motorized mounted C-Arm
(Carl et al.,2019), [3]	Spine lesions Surgery	CT X-Ray MRI positron emission tomography (PET) intraoperative ultra-sound (iUS)	A: the tumour extent, Registration accuracy is measured D: delineate the 3-dimensional outline of the vertebra PK: N/S	Intraoperative computed tomography (iCT) A registration arrays Auto-segmentation,	P	HMD	Operating microscopes
(Elmi-Terander etal.,2019), [4]	Spine Surgery	CT X-Ray XperCT Optical video input 3Dconebeam CT	A: virtual screw positions D:surface around the surgical field PK:	Continuous video detection of flat.	p	M	optical cameras mounted into the frame of the C-arm detector Hybrid OR, Robotic ceiling mounted C-arm, optical markers
(Pietruskia et al.,2019), [5]	mandibular resection	CT	A: angular deviation from the planned osteotomy trajectory, and registration error D: position and angulation of the blade in real time PK:	Intraoperative navigation system	EM	HMD	Virtual planning software of the mentor eye system.
(MA, et al.,2017), [1]	pedicle screw placement surgery	CT MRI US Image	A: targeting error and angle error D:naked-eye3Dimages of the planning path PK:	Ultrasound (US) Assisted Registration	p	M	Ultrasound probe Optical tracker IV overlay device
(Hajek et al.,2018), [6]	Orthopedic Surgery	CT X-Ray	A:residual error of our Hand-Eye calibration and Target Registration Error D: PK	optical see-through head-mounted display (OST HMD)-based AR Microsoft HoloLens	p	HMD	Microsoft HoloLens
(Wu, et al., 2017), [7]	lumbar spondylolisthesis	CT	A: Compare MISS-iCT and MISS-FS D: The demographic and preoperative data were analysed PK: gender, age, body mass index.	intraoperative computed tomography integrated navigation	P	M	Registration pointer
(Elmi-terander et al.,2018), [2]	thoracolumbar surgical	CT Video input	A: Technical accuracy and processing time D: Distance between the tip of needle and its planned path PK:	Optical camera mounted into the frame of the flat detector.	p	M	motorized ceiling-mounted C-arm on Hybrid operating room

the paper. Our inclusion criteria include feasibility of the method, importance of hybrid operating room on our domain, criteria for measuring the feedback, how ARSN improves feedback on the domain, etc. We classify ARSN based on three factors data acquired, instrument navigation and tracking and feedback.

3.1 Data Acquisitions and Registration

The purpose of classifying data as a component is to provide information on which type of data is needed, and which data is to be obtained at every phase of the surgical procedure. Two subclasses of data were considered: animal cadaver/patient data and visual data. The animal cadaver data gives information on what kind data needs to be collected and assessed before and during surgery. Crucial subcomponents of the data necessary for flexibility and accuracy are image calibration, and intraoperative verification. In addition, data in the context of our proposed system is in three sub-categories, namely:

raw data, processed data, and derived data. This data is obtainable from the patient, (or the phantom or models) and the navigation systems before and during the surgery, with the characteristics and dimensions and sensors can be representative of real or virtual data objects.

3.2 Instrument Tracking and Surgical Navigation

Tracking, imaging, navigation etc. These are not just terminologies you hear in the operating room. In recent years, they have had a lot of focus in improving these techniques and integrating them to achieve an accurate surgical procedure. These components, when integrated make a complex surgical procedure less complex and safer [8]. The purpose and benefits of instrument tracking and surgical navigation is that it offers surgeons the opportunity to pre-operatively plan and carry out accurate surgical operation. Since this is an integral component of computer-assisted surgery, the concept is to reduce or eliminate surgical errors and improve patient safety.

3.3 Navigation Feedback

The purpose of using feedback as part of our classification is to demonstrate the relevance of displaying the much-needed information. It can facilitate or hinder the entire process during an operation. The display is part of the needed technologies that project the information as output to the surgeons. Feedback helps the user to understand steps that have been taken, identify the next step, evaluate the options, and achieve their aim. The interaction tools are made up of various virtual tools for interaction.

4 System Classification and Evaluation

We got 1452 results when we did our initial search; eight of them were selected to be best solutions as summarized in Table 1. In our proposal, the need for an objective evaluation and validation method to prove its relevance was also borne in mind. Although they sound very similar, the terms "validation" and "evaluation" are different though interwoven. In the context of its usage in this study, validation is the confirmation of whether a given system is accurate, or valuable and fit for the purpose of surgical navigation and tracking, while evaluation implies the actual value, mostly in quantifiable terms.

Most of the papers used this as their input data and the data are inform of CT, MRI, X-ray, sensors, video input, ultrasound images etc. CT and MRI are input data that is most used by several authors. Carel et al. [3] and Ma et al. [1] combined MRI with one or two raw imaging data for processing. Elmi-terander et al. [2] and [4] used video input combines with other imaging data for processing. While all of the papers used CT data, some like Wu et al. [7] used only CT data in their processing and full details are shown in the table above. Visually processed data is further grouped into analysed data, derived data and prior knowledge data. Almost none of the papers specified prior knowledge data but they stated their analysed and derived data. Some works, like [1–3, 6] analysed accuracy by measuring several parameters in their works. In all the papers we looked at, we were able to take notice of three key components, which is perception

Table 2. Validation/evaluation of AR and VR aided tracking and navigation of spine surgery

REF	CLINICAL CONTEXT	COMPONENT VALIDATED OR EVALUATED	STUDY CRITERIA	VALIDATION/ EVALUATION METHOD AND/OR DATA SET	RESULTS
(Burstrom et al.,2019), [8]	Spine surgery	Whole System	Accuracy of the tracked needle	AC	The technical accuracy at the tips is 0.80 The technical accuracy at bone entry is 0.88, while the navigation time is 0.30 proven to have accuracy of 97.4% – 100%
(Carl et al.,2019), [3]	Spine lesions Surgery	Navigation Feedback	accuracy Radiation Exposure Registration Error	Patient	a mean registration error of only about 1 mm. There was a reduction in radiation exposure of 0.35–0.98 mSv for cervical, 2.16–6.92 mSv for thoracic, and 3.55–4.20 mSv for lumbar surgeries, which is a decrease in the effective radiation dose by 70%.
(Elmi-Terander etal.,2019), [4]	Spine Surgery	Whole System	Accuracy Navigation time Screw placement time virtual screw position surface around the surgical field	patient	navigation time was measured to be less than 4.0minute Screw placement time was of lower value of 3.1 The solution further prove the accuracy of 94.1% in using augmented reality for navigation in a larger sample.
(Pietruskia et al.,2019), [5]	mandibular resection	Whole System	Angular deviation from the planned osteotomy trajectory, Registration error position and angulation of the blade in real time Point displacement	Experimental model	His solution provided has an mean angular deviation of 4.94±4.62 and mean control point displacement of 1.65±0.88 mm.
(MA, et al.,2017), [1]	pedicle screw placement surgery	Navigation and tracking error	targeting error and angle error Naked-eye 3D images of the planning path	patient	(Ma et al.,2017) provide a mean targeting and angle errors in K-wire insertion by means of skin markers-based registration and US-assisted registration were 5.18mm and 5.89°, and 2.41mm and 3.13°, respectively
(Hajek et al.,2018), [6]	Orthopedic Surgery	Feedback Navigation and tracking	Residual error of our Hand-Eye calibration and Target Registration Error Achieving "Bull's Eye" View	patient	An average residual error of 6.18°,5 .82°, and 5.17° while for translation the root mean-squared residual was 26.6mm The point-to-line Target Registration Error averaged over all points and users was 11.46mm.
(Wu, et al., 2017), [7]	lumbar spondylolisthesis	Whole system	Operation time Accuracy Patient satisfaction	Patient	hospital stay was shorter for the MISS-iCT group with 7.32±2.96 days and the MISSFS group with 7.53±1.43 days compared with the OS group with 8.78±2.05 days (p=.01). Blood loss was lower in MISS-iCT (390.91±139.42mL) and shorter operation time (247.55±26.48 minutes)
(Elmi-terander et al.,2018), [2]	thora-columbar surgical	Feedback Navigation and tracking	Technical accuracy and processing time Navigation time Distance between the tip of needle and its planned path	patient	The study provides technical accuracy of 2.2 ± 1.3 mm and Navigation time per insertion of 90 ± 53 seconds

location, display, and interaction tools. Perception location in this work focused on where the experiment is conducted. Elmi-terander et al. [8] used animal cadaver to test their algorithm while the others use a model of human parts to conduct their experiment. The rest of the papers stated patients in their research. We are also concerned on how the technology with the technique gives feedback to the operators (surgeons). Hajek et al. [6] and Carel et al. [3] used head mounted displays (HMD). In Table 2, we have provided a summary of examinations of the components that were validated and evaluated in the journals reviewed. In the table that follows, we have provided a summary of examination of the papers that have their Validation/evaluation method and/or data set and results clearly shown.

Most of the papers had their focus on accuracy as the major component being validated and evaluated, most likely because the major tracking and navigation is about the most needed attribute of every AR system. A few papers also considered navigation time, apart from accuracy. Burström et al. [8] measured the navigation time, registration time and displacement errors. Furthermore, while many of the papers validated only the registration factor of their system, only a few validated the whole system. All the papers validated their system, however only a few did validation and evaluation at the same time. Others that did validation only include Carl et al. [3]. Some works expressed the usefulness of their proposed systems via quantitative measurements, like [1–3].

While we recommend this limitation to be a focus for future research, there is nothing suggesting that verification and calibration of the 3-D images obtained during data acquisition is unimportant. This was lacking in virtually all the papers reviewed. All the papers reviewed made efforts to emphasize that their systems had pre-operative usefulness/ completeness by using certain related words to an appreciable degree. However, the most frequent terminology used by the authors to show that their system met the completeness criteria was "accuracy" and its adjectival form "accurate". Other words frequently used included "adaptable" and "low mean score error".

5 Discussion

About one-quarter of the papers reviewed presented components that factored in data as their components. However, the extent of the consideration for data is little. Wu et al. [7] for instance, described a stage of data in the preoperative stage. The extent of such data, and the mode of translating it into the intraoperative situation is rarely mentioned. On the other hand, the ARSN model proposed by Elmi-Terander et al. [4] and Burstrom et al. [8] did not make an extensive mention of preoperative data, and this may imply that it was not considered in their model. The intraoperative computed tomography (ICT) proposed by Carl et al. [3] had a place for data acquisition, but the extent of information collected, and how such data became usable was not thoroughly discussed. Furthermore, the type and stage of data (prior knowledge or derived) was not clearly differentiated in any of the publications, except that of Burstrom et al. [8], and so, it was not clear whether atlas or reference anatomies were involved. The most crucial omission that exists in the reviewed systems under the data acquisition component is image verification and calibration. The fact that only 1 of the reviewed papers made mention of this important sub factor means that quality assurance purposes is preoperatively missing in them. Due to a difference in word choice, the majority of the publications used the expression "visual processing" to mention feedback.

6 Conclusion

We introduce ARSN which consists of the Data acquisition, Automated tracking and navigation, and navigation feedback, which we consider the necessary factors for seamless, accurate, precise, and flexible operation during spinal surgery. We propose that these system components should become a yardstick for evaluating and validating the applicability and appropriateness of any navigation and tracking systems that have existed or that will exist. This is crucial as it will create awareness on what is expected of any augmented reality navigation system and will provide insight into the reasons for the perceived inaccuracies and inflexibility of the existing systems. This will assist designers of augmented reality algorithms to be able to provide suitable systems thereby increasing the use of future augmented reality systems in spinal surgery theatres for the ease of surgeons and safety of patients. Several findings were obtained from the papers reviewed, and they provided a framework for comparing the proposed model with existing ones. The proposed system sought to find out and incorporate missing sub factors in existing models, which are crucial for a successful navigation. One of the questions that the research sought to answer is whether the existing state-of-art solutions placed importance in evaluating and validating the accuracy and precision for spinal surgery and the steps taken to prove its flexibility. Majority of the authors understood the importance of evaluating and validating the systems that they have proposed. While many of them carried out experiments on phantoms and models, the others conducted clinical trials on live patients and reported quantitative results on various aspects of their solutions such as mean positional errors, root mean squares, displacement errors, etc. This shows that the fitness of purpose of any proposed solution could be considered only based on what steps have been taken to evaluate it. Furthermore, determining whether the factors in the existing solutions complete enough to guarantee the needed level of flexibility during spinal surgery is also important.

References

1. Ma, L., Zhao, Z., Chen, F., Zhang, B., Fu, L., Liao, H.: Augmented reality surgical navigation with ultrasound-assisted registration for pedicle screw placement: a pilot study. Int. J. Comput. Assist. Radiol. Surg. **12**(12), 2205–2215 (2017)
2. Elmi-Terander, A., Nachabe, R., Skulason, H., Pedersen, K., Soderman, M., Racadio, J.: Feasibility and accuracy of thoracolumbar minimally invasive pedicle screw placement with augmented reality navigation technology. Spine **15**, 1018–1023 (2018)
3. Carl, B., Bopp, M., Saß, B., Voellger, B., Nimsky, C.: Implementation of augmented reality support in spine surgery. Eur. Spine J. **28**(7), 1697–1711 (2019)
4. Elmi-Terander, A., et al.: Pedicle screw placement using augmented reality surgical navigation with intraoperative 3D imaging. Spine **44**(7), 517–525 (2019)
5. Pietruski, P., et al.: Supporting mandibular resection with intraoperative navigation utilizing augmented reality technology - a proof of concept study. J. Cranio-Maxillo-Facial Surg. **47**, 854–859 (2019)
6. Hajek, J., et al.: Closing the calibration loop: an inside-out-tracking paradigm for augmented reality in orthopedic surgery. In: Frangi, A., Schnabel, J., Davatzikos, C., Alberola-López, C., Fichtinger, G. (eds.) MICCAI 2018. LNCS, vol. 11073, pp. 299–306. Springer, Cham (2018). https://doi.org/10.1007/978-3-030-00937-3_35
7. Wu, M.-H.: Comparison of minimally invasive spine surgery using intraoperative computed tomography integrated navigation, fluoroscopy, and conventional open surgery for lumbar spondylolisthesis: a prospective registry-based cohort study. Spine J. **17**(8), 1082–1090 (2017)
8. Burström, G., Nachabe, R., Persson, O., Edström, E., Terander, A.E.: Augmented and virtual reality instrument tracking for minimally invasive spine surgery: a feasibility and accuracy study. Spine **44**(15), 1097–1104 (2019)

GPS Navigated Drones to Deliver Emergency Medical Aid Post Catastrophic Event

Ankit Shrestha[1], Shayma Ismail Ali[2], Ali A. Alwan[3](✉), AB Emran Salahuddin[4], Muhammad Siddiqi[4], and Tarik A. Rashid[5]

[1] Study Group Australia, Darlinghurst, Australia
Ankit.shrestha47@gmail.com
[2] Cihan University Duhok, Duhok, KRG, Iraq
shayma.ali@duhokcihan.edu.krd
[3] Ramapo College of New Jersey, Mahwah, New Jersey, USA
aaljuboo@ramapo.edu
[4] Kent Institute Australia, Melbourne, Australia
{emran.salahuddin,msiddiqi}@kent.edu.au
[5] University of Kurdistan Hewler, Erbil, KRG, Iraq

Abstract. The use of GPS navigation systems for drone delivery in a dynamic environment has grown significantly in recent years. The potential of GPS navigation techniques in such a context for emergency purposes has not yet been fully explored. This paper presents a taxonomy for GPS-based navigation Unmanned Aerial Vehicles (UAVs) that identifies the major components of a navigation system for UAVs to deliver emergency medical aid. We demonstrate that these components are crucial and serve as a validation criterion when introducing a navigational routing algorithm into UAV delivery applications. The proposed taxonomy is a step toward developing a robust routing strategy that helps vendors and receivers understand and discuss the components of GPS navigation of UAVs for delivering emergency medical aid. We demonstrate the utility of the proposed taxonomy in the field of UAV/drone delivery utilizing GPS navigation. The proposed taxonomy facilitates an understanding of the classification groups, validation criteria, and future trends in drone applications aiming at reducing the time and cost of drone delivery systems.

Keywords: Taxonomy · Healthcare · Delivery · Rural health · UAV (Unmanned Aerial Vehicle)

1 Introduction

The GPS navigated drones' systems have become a common facility for delivering medical aid and food in unreachable areas during emergencies. The main concern of these GPS navigated drones is to improve the routing solutions of the path in which the drones fly [1, 2]. This is typically achieved by collecting some essential modalities such as the estimated distance between the two points, the altitude of the drone, the payload of the drone, the capacity of the battery for the drone. The navigational plans,

K. Daimi and A. Al Sadoon (Eds.): ICR 2022, AISC 1431, pp. 84–92, 2022.
https://doi.org/10.1007/978-3-031-14054-9_9

the pre-defined route and the graphical representation of the *drone's routed path* and its performance including the real-time estimated arrival time and cost are crucial during the flight to guide people in their task [2, 3]. From the literature, it has been found that few GPS systems are used for drone navigation. Moreover, a limited number of these GPS systems have been developed for commercial purposes. Although it is becoming more common for commercial drones to make GNSS-based navigations available [1, 2]. For instance, real-time vision-based, sound-based, and gas sensor-based navigations are not common to use in non-commercial drones. Several reasons cause these GPS systems not to be widely used. First, most of these GPS systems are developed as proof-of-concept prototypes and therefore may not take into account the direct navigational needs for drone routing. Second, the added benefit in case of a GPS spoofing attack, the drone can easily fight against the attacker. Third, the systems are not sufficiently evaluated [3–5]. Thus, it is still rare to see the integration of GPS navigation systems into a real dynamic environment and workflows.

This paper aims at developing a taxonomy of GPS navigation techniques used for drone delivery based on the types of the data set and how these data are processed before being presented to the end-user. The role of each major component of the GPS-based navigation UVA for emergency delivery taxonomy has been explained. The proposed taxonomy is beneficial by introducing a framework in which GPS navigation systems may be discussed, analyzed, and evaluated. Besides, it also allows a better understanding of the most relevant and important components to be considered for GPS navigation systems in drones. We also define and discuss each of the major components that should be considered to facilitate the discussion. Proper analysis and validation of the major entities of current systems allow developers to easily recognize which components can be reused. We demonstrate the usefulness of the GPS navigated UAV taxonomy by classifying 12 state-of-art remarkable publications which describe navigation via GPS in drone delivery.

The rest of the paper is organized as follows. A discussion of previous works on navigation taxonomies is presented in Sect. 2. In Sect. 3, the proposed taxonomy is discussed. The system classification is introduced in Sect. 4. The validation and the evaluation of the system components are elaborated in Sect. 5. In Sect. 6, we describe the components that were not well examined in the chosen publications and point out avenues of future research efforts in GPS navigated UAV systems for delivering goods during disasters. Conclusions are given in Sect. 7.

2 Literature Review

Previous navigation taxonomies and models have typically focused on only one or two aspects of navigation such as route, altitude, and obstacles [2]. In the following section, we discuss several proposed navigation taxonomies and the aspects of the navigation processes they emphasized.

2.1 Navigation for Drones in Urban Area

The work in [1] has introduced a system that helps in reducing the GPS positioning errors exploiting the offline path planning feature to input information about obstacles and GPS issues. Satellite clock/orbit bias, atmospheric delays, receiver thermal noise multipath delays, and others are calculated to identify the exact issues that could arise in terms of positioning errors. However, the proposed solution does not resolve the issue of positioning errors, but it only attempts to avoid them during high traffic congestion. Nevertheless, changing paths for long flights is undesirable. The work proposed in [6] has devised a solution that helps people with chronic disease in rural areas to receive medication on regular basis with the help of UAVs. The main feature of the proposed system is the introduction of operational planning that assists in identifying the locations of each centre and the number of drones to be deployed per centre based on the number of patients served and several patients in the route. The proposed system results in a significant saving in time and money. However, since the patients are divided into subzones and if the nearby location is divided into different zones, multiple drones would be taking the same path.

2.2 Delivery of Emergency Medical Aid

The work reported in [2] discusses the issue of facilitating early emergency medical services (EMS) in the event of out-of-hospital cardiac arrest (OHCA). The work aims to shorten the time from collapse to defibrillation which is the most important time for a patient's survival. The purpose of the work is to design a UAV drone system that reduces the time it takes for a person who collapses due to fibrillation in an event of OHCA to obtain immediate assistance. The proposed approach has been evaluated based on time constraints. Having said that, there is a time difference between a person collapsing and an AED being attached to the patient and the ambulance and drone getting to the location of the incident. The bystander, who makes the call, must performs all of the major tasks as soon as the package is delivered. He performs T-CPR, and then connects the package to the patient.

2.3 Persistent UAV Delivery Logistics: Delivery Scheduling and Routing

The work introduced in [3] has developed a path scheduling model for a UAV system to provide a better delivery service. The proposed model emphasizes offering services relying on two major components, namely: a fully functional service station to charge and load the UAV, and a control centre to control and monitor each UAV. The proposed system incorporates multiple service stations for drones that facilitate the recharging services for drones and load/unload them whenever needed. The proposed model achieves a significant reduction in battery consumption when the drone is operating. The work contributed by [4] tackled the issue of control centres when drones are operating. The idea of the work relies on collecting the information required by drones under their services. The idea of the service centre in the middle of the service for battery recharging purposes is beneficial to expand the area covered by the drones. Nevertheless, the service stations need to be placed in every corner whenever the drone's battery life reduces.

3 Proposed Taxonomy

The multi-depot vehicle routing was developed based on strategic and operational planning. It also builds on the solution approach and cost-benefit analysis methodology. With the help of numerical experiments in vehicle routing and developing GPS navigation of the routes, we iteratively refined a taxonomy that would consider the most relevant factors for the development, validation and evaluation of such a system.

We found 105 research publications on the topic, out of which 12 met our inclusion criteria as follows: the publications that described an entire visualization system for use in the drone delivery, even if the focus was only on one aspect of the system, e.g., only on GPS navigational process or only on the navigational technology used. Some results were excluded: 32 were rejected as they were not relevant to the domain. 13 papers were discarded because they described drones for military rather than for delivery. 15 papers were neglected because they described only one aspect of a system or were review papers. Finally, 16 papers were rejected because these papers were written in a foreign language.

Based on our review, we believe that in order to provide pilots with a tool to effectively assist them during the flight, three main points should be considered, namely: (1) the current positional data of the drone, (2) how it can be effectively routed and obstacles can be avoided, and (3) delivery of the goods to customers. We classify a GPS navigated drone delivery system based on three factors: delivery area, load capacity and dynamic drone routing. The first factor that is used in the GPS navigated UAV taxonomy is positional data. It includes GPS coordinates and navigational data classes with the properties of altitude and speed, whether the data are acquired preoperatively or intraoperatively, and whether it represents a real of the virtual object in the end view of the navigational process. Second, the routing algorithms that are used to transform the data to create a numerical representation of the data are used for classification. Lastly, we classify the papers based on the delivery of the goods to customers and the navigation is measured according to the delivery time and cost consumption. These three components are elaborated in Fig. 1.

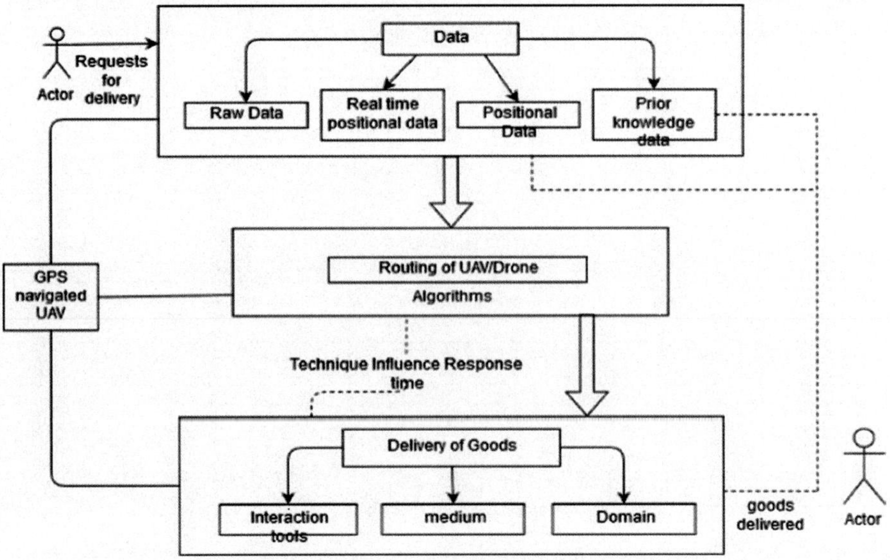

Fig. 1. The GPS navigated drones and their components.

Two main subclasses of positional data have been considered. This encompasses the exact coordinates of the drone and the graphical representation of the drone. The purpose of using data as part of our classification is to highlight the importance of deciding which of the available data should be shown to the end-user. As the number of possible data sets that can be acquired increases, there is a stronger demand for integration of the different modalities and numerous visually processes data sets into coherent navigation. For example, numerous data sets may be gathered in drone delivery, including both structural data (altitude, speed, payload capacity) and functional data (time consumption, performance), and used for routing and path planning. The problem of which data and information should be used, and how data should be graphically represented to give a useful representation for a given navigational delivery is nontrivial. Showing too much or all the available data is not always desirable as it may confound the viewer and makes it difficult to highlight the most important features. Therefore, it is important that careful consideration is given to what type of data should be calculated and at what point during the flight or delivery it was useful.

4 System Classification

This section presents and discusses the research publications that met our inclusion criteria. To get an overview of the current work that is done in the area, we chose the research groups or authors that had two or more publications in the database since the year 2000. From the research groups and authors, we chose the most recent publications. However, if that publication did not describe the developed GPS navigation in drones in enough detail, we chose the next most recent publication. A detailed description of the selected papers is summarized in Table 1. The table illustrates the taxonomy components and discusses the proposed solution for each work.

Table 1. System classification based on (Data, GPS module information, routing, and application)

Ref	Types of Navigation	Data			GPS module information	Routing	Application/delivery	
		Raw data	Real-time data	Significant data			Device	Interaction tools
[7]	3D path planning navigation	Image 3D camera	Live video data	Graphical representation, 3D path and obstacles display	Location, positional data	Path planning algorithm	Situation awareness system, UAV, On-Board computers	Drone simulator, Ground control system
[5]	Automated navigational delivery	N/A	target location, obstacles, time calculation	Flight ready loaded drone, path planning, obstacle avoidance	Target location coordinates, home base location coordinates.	A quasi-experiment methodology approach	Drone, AED, Manikin	Drone simulator, computational devices, Ground control system, delivery materials
[8]	Reinforcement learning framework	Target area, environment, obstacles	Audio, video, obstacles, battery calculation, route planning	Route planning, search and rescue mission	The target search area, home base location	Feature extraction, situation awareness system	UAV, Onboard computer, Barometer, Magnetometer, Exteroceptive sensors RGB fish-eye lens	Drone simulator, ground computing systems
[9]	Target Positioning Algorithm	Subject identification, target area, obstacles	Video, path allocation, search area, search object	Search and rescue mission, service area allocation and division	Search area, home-base location	Target positioning algorithm, gas sensor system	UAV/drone, Onboard sensors, Onboard computer, gas sensor system	Drone simulation system, ground computing systems
[1]	Ray-tracing navigational technique	Target position, payload, route distance	Routing processes, video, environment, obstacles	Path routing, obstacle avoidance	Drone's location, path navigation, target position	Offline path planning, Prediction of GPS positioning error	Multirotor UAV, on-board computer. GPS module	Cameras, UAV simulator, computing and comparing devices.
[10]	Hybridized fall detection algorithm (FDB-HRT)	N/A	Fall detection, target location, obstacles, time calculation	Flight ready loaded drone, path planning, obstacle avoidance	Drone's location, target location	Hybridized fall detection, UAV navigational algorithm	Advanced First Aid System, Fall Detection Device, Unmanned Aerial Vehicle, Heartbeat sensor, GPS sensor, onboard computers	Drone simulator, computational devices, Ground control system, delivery materials
[11]	Multi-depot vehicle routing, set covering approach	Patient's location, payload, route	Video, obstacles, dynamic routes	Route division, set covering	Drone's location, customer's location, routing, route planning	Pre-process algorithm, bound generation method	Multirotor UAV, on-board computer, GPS module	Cameras, UAV simulator, computing devices
[12]	Covert spoofing algorithm	Customer's location, payload, battery	Video, audio, battery consumption, security problem	Covert spoofing, safety, reliability	Target location, drone's location, home-base location	Spoofing algorithm of UAV based on the GPS/INS Integrated Navigation systems.	UAV, microprocessor, camera, GPS module	Cameras, UAV simulator, computing devices
[13]	Obstacle detection and sensing algorithm	Flight route, source, destination, payload, distance, battery	Obstacles, rerouting, video, location	Accuracy, reliability, cost-effective, less time	Drone location, target location, real-time routing	Traffic Collision Avoidance System	GPS, TACAS transponders, RADAR, UAV, on-board computers	UAV simulator, module installer, ground computer, onboard computer
[14]	Follow-me tracking system	Target subject	Subject's route, location, environment, obstacles, video	Following system, tracking system	Real-time location of the drone, target location	Hybrid GPS-Visio algorithm for tracking.	Onboard camera, GPS, Obstacle sensors, On-board computer	Computing devices, simulation device, module installer, sensors
[2]	Vehicle Routing algorithms with Drones	Source, destination, target, payload, battery, distance	Route, obstacles, environment, video	Time consumption, reliability	Source, destination, depot, drone location	Vehicle routing algorithm	UAV, Onboard camera, GPS, Obstacle sensors, On-board computer, Navigation module	UAV simulator, modules, ground computer, on-board computer, particle filter
[15]	GPS restoring and routing algorithm	Target location, route, payload, battery	Video, environment, obstacles, GPS threat, battery consumption	Backup navigation source, custom hardware	Target positioning, drone positioning, GPS jamming	The direction of arrival method.	UAV: Phantom 4, GNSS receiver, STMicroelectronics microcontroller, IEEE 802.15.4 compatible radio.	Drone simulator, micro controlling device, ground control unit.

5 System Components Validation and Evaluation

In determining the most relevant factors of a GPS navigated drone delivery system, we also determined the components which must be evaluated and validated to demonstrate whether there is added value in using the system. We differentiate between validation and evaluation in the following way: validation proves the accuracy of the system and shows if the right system was built, and evaluation is converted by showing the usefulness and value of the system. In the following section, we look at which components, described in the selected publications, were validated or evaluated. Table 2 summarizes these validations and evaluations.

Table 2. Evaluation and validation of the components of the proposed taxonomy

Ref	Context of study	Component validated or evaluated	Study criteria	Validation/ evaluation method and or data set	Results
[7]	Drone delivery	Routing and navigation	Cost function	Compare and path determination	Cost function checked frequently by C (p_j, p_{j+1}). If the value is ≤ 0, then it is known as the path is collision-free. Otherwise, searches for an alternative path.
[5]	Emergency drone delivery	Delivering and Routing	Time is taken for delivery and transportation	Calculation and comparison	Time taken by standard EMS to reach the site was 22 minutes, but for the drone, its 5 minutes and 21 seconds. Time taken from collapse until AED attached to the patient is 9 minutes 47 seconds when using a drone and it is 37 minutes when using the standard EMS.
[8]	Drone routing	Search, rescue and delivery	Accuracy, versatility	Direct calculation	The landing accuracy of the UAV is 83%.
[9]	Tracking and positioning	Target positioning, navigation	Errors, time	Direct calculation	The error with gas sensors is 3 meters from the target. The time duration taken by the model which has a gas sensor is lesser than models equipped with cameras and sensors.
[1]	Drone delivery in an urban area	GPS positioning and path planning	GPS Positioning error of the UAV	Direct calculation	The positioning error of the drone has been reduced from 50 meters to 32.62 meters.
[10]	Emergency Drone delivery	Delivery of medical services	Time, accuracy	Direct calculation	Time-saving of 31.81% was achieved when using a UAV to transport a first aid kit to the patient compared to an ambulance. The accuracy of the algorithm is 99.2% when detecting the fall of a patient.
[11]	Drone delivery in rural areas	Drone routing, partition method	Cost, time consumption	Direct calculation	The cost of travelling is reduced as low as $0.58/mile.
[12]	Drone safety and security	Covert spoofing	Position of the drone, velocity of the drone	Direct calculation	The positional shake deviation of the UV tracking spoofing trajectory is up to 20 m. The velocity shake deviation is up to 2 m/s.
[13]	Drone navigation	Obstacle detection and sensing	distance between the drone and the obstacle	Direct calculation	The detection of an obstacle is very high and sensitive.
[14]	Drone navigation	Tracking and following	Accuracy, path recovery	Direct calculation	The drone has 50% higher accuracy than the previous systems. The system can recover any kind of failure within 3-7 seconds.
[2]	Drone delivery	Routing errors	Completion time of the mission	Mathematical calculation	The completion time is 75% better than the previous systems.
[15]	Drone safety and security	GPS jamming	Calibration, angular errors	Mathematical calculation	The standard calibration median is 0.6745

6 Results and Discussion

The following section explores the components of GPS navigated UAV taxonomy that is not clearly described in the selected 12 publications. In this paper, we use examples from the literature to demonstrate that GPS navigated GPS components are present in drone delivery and navigation systems for drone delivery and are therefore relevant to such a taxonomy. Additionally, we emphasize the need to carefully consider solution options for the components.

6.1 Data: Prior Knowledge Data and Real-Time Positional Data

Several publications featured in this work include prior knowledge data. Drones must fly to the desired target location for navigational purposes, usually following the target location described in prior knowledge data. Routing is the key component of UAV GPS navigation. In GPS-navigated UAVs, prior knowledge of target location helps us determine how to get from a source to a destination depending on obstacles and the environment. Position data in real-time are the types of information that are communicated from the drone to the Ground Control System or a Home Depot. For further routing and pathfinding purposes, this data indicates the position of the UAV on the graphical map. The use of deviation of the target position of the drone's landing position was not mentioned in the systems presented in the selected publications because the deviation of the target position and actual landing position is not a novel concept. Finding the prior knowledge data position and real-time positional data position is a must to find out the actual location and fault of the drone. The work contributed by [16] proposed a system where there is a need for prior knowledge data of the target location of the customers. The lack of prior knowledge data and real-time positioning data might suggest that the presented taxonomy does not need to include these types of data to classify systems. However, we believe that the prior knowledge of the positioning of the customers, route calculation, and the real-time positioning of the drone and obstacles are helpful in guidance and require further study.

6.2 Drone Routing: Vision-Based Routing

Few publications described or included vision-based routing. The vision-based routing algorithm that was described, for the most part, consisted of how the drones were routed for navigation and guidance. In general, vision-based navigation is the key part of the drone routing algorithm in these taxonomies. In these taxonomies, the drone senses the obstacles and uses a vision-based algorithm for finding the path avoiding those obstacles in a dynamic environment. The camera shows real-time footage on the screen of the pilot in the Ground Control Unit (GCU), and the pilot can manually fly the drone or can make it fly on autopilot based on vision-based maneuverability. However, this technique may be problematic when it comes to navigation and routing, because only seeing the locality, we cannot be able to detect the whereabouts of the drone, and during the night it will be almost impossible to fly the drone manually.

6.3 Delivery of Goods

Although delivery of goods to those in need was well described in the 12 selected publications, few publications referred to it or didn't mention it. Other taxonomies were more concerned with navigating and directing the drones, rather than delivering goods to the people in need. Moreover, other taxonomies used advanced technologies to navigate the drone, including gas-emitted, vision-based, or GPS-based techniques, but there were no algorithms available for delivering the goods.

7 Conclusion

This paper presents a taxonomy for GPS-guided drones to deliver medical assistance after disasters. Three major components were identified in the taxonomy for the development of drone systems to deliver medical supplies during catastrophes. The study found that drone data, drone routing, and the delivery of goods are the three main components that should be taken into account when designing a drone system. The study found that most of the proposed algorithms and ideas for routing drones to their destinations failed to improve accuracy, reduce costs, or time. The work can be extended by incorporating more training data into the analysis to improve the accuracy of GPS navigated drones to work under different conditions and ensure maintaining a higher performance of these GPS drone systems.

References

1. Sundar, K., Rathinam, S.: Algorithms for routing an unmanned aerial vehicle in the presence of refueling depots. IEEE Trans. Autom. Sci. Eng. **11**(1), 287–294 (2014)
2. Song, B.D., Park, K., Kim, J.: Persistent UAV delivery logistics: MILP formulation and efficient heuristic. Comput. Ind. Eng. **120**, 418–428 (2019)
3. Sanfridsson, J., et al.: Drone delivery of an automated external defibrillator – a mixed method simulation study of bystander experience. Scand. J. Trauma Resusc. Emerg. Med. **27**(40), 1556–1561 (2019)
4. Zhang, G., Hsu, L.T.: A new path planning algorithm using a GNSS localization error map for UAVs in an urban area. J. Intell. Rob. Syst. **94**(2), 219–235 (2019)
5. Cordeau, J.F., Laporte, G., Mercier, A.: A unified tabu search heuristic for vehicle routing problems with time windows. J. Oper. Res. Soc. **52**(8), 928–936 (2001)
6. Caffrey, S.L., Willoughby, P.J., Pepe, P.E., Becker, L.B.: Public use of automated external defibrillators. N. Engl. J. Med. **347**(1242), 1–7 (2002)
7. Sanchez, J.L., Wang, M., Olivares, M.A., Molina, M., Voos, H.: A real time 3D path planning solution for Collision free navigation of multirotor aerial robots in dynamic environments. J. Intell. Robot. Syst. **93**, 33–53 (2019)
8. Sampedro, C., Rodriguez, A.R., Bavle, H., Carrio, A., Puente, P., Campoy, P.: A fully-autonomous aerial robot for search and rescue applications in indoor environments using learning-based techniques. J. Intell. Rob. Syst. **29**, 601–627 (2019)
9. Yuan, H., et al.: Target detection, positioning and tracking using new UAV gas sensor systems: simulation and analysis. J. Intell. Rob. Syst. **94**, 871–882 (2019)
10. Fakhrulddin, S.S., Gharghan, S.K., Naji, A.A., Chahl, J.: An advanced first aid system based on an unmanned aerial vehicles and a wireless body area sensor network for elderly persons in outdoor environments. Sensors **19**(13), 1–28 (2019)
11. Kim, S.J., Lim, G.J., Cho, J., Cote, M.J.: Drone-aided healthcare services for patients with chronic diseases in rural areas. J. Intell. Robot. Syst. **88**(13), 163–180 (2017)
12. Aswini, N., Krishna, E.K., Uma, S.V.: UAV and obstacle sensing techniques – a perspective. Int. J. Intell. Unmanned Syst. **6**(1), 32–46 (2018)
13. Tuan, D.T., Anh, H.: Visual-GPS combined 'follow-me' tracking for selfie drones. Adv. Robot. **32**(19), 1047–1060 (2018)
14. Peng, K., et al.: A hybrid genetic algorithm on routing and scheduling for vehicle-assisted multi-drone parcel delivery. IEEE Access **7**(1), 2169–3536 (2019)
15. Pollin, S., Bergh, B.V.: Keeping UAVs under control during GPS jamming. IEEE Syst. J. **13**(2), 2010–2021 (2019)
16. Chiang, W.C., Li, Y., Shang, J., Urban, T.L.: Impact of drone delivery on sustainability and cost: realizing the UAV potential through vehicle routing optimization. Appl. Energy **242**(2019), 1164–1175 (2019)

Nanotechnology Based Photodynamic Therapy for Cancer Treatment

Bindu Bashyal[1], Shahad Ahmed[2], Anchal Shrestha[3], Nada AlSallami[4](✉), Nawzat Sadiq Ahmed[5], Omar Hisham Alsadoon[6], and Shaymaa Ismail Ali[7]

[1] Study Group Australia, Darlinghurst, Australia
[2] The University of Duhok, Duhok, KRG, Iraq
[3] Kent Institute Australia, Sydney, Australia
anchal.shrestha@kent.edu.au
[4] Worcester State University, Worcester, MA, USA
nada.alsalami@yahoo.com
[5] Duhok Polytechnic University, Duhok, KRG, Iraq
nawzat.ahmed@dpu.edu.krd
[6] Al Iraqia University, Baghdad, Iraq
[7] Cihan University, Duhok, KRG, Iraq
shayma.ali@duhokcihan.edu.krd

Abstract. The application of Nanotechnology based photodynamic therapy (PDT) in the medical area is considered as a promising alternative treatment modality to others current treatments against different types of cancer. The targeted treatment method has not been considered yet for the effective treatment for the cancer cell. The aim of this research is to propose a new taxonomy that can be used to implement nanotechnology-based photodynamic therapy for cancer treatment which is based on a targeted treatment method. The components that we have considered in this system are data, delivery of nanoparticles, and laser light emission (LLE). These components are used to determine the side effects of the therapy. Based on the review of numerous articles and publications, we found synergic effects of nanotechnology and photodynamic therapy by providing focused treatment without side effects to the therapist during treatment. This work demonstrates the synergic effects of light and nanoparticles in the field of cancer treatment through the critical analysis of different research. Furthermore, the therapist will learn more about tumour targeted therapy systems, and cancer patients will get fewer side effects.

Keywords: Nanotechnology · Photodynamic therapy · Taxonomy · Monitoring · Synergic effect · Cancer

1 Introduction

Nanotechnology is a novel technology which offers the way for tumor targeted therapy and enhances the radiation based therapeutic efficacy. Sending drug through nanotechnology is used in Photodynamic Therapy (PDT) to give a clear vision of the tumor cells

K. Daimi and A. Al Sadoon (Eds.): ICR 2022, AISC 1431, pp. 93–101, 2022.
https://doi.org/10.1007/978-3-031-14054-9_10

so that therapist can send drug on targeted area. This is typically obtained by monitoring the features from raw data of light emitter in photodynamic therapy. As a result, clear view of release of drug, graphical representation of therapeutic tools and instruments is obtained which guides the therapist to do focused treatment without affecting neighbor healthy cells [1]. The aim of this research is to introduce and analyze different components to perform focused therapy having less side effects on healthy tissues. To satisfy this, some articles have been chosen based on our inclusive criteria. We propose that the defined components should be discussed and compared to those which were developed on previous works. We also discuss about the efficacy of output of photodynamic therapy based on nanotechnology and compared with previous results. From this analysis and validation of important entities, future researchers can easily recognize components that can be reused. Thus, this research will address all the possible issues on developing such technology and technique on medical domain. The rest of the work is organized as follows. In Sect. 2, the selected papers are discussed by categorizing them based on technology and techniques. In Sect. 3, taxonomy components are developed and discussed based on their subcomponents and instances. Section 4 includes the validation and evaluation of proposed taxonomy components. The discussion is given in Sect. 5. At last, the conclusion of the study and the future work are given in Sect. 6.

2 Literature Review

In this section, we discussed various number of drugs deliver techniques and specific aspects of delivery procedure that they emphasized. These articles are classified based on the type of materials used and methodology proposed. Calixto et al. [1] described three components which act simultaneously in PDT. First is photosensitizer (PS), second is light source and third is oxygen molecule. This research provided the information to generate singlet oxygen. This phenomenon is also called triplet-triplet annihilation. Li et al. [2] offered a solution to the problem by combining phototherapy with the immunotherapy to increase the effectiveness of the phototherapy against cancer. They provide the combination of three technologies such as phototherapy, immunotherapy, and nanomaterials to treat metastatic cancer. Liange et al. [3] investigated the efficiency of drug delivery and bio effectiveness of a new photodynamic therapy (PDT) matrix drug delivery system. The research offered a solution to the problem by using of triple layered photofrin-releasing membrane. This solution provides a multiple layered stent based on PDT with dual release mechanism which can be novel therapy technique for cholangiocarcinoma and other type of lung cancer. Kruger and Abrahame [4] upgraded the PDT by using photosensitizer (PS) drug which accumulate within the damaged cells site and once exposed to certain wavelength of light then it successively produces ROS which finally damage the tumor tissues. Xaia et al. [5] developed a cancer-cell specific photosensitizer nano-delivery system by synthesizing protoporphyrin IX (PpIX)-conjugated pullulan (P) with reducible bonds. This provides an acceptable range of quenching effect between photosensitizer moieties in the core of nanoparticle, which minimize the potential side effects of PDT. Gao et al. [6] proposed Single-walled carbon nano horn Indocyanine green (SWNH-ICG) technique by coating Indocyanine green (ICG) on the surface of single-walled carbon nano horns (SWNHs) through p–p stacking to get SWNH-ICGs with high solubility and stability below physiological. Liposome-based nanomedicine was highlighted by Guo et al. [7] as that would successfully deliver oxygen to tumors and reduce tumors hypoxia state and demonstrate the ability of nanotechnology to overcome drawbacks of traditional cancer therapy. Bagloa et al. [8] proposed the porphyrin-lipid nanovesicles technique to overcomes the problem of developing multidrug resistance in cancer treatment. This research shows that the in tumors expressing ABCG2 and P-gp, intracellular photosensitizer's levels could be maintained when using 'lipid-anchored' BPD and its liposomal formation.

3 Proposed Taxonomy Components

The search returned 124 results, of these 8 met our inclusive criteria as follows: The journals described about the entire process of photodynamic therapy. The articles that were included in our study were selected because of description of the process of photodynamic therapy combining with nanotechnology for drug targeted cancer treatment. Also, these papers describe the strategies to enhance the effectiveness of photodynamic therapy (PDT) by selecting proper photosensitizer and nanoparticles and treatment focusing on cancerous tissues to reduce the side effects on healthy cells. Based on our review, we classified the photodynamic therapy based on three factors: data, monitoring processing and delivery of nanoparticles, and laser light emission. The first factor includes various types of data in image and graphic form. These data have various properties like semantic, length of trajectories, whether used on in vivo and in vitro study, patterns and so on. This data also provides information about drug delivery system with and without presence of laser light. The second factor is delivery of nanoparticles with various algorithms such as tumor targeting nanoparticles, redox responsive Porphyrin-Based nanoparticles, bio reducible self-assembled nanoparticles, multifunctional theragnostic Nano platform etc. These algorithms and monitoring processes are used to modify data to provide more accurate and pictorial view of the data for classification. At last, our classification is based on the emission of laser light which gives the efficacy of focused therapy of cancer cells without effecting on healthy cells and it is the final result of photodynamic therapy, as shown in Fig. 1. Figure 1 represents three factors of nanotechnology based photodynamic therapy along with its subcomponents and relationship among them. In the below sections, an explanation is given to each of the components and their subcomponents by providing reasons of using each factor for classification. The main reason of considering these components is to describe how the information is suggested to the therapist so that correct choice of laser light could be made for side effect less therapy.

A. **Data:** Four main subclasses are considered which are raw data, laser emitting information, analyzed data, and derived data. Generally, different classes of data may be viewed and goes through one or more transition for monitoring process of data. Raw data are obtained as direct output of the acquisition system. These data are obtained during the photodynamic therapy task. Raw data are transformed into analyzed data and then visualized. Laser emitting information is data which are obtained after using algorithms or frameworks of photodynamic therapy technique. Analyzed data are obtained from camera, video and UV spectrometer used during the process, that

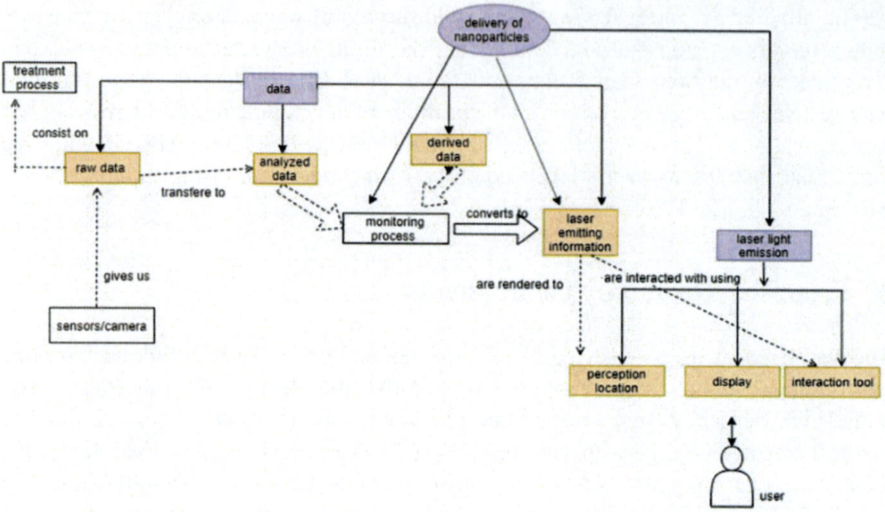

Fig. 1. The proposed taxonomy of nanotechnology based photodynamic therapy for cancer treatment

are analyzed to provide specific result from raw data. Derived data are data which are obtained from the specified source of the nanotechnology system and obtained from prior knowledge data as well.

B. **Delivery of nanoparticles:** This technique represents transformation of data used to show best pictorial representation of data for certain task during treatment process. For drug delivery, various algorithms have been considered which consist of polyethylene glycol Pyro-loaded nanoparticles, Nanoaminolevulic acid photodynamic therapy (NanoALA-PDT) etc. the major function of this technique is to transfer raw data into pictorial form to analyze it.

C. **Laser light emission (LLE):** This is the product of data where result of photodynamic therapy is obtained from analyzed data and the set of data in treatment process room. It described the system to the end users so they can analyze comparatively and interact with the system.

4 System Classification and Evaluation

Eight articles are selected depending on our selection criteria as explained in Sect. 1. These articles are published between 2016 and 2019 in high ranked journals. These articles are summarized in Table 1. The columns represent system components which are data, delivery of nanoparticles, and laser light emission. These components are further divided into subcomponents. From Table 1, most of the articles have used raw data obtained from the UV-vis spectrometer used by therapist during the process of tumor targeted photodynamic therapy. Some of the articles have used raw data to get final result of their research. Whereas some of the articles have used analyzed data obtained from cameras and videos to find efficacy and side effects of such therapy from cell viability. Some of the articles have used analyzed data to get end product.

These analyzed data include subdivision which further passed through an algorithm of photodynamic therapy to get desired result. Most of the articles provide the information about the laser light which was emitted during the process of therapy. Such information would be the wavelength of light, power and nature of light, source information etc.

In this section our proposed taxonomy is validated and evaluated. The validation process is used to verify the accuracy of the system and confirm that the system is correct. On the other hand, the evaluation process is involved to show the usefulness and the advantages of the proposed system. To determine the most relevant factors of feature monitoring technique of nanotechnology based photodynamic therapy, we discover the components which must be evaluated and validated to show whether there is additional value in using the system. We also distinguish between validation and evaluation as follows: validation verify the accuracy of the system and confirm that the built system is right, and evaluation involved to shows the usefulness and value of the proposed system. After analyzing all the selected articles, we have concluded that, all these articles were described some sort of validation and evaluation of their systems. Most of the articles focused on enhancing the photodynamic therapy (PDT) as major factor to validation and evaluation All the reviewed articles are describing some sort of validation and evaluation of their system. Most of the articles focused on enhancing the photodynamic therapy (PDT) as major factor to validation and evaluation.

Table 1. System classification

Ref	Type of nanoparticle used	Data			Emission of laser light		
		Raw data/analyzed data	Laser emitting information	Delivery of nanoparticles	Location	Display	Interaction tool
[1]	Reviewed others work	Not specified	600–800 nm	N/A	Several types of cancer	Screen	Camera
[2]	Polymeric nanoparticles	Laser scanning microscope	NIR laser	Immunological response created by nano phototherapy	Not specified	Screen	Laser light emitter
[3]	Photofrin layered stent	UV/VIS spectrometer	630 nm	Photodynamic (PDT) matrix drug delivery system (DDS)	Lung cancer	Screen	Cell Counting Kit-8
[4]	Organic and non-organic NPs	Transferrin receptors (TfR)	Not specified	Surface functionalized tumour-targeting moieties NPPS drug delivery systems	Skin cancer	Monitor	Screen
[5]	P-s-s-PpIX NPs and P-PpIX NPs	Fluorescence spectrophotometry	448 nm	Bio reducible self-assembled P-s-s-PpIX NPs with self-quenchable photoactivity	Breast cancer cell	Monitor	Cell Counting Kit-8

(*continued*)

Table 1. (*continued*)

Ref	Type of nanoparticle used	Data			Emission of laser light		
		Raw data/analyzed data	Laser emitting information	Delivery of nanoparticles	Location	Display	Interaction tool
[6]	Single-walled carbon nanohorns	UV/Vis spectrophotometer	650–900 nm	Single-walled carbon nanohorn Indocyanine green (SWNH-ICG)	Triple-negative breast cancer 4T1 cells	Screen	Camera
[7]	Lipsomes loading indocyanine green, ICG and Hb (LIH)	Malvern Zetasizer	NIR light	N/A	Not specified	Monitor	Spectrometer
[8]	p-glycoprotein	Zetasizer NanoZS	488 nm and 405 nm	Porphyrin-lipid nanovesicles technique	Breast cancer cell	Screen	Camera

The set of articles which are worked to enhance PDT are: Calixto et al. [1], Kruger and Abrahamse [4], Guo et al. [7] and Gao et al. [6]. Similarly, some of articles has taken novel drug delivery agent as a factor of validation and evaluation because this gives therapist novel strategy to make side effect less therapy for different type of cancer treatment. These articles are Xia et al. [5] and Gao et al. [6]. In most of the article, delivery of nanoparticles and laser emission was validated and evaluated. Among them, most of articles validate the whole system whereas few validated some factors instead of whole system. In the evaluation process, we have used both qualitative and quantitative methods to evaluate the components of our taxonomy.

Table 2. System validation and evaluation

Ref	Type of nanoparticle used	Component validated or evaluated	Study criteria	Validation/evaluation method and/or data set	Mathematical formula	Results
[1]	Reviewed others work	Whole system	Enhanced PDT	Reviewed and comparison	N/A	This nanotechnology-based drug delivery system enhances the transcytosis of PS and offer the simultaneous delivery of two or more drugs

(*continued*)

Table 2. *(continued)*

Ref	Type of nanoparticle used	Component validated or evaluated	Study criteria	Validation/evaluation method and/or data set	Mathematical formula	Results
[2]	Polymeric nanoparticles	Whole system	Strong preclinic promise	Comparison based	N/A	Provide a strong pre-clinical promise to deal cancer from metastatic phase which provides therapists a new way of treatment with minimum death rate of cancer patients
[3]	Photofrin layered stent	Release rate	Novel drug delivery method	Physical phantom	N/A	The released rate of photofrin reached ~80%
[4]	Organic and non-organic NPs	Whole system	Enhanced PDT	Comparison based	N/A	Drug was absorbed only by cancerous cell which gives focused treatment with no side effect
[5]	P-s-s-PpIX NPs and P-PpIX NPs	Cell viability	Enhanced PDT	Comparison and analysis	N/A	Cell viability decreases
[6]	Single-walled carbon nanohorns	Volume of cancer cells after injecting nanohorns	Enhanced PTT and PDT	Mice (5 different classes of mice)	Volume of tumour = $\frac{\text{length}*(\text{width})^2}{2}$	Volume of cell after treatment using carbon nanohorn was not increased as compared to cell not using nanohorn
[7]	Lipsomes loading indocyanine green, ICG and Hb (LIH)	ROS release rate	Enhanced PDT	Direct observation of mice	Volume of tumour = $\frac{\text{length}*(\text{width})^2}{2}$	ROS generation by LIH shows decrease on tumor growth and 100% survival of mice
[8]	p-glycoprotein	Algorithm	Novel technique	Comparison and analysis	N/A	Attachment of galactose to HPPH also reduced the HPPH efflux by ~50% in the RIF-1 murine radiation-induced fibrosarcoma cell line

The common way of evaluating the system components is the direct observation and comparison method where cell viability and drug release rate is evaluated by using different sort of nanoparticles. In the process of qualitative method of evaluation, system is compared with the state of art technique. In the process of quantitative measurement, some of the articles have used numerical method to calculate drug release rate and volume of tumor cell to find out the side effects of therapy with the help of various algorithms. To evaluate the photodynamic therapy monitoring technique, we focus on the overlapping terms in between the taxonomy and the literature. As given in Table 2. Although, it is not feasible to fully automate this system because the terms we consider in our taxonomy are dependent on the context. For an instance, the analyzed monitoring data might represent the volume, length and weight of tumor cell after therapy. However, the term volume can be used to represent different context that have no relation with volumetric data as that may be derived data like initial volume of cell, volume of drug etc.

5 Discussion

The above taxonomy shows that nanotechnology-based drug delivery enhanced the photodynamic therapy. One of the important tasks before starting therapy is correct selection of NPs, PSs and wavelength of laser light because efficacy of therapy depends upon these three factors that we have described above. Hence, research need to start exploring further function of nanoparticle-based drug delivery system on photodynamic therapy of various cancer by performing more effective theoretical and mathematical models to get more accurate result. The major contribution of this research paper is to demonstrate the synergic effects of light and nanoparticles in the field of cancer treatment through the critical analysis of different research. Furthermore, the therapist will learn more about tumour targeted therapy systems, and cancer patients will get fewer side effects. The objective of this research is to identify various approaches related to photodynamic therapy to find the advantages which could be used for successful and efficient therapy of cancerous cells. The purpose of defining such classification is to point out the best method to perform photodynamic therapy by using nanoparticles as a drug deliver for focused cancer treatment. The importance of considering the components is to analyze the interaction with each other to deliver specific patterns to the therapist so that they can processed treatment without affecting healthy cells. In general, selection of nanoparticles and wavelength of laser light is key element in this system. Most of the articles select near infrared (NIR) laser light for photodynamic therapy which have wavelength of range 600 nm to 1 mm. Li et al. [2] and Guo et al. [7] have used NIR light for treatment of cancerous cells. Very few articles such as Guo et al. [7] has used visible light having wavelength range 400 nm to 600 nm. The use of laser light depends upon the nature of nanoparticles and photosensitizers, type of tumor cell and the environment of therapy. All selected articles have clearly described about the drug delivery mechanism by using nanoparticles for targeted therapy. Some articles are used Solid lipid nanoparticles (SLNs) as drug deliver for treatment of various cancerous cells, like Guo et al. [7] and Gao et al. [6]. All selected articles have discussed about the photodynamic therapy but have used different algorithms of it. Some of the algorithms used in the photodynamic therapy are Nanoaminolevulic acid photodynamic therapy (NanoALA-PDT), polyethylene glycol Pyro-loaded nanoparticles, photodynamic (PDT) matrix drug delivery system (DDS), indirect photodynamic therapy; Uconversion nanoparticle (UCN) based PDT technology etc. However, these techniques monitor data very precisely, they have some drawbacks too. Kruger et al. [4] mentioned that the photothermal conversion effect of SWNH-ICG cannot appear above 808nm laser irradiation. Sometimes, NIR laser can decrease the sensitivity of targeted surface and small difference in wavelength used to irradiate laser can affect the tissues [4].

6 Conclusion and Future Work

The main objective of this research is to address the drawbacks of traditional photodynamic therapy by using nanoparticles as a drug deliverer to obtain side effect less targeted therapy by reviewing and analyzing the various articles published recently. In this work, we have considered three components: data, delivery of nanoparticles, and laser light emission and their respective subcomponents as well. Based on the research that we have done; it can be said that the PDT is undoubtedly a very successive solution and alternative to cancer treatment. In this review, it has been concluded that nanotechnology-based drug delivery enhanced the photodynamic therapy. One of the important tasks before starting therapy is correct selection of NPs, PSs and wavelength of laser light because efficacy of therapy depends upon these three factors that we have described in our work. Hence, further research needs to be conducted to identify the other features of nanoparticles-based drug delivery system on photodynamic therapy of various cancer by performing more effective study on theoretical and mathematical models to get more accurate result. In the future, photodynamic therapy will be accepted as one of the finest methods for cancer cell treatment due to its less side effects and accuracy. The findings of this study allow further research if there are any unforeseen limitations for this type of cancer treatment to push application of targeted photodynamic therapy using nanoparticles in the field of oncology.

References

1. Calixto, G.M.F., Bernegossi, J., de Freitas, L.M., Fontana, C.R., Chorilli, M.: Nanotechnology-based drug delivery systems for photodynamic therapy of cancer: a review. Molecules **21**(3), 342–360 (2016)
2. Li, Y., et al.: Nanotechnology-based photoimmunological therapies for cancer. Cancer Lett. **442**(12), 429–438 (2019)
3. Liang, P.-C., et al.: A novel photodynamic therapy-based drug delivery system layered on a stent for treating cholangiocarcinoma. Biomed. Microdevice **20**(3), 105–113 (2018)
4. Kruger, C.A., Abrahamse, H.: Utilisation of targeted nanoparticle photosensitiser drug delivery systems for the enhancement of photodynamic therapy. Molecules **23**(2628), 203–224 (2018)
5. Xia, J., Zhang, L., Qian, M., Bao, Y., Wang, J., Li, Y.: Specific light-up pullulan-based nanoparticles with reduction-triggered. J. Colloid Interface Sci. **498**(12), 170–181 (2017)
6. Gao, C., et al.: Near-infrared light responsive imaging-guided photothermal and photodynamic synergistic therapy nanoplatform based on carbon nanohorns for efficient cancer treatment. Chem. Eur. J. **24**(1), 12827–12837 (2018)
7. Guo, X., et al.: Synchronous delivery of oxygen and photosensitizer for alleviation of hypoxia tumor microenvironment and dramatically enhanced photodynamic therapy. Drug Delivery **25**(1), 585–599 (2018)
8. Bagloa, Y., Barry, J.L., Robert, W.R., Suresh, V.A., Michael, M.G., Huang-Chiao, H.: Porphyrin-lipid assemblies and nanovesicles overcome ABC transporter mediated photodynamic therapy resistance in cancer cells. Cancer Lett. **457**(10), 110–118 (2019)

Artificial Intelligence-Based Image Classification Techniques for Clinician Diagnosis of Skin Cancer

Shreyanth R. Chamakura[1], P. W. C. Prasad[2], Ali Abas Albabawat[3](✉), Hanspreet Kaur[2], Qurat Ul Ain Nizamani[2], and Razwan Mohmed Salah[3]

[1] Study Group Australia, Darlinghurst, Australia
[2] Kent Institute Australia, Sydney, Australia
{chandana.withana,hanspreet.kaur,qurat.nizamani}@kent.edu.au
[3] University of Duhok, Duhok, KRI, Iraq
ali.abas@uod.ac

Abstract. Skin cancer has become one of the common forms of malignancy in humans. The early and effective detection of these malignancies is essential for the effective treatment of the patients. However, accurate diagnosis of these lesions by visual examination of images is tedious, laborious, and fault-prone. Many computer-aided diagnosis methods have been devised for the diagnosis and detection of lesions, but these existing techniques perform poorly on challenging features of the lesions. The main aim of this work is to review different Artificial-intelligence (AI) dependent lesion classification techniques for the prognosis of skin cancer. Further, this study will help in determining the essential components required by a system for the diagnosis of skin lesions. For this purpose, secondary research was performed with the help of latest research articles. A literature review of collected papers was conducted to identify the technique used and the merits and demerits of each approach or study. On the basis of this review, system architecture with essential components has also been suggested. This study will provide a comprehensive insight into the already existing techniques for the categorisation of skin-related lesions.

Keywords: Algorithm · Convolutional Neural Networks (CNN) · Deep learning lesions · Melanoma · Classification

1 Introduction

Cancer is one of the fatal diseases witnessed by human beings. Even today, no proper cure is available for the treatment of cancer. Among different types of cancer, cases of skin cancer are on rise in recent times, in fact it is the most common type of cancer in the United State according to CDC. Many different factors such as genetics, environmental factors, ultraviolet (UV) radiation, exposure to mutagenic chemicals can contribute to the development of the disease [1]. The diagnosis and classification of these diseases are generally done by the dermoscopic techniques. It enhances the image and reduces

K. Daimi and A. Al Sadoon (Eds.): ICR 2022, AISC 1431, pp. 102–111, 2022.
https://doi.org/10.1007/978-3-031-14054-9_11

the chances of error, but the success of these techniques is greatly dependent on the experience and knowledge of the dermatologist. Also, the visual inspection of dermoscopic images for diagnosis and detection of lesions employs ABCD (asymmetry, border, color, and diameter) rule, 3-point and 7-point checklist rule. But these procedures are fault-prone and require years of experience [2]. Thus, a computer-aided diagnosis system utilizing artificial intelligence for the determination and diagnosis of skin cancer is essential for the correct diagnosis of skin cancer [3]. However, the currently available AI-based classification solutions for detection of skin lesions face some major challenges. These systems perform poorly on lesions with artifacts, fuzzy boundaries, low contrast with the background, the visual similarity in lesions, pigmentation and other complex conditions.

The aim of this work is to review and analyze the research done in the field of AI-based image classification techniques for the diagnosis of skin cancer. This study will help in better understanding of different classification techniques used for prognosis of different type of skin lesions. This research only considers image classification procedures used to determine skin cancer.

2 Literature Review

This study aimed at most recent journal articles in order to draw information about image classification techniques for the diagnosis of skin cancer using deep learning technologies. Deep learning is a branch of machine learning used for the automation of the different processes and is being applied in the field of healthcare to improve the detection and diagnosis of the patients. Detection and classification of various skin lesions is significant for the prognosis of skin malignancy. Many computer-aided diagnosis technologies have been applied for the classification of images, but these techniques lag in some aspects. Adegun and Viriri's [4] framework for automatic identification of skin cancer uses an encoder-decoder for feature extraction and a DenseNet framework for the classification of the images. The approach was found to outperform the other methods after being evaluated on different datasets and metrics. Liu et al. [5] stated that due to the similarity between the various lesions and the typical skin state, techniques that use the visual characteristics as input are not discriminative enough. The authors have proposed a Convolutional Neural Network (CNN)-based mid-level feature learning method to overcome these issues. The method detects the region of interest and obtains mid-level features. This model cannot process high-resolution images, which is one major drawback of this study. Tang et al. [6], utilized the G-CNN to withdraw the information from the downscaled images to form the Classification Activation Map (CAM). The P-CNN is educated with this CAM to recognize the local information of lesions. This model was analyzed on the International Skin Imaging Collaboration (ISIC) 2016 and ISIC 2017 datasets and achieved high classification performance. However, the system only uses a single modality of the dermoscopic images, which does not give enough information for the categorization of melanoma. To overcome the challenges of complicated network structure, limited training samples, and high computational cost, Zhou et al. [7] proposed the use of Spiking Neural Networks (SNNs) and Spike-Timing-Dependent Plasticity (STDP) to achieve efficient identification and classification. It was found that this method faces difficulty in encoding the visual features, and it does not include multi-classification of lesions after it was evaluated on ISIC 2018 dataset and compared with other techniques. The work of Almasni et al. [3] aimed on utilizing the CNN classifier for the classification of the segmented images but requires data preparation for each of the cascade network stages. Also, the augmented data used in the study have a correlation with the original data. As stated earlier, an early and efficient detection of the lesions is essential for the treatment of the disease and many computer-based techniques have been developed for accurate and efficient detection of the lesions. Some of those have been cited above, however, the cited techniques have certain limitations, such as the use of complex models, a restricted performance due to the complex visual properties of lesions, similarities between different lesions, and complex training techniques. State of the art work is discussed in this paper to form a sophisticated system architecture and compare different approaches to address best practices and challenges.

3 System Components and Proposed Model

This section presents components that have been identified from various research articles to conduct the study and are presented in Table 1. This table specifies factors, attributes, and instances. These factors have been formulated on the basis of major factors such as input used in the research processing, the final output of the research, and its evaluation. These factors are further sub-divided into several attributes, which demonstrate the major elements contributing to the components. The final column of instances represents the examples of these attributes used in different research articles. Figure 1 describes the basic architecture of the system developed on the basis of the review study of selected 12 articles. This architecture was developed with the help of the major factors required for the classification of images for the diagnosis of skin cancer. These factors include lesion images, image segmentation, classification of lesions, diagnosis, and evaluation. Further, emphasis was laid on considering the different attributes of these factors such as dataset, type of lesions, characteristics, techniques, algorithms, networks, models techniques, performance parameters, and metrics. The skin lesion images collected from the different datasets were used as input for the system. These images were then fed to the model to perform the segmentation and classification tasks with different techniques, networks, and algorithms. After this processing, the final outcome of the diagnosis of lesion was obtained in the form of classification of disease.

4 Evaluation of the Components

Table 2 describes the quantitative data of the 12 most-relatable journal articles used for this review study. This table consists of the numerical data which is associated with the respective components of the system. These components include lesion images, segmentation, classification, and diagnosis. These factors have been categorised in different columns depending on the numerical data associated with them. Some authors have used only 2 types of lesions, while other authors have used 7–8 types of lesions, which enhances the performance of the main systems. The authors of [1] have used around 22000 samples to train and test their model, which enhances the authenticity of

Table 1. Classification table

	Lesion images				Image Segmentation			Classification of lesions			Diagnosis		Evaluation
Author	**Datasets**	**Types of skin lesions**	**Characteristics/artefacts**	**Image dimensions**	**Technique**	**Technique**	**Tools**	**Technique**	**Network**	**Algorithm**	**Disease classified**	**Analysed features**	**Performance parameters**
[1]	Dermquest	melanoma	Body hairs	28 × 28	CNN	Lévy flight	N/A	NA	Optimized CNN	Whale optimisation algorithm	Skin lesions	Pixel color features	Accuracy
[2]	HAM10000	Basal cell carcinoma	Fuzzy boundaries	NA	FCN	DenseNet	Softmax classifier	DenseNet	CNN	SGD	Basal cell Carcinoma	Discriminative features	Confusion matrix
[3]	ISIC2016	melanoma	Boundaries	192 × 256	full resolution convolutional network (FrCN)	Deep segmentator	Dermoscopy imaging tool	Deep learning	Inception-V3, ResNet-50	bilinear interpolation	Benign or malignant	Skin lesion boundaries	F1- score and sensitivity
[4]	PH 2	Melanoma	bubbles	224 X 224	Deep learning	DCEDN	NA	Deep learning	DCEDN	Lesion classifier	Melanoma	boundaries	Accuracy
[5]	ISIC 2017	Seborrheic keratosis	Color inconsistency	224 × 224	CNN	Deep learning	Encoder and decode blocks	mid-level feature learning	ResNet	Adam optimisation algorithm	Seborrheic keratosis	Mid-level features	Area under curve (AUC)
[6]	ISIC 2017	seborrheic keratosis	NA	300 × 300	CNN	NA	SGD optimizer	DTEL	GPCNN	Shade of gray algorithm	Seborrheic keratosis	Fine-grained features	Sensitivity
[7]	ISIC 2018	Melanoma	Hairs	NA	NA	Deep learning	SVM classifier	STDP learning rule.	CSNN	Dullrazor algorithm	Melanoma	Visual features	Accuracy
[8]	MED-NODE	Melanoma	Noise	201 X 257	DNN	Deep learning	NA	Statistical image classification	DNN	Ensemble algorithm	melanoma	Asymmetry, border and color	Accuracy, precision
[9]	ISIC 2017	Nevus	Blood	224 × 224	Root-Seg-Net	NA	Adam optimiser	Multi-task learning	CKDNet	Multi-task learning algorithms	Nevus	Region of Interest	AUC and Dice coefficient
[10]	ISBI 2016	Skin lesions	Hairs	224 X 224	Lightweight CNN	NA	Adam optimizer	Ensemble learning	Lightweight CNN	TSNE	Skin cancer	Discriminative features	Jaccard index.
[11]	ISIC 2017	Melanoma	Symmetry, colour	500 X 375	RCNN	Ensemble method	Momentum optimizer	NA	NA	Shades of gray algorithm	Skin lesions	noise	Jaccard similarity index
[12]	ISIC 2018	Benign Keratosis	Hairs	224 × 224	Deep networks	Transfer learning	NA	Transfer learning	Convolutional Neural networks	grayworld colour constancy	Skin lesions	Colour-constancy	ISIC 2018 challenge test set

the study. It was observed that images were resized in most of the studies to a suitable pixel ratio. Different batch sizes have been used in these works to train and evaluate the model. The authors have set the learning rate to 0.0001 for their systems, excluding [1]. It was also found that all authors used the detection accuracy along with a combination of sensitivity, specificity, and/or AUC as performance parameters for the evaluation of their systems. The system proposed by [5] achieved the lowest accuracy of 87.25%, while the model proposed by [2] achieved the highest detection accuracy of 98.3%. This table helps in comparing the different recent studies on the topic, which have been used for this study. It also provides a comparative analysis of the different works, which can help in designing future study.

5 Discussion

This work focuses on the subject of diagnosis and detection of skin cancer and associated lesions with the application of Artificial Intelligence (AI) based image classification techniques. Artificial intelligence (AI) technology is applied in various fields to solve problems and dilemmas that are beyond human capabilities. According to WHO, 3–4 million people are diagnosed with skin cancer, non-melanoma and melanoma, globally every year wherein late detection or false diagnosis forms the number one reason for deaths. This is where AI techniques become useful for early and accurate diagnosis. In this study, a literature review of the recent journal articles related to the topic was performed. In this section, discuss the key findings of this work, and also the work of the

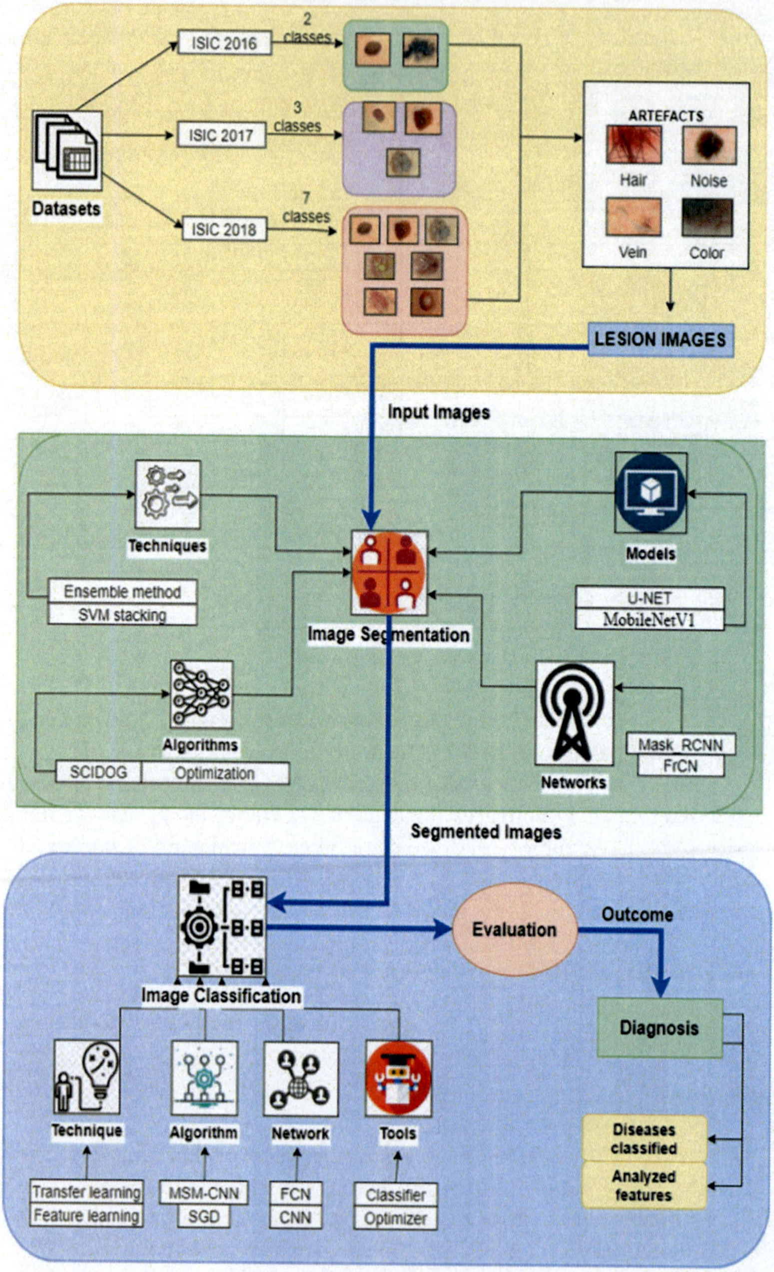

Fig. 1. System architecture

previous authors is discussed. [2], have contributed to the segmentation and diagnosis of the lesion with the help of a deep convolutional neural network.

Table 2. Evaluation of components

Authors	Type of lesions	Number of samples	Size of image	Batch size	Epochs	Learning rate	Accuracy	Sensitivity	Specificity	AUC	Precision	Recall
[1]	1	22000	28X28	-	45	-	.96	.98	.95	-	.88	.92
[2]	8	10030	768X560	128	800	0.0001	98.3%	98%	97%	98%	98%	98.5%
[3]	7	10015	450X600	20	100	$1e^{-4}$	89.28%	81%	87.16%	73.94%	-	81%
[4]	3	2000	224X224	-	250	0.0001	95%	97%	96%	-	-	97%
[5]	3	2000	224X224	24	100	0.0001	87.25%	-	-	89%	-	-
[6]	2	900	384X384 X3	32	150	0.01	0.935	0.722	0.965	0.926	0.728	0.722
[7]	2	7818	-	-	20	-0.01	0.877	0.903	0.847	0.936	0.846	0.903
[8]	2	170	201X257	288.0	300	0.01	0.91	0.89	0.93	0.92	0.92	0.93
[9]	3	2000	224X224	32	100	0.0001	0.946	0.700	0.925	0.738	0.738	0.700
[10]	2	900	1024X1024	32	50	0.0001	0.876	0.934	0.974	0.854	0.724	0.934
[11]	2	200	500X375	1	100	0.001	0.938	0.987	0.929	-	-	0.987
[12]	7	1512	450X600	50-100	70	0.0001	96.3%	-	-	98.1%	91.3%	86.2%

5.1 Lesion Images

This review provides insights into the skin cancer-related datasets, different AI-based techniques, algorithms, networks, models, and tools used for the diagnosis of skin cancer. It was observed that most of the authors had used the International skin imaging collaboration 2016, 2017, or 2018 dataset for their studies. The ISIC 2017 dataset, which only consists of images of three types of skin lesions, was used [12]. The ISIC 2018 dataset with seven types of skin lesions, was used to overcome the issue of a limited type of skin lesions. These datasets consist of images of different types of skin lesions such as Seborrheic keratosis, basal cell carcinoma, melanoma, vascular lesions, and others. However, it was found that the other datasets such as Dermquest and PH2 datasets have also been used by some authors. It was observed that the images in these datasets had some artifacts, for example, hair, bubbles, irregular boundaries and blood vessels [4]. These input images were of variable pixels, so most of the studies first resize these images in suitable pixels and then feed them as input. The authors have used 7 different types of lesions to train the model and achieved an accuracy of 89.28% [3]. However, the accuracy of 96.3% was achieved by a model which used the 7 different types of samples from ISIC 2018 dataset [12]. It was also seen that a deep learning model could achieve an accuracy of 91%, but the model was only trained on 2 types of samples [8]. Compared to all these models, an efficient skin cancer detection model, trained on 8 different types of lesions attained detection accuracy of 98.3% [2].

5.2 Segmentation

These input images undergo two major processes of segmentation and classification, which are related tasks [5]. The segmentation of the boundaries of the lesion is a crucial task for accurately localizing the lesion in dermoscopic images and diagnosis of different skin lesions. Different techniques, models, algorithms, and tools have been used for the purpose of both segmentation and classification of lesions. Deep learning (DL) approaches such as Ensemble deep learning, and Full resolution convolutional networks (FrCN) were applied for the image segmentation [3]. A deep learning ensemble technique was used to obtain high sensitivity and specificity for the segmentation of lesion boundaries [11]. This method attained a specificity of 97.94% and sensitivity of 89.93% on ISIC 2017 training set. The existing DL based approaches utilize multiple sub-sampling layers, which result in loss of resolution of the features extracted from images. To address this problem, [3] used an FrCN segmentation that learns the features from the dermoscopic images with minimum resolution loss. The single task-driven models for segmentation of images do not use the provided knowledge, while multi-task learning techniques utilize costly annotation of lesions. A cascade knowledge diffusion network was introduced that can use the abandoned knowledge for segmentation purpose [9]. This model achieved an accuracy of 94.6% for segmentation. The previous segmentation methods still face many issues such as the requirement for removal of artifacts, manual annotations, and they cannot process low contrast lesion images. A segmentation algorithm; SCIDOG & PECK, which achieved accuracy of 91% was proposed [8]. The deep learning technique trained on 7 different types of samples forms the ISIC datasets achieved segmentation sensitivity of 81% and specificity of 87.1% [3]. As compared to this system, the ensemble learning-based algorithms for the segmentation of the images achieved higher specificity of 93% [8].

5.3 Classification of Lesions

The classification of skin lesions is a significant task for efficient diagnosis of skin associated malignancy. These days several different computer-aided skin lesion classification methods are being used. The role of image size in the classification of these lesions was determined [12]. For this purpose, the authors used a transfer learning approach along with deep CNN and developed a MSM-CNN method for the classification purpose. However, the models used in this method require a large amount of training time. The existing classification methods based on deep learning often face the challenge of limited training sample and high computational cost. These challenges were addressed by using a spiking neural network with STDP learning rule [7]. The authors observed that this model was able to achieve better classification accuracy, have better run time, and it is much easier to use as compared to the CNNs. The traditional methods for classification fail in cases of similar lesions and typical skin conditions [5]. To resolve this problem, the authors introduced a model based on CNN that uses mid-level feature learning for classification of images. The existing classification techniques suffer from different similarities and variation in lesions and generalization of a model trained on limited data [6]. The authors used Deep learning approach and CNN to treat information with importance. This model achieved an accuracy of 93.5% and specificity of 96.5%

for the classification of lesions on ISIC 2016 and ISIC 2017 dataset. The feature extraction module and feature discrimination network was employed for the categorization of lesions [10]. It was found that the method can enhance the identification performance of a model by determining more discriminative features of malignancy. Also, it achieved precise segmentation of lesion area without the need for image pre-processing step. As per [4], existing computer-aided methods for diagnosis of skin lesions does not perform well on lesions with typical features such as artefacts and low contrast. The authors proposed a system with fully convolutional network and FCN based-based DenseNet for segmentation & classification tasks. This model achieved 98% accuracy and 99% AUC score on HAM 10000 dataset.

5.4 Diagnosis

Various features of lesions such as symmetry, border, color, artefacts, texture, etc. are analyzed for the efficient diagnosis of the skin lesions [2]. The early detection and diagnosis of these malignancies can save the life of a patient. A model for the detection of skin cancer was developed by using CNN and whale optimization algorithm [1]. The authors used accuracy and specificity as evaluation parameters. This model was able to detect skin cancer with an accuracy of 96% and specificity of 98%. Albert [8] determined the melanoma and nevi lesions. These lesions have a high similarity, and classifying them is a challenging task. This model achieved significant success in the classification and diagnosis of these diseases. An architecture for the diagnosis of melanoma was introduced using a deep convolutional neural network [2]. It was found that this method improved the ability for the diagnosis of melanomas from dermoscopic images. Many different parameters were used for the assessment of these models. The authors have used precision, accuracy, sensitivity, specificity and F1-score for evaluation of these systems. These parameters helped in determining the overall diagnosis efficiency of these models. A model which considers the differences and similarities in the images by applying discriminant analysis was developed [10]. This model only achieved the detection accuracy of 87.6%. A deep learning-based CNN method for the categorization of lesion images was proposed [6]. This system was able to classify the images and attain 93.5% detection accuracy. The framework for the automated classification of images could detect the patients with 95% accuracy [4].

6 Conclusion

Cancer accounts for a large proportion of deaths every year. However, the early detection of cancer can save the life of the patients. The classification of the dermoscopic images is essential for the identification and diagnosis of skin cancer in the patients. The classification based on the examination of dermoscopic images is challenging and fault-prone. Thus, many automated techniques based on machine learning have evolved to improve the detection accuracy. This study focusses on the AI-based image classification techniques for the prognosis of melanoma in patients. In this project, several different articles on deep learning-based techniques for classification of skin lesion image were reviewed and analyzed. It can be concluded that these techniques can be used for the detection and diagnosis of lesions, and they can assist the physicians in making decisions. Analyzing the ISIC 2018 dataset which contains 8 types of lesion while considering various features such as symmetry, border, color, artefacts, texture, etc. learning these features from the dermoscopic images with minimum resolution loss, [2] managed to acquire the highest accuracy, 98.3%, with the help of FCN. the techniques discussed in this work provide high detection accuracy, consume less time and are cost-efficient. However, these techniques face some limitations namely i) pre-processing of the images needed, ii) poor identification of lesion with similar properties, iii) poor performance due to complex skin conditions and iv) artefacts and limited training data for training these systems. Further improvements are required to tackle these issues such as reducing time and effort needed for pre-processing through producing standardized images thus improving classification and identification. Using datasets with large number of skin cancer types would also have better impact on the identification accuracy. In future, a model that can address these issues of pre-processing can be trained with enough data, have easy implementation, can differentiate between different lesion should be formed.

References

1. Zhang, N., Cai, Y.-X., Wang, Y.-Y., Tian, Y.-T., Wang, X.-L., Badami, B.: Skin cancer diagnosis based on optimised convolutional neural network. Artif. Intell. Med. **102**, 101756 (2019). https://doi.org/10.1016/j.artmed.2019.101756
2. Adegun, A.A., Viriri, S.: Deep learning-based system for automatic melanoma detection. IEEE Access **8**, 7160–7172 (2020). https://doi.org/10.1109/access.2019.2962812
3. Al-masni, M.A., Kim, D.-H., Kim, T.-S.: Multiple skin lesions diagnostics via integrated deep convolutional networks for segmentation and classification. Comput. Methods Programs Biomed. **190**, 105351 (2020). https://doi.org/10.1016/j.cmpb.2020.105351
4. Adegun, A.A., Viriri, S.: FCN-based DenseNet framework for automated detection and classification of skin lesions in dermoscopy images. IEEE Access **8**, 150377–150396 (2020). https://doi.org/10.1109/access.2020.3016651
5. Liu, L., Mou, L., Zhu, X.X., Mandal, M.: Automatic skin lesion classification based on mid-level feature learning. Comput. Med. Imaging Graph. **84**, 101765 (2020). https://doi.org/10.1016/j.compmedimag.2020.101765
6. Tang, P., Liang, Q., Yan, X., Xiang, S., Zhang, D.: GP-CNN-DTEL: global-part CNN model with data-transformed ensemble learning for skin lesion classification. IEEE J. Biomed. Health Inform. **24**(10), 2870–2882 (2020). https://doi.org/10.1109/jbhi.2020.2977013
7. Zhou, Q., Shi, Y., Xu, Z., Qu, R., Xu, G.: Classifying melanoma skin lesions using convolutional spiking neural networks with unsupervised STDP learning rule. IEEE Access **8**, 101309–101319 (2020). https://doi.org/10.1109/access.2020.2998098
8. Albert, B.A.: Deep learning from limited training data: novel segmentation and ensemble algorithms applied to automatic melanoma diagnosis. IEEE Access **8**, 1 (2020). https://doi.org/10.1109/access.2020.2973188
9. Jin, Q., Cui, H., Sun, C., Meng, Z., Su, R.: Cascade knowledge diffusion network for skin lesion diagnosis and segmentation. Appl. Soft Comput. **99**, 106881 (2021). https://doi.org/10.1016/j.asoc.2020.106881
10. Wei, L., Ding, K., Hu, H.: Automatic skin cancer detection in dermoscopy images based on ensemble lightweight deep learning network. IEEE Access **8**, 99633–99647 (2020). https://doi.org/10.1109/access.2020.2997710

11. Goyal, M., Oakley, A., Bansal, P., Dancey, D., Yap, M.H.: Skin lesion segmentation in dermoscopic images with ensemble deep learning methods. IEEE Access **8**, 4171–4181 (2020). https://doi.org/10.1109/access.2019.2960504
12. Mahbod, A., Schaefer, G., Wang, C., Dorffner, G., Ecker, R., Ellinger, I.: Transfer learning using a multi-scale and multi-network ensemble for skin lesion classification. Comput. Methods Programs Biomed. **193**, 105475 (2020). https://doi.org/10.1016/j.cmpb.2020.105475

DTR Taxonomy on 3D Computer Aided Simulation of Image Processing Expansion in Facial Maxillary Surgery: An Extensive Review

Kristina Tandukar[1], Razwan Mohmed Salah[2], Nada AlSallami[3](✉), Syed Altaf[4], Shahad Ahmed[2], and Guninder Sandhu[4]

[1] Study Group Australia, Darlinghurst, Australia
[2] The University of Duhok, Duhok, KRG, Iraq
razwan.mayi@uod.ac
[3] Worcester State University, Worcester, MA, USA
nada.alsalami@yahoo.com
[4] Kent Institute Australia, Sydney, Australia
{syed.altaf,guninder.sandhu}@kent.edu.au

Abstract. Background and Aim: Three-Dimensional Computer Aided Simulation (3D-CAS) in Expansion have been a vast section for use in Maxillary Surgery (MS). However, it has some limitation in practical operation due to less evaluation in the technical area. Methodology: This research introduce a new taxonomy called Data, Transverse Image Processing in Expansion, and Response to Processed Outcome (DTR) which define the major components that are required to implement computer aided simulation in 3D maxillary surgery. We propose and consider these components focusing on validation criteria for simulation modelling in maxillary surgery during operation. DTR taxonomy of MS expansion is a forward step that will help the end users and the surgeons to analyze and understand constraints of simulation modelling in expansion focusing on its use in operating system. Results: We evaluated DTR taxonomy based on position accuracy, stress distribution and stress displacement with minimum processing timeframe. We demonstrated the effectiveness of DTR taxonomy by classifying nine state-of-the-art research papers in the domain of 3D-CAS expansion in MS systems. Conclusion: Our classification shows that components of maxillary surgery expansion have been validated and some of them are evaluated. This article reviews the image processing in the surgical room for pre-operative and intra-operative scenario in terms of position accuracy, operation time, stress distribution and stress displacement to ease the surgical procedure.

Keywords: Maxillary expansion · Taxonomy · Image processing · Expansion · Three-Dimensional Computer Aided Simulation · Finite element method analysis

K. Daimi and A. Al Sadoon (Eds.): ICR 2022, AISC 1431, pp. 112–120, 2022.
https://doi.org/10.1007/978-3-031-14054-9_12

1 Introduction

The purpose of 3D-Computer Aided Simulation in maxillary expansion surgery is to improve the understanding in oral biomechanics based on computational simulation. It takes account into bone structures like maxilla analyzing interdigitation influence on behavior with Midpalatal Suture (MPS) exposed in maxillary expansion defined by Guerrero et al. [1]. New advanced computer aided simulation with various expansion techniques have been proposed from tooth-borne to hybrid-borne palatal expanders. However, only few systems are used for maxillary surgery and even less are developed for commercial use. The objective of this work is to propose a new taxonomy of expansion techniques used in maxillary surgery and used by the end users and the surgeons. The purpose of significant taxonomy is twofold: First is to define framework with finite element analysis for discussing, evaluating, and validating. Second for better understanding with components defined in computer aided simulation with expansion in three-dimensional state. The papers were selected to demonstrate maxillary surgery in 3D computer aided simulation focusing on finite element analysis in expanders. The verification of DTR taxonomy is based on position accuracy, stress distribution and stress displacement. The rest of the work is organized as follows. In Sect. 2, the selected papers are discussed by categorizing them based on technology and techniques. In Sect. 3, taxonomy components are developed and discussed based on their sub-components and instances. Section 4 includes the validation and evaluation of proposed taxonomy components. The discussion is given in Sect. 5. At last, the conclusion of the study and the future work are given in Sect. 6.

2 Literature Review

Knoops et al. [2] proposed finite element modelling using Iterative Closest Point (ICP) algorithm. This model determines and evaluates preoperative CBCT with image processing to visualize the colourmaps and error value. Kayalar et al. [3] defined the 3D-finite element model generation defines transient thermal finite element analyzes, the research proposed various tooth-borne and hybrid-borne techniques for palatal expansion. Blaehr et al. [4] stated that that these tooth-borne, bone-borne appliances with skeletal and dental arch expansion shows statistically significant changes based on the patients' results. Gul et al. [5], proposed Surgically Assisted Rapid Maxillary Expansion (SARME) to determine the downward displacement with automatic facial land-marking algorithm. Also, it processed the mechanism based on automatic stereophotogrammetry analysis. Fındık et al. [6] defined two approaches for SARME with surgical technique and analysis on surgical images with 3DMD stereophotogrammetry facial system. Cantarella et al. [7] defined novel 3D method for cone beam computed tomography imaging based on micro-implant supported skeletal expander with OnDemand Software and Digital Caliper. Guerrero et al. [1] defined the expansion technique based on computed tomography image of maxilla defined with the expansion displacement with less analysis on computational simulations into account of bone structures. The expansion is further defined with finite element model with the raw data instantiated. Ismail et al. [8] defined propagation of interface during image processing with geometric characteristics lengths with creation of trans palatal arch wire. Asan et al. [9] defined the use of Cone Beam Computed Tomography (CBCT) images of a formal patient with various types such as coronal, axial and sagittal images then further converted into Digital Imaging and Communications in Medicine (DICOM) format.

3 System Components

The proposed DTR taxonomy is based on three factors: Data (along with subclasses data in maxillary surgery), Transverse Image Processing in Expansion (along with various software used to process), and Response to Processed Outcome (outcome of formatted image). The DTR taxonomy has been developed based on change in computer aided simulation over time in medical sector specifically in maxillary surgery. It helps to improve practical experience for experts in both surgery and information technology sectors. The taxonomy mainly determines the relevant factors for developing, analyzing and evaluating the entire system. Based on inclusive criteria defined, 9 papers were refined and selected which met the criteria and are published in high levels journals from 2017 to 2019. Our major considerations are based on how surgeons assist with the help of expanders simulating the 3D images. The classification of system is based on expansion in computer aided simulation for maxillary surgery during operation with three factors and they are: data, image processing and display. The first factor used in DTR taxonomy is data. It includes patients' classes and instances based on dimension, measurements, bone-force application in virtual or real object. The data acquired may be pre-operative for segment orientation or intra-operative for operation. These classes help to divide the type of data for palatal expanders. We consider data as two major subclasses: patient data (with all the personal and specific information) and visualizable data (based on processed data). The patient data includes raw data that needs to be formatted for processing using software. The raw data includes dimension, types of sensor and acquisition time. In addition, other relationship is shown such as medical store and demographic information. The visualizable data include processed data based on analyzed data, derived data, and prior knowledge data. The importance of data is to display to end user with pre-operative data such as CBCT scans that are processed in various dimensions as per the requirement. The second component of DTR is Transverse Image Processing in Expansion, the expansion technique emphasizes the procedure based on obtained data to provide image processing information for 3D computer aided simulation. The purpose of using image processing as a part of our classification is to navigate the processed data to maintain position accuracy to surgeon. This is to provide stress distribution and displacement as there are many scenarios where these are not noted. Moreover, it helps to minimize complications during surgery with all pre-processed outcomes. The images of formal patient are used for ease and to overcome the previous complications to determine actual distractor size and further detailing processes. For instance, various computed tomography (CT) matrix data are converted into 3D-CT images used for simulation. Therefore, the quantification of 3D image data is carried out to analyze the system systematically. The third component of DTR is Response to Processed Outcome. The display provides the overall outcome of the processed data in various formats. The perception location, tools and devices that are used for surgeons helps them to interact with the entire system. The purpose of response to processed outcome as a part of our classification is to use the processed data as an outcome and view them using various devices. The components are defined with their classes, attributes and instances in Table 1 and the relationship between components with subclasses in Fig. 1.

Table 1. DTR taxonomy classification

Author	Domain	Data				Transverse Image Processing in Expansion	Response to Processed Outcome		
		Raw	D	VPD	DDP		PL	Device	INT
(Guerrero-Vargas et al., 2019)	Maxillary Surgery	CT image	3D	Real object	Accuracy (MPa), dispersion (mm)	Dental anchorage and Dnt-skeletal anchorage	P	Hyrax, distractor and expander devices	Geometric model
(Ismail et al., 2019)	Maxillary Surgery	CBCT	3D	Real object, virtual object	Operative time, effective execution time	Creation of Transpalatal Archwire (TPA)	P	Transpalatal archwire, Palatal strap	Surgical and measurement tools (archwire)
(Kayalar etal., 2019)	Maxillary Surgery	CBCT	3D	Real object	Age group, operation success rate	Le Fort I osteotomy with pterygomaxillary dysjunction, midline osteotomy, and no down-fracture	SR	Hybrid Hyrax (HH)	Baseline and participation flow
(Blæhr et al., 2019)	Bone-borne and tooth-borne expand-ers	Coronal CBCT	2D radio-graphs	Real object	Eligibility, inclusion screen	Skeletal and Dentalarch expansion	P	N/S	Protocol and Registration
(Gul, et al., 2019)	Maxillary Expan- sion	Radio-graphs	2D,3D	Real object	Efficiency (P-significan't value), accuracy (landmark set)	Mandibular midline distraction, SARME	P	N/S	automatic stereophoto-grammetry, automatic landmarking
(Knoops, etal., 2019)	Orthognathic Sur-gery	CBCT	3D	Virtual object	Position Accuracy, operating time, displacement, percentage of efficiency	Finite Element Models (FEM), Mass Tensor Models (MTM), or Mass Spring Models (MSM), Landmark Based Algo- rithm	P, SR	Scanner	DICOM, STL file
(Asan et al., 2018)	Maxillary Surgery	CBCT	3D	Real object, virtual object	Displacement, scanning time, distractor dimension	Three-Directional (3D) design of the distractor, Finite Element Method (FEM) analyses	P	Scanner, Rigid External distractor (RED)	Solidworks Premium, Software Rhi-noceros 4.0
(Fındık et al., 2019)	Maxillary Surgery	CBCT	3D	Real object	Operating time, cost, variance (mean value)	Le Fort I osteotomy, Surgically Assisted Rapid Maxillary Expansion (SARME)	SR	Distractor device	3DMD stereo-photogram-metry
(Cantarella etal., 2018)	Maxillary Surgery	CBCT imaging	3D	Real object	Reliability, position accuracy	Novel three-dimensional (3D) method Cone Beam Computed Tomography (CBCT) imaging, Micro-implant sup-ported skeletal expander	SR	RPE device	OnDemand software, Digital Caliper

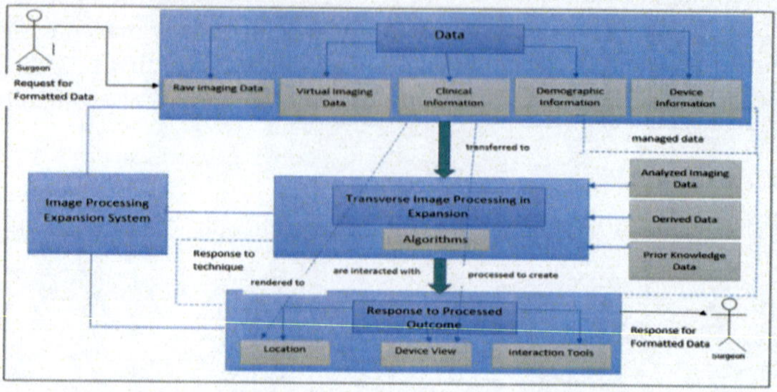

Fig. 1. The component of DTR taxonomy, the solid line represents classes and subclasses whereas dashed line represents their relationship.

4 System Classification and Evaluation

The accuracy is determined for validation and shows that right system was built with it, and evaluation proves usefulness and value to the system. The summarization of these validations and evaluations are depicted in Table 2. All the papers that are analyzed have different validation and evaluation ways in the system. Most of the papers focused on position accuracy, as one of the major factors in validation and evaluation. Since the major goal of a system is based on image processing, the publications prioritize in position accuracy. However, there are papers that focuses on other factors. Few publications focus on overall accuracy, whereas other focuses on stress displacement and distribution. In addition, other few papers focus on reliability, scalability and effectiveness as validation and evaluation factors. The major components of image processing in the system have been validated and evaluated in different publications. Here, we present some papers that validated and evaluated the system. Whole system has been validated in many of the publications whereas others have just evaluated the system. Asan et al. [9], and Guerrero et al. [1] considered whole system for validation and evaluation based on correction to maxillary transverse in response to midpalate suture during maxillary expansion. The consideration of maxillary surgery is based on pre-operative and intra-operative scenario focusing mainly on hard-tissues and their complications during surgery. Knoops et al. [2], and Ismail et al. [8] validated the system based on position accuracy and the entire system built. In addition, it shows accuracy of the whole system, stress displacement and distribution during maxillary surgery. Cantaerlla et al. [7], and Findik et al. [6] evaluated the system based on the patients that underwent surgery with preoperative and intraoperative data. The outcomes are based on successful rates the overall system has shown and its value to the system. The best solution for image processing component is based on position accuracy of maxilla, accuracy of the whole system, system displacement and distribution. For evaluation process we have analyzed and provided both qualitative and quantitative methods. This includes measuring domain experts based on certain criteria (e.g., completeness, consistency, accuracy, reliability, and scalability). In addition, some authors have used the approaches of data driven cases. Knoops et al. [2] suggested that taxonomy can be evaluated using a "position accuracy" measure.

Table 2. Validation and/or evaluation of DTR taxonomy

Author	Clinical Context	Compo-nent Vali-dated or Evaluated	Study Criteria	Valida-tion/ Evalua-tion method and/or data set	Mathematical Formula	Results
(Guerrero-Vargas et al., 2019)	Maxillary Surgery	Interdigita-tion model-ling	Position accuracy, stress distri-bution anddisplace-ment	Compu-tational sim-ulation	N/A	Influence of interdigita-tion on midpalatal suture (MPS) with mechanical be-haviour is more than that ofreal bone geometry.
(Ismail et al., 2019)	Maxillary Surgery	Whole system	Opera-tive time, execution time	Direct measure-ment	$\gamma = tan^{-1}(4A/\lambda)$ where, $\gamma = kink\ angle$, A = amplitude, $\lambda = wavelengt$	Skeletal expansion is as-signed as (>5mm) and 26-gauge circum-dental wiresis secured.
(Kayalar et al., 2019)	Maxillary Surgery	Whole system	Age group, oper-ation suc-cess rate	20 skele-tally mature patients (mean age 19.4) ran-domly as-signed to hy-brid or tooth-borne devices.	N/A	There was a positive cor-relation (63.6%) between the changes in skeletal val-ues.
(Blæhr et al., 2019)	Bone-borneand tooth-borne ex-panders	Whole system	Eligibil-ity, qualita-tive synthe-sis	Phantom and patient	N/A	Dental arch expansion is significantly greater than the skeletal expansion with treatment modalities.
(Gul, et al., 2019)	Maxillary Expansion	Whole system	Effi-ciency, accu-racy	20 pa-tients under-went maxil-lary surgery (12 of them went bimax-illary expan-sion); age (16 to 47 years)	N/A	Increase in significant mean of 2.20 mm in inter-alar width and non-signifi-cant mean of 1.17 mm in in-ter-alar curvature point.
(Knoops, et al., 2019)	Orthog-nathic Sur-gery	Whole system	Position accuracy, operating time, effi-ciency	Phantom and Patient (7 patients: 5 females, 2 males under-went Le FortI osteotomy; mean age: 18 years)	$G = \frac{(1-c^2)}{Ex}\overline{(a^2 + b^2)}$ $\varphi = tan^{-1}(b/a)$ where, G = phase depend-ent rate, $\varphi = phase\ angle$ a,b,c,x = intensity factors, E = efficiency	Accurate predictions with root mean square dis-tances (RMS = 1.3 ± 0.4 mm).
(Asan et al., 2018)	Maxillary Surgery	Whole system	Scanning time, dis-tractor rate	Physical Phantom and patient	$UK_m = \frac{\sum_{i=1}^{n} K_{mi}\,\mu(\Delta K_{mi})}{\sum_{i=1}^{n}\mu_i}$, $m = p, i, d$ where, UK_m: stress distribution, μ_i: subjection function, ΔK_{mi}: the output parameter, p: proportion, i: integral, d: differential out-put.	Maximum stress distri-bution on maxillary bone is found under 234 N and 93 Nbased on biomechanicaltest results.
(Fındık et al., 2019)	Maxillary Surgery	Whole system	Effec-tiveness, op-erating timeand cost	32 pa-tients under-went surgery	N/A	Timepoints determined with preoperative and dis-traction phases are meas-ured based on dimensions for effectiveness.
(Cantarella et al., 2018)	Maxillary Surgery	Whole system	Position accuracy, re-liability	15 pa-tients under-went sur-gery; aver-age age: 17.2 years	N/A	Zygomatic bones with 1.4 mm with cast cap splint expander was used in ado-lescents.

5 Discussion

The major considerations are based on how surgeons assist with the help of expanders simulating the three-dimensional images. Therefore, the first main point to consider is what kind of data are available for further processing. The second point is how the images are processed using computer aided software with transverse expansion, and the third point to consider is how it should response to processed outcome based on patients' scenario and the interaction among the system. The classification of system is based on expansion in computer aided simulation for maxillary surgery during operation with three factors and they are: data, image processing and display. All chosen 9 publications have presented well defined discussion over analyzed imaging data and derived data; however, there are only few publications that defined prior knowledge data. There are few papers which defined about prior knowledge data but not clearly discussed. As defined by Guerrero et al. [1], various considerations should be analysed to provide best representation to improve image processing visually rather than less localization. The use of prior knowledge data based on underlying model were not mentioned in some selected publications. However, underlying model such as details of formal patient records used in surgery preoperatively and intraoperatively haven't been considered in few publications. Asan et al. [9] defined maxillary surgery with the help of prior formal patient records in real and virtual object for three-dimensional object. The visually processed data and analyzed imaging data help to determine the relevant processed outcome. These analyzed data act as an input for another component. Furthermore, it helps for transverse image processing in expansion. The overall processed data helps to develop the system and enhance the image processing methods. It further needs more study in detail to define overall scenario. Various papers mentioned different methods for image processing in maxillary expansion surgery. However, some of the publications haven't described clearly over image processing and its real impact to the system. Blaehr et al. [4] described skeletal and dental arch expansion but has not explained the overall system expansion techniques. Ismail et al. [8] mentioned creation of trans palatal arch wire but hasn't considered the methods to operate the system such as finite element analysis, SARME or SARPE. Therefore, proper consideration of various techniques is required to maintain the system in advanced way. The algorithms that are used for transverse image processing help to determine the appropriate methods for operation in surgical room and the benefits for end users. Perception Location and Interaction tools were well defined in all publications whereas the devices are unclear in few. Interaction tools are well defined in terms of hardware, virtual and software tools and they act as an intermediate in the system. However, the use of devices might be defined in few papers, but the detail discussion is further required and further access to it in order to minimize the complications. Kayalar et al. [3] defined device as hybrid hyrax but has not mentioned the detail of the devices. Devices help to direct the flow in the system such that it plays a vital in the system. However, few publications lack defining the devices and how these devices assist to obtain the response to processed outcome. Various outcomes are based on the perception location, devices and interaction tools interlinked to develop a system. However, some publications haven't considered the exact device used to determine the scenario. Gul et al. [5] defined the maxillary expansion with radiographs but didn't consider the exact devices for the patient's surgery. Interaction tools are further based on hardware, software, and virtual tools. The exact perception location helps to determine the overall system and the devices used for the surgery. The accurate use of various interaction tools in perception location help to achieve the best result in operating room.

In addition, the lack of proper use of devices might suggest that presented taxonomy doesn't include the system to operate vividly.

6 Conclusion and Future Work

This paper focuses on three-dimensional computer-aided simulation as DTR taxonomy for image processing expansion. All the analysis and research on this review are based on position accuracy, stress distribution and stress displacement with minimum processing timeframe. The journals are analyzed based on Q1 and Q2 levels and are reviewed on facial maxillary surgery through the computer-aided simulation. All the analysis and research on this review are based on position accuracy, stress distribution and stress displacement with minimum processing timeframe. There is an evolution in image processing mechanism in maxillary surgery since decades, in order to improve in terms of accuracy, stress distribution and stress displacement. In addition, to minimize the risks and complications with pre- and intra-operative scenario; various techniques should be taken into considerations. 3D computer-aided simulation helps to interlink the end users with data into processed and analyzed data with various software interaction tools with patient in the surgical room. This paper highlights three major components as data, transverse image processing in expansion, response to processed outcome setting a framework for maxillary surgery. The various input data are used and are processed for image processing in expansion and then used in response for processed outcome. DTR taxonomy shows a pathway for research in maxillary surgery as a domain which is then classified and validated based on the techniques used. In addition, interaction tools have been used to improve and modify technology during surgery. The overall research provides the steps in image processing with expansion with data and then outcomes in terms of display for maxillary surgery.

References

1. Guerrero-Vargas, J.A., Silva, T.A., Macari, S., De Las Casas, E.B., Garzón-Alvarado, D.A.: Influence of interdigitation and expander type in the mechanical response of the midpalatal suture during maxillary expansion. Comput. Methods Programs Biomed. **176**, 195–209 (2019). https://doi.org/10.1016/j.cmpb.2019.05.007
2. Knoops, P., et al.: Three-dimensional soft tissue prediction in orthognathic surgery: a clinical comparison of Dolphin, ProPlan CMF, and probabilistic finite element modelling. Int. J. Oral Maxillofac. Surg. **48**(4), 511–518 (2019). https://doi.org/10.1016/j.ijom.2018.10.008
3. Kayalar, E.S.-S.: Nasal soft- and hard-tissue changes following tooth-borne and hybrid surgically assisted rapid maxillary expansion: a randomized clinical cone-beam computed tomography study. J. Cranio-Maxillofac. Surg. **47**, 1190–1197 (2019). https://doi.org/10.1016/j.jcms.2019.01.005
4. Blæhr, T.L., Mommaerts, M.Y., Kjellerup, A.D., Starch-Jensen, T.: Surgically assisted rapid maxillary expansion with bone-borne versus tooth-borne distraction appliances—A systematic review. International J. Oral Maxillofac. Surg. **48**(4), 492–501 (2019). https://doi.org/10.1016/j.ijom.2018.12.010
5. Gul, A., et al.: Three-dimensional soft tissue effects of mandibular midline distraction and surgically assisted rapid maxillary expansion: an automatic stereophotogrammetry landmarking analysis. Int. J. Oral Maxillofac. Surg. **48**(5), 629–634 (2019)

6. Fındık, Y., Baykul, T., Yazıcı, T.: Nasal soft tissue changes after two different approaches for surgically assisted rapid maxillary expansion. Int. J. Oral Maxillofac. Surg. **48**(7), 957–961 (2019). https://doi.org/10.1016/j.ijom.2019.01.019
7. Cantarella, D., et al.: Midfacial changes in the coronal plane induced by microimplant-supported skeletal expander, studied with cone-beam computed tomography images. Am. J. Orthod. Dentofac. Orthop. **154**(3), 337–345 (2018). https://doi.org/10.1016/j.ajodo.2017.11.033
8. Ismail, M., Wessel, J., Farrell, B.: Maintenance of segmental maxillary expansion: the use of custom, virtually designed, and manufactured palatal appliances without the use of an occlusal splint. J. Oral Maxillofac. Surg. **77**(7), 1468.e1-1468.e8 (2019). https://doi.org/10.1016/j.joms.2019.03.013
9. Asan, C.Y., Kütük, N., Kurt, G., Alkan, A.: Development of a new three-directional distractor system for the correction of maxillary transverse and sagittal deficiency. J. Cranio-Maxillo-Fac. Surg. **46**(3), 424–431 (2018). https://doi.org/10.1016/j.jcms.2017.12.010

A Survey on Deep Learning Architectures in Human Activities Recognition Application in Sports Science, Healthcare, and Security

Basant Adel[1,2], Asmaa Badran[3], Nada E. Elshami[1,2], Ahmad Salah[1,4(✉)], Ahmed Fathalla[5], and Mahmoud Bekhit[5,6,7]

[1] College of Computers and Informatics, Zagazig University, Zagazig, Egypt
{Basant.anany020,nada.emad020}@fci.zu.edu.eg, {Basant.ali, Nada.hussien}@fue.edu.eg, ahmad@zu.edu.eg, ahmad.ibr@cas.edu.om
[2] Faculty of Computers and Information Technology, Future University, New Cairo, Egypt
[3] Faculty of Science, Arish University, Arish, Egypt
[4] College of Applied Science, University of Technology and Applied Sciences, Ibri, Oman
[5] Department of Mathematics, Faculty of Science, Suez Canal University, Ismailia, Egypt
fathalla_sci@science.suez.edu.eg, mahmoud.bekhit@kent.edu.au
[6] Kent Institute Australia, Sydney, Australia
[7] The Institute of International Studies, Sydney, Australia

Abstract. In a typical human activity recognition (HAR) system, human activities are recognized by collecting data from inertial sensors (i.e., Inertial measurement unit (IMU)) or visual sensors (i.e., cameras). Then, the collected data is labelled with human activities. In turn, the data is used to train machine learning (ML) or deep learning (DL) models. HAR systems are widely used in different applications such as security, healthcare, the Internet of Things (IoT), and sports domains. The highest accuracy rates are achieved by DL models. In this context, we review the recent advancements of HAR systems in three trendy domains, namely, 1) sports science, 2) healthcare, and 3) security. The aim of this review is to reveal the most widely used DL architectures alongside the highest achieved accuracy rates in each of these domains. Both the Convolution Neural Network (CNN) and the Long Short Term Memory (LSTM) architectures achieved the best performance in both fields of sports science and healthcare. In the security field, the best performance was achieved by the adapted VGG-16 model.

Keywords: Deep learning · HAR · Healthcare · Security · Sports science

1 Introduction

The HAR field is developing fast for both improving HAR models and HAR applications. Numerous approaches have been proposed throughout recent years, focusing on different HAR applications. Some approaches provide a solution for gesture recognition, while others provide tracking solutions; using image processing and/or machine learning techniques. Such approaches can be classified into three categories, namely, 1) device-free, 2) wearable, and 3) hybrid solutions. On the other hand, in terms of the employed

K. Daimi and A. Al Sadoon (Eds.): ICR 2022, AISC 1431, pp. 121–134, 2022.
https://doi.org/10.1007/978-3-031-14054-9_13

technologies, solutions may utilize RFID, Kinect, Infra-Red, Radar, Sensor Fusion, Wi-Fi, Hybrid (fusion of multiple technologies), etc. This survey has explored some aspects of the trendy HAR applications, typically utilizing deep learning techniques. One of the most intensely studied HAR applications is in sports science. The quality of the game, personal training, coach assistant, beginner's tutorials, perfect game analysis for future benefits, and even injury prediction and prevention are all hotly debated topics in the field, and many more are emerging. Although the scope of the activity being recognized in sports science is now confined to a specific game or a small group of related motions, that does not make it any less challenging to recognize human daily behavior and interaction in the surrounding environment. On the contrary, it is more complex as every game's motion pattern varies hugely from the others. Most of the games are outdoors, and they need continuous improvement as the state-of-the-art methods are constantly changing.

When it comes to healthcare, many researchers have discussed tracking abnormal natural changes such as Parkinson's Disease, autism, impaired speech, and movement, or specific abnormal changes caused by incorrect practice in sports activities or heavy labor such as construction or mining work. Many abnormal changes are easy to notice, while others are difficult to notice. The main benefit of using HAR is detecting abnormal changes in their early phases, preventing permanent disabilities. This process can be done by tracking the human body using images or videos of normal life activities to help the clinician, physical therapist, athletic trainers, and the general public at home detect changes using a variety of techniques, sensors, or programs. In general, it is a future because new diseases are discovered every day, making it ideal for developing models that can assist people in predicting diseases in a timely and accurate manner.

Recently, HAR has been widely used in public security areas such as automatic identification, video surveillance, early warning systems, patient monitoring, event analysis, intrusion detection systems, and indexing and abnormal activity detection [1, 2]. As part of public security, the integration between HAR and video surveillance systems is commonly used to improve safety and security in various areas such as marketplaces, shopping malls, hospitals, banks, streets, educational institutions, city administration offices, and smart cities. Moreover, monitoring the movements of crowds and HAR can be used to detect violent and criminal behaviors. Besides, HAR plays an important role in detecting terrorism activities and security monitoring in public areas like airports, subways, high-speed rail stations, and stadiums.

Recent years have seen a lot of progress and development in deep learning architectures and applications, for instance, HAR and various forecasting applications [3–5]. In contrast to traditional machine learning models, deep learning can mitigate the burden of designing features and learn many more high-level and meaningful features by training in an end-to-end approach. Hence, deep learning is ideally suited for HAR as investigated and widely explored throughout the paper sections. For deep learning HAR models, achieving state-of-the-art results mostly relies on increasing model size or the ability to scale to huge datasets [6]. HAR applications using deep learning models mainly employ recurrent neural networks (e.g., LSTM and gated recurrent units (GRU)) and/or CNN. Generally, no specific model outperforms others in all situations. Therefore, researchers aim to adapt different deep learning architectures to fit the utilized data best.

Figure 1 illustrates the role of DL models in HAR systems, with various types of DL models included. First, raw signals are collected from a variety of sources (e.g., smartphones, watches, Wi-Fi, Bluetooth, and video cameras). Second, the collected data is used to train and validate the DL models. Finally, these trained DL models predict different human activities.

The aim of this article is to explore the recent advancements of the DL-based HAR systems in the fields of sports science, healthcare, and security. Thus, this work aims to outline the most used DL architecture in each field and the reported hyperparameters of the DL architectures, e.g., learning rate and activation functions.

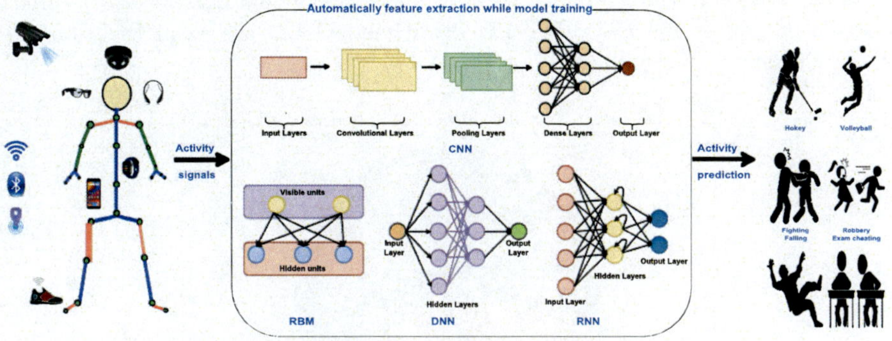

Fig. 1. A diagram of activity recognition using different models.

The rest of this paper is organized as follows. Several HAR systems in the field of sports science were discussed in Sect. 2. In Sect. 3, several healthcare applications that utilized DL-based HAR systems are reviewed. Examples of HAR applications in the security field are exposed in Sect. 4. Finally, the paper is concluded in Sect. 5.

2 HAR in Sports Science

In this section, we discuss the recent advances in applying DL-based HAR systems in the field of sports science. For instance, there are 19 papers related to using HAR system in sports science which are published in the Web of Science database from the period 1-January-2021 to 1-May-2022. Figure 2 depicts the distribution of these methods based on the used architecture. Apparently, the most dominant method is hybrid methods (i.e., more than one DL architecture is integrated in one Har model). Then, the most dominant single used architecture was CNNS. In the following, we discussed in detail samples of the proposed DL-based HAR systems, which are applied in the field of sports science.

The authors in [7] proposed an indoor analytic system for the localization of ice hockey players. The proposed system includes recognizing six activities, four-shot types, handling of the stick, and hockey stance; the data collection is achieved using wearable stick IMU and ultra-wideband (UWB) positioning technology. Four campaigns were used to collect data in a controlled lab or ice rink, yielding 1,742,280 data points. The proposed system utilized a sequential CNN consisting of multiple multi-dimensional pooling convolution layers with different kernel sizes, a rectified linear unit activation function, and an Adam optimizer. The proposed method performance is examined using 5-fold cross-validation, and the confusion matrix shows an average of 76% accuracy, with the maximum player accuracy of 90%. In [8], the authors proposed a deep-learning pose estimation system for kumites (Karate combats) using computer vision OpenPose [9] algorithm, modeling psychomotor performance, which means the interaction of the joints of two players rather than one. Dataset was collected by statically recording several videos of a green belt player posture in of three classes of attacking and defensing. Four data-mining algorithms were used to classify the movement, J48, BayesNet, MLP, and DeepLearning4J all with 10-fold cross validation. The four algorithms results in correct classification results of 99.95%, 99.94%, 99.95% and 99.97% and recall results of 1.00, 0.99, 1.00, and 1.00 respectively.

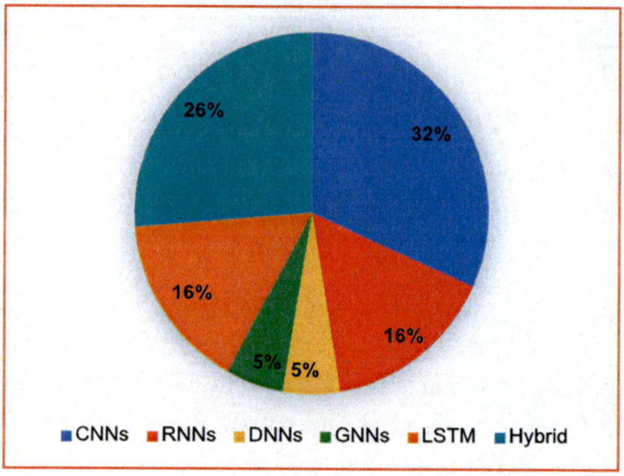

Fig. 2. The distributing of DL-based HAR models in sports science by the utilized architecture.

In [8], the authors proposed a deep-learning pose estimation system for kumites (Karate combats) using the computer vision OpenPose [9] algorithm, modeling psychomotor performance, which means the interaction of the joints of two players rather than one. The dataset was collected by statically recording several videos of a green belt player's posture in each of three classes of attacking and defending. Four data-mining algorithms were used to classify the movement, J48, BayesNet, MLP, and DeepLearning4J all with 10-fold cross validation. The four algorithms result in correct classification results of 99.95%, 99.94%, 99.95% and 99.97% and recall results of 1.00, 0.99, 1.00, and 1.00, respectively.

Pre-trained deep learning model, VGG-16 [10], is proposed in [11], for the recognition of four hockey activities, long and penalty corner, free hit, and goal. There's no publicly available hockey dataset, so a new one has been constructed from Youtube video game broadcasts, 400 frames were extracted at a 25 fps rate from 12 matches, 100 frames per activity, and then the activities were manually annotated. Extracted Red, Green, and Blue (RGB) frames are resized to an image of 224 × 224 pixels and fed to VGG-16, a pre-trained transfer learning model with 16 convolution layers, three fully connected layers, and a softmax layer. The single hyper-parameter of the epoch is changed and examined three times, 100, 200, and 300 epoch sizes; using 300 epoch size, the higher accuracy of 98%, where 200 and 100 show 95% and 90% respectively. The accuracy is calculated from three metrics: precision, recall, and F1-score.

A HAR system is proposed in [12] for more gym physical activities (GPAs) in addition to the traditional physical activities (PAs) for the expansion of the areas of application in IoT healthcare. The system has two main components: first, a preliminary classification model OC-SVM classifies free and non-free weight PA. Then, a fine-grained classification model passes free-weight to Neural Network (NN) classification and non-free-weight to LVQ-HMM (Linear Vector Quantization-hidden Markov model) classification. A dataset was collected from ten subjects (seven males, three males, and four professional trainees) wearing an on-chest Shimmer wireless sensor in addition to subject profile data such as age. Preliminary classification results in an average accuracy of 85%, NN classification results in 95.2%, and HMM recalls the highest score of 91.4% and the lowest score of 80.5%.

A deep-learning squat monitoring system is proposed in [13] for self-training to prevent possible musculoskeletal injuries. The system used five worn IMUs (tri-axis accelerometer and gyroscope) on lower body parts (thighs, clafs, and lumber). For the classification, two modules were used: convolution machine learning (CML) with random forest trees and deep learning with Convolution Neural Network CNN-LSTM, for a purpose of comparison. The convolution network is made up of three convolution layers: a recurrent, dense, and softmax layer, each with a 3×3 ***N*** kernel size and ReLU activation function. Data was collected from 39 subjects, with six correct and five incorrect squat exercises performed by each. The accuracy changed as the number of IMUs employed changed. Five, two, and one IMU resulted in accuracy rates of 91.7%, 88.7%, and 80.9%, respectively, for three DL models, and 75.4% and 58.7% for two ML models. In [14], the authors proposed a deep-learning recognition system for basketball shooting activities based on a fusion of two independent wireless sensor technologies: a sensing module on the force hand and one on the force foot (e.g., right hand and left foot) that passed through a fusion strategy. Every sensing module is composed of an IMU, an accelerometer, and a gyroscope, and the data collected by them is transferred to the MCU (micro-controller unit). A classification model VGG-16 network is used with a convolution layer, max pooling, and a fully connected layer. A total of 12,210 entries were collected from 13 Chinese right-handed male subjects who performed five basic shootings and five composite ones 50–150 times. The classification model showed a 98.6% average recall rate, while some postures showed a 100% rate, and the minimum rate was 96%.

The authors in [15] proposed a deep learning five football activity recognition system that considers replacing the highly-priced and challenging-to-transport current video technologies with acceleration sensor collected data followed by CNN and LSTM classification models. Three deep-learning models were constructed: CNN, Recurrent Neural Network (RNN), and a combination of both of them. The dataset used is from a previous literature work with 11 male subjects, with five IMUs on different body segments, and each subject performed different soccer activities. The deep-learning models show higher accuracy rates than machine learning ones; the accuracy was 98.5%, whereas the rest of the models result in inaccuracy rates of between 40% to 90%.

Finally, the discussed methods are summarized in Table 1. Table 1 lists the accuracy of the proposed method with the used hyperparameters. Of note, some papers didn't provide the source code or the hyperparameters of their proposed method. This makes the process of reproducing their results an infeasible task.

Table 1. Summary of DL-based HAR models in sports science

Ref.	Model	Accuracy	Hyper parameters
[7]	CNN	76.0%	ReLU, Adam optimizer
[8]	DeepLearning4J	99.9%	–
[16]	I3D network	75.0%	–
[11]	VGG-16 model	98%	300 epoches
[12]	NN and LVQ-HMM	85.0%	Radial basis function kernel function
[13]	CNN	91.7%	ReLU
[14]	VGG-16	98.6%	One-dimensional convolution kernels
[15]	CNN + LSTM	98.5%	ReLU

3 HAR in Healthcare

In this section, we review the most recent methods. For instance, the number of published papers in the period of 1-January-2021 to 1-May-2022 in the Web of Science database which utilized the DL-based HAR system in the field of healthcare was 16. These 16 methods are classified by the utilized the DL architecture in Fig. 3. Half of these papers (i.e., eight papers) used the hybrid DL architecture. In the following, several recent methods of HAR systems in the field of healthcare are discussed in detail.

Body movement data is utilized in healthcare to detect abnormal changes and determine the disease to which they are related. A summary of recent applications that predict diseases in infants, adults, construction workers, and mining workers will be discussed in this part.

With the growth of wearable and mobile devices, sensors are used to gather healthcare records that could be a remarkable change in HAR. However, there are outcomes which include a massive lack of records even as saving it as weakly labeled records while managing it takes extensive time and cost. The authors in [17] designed a semi-supervised deep learning framework consisting of an auto labeling schema using Deep Q-Network (DQN) to analyze the weakly labeled records and send them to the LSTM neural network connected with multi-sensors-based data fusion to train the model and get excessive accuracy of HAR healthcare collected records. They used two free sensor datasets [18, 19] that collect daily life activities using smartphones and on-body wearable sensors, and the dataset is split into 60% training, 20% validating, and 20% testing. For overall performance evaluation, the authors evaluate their model with DNN, RF, and SVM-based classifiers and find that their proposed model has excessive achievability and effectiveness with a 97% accuracy rate.

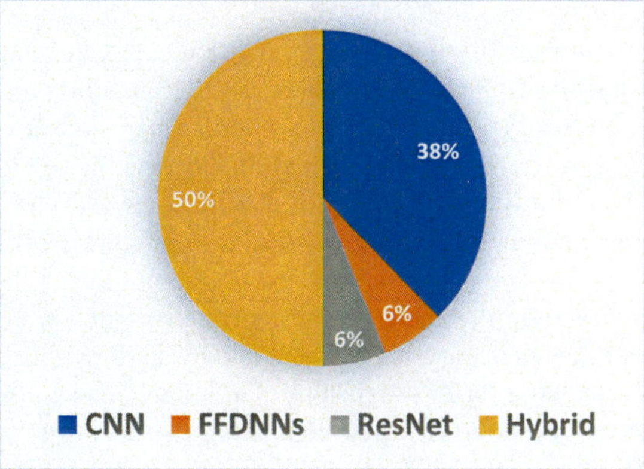

Fig. 3. The distributing of DL-based HAR models in healthcare by the utilized architecture.

The authors in [20] are focused on recognizing and classifying awkward working postures for workers' construction. The proposed model consists of an RNN with a wearable insole sensor to determine feature extraction, which is consequently used for classifying the data. The classification consists of three RNNs: LSTM, bidirectional LSTM, and GRU [21]. Plantar pressure data, collected on-site, is used to assess the model. After testing the model for the 100th epoch, the GRU model shows an accuracy of 99.01% and an F1-score of between 93.19% and 99.39%, confirming that GRU exceeds other models. This paper discussed how to prevent any risks for workers during construction and decrease the consequences of these risks using the proposed HAR model.

In [22], the authors propose their own dataset, which is called MMC-PCL-Activity. It contains 6,499 activity samples of daily activities for 14 participants. These activities are labeled as events, activities, and physical and mental states. The system consists of a smartphone (i.e., an Android or iPhone), a Database Management System web page, Mi-Band 3, participants, and a supervisor. The participant wears a Mi-Band 3 and connects it to their smartphone via Bluetooth after installing the Health Mate application. Next, choose from the labeled list which activity to do and record data via the sensor in the band and supervisor on the other side. Start taking images of the participant while the participant at the end uploads a record that is at least 30 s long for the activity to the application. To evaluate the dataset, they split it into 70% and 30% for training and testing sets, respectively. Then, the model is trained on single-modal HAR (CNN and LSTM) and multi-modal HAR (Early Fusion and Late Fusion). They concluded that multi-modal fusion gets a high advantage with an accuracy of 65.1%, recall of 51%, precision of 50.5%, and an F1 score of 51.5%.

Physical recovery exercises go in two steps; gaining proficiency with the essential procedures with your clinician and proceeding with training alone in your home, which demands tremendous time and effort to practice accurately. It doesn't make any difference in the number of exercises you do and how much advantage you get from these exercises. For that, the authors in [23] proposed a model to assist the quality of physical rehabilitation exercises using DNN. The model consists of metrics to determine movement performance and a scoring function to map the metrics into numerical scores. Deep neural networks produce quality scores for inputs to movements. The model has been approved by utilizing the College of Idaho–Physical Rehabilitation Exercise Dataset (UI-PRMD) [24]. Contrasting the model with several other models such as Euclidean, Mahalanobis, DTW distance, and Gaussian mixture models (GMM), log-likelihood supports that it beats the cutting edge of DNN for moving analysis. The authors will focus on connecting the validation data with ground truth for future work, which clinicians endorse.

In [25], the authors used the same strategy for their model, which is a hybridized hierarchical DCNN but with supervised learning and by starting with an image segmentation algorithm. Depending on this algorithm, the model shows a high accuracy rate of 98.9% for recovery sports exercise, strengthening the network speed and reducing training time. The authors used 1,900 pieces of training and validation data to analyze the model. The contributions of this work are two-fold; first, the authors created their own data set for sports athletes; second, the proposed model supports doctors in their diagnostic process, which reduces error rates and doctor tasks to increase their capacity to help more patients.

In [26], the authors used the same dataset as SisFall but tested it with a different algorithm using the CNN-Casual LSTM network. This network was composed of three layers of decoders and encoders with the ResNet18 classifier to indicate if the person falls or not. Compared with RNN, FD-CNN, CNN Causal LSTM, and LSTM, the CNN Casual LSTM outperforms the other models with an accuracy of 99.79%, a sensitivity of 100%, and specificity of 99.73%.

As we discussed fall detection and physical fatigue analysis, there is a significant point in HAR to analyze human gait to determine if there are any abnormal changes in their walking that might prompt anticipating osteoarthritis in the beginning phases. The authors in [27] proposed a framework that begins with preparing CNN utilizing CASIA-A [28] and CASIA-B [29] gait datasets, followed by feature selection utilizing

Table 2. Summary of DL-based HAR models in healthcare

Ref.	Model	Accuracy	Hyper parameters
[17]	LSTM with DQN	97.0%	Dropout 0.4, learning rate 0.05, batch size 25, sigmoid activation function, SoftMax function
[20]	RNN	99.0%	Epoch, dropout = 0.5, batch size = 64, and learning rate = 0.001
[22]	Early fusion	56.1%	Learning rate = 0.001 and SoftMax function
[23]	DNN	–	Batch size = 5 and the Adam optimizer
[25]	DCNN	98.9%	ReLu
[26]	CNN-Casual with LSTM	99.8%	Sigmoid function
[27]	CNN	96.0%	Batch size = 64, learning rate = 0.006, and Sigmoid function

probabilistic techniques made out of Euclidean Norm and Geometric Mean Maximization along with Conditional Entropy (ENGMwCE), and feature aggregation consisting of Canonical Correlation Analysis (CCA) and Kernel Extreme Learning Machine (KELM) to finally recognize the data. Compared with traditional classifiers, the proposed framework shows the most elevated accuracy beyond 96% with the least error rate, however, with high computational time. Finally, the exposed methods of healthcare, in this section, are summarized in Table 2.

4 HAR in Security

For many reasons, the classic security and surveillance method is to have an observer keep guard and monitor. For example, humans have limitations (e.g., they cannot continuously focus for 24 h). Thus, such limitations are overcome by conducting research on human activity recognition. In this context, various applications of HAR have been implemented in public security, including automatic identification, early warning systems [30], video surveillance, etc. Video surveillance can be used to monitor human activity in public and sensitive areas, including elevators [31], campuses [32], ATMs [33], and other areas to prevent crime, theft, terrorism, and other suspicious activities. And monitoring the exam for cheating behavior is critical to ensure maintaining the assessment's sanctity. On the other hand, home-care surveillance plays a critical role in the lives of the elderly, and handicapped [34, 35]. Figure 4 shows that there are 23 papers published in the period of 1-January-2021 to 1-May-2022 in the Web of Science database that apply HAR methods in the field of security. The vast majority of these methods utilized the CNNs architecture (i.e., six out of 23 papers). Then, the second most used architecture was the hybrid DL architecture. In the following, we explore some of the security-wise applications using HAR techniques throughout this section.

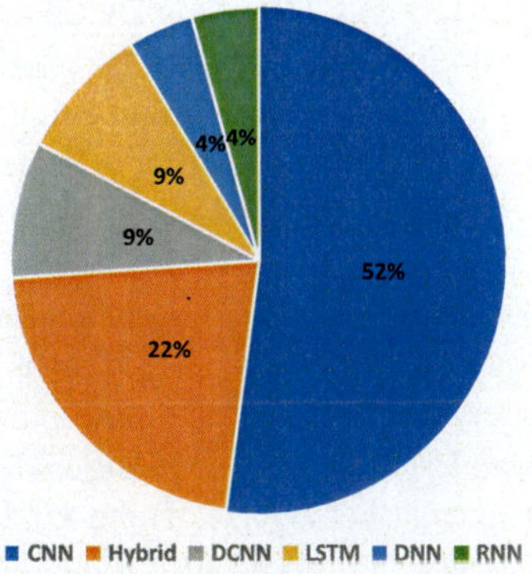

Fig. 4. The distributing of DL-based HAR models in security by the utilized architecture.

The authors in [32] proposed a monitoring approach for students' activities using campus CCTV cameras. Typically, an LSTM model architecture is used to classify the frames as suspicious or normal. For normal behavior (running and walking), the model is trained based on the KTH dataset [36]. While for suspicious behavior (using mobile phones inside the campus, fighting, and fainting), the model is trained based on the CAVIAR dataset [37], videos taken from campus, and YouTube videos. Whenever suspicious activities are detected, a message is sent with the predicted class to the corresponding authority. The classification accuracy achieved by the proposed system is 87.15%.

In [38], the authors implemented a deep learning model which is capable of classifying and localizing activities. This model has been trained on the COCO dataset [39], and the task of activity detection and recognition has been achieved using the single-shot detector (SSD) algorithm. The proposed model can detect four usual activities (jumping, running, drinking, and cycling), four unusual activities (climbing, kicking, punching, and vandalizing), and two weapons (a knife and a gun). Moreover, the model classification accuracy for running, climbing, and jumping is 0.93, 0.26, and 0.59, respectively, while the gun detection accuracy is 0.99.

Shi et al. [31] proposed S-LRCN (S-Long-term Recurrent Convolutional Network) for identifying abnormal behavior (i.e., door picking or door blocking) in actual elevator cabs and improving their safety. The proposed study utilized a dataset of 500 video clips from real elevator cabs. The model recognition accuracy is 85%.

In [40], the authors presented a deep learning-based approach for identifying normal (i.e., walking, sitting, standing), abnormal (i.e., fighting, chasing, crowd running), and suspicious human behavior (i.e., loitering, hiding faces, leaving a bag unattended for a long time) from a combination of skeleton activity forecasting (SAF) and a Bi-LSTM network. The model is trained using the MSR Action Recognition dataset [41], the MPII Human Pose Dataset [42], and the IIT-B Corridor Dataset [43]. The system achieves a recognition accuracy of 97.2%, and precision of 85.6%.

In [34], a real-time abnormal human activity detection method is proposed, using skeletons to detect falls. It combines one-dimensional CNNs and LSTMs. Two datasets are utilized in this method: the TST Fall Detection Dataset v2 [44] and a custom subset of NTU-RGB+D [45]. There are two types of actions: activities of daily living (ADL) include sitting, grasping, walking, laying, picking up, standing up, and answering the phone; and falling is split into (falling to the front, side, back, and ending up sitting). The method achieves a precision of 96.6% and an accuracy of 91% on the TST Fall Dataset v2.

A three-dimensional spatiotemporal convolution neural network is proposed for the recognition of crowd abnormal behavior in [33]. It is used to classify abnormal behavior (double fights, robbery, multi-fights, and other abnormal behaviors) and normal behavior (single withdrawal, double queue withdrawal, double close conversation, multi-withdrawal, and other normal behaviors). Three kinds of data sets are used: the Behave dataset [46], Caviar dataset [37], and the simulated ATM data. The proposed method suffers from human occlusion and dim light issues. The classification accuracy of the proposed method can reach more than 91%.

Detecting suspicious activity automatically and instantly will reduce financial costs and improve human security. Saba et al. [30] proposed L4-Branched-ActionNet, a 63-layer deep CNN model, to distinguish suspicious activities (falling on the floor, fighting, fire or smoke, a person firing, a person running) for surveillance environments. The proposed model is trained on a dataset called CIFAR-100 [47]. The classification accuracy of the proposed model is 99.24%.

One of the security-wise concerns inside a home or a building is how it is done to ensure people's safety inside it. In this context, anomalies in daily living activities are a good indicator of cognitive decline. Therefore, home care supervision is essential, especially for the elderly and handicapped, at even more significant health risks. It creates a need for online and distance-based alternatives for human interaction to ensure their safety. The authors in [35] proposed an approach that recognizes the activities performed in a smart home (e.g., chores, kitchen activities, reading, etc.). The proposed model distinguishes normal and anomalous activities by using a probabilistic neural network (PNN) for activity recognition. A comprehensive evaluation of the proposed approach is examined using two publicly available CASAS smart home datasets [48]. The proposed approach can recognize a majority of the activities with an overall classification accuracy and an F1-score of 90% and 74%, respectively. While reviewing HAR applications, almost all the solutions have ignored the security aspect, whereas the proposed solutions are more focused on accuracy, cost, scalability, etc. [49]. A summary of the discussed methods is listed in Table 3. The literature does not discuss how people can access, protect, and share information about their lives, and this area needs more investigation.

Table 3. Summary of DL-based HAR models in security

Ref.	Model	Accuracy	Hyperparameters
[30]	L4-Branched-ActionNet	99.2%	Activation function: SoftMax, learning Rate = 0.001, epochs = 30, mini batch = 128, optimization = SGD
[31]	S-LRCN	85.0%	Activation function: SoftMax
[32]	LSTM	87.2%	Activation function: ReLU, epochs = 10
[33]	3D CNN	91.0%	Activation function: ReLU
[34]	CNNs + LSTMs	91.0%	Learning rate = 0.001, epochs = 6
[35]	PNN	90.0%	Activation function: tanh
[38]	SSD	59.3%	–
[40]	SAF and Bi-LSTM network	97.20	Activation function: SoftMax, learning rate = 0.001, Stochastic optimization

5 Conclusions

This work proposes discussing three trendy applications of HAR systems, namely, sports sciences, healthcare, and security. The most dominant DL architectures for sports science are the CNN and hybrid CNN-LSTM in terms of accuracy rates and usage. Most of the HAR systems applications in the field of healthcare utilized the CNN architecture. Both

CNNs and RNNs architectures achieved very close classification accuracy rates. Finally, there is no dominant DL architecture in HAR system applications in security, while customized CNN models achieve the best results. Of note, transfer learning is widely used in sports sciences and healthcare HAR applications, while it is not commonly used in security applications of HAR. Besides, we discussed the utilized hyperparameters of the proposed methods. For the sake of reproducing the results of any DL-based HAR systems, both the description of the model architecture and the values of the hyperparameters should be known. Most of the reviewed models exposed the vales of the hyperparameters to different extents.

References

1. Dhiman, C., Vishwakarma, D.K.: A review of state-of-the-art techniques for abnormal human activity recognition. Eng. Appl. Artif. Intell. **77**, 21–45 (2019)
2. Zhou, K., Hui, B., Wang, J., Wang, C., Wu, T.: A study on attention-based LSTM for abnormal behavior recognition with variable pooling. Image Vis. Comput. **108**, 104120 (2021)
3. Eldesouky, E., Bekhit, M., Fathalla, A., Salah, A., Ali, A.: A robust UWSN handover prediction system using ensemble learning. Sensors **21**(17), 5777 (2021)
4. Ali, A., Fathalla, A., Salah, A., Bekhit, M., Eldesouky, E.: Marine data prediction: an evaluation of machine learning, deep learning, and statistical predictive models. Comput. Intell. Neurosci. **2021** (2021)
5. Fathalla, A., Li, K., Salah, A., Mohamed, M.F.: An LSTM-based distributed scheme for data transmission reduction of IoT systems. Neurocomputing **485**, 166–180 (2022)
6. Cheng, X., Zhang, L., Tang, Y., Liu, Y., Wu, H., He, J.: Real-time human activity recognition using conditionally parametrized convolutions on mobile and wearable devices. IEEE Sens. J. **22**(6), 5889–5901 (2022)
7. Vleugels, R., Van Herbruggen, B., Fontaine, J., De Poorter, E.: Ultra-wideband indoor positioning and IMU-based activity recognition for ice hockey analytics. Sensors **21**(14), 4650 (2021)
8. Echeverria, J., Santos, O.C.: Toward modeling psychomotor performance in karate combats using computer vision pose estimation. Sensors **21**(24), 8378 (2021)
9. Cao, Z., Hidalgo, G., Simon, T., Wei, S.-E., Sheikh, Y.: OpenPose: realtime multi-person 2d pose estimation using part affinity fields. arxiv 2018. arXiv preprint arXiv:1812.08008 (2018). 1812
10. Simonyan, K., Zisserman, A.: Very deep convolutional networks for large-scale image recognition. arXiv preprint arXiv:1409.1556 (2014)
11. Rangasamy, K., As'ari, M.A., Rahmad, N.A., Ghazali, N.F.: Hockey activity recognition using pre-trained deep learning model. ICT Express **6**(3), 170–174 (2020)
12. Qi, J., Yang, P., Hanneghan, M., Tang, S., Zhou, B.: A hybrid hierarchical framework for gym physical activity recognition and measurement using wearable sensors. IEEE Internet Things J. **6**(2), 1384–1393 (2018)
13. Lee, J., Joo, H., Lee, J., Chee, Y.: Automatic classification of squat posture using inertial sensors: Deep learning approach. Sensors **20**(2), 361 (2020)
14. Fan, J., Bi, S., Wang, G., Zhang, L., Sun, S.: Sensor fusion basketball shooting posture recognition system based on CNN. J. Sens. **2021** (2021)
15. Cuperman, R., Jansen, K.M., Ciszewski, M.G.: An end-to-end deep learning pipeline for football activity recognition based on wearable acceleration sensors. Sensors **22**(4), 1347 (2022)

16. Gerats, B., Bouma, H., Uijens, W., Englebienne, G., Spreeuwers, L.: Individual action and group activity recognition in soccer videos from a static panoramic camera. In: Proceedings of the 10th International Conference on Pattern Recognition Applications and Methods – ICPRAM, pp. 594–601. INSTICC, SciTePress (2021)
17. Zhou, X., et al.: Deep-learning-enhanced human activity recognition for internet of healthcare things. IEEE Internet Things J. **7**(7), 6429–6438 (2020)
18. Micucci, D., Mobilio, M., Napoletano, P.: UniMiB SHAR: a dataset for human activity recognition using acceleration data from smartphones. Appl. Sci. **7**(10), 1101 (2017)
19. Sztyler, T., Stuckenschmidt, H., Petrich, W.: Position-aware activity recognition with wearable devices. Pervasive Mob. Comput. **38**, 281–295 (2017)
20. Antwi-Afari, M.F., et al.: Deep learning-based networks for automated recognition and classification of awkward working postures in construction using wearable insole sensor data. Autom. Constr. **136**, 104181 (2022)
21. Cho, K., Van Merriënboer, B., Bahdanau, D., Bengio, Y.: On the properties of neural machine translation: encoder-decoder approaches. arXiv preprint arXiv:1409.1259 (2014)
22. Hu, M., et al.: Towards a multimodal human activity dataset for healthcare. Multimed. Syst. 1–13 (2022)
23. Liao, Y., Vakanski, A., Xian, M.: A deep learning framework for assessing physical rehabilitation exercises. IEEE Trans. Neural Syst. Rehabil. Eng. **28**(2), 468–477 (2020)
24. Vakanski, A., Jun, H.-P., Paul, D., Baker, R.: A data set of human body movements for physical rehabilitation exercises. Data **3**(1), 2 (2018)
25. Tang, D.: Hybridized hierarchical deep convolutional neural network for sports rehabilitation exercises. IEEE Access **8**, 118969–118977 (2020)
26. Wu, J., Wang, J., Zhan, A., Wu, C.: Fall detection with CNN-casual LSTM network. Information **12**(10), 403 (2021)
27. Khan, M.A., et al.: Human gait analysis for osteoarthritis prediction: A framework of deep learning and kernel extreme learning machine. Complex Intell. Syst. 1–19 (2021)
28. Zheng, S., Huang, K., Tan, T.: Evaluation framework on translation-invariant representation for cumulative foot pressure image. In: 2011 18th IEEE International Conference on Image Processing, pp. 201–204. IEEE (2011)
29. Zheng, S., Zhang, J., Huang, K., He, R., Tan, T.: Robust view transformation model for gait recognition. In: 2011 18th IEEE International Conference on Image Processing, pp. 2073–2076. IEEE (2011)
30. Saba, T., Rehman, A., Latif, R., Fati, S.M., Raza, M., Sharif, M.: Suspicious activity recognition using proposed deep L4-branched-ActionNet with entropy coded ant colony system optimization. IEEE Access **9**, 89181–89197 (2021)
31. Shi, Y., et al.: Recognition of abnormal human behavior in elevators based on CNN. In: 2021 26th International Conference on Automation and Computing (ICAC), pp. 1–6. IEEE (2021)
32. Amrutha, C., Jyotsna, C., Amudha, J.: Deep learning approach for suspicious activity detection from surveillance video. In: 2020 2nd International Conference on Innovative Mechanisms for Industry Applications (ICIMIA), pp. 335–339. IEEE (2020)
33. Cao, B., Xia, H., Liu, Z.: A video abnormal behavior recognition algorithm based on deep learning. In: 2021 IEEE 4th Advanced Information Management, Communicates, Electronic and Automation Control Conference (IMCEC), vol. 4, pp. 755–759. IEEE (2021)
34. Hristov, P.: Real-time abnormal human activity detection using 1DCNN-LSTM for 3D skeleton data. In: 2021 12th National Conference with International Participation (ELECTRONICA), pp. 1–4. IEEE (2021)
35. Fahad, L.G., Tahir, S.F.: Activity recognition and anomaly detection in smart homes. Neurocomputing **423**, 362–372 (2021)

36. Schuldt, C., Laptev, I., Caputo, B.: Recognizing human actions: a local SVM approach. In: Proceedings of the 17th International Conference on Pattern Recognition, ICPR 2004, vol. 3, pp. 32–36 (2004)
37. Bins Filho, J.C.: Context aware vision using image-based active recognition (2004). http://homepages.inf.ed.ac.uk/rbf/CAVIARDATA1/
38. Sunil, A., Sheth, M.H., Shreyas, E., et al.: Usual and unusual human activity recognition in video using deep learning and artificial intelligence for security applications. In: 2021 Fourth International Conference on Electrical, Computer and Communication Technologies (ICECCT), pp. 1–6. IEEE (2021)
39. Lin, T.-Y., et al.: Microsoft COCO: common objects in context. In: Fleet, D., Pajdla, T., Schiele, B., Tuytelaars, T. (eds.) ECCV 2014. LNCS, vol. 8693, pp. 740–755. Springer, Cham (2014). https://doi.org/10.1007/978-3-319-10602-1_48
40. Kumar, D., Sailaja, S.R.: Abnormal activity recognition using deep learning in streaming video for indoor application. In: 2021 ITU Kaleidoscope: Connecting Physical and Virtual Worlds (ITU K), pp. 1–7. IEEE (2021)
41. Li, W., Zhang, Z., Liu, Z.: Action recognition based on a bag of 3D points. In: 2010 IEEE Computer Society Conference on Computer Vision and Pattern Recognition-Workshops, pp. 9–14. IEEE (2010)
42. Andriluka, M., Pishchulin, L., Gehler, P., Schiele, B.: 2D human pose estimation: new benchmark and state of the art analysis. In: IEEE Conference on Computer Vision and Pattern Recognition (CVPR), June 2014 (2014)
43. Rodrigues, R., Bhargava, N., Velmurugan, R., Chaudhuri, S.: Multi-timescale trajectory prediction for abnormal human activity detection. In: The IEEE Winter Conference on Applications of Computer Vision (WACV), March 2020 (2020)
44. Cippitelli, E., Gambi, E., Gasparrini, S., Spinsante, S.: TST fall detection dataset v2. In: IEEE Dataport. IEEE (2016). https://doi.org/10.21227/H2VC7J
45. Shahroudy, A., Liu, J., Ng, T.-T., Wang, G.: NTU RGB+D: a large scale dataset for 3D human activity analysis. In: Proceedings of the IEEE Conference on Computer Vision and Pattern Recognition, pp. 1010–1019 (2016)
46. Blunsden, S., Fisher, R.: The BEHAVE video dataset: ground truthed video for multi-person. Ann. BMVA **4**, 04 (2009)
47. Krizhevsky, A., Hinton, G., et al.: Learning multiple layers of features from tiny images (2009)
48. Cook, D.J., Crandall, A.S., Thomas, B.L., Krishnan, N.C.: CASAS: a smart home in a box. Computer **46**(7), 62–69 (2012)
49. Hussain, Z., Sheng, M., Zhang, W.E.: Different approaches for human activity recognition: a survey. arXiv preprint arXiv:1906.05074 (2019)

Review of Performance Analysis Technique of High-Resolution Imaging in Mobile Telemedicine System

Farhan Khalid[1], P. W. C. Parsad[2], Qurat Ul Ain Nizamani[2](✉), Nectarios Costadopoulos[2], Nawzat Sadiq Ahmed[3], and Ahmad Alrubaie[4]

[1] Study Group Australia, Darlinghurst, Australia
[2] Kent Institute Australia, Sydney, Australia
{chandana.withana,Qurat.Nizamani, Nectarios.Costadopolos}@kent.edu.au
[3] Duhok Polytechnic University, Duhok, KRG, Iraq
nawzat.ahmed@dpu.edu.krd
[4] University of New South Wales, Sydney, Australia

Abstract. Mobile telemedicine system provides the facility of exchanging medical information from one location to another with information and communication technology. This work aims to review the performance analysis techniques implemented in a mobile telemedicine system for managing high-resolution medical imaging in order to improve the flexibility and accuracy of healthcare services. In this secondary review analysis, journal articles focused on high-resolution imaging and mobile telemedicine systems were reviewed. It was observed from this study that performance analysis of the high-resolution medical images provides efficient transparency as well as robustness in the information transmission.

Keywords: Medical imaging · Telemedicine · Performance analysis · High-resolution images · Image optimization

1 Introduction

The telemedicine platform efficiently offers healthcare services by maintaining a Communication Bridge between providers and patients. Mobile telemedicine is a computer network-based healthcare facility system that helps patients with improved accuracy and reliability. High-resolution imaging plays a significant role in computer-vision applications for pragmatic clinical trials and image-guided surgery. Medical imaging technology used in telemedicine provides the accessibility of the medical records in remote locations and provides accurate detection and diagnosis to the patients [1].

In this paper we review the performance analysis techniques and approaches recommended by different authors to implement in mobile telemedicine for efficient image processing and transmission. This study does not include any disease diagnosis method.

The following research questions will be addressed in this work by conducting the secondary analysis. Firstly, we ask which types of algorithms are used to enhance the

K. Daimi and A. Al Sadoon (Eds.): ICR 2022, AISC 1431, pp. 135–143, 2022.
https://doi.org/10.1007/978-3-031-14054-9_14

efficiency of the imaging and resolution process? and secondly what can performance analysis parameters be used in the mobile telemedicine system for image resolution study?

The paper is organized with the following sections. The literature review analysis that helps answer research questions, the central system component, classification and system architecture is discussed in Sect. 2. Section 3 discusses the usefulness of system evaluation components. The final section includes the conclusion of this work and future research directions.

2 Literature Review

In this study, secondary sources have been used for collecting the data required for conducting the review. The most recent and relevant articles focused on high-resolution medical imaging and telemedicine review are used to do performance analysis approaches.

The image pyramid scheme uses a practical query approach to obtain efficient telemedicine system transmission. This architecture uses a typical image pyramid scheme (TIPS) to encompass the features of novel images obtained from the image layering method. This approach is significant in telemedicine, reducing medical images' average image generation time. However, 4G and 5G mobile networks can cause network instability due to bandwidth differences that affect the medical images' transmission accuracy in rural and remote areas. Accessing, retrieval of pyramid structure's performance helps balance the medical images. In the future, the storage space required for high-resolution photos can be further reduced by improving the query and indexing efficiency [2].

The double random phase encoding (DRPE) framework is efficient in decomposing the medical image into sub-images for transforming the pixel positions of the photos Scrambling and sub-images of the pixels are synthesized into a single image that improves the images' encryption accuracy [3].

The interactive medical image segmentation technique is efficient in segmenting different medical imaging objects. The proposed approach of medical image segmentation is efficient in segmenting the medical images using sequential patches during the manual delineation process. The innovative segmentation method efficiently represents the bi-directional sequential patches that reduce the image segmentation time. Input sequencing of the foreground region at the image's background can propagate the memory forward and backward. However, predicting the predictive boundary's location is challenging in this interactive image segmentation approach. Efficient compression schemes can be used to eliminate the redundancy of data for optimizing the storage pace [4].

3 Findings

This secondary review is focused on the performance analysis technique for maintaining the quality of high-resolution images in mobile telemedicine systems. Performance analysis techniques are efficient in processing high-resolution images with appropriate

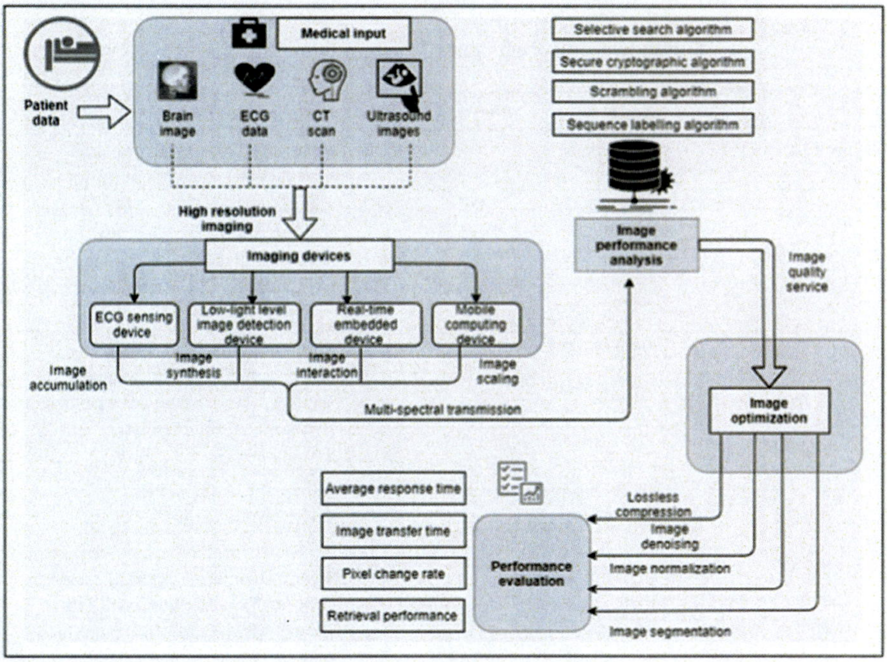

Fig. 1. System architecture performance of image quality and service is evaluated using average response time, pixel rate and image transfer time, by implementing image normalization, denoising, and lossless compression method.

security. However, this study does not focus on the privacy-preserving methods that help secure the mobile telemedicine network from external security attacks.

The diagram in Fig. 1 demonstrates the architecture of performance analysis of high-resolution medical images obtained from different imaging devices in mobile telemedicine systems. Other types of patient data, such as CT scan, ECG data, ultrasound images, brain images, is collected and transmitted in the telemedicine network using sensing devices. Performance analysis techniques and algorithms are implemented to optimize the images and preserve the quality of telemedicine services.

Classification of the major components of this review study identified in Table 1 is demonstrated in Fig. 2. Medical images are classified into input image, input image feature, input image format, input image dataset and imaging devices that different authors use for collecting the high-resolution images. Figure 2 classifies the instances of major components used by different authors considered in this review study. This table includes different high-resolution imaging methods used by different authors that help analyses the imaging method's performance. Performance analysis is further classified into parameters such as technique, algorithm, and models used to evaluate image optimization's performance. Evaluation of the performance parameter is performed with the help of different parameters considered by authors such as response time, sensitivity, mean square error, pixel change rate, peak signal to noise ratio, retrieval, and detection accuracy.

Table 1. Component table of factors outlined in Fig. 1.

Factor	Attributes	Instances
Medical images	Input image	Radiological, MRI, CT images, Weighted brain image, Positron emission tomography (PET) image, Digital mammography (DM) Image, Digital radiography (DR) image, CT scan images, Ultrasound images, X-ray images, Brain MRI image
	Input image feature	Scaled, Interpolated, Interactive, Dermatoscopic, Macroscopic, Multi-spectral, frame-accumulated, synthesized, Bidirectional, low-light-level
	Input image format	JPEG, JPEG2000, PNG, OPT_JPEG-XT, JPEG-XT
	Input image dataset	MIT-BIH ECG arrhythmia dataset, Public UCI dataset, NSCLC dataset, VOC2007 dataset, PROMISE12 dataset, IRMA dataset, ImageNet dataset
	Image devices	ECG sensing device, LLL (low-light-level) image detection device, Real-time embedded device, mobile computing device, Medical imaging software
High-resolution Imaging	Imaging type	Multi-spectral transmission imaging, Biological tissue imaging, Optical, Computed tomography (CT) imaging, Near-infrared fluorescence optical imaging, Non-invasive optical imaging, Magnetic resonance imaging
Performance analysis	Technique	Standardized evaluation technique, Lossless compression technique, Image watermarking technique, Hash code generation technique, Irreversible image coding technique, Medical imaging technique, Modulation-demodulation-frame accumulation technique (MDFAT) technique, Image processing technique, the Imaging technique

(continued)

Table 1. (*continued*)

Factor	Attributes	Instances
	Algorithm	Indexing algorithm, Particle Swarm Bacterial Foraging Optimization algorithm (PSBFO), Secure cryptographic algorithm, Coordinate descent algorithm, Selective search algorithm, Scrambling algorithm, Image compression algorithm, Sequence labelling algorithm, Synthetic minority over-sampling technique algorithm
	Model	Tile-pyramid model, Optimal predictive model, Radiomics model, Multi-modality predictive fusion model, Spatial pyramid matching model, Probabilistic graphical model, Independent image translation model, Pulse coupled neural network (PCNN), model
Image optimization	Quality service	Lossless compression, Image storage space reduction, Tamper detection, Reduced computational time, Image feature modality, Image clarity, Image denoising, Image encryption, Image filtering, Image normalization, Image segmentation, Image post-processing
Evaluation	Performance measurement parameter	Mean average precision, Retrieval accuracy, Precision, Detection probability, Compression rate, Sensitivity, Detection accuracy, Room mean square error, Dice Ratio Score, Centroid Distance, Peak signal-noise-ratio, Mean-square-error, Signal compression
	Evaluation metrics	Average response time, Standard deviation, Reconstruction quality, Pixel change rate, Average changing intensity, Correlation coefficient, Retrieval performance, Image transfer time

High-resolution imaging used in mobile telemedicine should have the appropriate performance for maintaining the telemedicine system's efficiency. High-resolution images are considered as input in the system. Image block size demonstrated in Fig. 2 denotes the size of image blocks considered by different authors as input along with the quantity of these input attributes. Image storage size denotes the storage space consumed in the network by input images. Image dimension denotes the dimensionality of medical images used in mobile telemedicine system. Image compression ratio denotes the reconstruction ratio of the medical images implemented in telemedicine that reduces the statistical value of the images without affecting the relevancy of images. Value of image compression ratio is different for PNG and JPEG images.

Image resolution denotes the pixel size of images considered by different authors. Processing time of imaging includes the time required for completing the predefined procedure of imaging in telemedicine. Standard deviation indicates the representation of values spreading over the range of mean values. Mean average precision considers the output parameter and metric that helps measure the average of all the values categorised in the classification. Peak signal to noise ratio is denoting the ratio of signals to the noise ratio affecting the quality of signals in transmission. Mean square error denotes the difference between estimated values and actual values, and this difference of values is considered an error in the outcome.

Author	Input image feature	Input image format	Input image dataset	Image block size	Image storage size	Image dimension	Image compression ratio	Image resolution pixels	Processing time
[5]	Dermatoscopic	JPEG2000	IRMA	66 KB (JPEG)	40% of storage space	Multi	0.401	2157×2928	2293 ms
[6]	Bidirectional	OPT_JPEG-XT	MIT-BIH ECG arrythmia	330 KB	4-15% of XML files	1-D	1.0-2.0	128×128×3	4.18 sec
[7]	MS	JPEG-XT	NSCLC	4 words of 32 bits	39% of JPEG images	Multi	0.9772	160×240	2.2180 ms
[8]	Interactive	PNG	ImageNet	128 bits	12 MB	1-D	0.9408	180 × 20	5-10 ms
[9]	Macroscopic	JPEG2000	Public UCI	8 bits	40% of CT images	2-D	NA	734 × 89	0.5-3 sec
[10]	MS	OPT_JPEG-XT	PROMISE12	32×32pixels	90% of encode files	1-D	0.35015	512×512	28.87 min
[11]	Interactive	PNG	IRMA	256 bits	35.1 MB	2-D/3-D	0.5-2.0	2800 × 3408	18.83 sec
[12]	Interpolated	PNG	Public UCI	192 bits	30% of MRI images	4-D	0.519	296 × 296 × 40	3.89 sec
[13]	Synthesized	JPEG2000	ImageNet	128 bits	20% of sub-images	Multi	0.9338	193 × 153 × 60	10 sec
[14]	Scaled	OPT_JPEG-XT	ImageNet	8×8 pixels	92% of JPEG-XT	2-D	1-100	1788 × 3001	17 us

Fig. 2. Classification of the major components.

High-resolution medical images are used as input in mobile telemedicine systems. [6, 10] and [9] used MRI images as input while [11] and [2] used CT images for performance analysis. The authors consider CT scan images as it provides clear pictures of tissues, skeletal and organ structures. MRI images detect abnormal tissues within the human body. However, MRI does not provide as detailed detection as compared to CT scan images. Network storage size consumed by medical images depends on image block size and dimension. ECG images are considered by [9, 12] and [13] as input due to its multi-swarm features. Image block size and image storage size are considered by most of the authors for input variations.

Authors such as [8, 12] and [9] consider digital radiography images as input as these images have effective image block sizes. Images considered by [13] consume 40% of storage space and images considered by [7] consumed 30% of the storage space approximately. [8] and [6] consider image block size in 32 × 32 pixels and [13] consider 8 × 8 pixels. However, it consumes the enhanced image storage size in the telemedicine system. Image dimension is considered by most of the author's input quantity as it affects input image features' performance. Authors such as [6] considered mean average precision up to 82.16%, [7] considered 94.78%, [10] considered 92.97% and [9] considered 94.16%. Peak signal to noise ratio is considered by [7] in range 35.18 dB, 252.87 dB by [9], <32 dB by [13] and 32–35 dB by [6]. In terms of input image formats, [12], and [11] considered JPEG2000 due to its multi-dimensional features that enhance the image resolution performance. Authors such as [9, 13] and [7] used the ImageNet as input image dataset as it is obtained with the use of real-time embedded computing devices. However, these input image datasets consume much space on network storage, affecting the image compression ratio and image resolution.

High-resolution imaging performance is evaluated based on the type of imaging performed on these images by using different techniques and algorithms. [5, 6] and [2] implemented Particle Swarm Bacterial Foraging Optimization algorithm for high-resolution medical imaging as this method provides the least standard deviation in image optimization. However, this method consumes more processing time in performing medical imaging. Image resolution obtained by [5] is 2157×2928 pixels, [9] considered 512×512, [7] considered 180×20 and [13] considered 1788×3001. Resolution of the medical images needs to be evaluated by maintaining the image compression ratio.

Authors including [7, 8] and [5] used the sequence labelling algorithm for performance analysis of high-resolution imaging as it is effective in reducing the processing time that is 10 s. However, it increases the peak signal to noise ratio in performance analysis of mobile telemedicine system. Image translation model are considered by [9, 11] and [12] for high-resolution imaging as it is effective in maintaining the image resolution efficient that is in range 734×89 and 512×512 pixels. However, both of these models increase the standard deviation range that is 1.98E−02/3.1E−03 and 20–1000. Image watermarking technique is used for medical imaging as it is effective in obtaining the efficient value of mean average precision that is 100% and 83.57% respectively and peak signal to noise ratio in range <0.9 and 0.008 respectively [11].

Medical imaging performance in mobile telemedicine is evaluated based on different parameters, including average response time, reconstruction quality, pixel change rate, image transfer time. [5] and [7] evaluated the system's performance based on the average response time of the images in the telemedicine system as efficient and fast responses are required for accurate prediction in telemedicine. [9] evaluated the performance of the telemedicine system based on image retrieval accuracy as images obtained from different imaging devices need to be retrieved with proper efficiency to maintain the quality of services.

Image optimization is considered the outcome of mobile telemedicine system as it helps maintain the quality of services. In terms of quality evaluating factors, [8] considered image filtering as the quality-of-service parameter as it is essential in telemedicine for maintaining the accuracy of disease detection rate. However, image filtering can affect the results of image optimization in telemedicine. [13] considered the peak signal to noise ratio for performance evaluation of medical imaging as it provides the accurate ratio of signal to the noise factor. [5] considered Image Denoising as quality service parameter, Image normalization is considered by [6, 11] as quality service parameter and image feature modalities are considered by [5, 7] and [13] as image optimization service parameter.

4 Conclusion and Future Direction

This work focused on reviewing the performance analysis techniques that can be implemented in a mobile telemedicine system. Image compression schemes are efficient in compressing the medical images for maintaining the quality and features of the images by performing lossless compression. It has been observed that the medical image segmentation methods include sequential patches for obtaining efficient image propagation. Multi-classifiers used in the fusion model are efficient in getting the image modality features that help assist the decision-making of image feature determination by estimating the weighting factors.

In terms of future directions of this work, the efficiency of the high-resolution medical images can be maintained by implementing mobile technologies. Effective guidelines related to the imaging parameters can be developed for obtaining effective performance of telemedicine system. Effective monitoring strategies can be implemented in mobile telemedicine to improve the efficiency of performance analysis techniques. Ambient assisted living programs can be developed for resolving the challenges of wireless body area network. Image optimization performance can be improved by improving the image features.

References

1. Alli, A., Alam, M.: The fog cloud of things: a survey on concepts, architecture, standards, tools, and applications. Internet Things **9**, 100177 (2020). https://doi.org/10.1016/j.iot.2020.100177. Accessed 1 Feb 2021
2. Hameed, M., Ibrahim, M., Manap, N., Mohammed, A.: A lossless compression and encryption mechanism for remote monitoring of ECG data using Huffman coding and CBC-AES. Future Gener. Comput. Syst. **111**, 829–840 (2020). https://doi.org/10.1016/j.future.2019.10.010. Accessed 1 Feb 2021
3. Liu, Y., et al.: Robust spiking cortical model and total-variational decomposition for multimodal medical image fusion. Biomed. Signal Process. Control **61**, 101996 (2020). https://doi.org/10.1016/j.bspc.2020.101996. Accessed 1 Feb 2021
4. Sabol, P., et al.: Explainable classifier for improving the accountability in decision-making for colorectal cancer diagnosis from histopathological images. J. Biomed. Inform. **109**, 103523 (2020). https://doi.org/10.1016/j.jbi.2020.103523. Accessed 1 Feb 2021
5. Liu, L., Cheng, J., Quan, Q., Wu, F., Wang, Y., Wang, J.: A survey on U-shaped networks in medical image segmentations. Neurocomputing **409**, 244–258 (2020). https://doi.org/10.1016/j.neucom.2020.05.070. Accessed 1 Feb 2021
6. Swaraja, K., Meenakshi, K., Kora, P.: An optimized blind dual medical image watermarking framework for tamper localization and content authentication in secured telemedicine. Biomed. Signal Process. Control **55**, 101665 (2020). https://doi.org/10.1016/j.bspc.2019.101665. Accessed 1 Feb 2021
7. Chen, J., et al.: Medical image segmentation and reconstruction of prostate tumor based on 3D AlexNet. Comput. Methods Programs Biomed. **200**, 105878 (2020). https://doi.org/10.1016/j.cmpb.2020.105878. Accessed 1 Feb 2021

8. Karani, N., Erdil, E., Chaitanya, K., Konukoglu, E.: Test-time adaptable neural networks for robust medical image segmentation. Med. Image Anal. **68**, 101907 (2021). https://doi.org/10.1016/j.media.2020.101907. Accessed 1 Feb 2021
9. Wen, T., et al.: Multiswarm Artificial Bee Colony algorithm based on spark cloud computing platform for medical image registration. Comput. Methods Programs Biomed. **192**, 105432 (2020). https://doi.org/10.1016/j.cmpb.2020.105432. Accessed 1 Feb 2021
10. Li, H., et al.: Edge detection of heterogeneity in transmission images based on frame accumulation and multiband information fusion. Chemometr. Intell. Lab. Syst. **204**, 104117 (2020). https://doi.org/10.1016/j.chemolab.2020.104117. Accessed 1 Feb 2021
11. Zhang, J., et al.: Interactive medical image segmentation via a point-based interaction. Artif. Intell. Med. **111**, 101998 (2021). https://doi.org/10.1016/j.artmed.2020.101998. Accessed 1 Feb 2021
12. Urbaniak, I., Wolter, M.: Quality assessment of compressed and resized medical images based on pattern recognition using a convolutional neural network. Commun. Nonlinear Sci. Numer. Simul. **95**, 105582 (2021). https://doi.org/10.1016/j.cnsns.2020.105582. Accessed 1 Feb 2021
13. He, Q., et al.: Feasibility study of a multi-criteria decision-making based hierarchical model for multi-modality feature and multi-classifier fusion: applications in medical prognosis prediction. Inf. Fusion **55**, 207–219 (2020). https://doi.org/10.1016/j.inffus.2019.09.001. Accessed 1 Feb 2021

Data Science

A Case for Exploration: Exploratory Data Analysis in Neural Networks for Renal Tumor Classification

Mikkel Pedersen(✉) and Henrik Bulskov

IMT, Roskilde University, Roskilde, Denmark
{mikkped,bulskov}@ruc.dk

Abstract. Exploratory data analysis provides insights into the structure and representation of data. By understanding data, more representative networks can be created without total reliance on implicit processes to match internal representations with expectation. The aim of this paper is to demonstrate how the usage of exploratory data analysis combined with knowledge from subject matter experts can increase the performance of networks and reduce reliance on mechanics. We use manual transformations based on data analysis to represent our data in a way that resembles the abstract processes that experts use to classify renal tumors. Compared to a baseline network, we achieved a significant increase in accuracy, 93.3% to 98.64%, without loss in external validations, while reducing the network size considerably. The reliance on internal mechanics to achieve the expected representation is flawed and exploratory data analysis can mitigate some of the pitfalls of this approach, leading to increased performance and a reduction in required compute power.

Keywords: Deep learning · Neural networks · Renal tumor · Exploratory data analysis · Classification

1 Introduction

The use of iterative development is essential to developing deep neural networks. Using iterative knowledge and results to change the network architecture and parameters in ways that increasingly align itself to the expected performance is seen all over the deep learning community and academia. But this approach is still heavily reliant on the full process of the network training and its implicit processes to show themselves in the evaluation, meaning there is not necessary any real knowledge of the alignment to expectation before or during the construction and training of the network. We rely on the network to show in the output results the use of its processes and context, which we evaluate in a given situation at the end of the training life cycle, independent of any representation that could misalign with the labeling of the data itself. It has come to be expected that the network will sort any faulty representations or transformations itself based on the given labeling of the problem at hand. But there is no insurance that the network will represent any problem in the same abstract way humans do, which can

K. Daimi and A. Al Sadoon (Eds.): ICR 2022, AISC 1431, pp. 147–156, 2022.
https://doi.org/10.1007/978-3-031-14054-9_15

lead to misconceptions about results and input parameters, or simply how to evaluate the results when the output of the network is the only interaction point of the network architect.

In the greater context of big data and general machine learning it is understood that data can be understood and represented in many different way, which may lead to completely different outcomes in models and labeling. This prompts the architect to explore the data in order to clarify how the data is represented and what it can and cannot represent, but also how to understand what problem is to be solved and most importantly how we expect it to be solved. How we want the problem to be solved sets the constrains on the evaluation of the network and how any result should be interpreted. Evaluation needs to be done in the context of the user or use-case, rather than in objective metrics, i.e. evaluation is inherently subjective. Thus, the data and network need to be shaped to produce actionable results in the expected context, otherwise the evaluation could be misaligned from the initial expected context of the results.

Although, the network will still be able to produce outputs without the data being manually explored and tailored to the expected representation, there is no insurance that transformations are correctly applied inside the network. Hence, we rely on the iterative application of changes from the resulting evaluation in order to mitigate any misrepresentation that might come from the internal representation of the data. The current deep learning literature focuses on implicit processes for correct representations of data, and not so much on the possible benefit of including data exploration.

In the medical literature some exploration of data already exists. Dey et al. [2] uses exploratory data analysis to analyses data from the first outspread of COVID-19 in Wuhan, China. They argue that by compiling data from multiple sources and analyzing numbers such as infected, dead, and recovered, they can understand the data better in an overall context. A visual overview is presented from the compiled data that removes the constrains of separate numerical values and moves the abstraction of the numbers into a realm that is understandable for any layman. Using these enhanced visualizations Dey et al. provides an actionable understanding of the data that can be implemented to understand and evaluate things such as containment procedures, infection rates, and spread predictions.

Gupta et al. [4] uses data analysis in another context and analyses images used to classify cancerous tissue based on performance when splitting the image into separate color channels before extracting features. Each color channel is then processed and the extracted features are fused together for the final prediction of the image. They observed an increase from 93.14% to 98.85% accuracy from the non color separation model compared to the color separation and fusion model. But their work does not contain any specific exploration of the data itself. There is no insurance that all color channels contribute with classification specific features. They only insure that the features contained within the color channels are not corrupted by other color channels. Meanwhile they rely on the classification part of the network to filter out non class specific features by not activating neurons after the feature fusion. Exploratory data analysis could have revealed which color channels contains features relevant to the classification, and subject matter experts could have provided relevant information to the classification understanding.

Lai et al. [7] proposes another method of separating color channels in order to remove non class specific features and noise. They use deep neural networks to detect polyps in the colon by not only separating but also mixing different color channels to gain an increase in accuracy. Using a full color image resulted in an accuracy of 95% which was the baseline for testing single color channel images. Lai et al. found that although each color channel performed worse than the baseline, red and green had 89% accuracy, the blue color channel had a significant drop in accuracy, 79%, compared to the red and green images. Removing the blue color channel and keeping the green and red channels were found to have an accuracy of 95%. They argue that the addition of the blue color channel might mask or add noise to the image with non class distinct features. It is clear that the use of exploratory data analysis for Lai et al. not only improved their network performance, but also revealed knowledge about colonoscopy imaging and how polyps behave in imaging. This could allow for either camera or image capturing software to be optimized for detecting polyps with either greater accuracy or lower cost depending on the criteria for the output.

The aim of this paper is to showcase the use of exploratory processes in deep learning to not only improve the performance of the deep neural networks, but also to improve the understanding and representation of the data and labeling in order to increase the insurance of the expected representation in the output results. Through the use of exploratory data analysis we reassess the raw data to gain an understanding of how closely the data is representing the features in regards to our expectation and in relation to the chosen truth labels. By using the knowledge gained from exploring the data, we showcase how the use of manual transformations can change the architecture of the networks as well as provide the correct context for the output of the network and its subsequent evaluation.

The base network and data is a continuation of a previously developed and published work that regarded the use of deep neural networks to classify renal oncocytoma and malignancies [10, 11]. The work showed great performance but required the use of a majority vote system to mitigate variation of performance in the area under the curve. This article aims to improve the stability of said network to further improve the efficiency in a clinical setting.

2 Experimental Setup

The focus of the experimental setup is to be consistent to the continuation of our previous work in order to separate variable changes from a hardware and software side to the performance and stability gains from the exploratory data analysis, modified data transformations and representations, and the subsequent architecture modification. Therefore the baseline network is a direct continuation of our previous work with the weights gained from training previously along with the reported performance. Any subsequent network architectures developed or any transformations done to the data will require a full reset of the weights to the initial state of imagenet weights for the convolutional block using transfer learning [6], with the dense classifier block being randomly initialized, unless otherwise stated. The partitioning schema and the choice of not using of k-fold is described in Sect. 2.2.

Using exploratory data analysis as well as subject matter experts, our goal is to create an understanding of how the data is supposed represented in relation to the abstract representation of the subject matter experts and how it is represented without the exploratory data analysis. This will allow us to understand how the truth labeling of the data is constructed and how the output of the network is to be evaluated in the given context rather than blind reliance on a binary answer.

Understanding of the context and labeling enable transformation of data to better represent the expected context at ingest and output. For medical imaging this could be use of the gray-scale color spectrum, segmenting the image into regions, using heatmaps as outputs, relying on relations between multiple images, augmentations, or transforming the data into another data representation. We will provide further detail for any given transformation of the data or any exploratory understanding obtained in Sect. 3 as they are used to optimize our network.

We expect the transformations to mainly impact the stability of the network performance on the single image evaluation as opposed to the majority vote performance for a single patient. Furthermore, we expect that this will allow us to reduce the size of the network considerably as we remove more and more non significant data while relying less on implicit network processes. This will in turn require less computing power allowing for cheaper and easier clinical implementations as specialist hardware might not be needed. Lastly, we also expect to gain insights into the internal transformations and representations of the original network based on the performance of given transformations and network architecture changes. By comparing the performance, stability, and output in relation to the expected representation, we gain insights into what abstract choices the original network made in order to represent the problem. We also expect this knowledge to shape how we represent and understand our data labels as well as how these are presented to any user or subject matter expert.

2.1 Network

The baseline network was developed in Keras [1] with the RMSprop optimizer, a learning rate of 0.000002, with ResNet50V2 [5] as the convolutional baseline using transfer learning [6] from imagenet weights. A total of 10 epochs for training were performed to gain the reported performance. All weights were available for the network to train (Fig. 1).

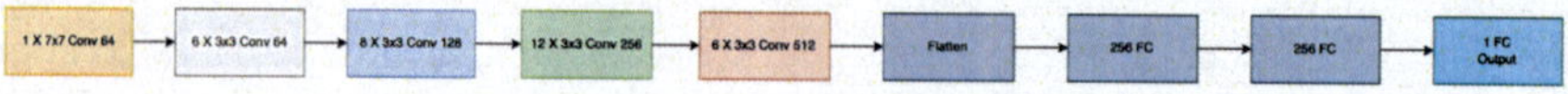

Fig. 1. Original network used. Notice the ResNet50V2 convolutional block with a Modified classifier in the fully connected layers.

2.2 Dataset and Partitioning

The dataset consist of CT scans of 369 patients with a renal tumor that is either benign or malignant, collected from the Zealand and Capital region hospitals in Denmark. More details of data capture is provided in [10]. For each scan of a patient the tumor was identified and the resulting images exported to a 512 $\times$ 512 color JPG image, with 10–100 images per patient based on the tumor position and size. As people mostly contact a hospital when they are sick, the dataset is skewed towards malignancies with a ratio of 80–20%. This bias is being mitigated with oversampling of the under-represented class to match the over-represented class by simple copying of images [3]. An argument for data augmentation could be made, but because of the high performance achieved in our earlier work [10, 11], we did not need to employ data augmentation. The use of basic data augmentation would most likely not produce any new data variation, partly because of the high similarity of image layers, but also because of the constraints of the image parameters from CT scans. Using rotation would not align itself to the image parameters of a CT scan which is always in the same orientation and size, which would require the network to develop transformations to handle the rotation towards the normality of CT scans for an input image. Mirroring of images would again require the network to develop transformations to handle the augmentation that does not occur in reality. A renal tumor will always occur in the kidney, in mostly the same orientation, and have specific development parameters. We refer to our earlier work for details of tumor constraints [10]. Mirroring the image will extend the parameters in unusual ways requiring network complexity and transformations that are not guarantied to be developed during training. We also regard data augmentation as part of data extension rather than understanding or exploration of data. Though, we do recognize that using advanced methods of data augmentation (GAN's and style transfer) as seen from Mikolajczyk et al. [8] could provide interesting results, but would ultimately not be part of data exploration.

Normally, a dataset has precise data-points that are constrained to a single observation without any overlap in data variance, such as a single picture of an object in an instantaneous moment or a whole CT scan with 20000 image slices being used as a single data-point. Since our dataset consists of multiple images all consisting of micro movements in slice length, they do not provide enough data variance in their singular form to be used as a separate observation across partitions. If two CT scan images of the same patient with only the image slice length as their variance are positioned with one image in the training partition and the other in the validation partition, memorization is likely to occur because of the very limited variance. Hence, we have chosen to manually partition the dataset with the patient as the data-point (or observation) rather than single images, meaning all images of a patient is constrained to either the training, validation, or test partition. This insures that we do not have cross partition memorization in our validation and test results. In effect we have two sets for evaluating the network performance. The first set is the partitioned test set that is part of the original data collected. The second set is the external validation set which is collected individually from other hospitals than the original data consisting of 49 patient observations. Differences such as operators, CT scanners, and imaging protocols, is present in the external validation set hence showing the ability of the network to generalize more clearly.

While we gain partition independence we also remove the possibility of using k-fold validation as our data-points based on patients would make wildly imbalanced partitions without insuring the null possibility of cross partition memorization. Therefore we have made manual partitions that are used for the training, initial validation, and evaluation, which contains 369 patients, while also collecting external validation datasets from other hospitals and CT Scanners to increase the data variance in the validation sets.

3 Results

Previously [10, 11] we have observed that our baseline network performs quite well with an accuracy of 93.3% for the test set and 90.4% for the external validation. While this performance is satisfactory it came with a cost of instability of the network during training and a very high compute cost. The images were already re-scaled from 512 × 512 down to 224 × 224 but because of the color channels and the massiveness of the ResNet50V2 network the complexity was still high. The compute cost could be justified during training as this is a one time event, but the compute cost of prediction is still high enough to require specialist hardware in a clinical implementation. This is not feasible in a clinical context as concerns about data security is raised. Further more our data was clearly showing text and information artifacts. Although, as discussed in Sect. 3.1, this text did not interfere with the prediction, we theories that the network will have to use complexity to remove the noise added. Therefore, we chose to use the exploratory data analysis together with knowledge from subject matter experts to analyses our data with the goal of doing manual transformations before ingest.

3.1 EDA Processes

As described in Sect. 1, multiple papers have had success with analyzing the effects of transforming color channels of their networks combined with specific domain knowledge for the medical field. In the case of CT scans specifically showing renal tumors, some points are to be understood.

Comparing the process to how a subject matter expert would analyses a CT scan we can conclude that the colors of the image is of little significance to the classification. The contrasting lines, clarity of objects, size of the tumor, and the flow of certain fluids through veins and arteries are the basis of malignancy classification in renal tumors. The colors produced from the image storage format would most likely not add any significant value to anything other than the JPG storage representation. Furthermore, we rely on the implicit transformation mechanics of the network when using the color representation of the JPG format in the neural network. Therefore, our understanding of the ingested data, internal transformations, and the output of the network may be misaligned.

CT scans are produced from x-rays and the resulting capture of said x-rays is computed to show tissue in the body. This computed representation is not reliant on the use of colors. Instead, it is reliant on the penetrative representation computed from the x-rays, meaning the intensity of the pixel value in the resulting image. Converting this representation to the JPG format just distributes the representation into multiple color channels that represents the gray-scale format. In other words, the colors seem irrelevant from a representational standpoint.

Based on these points it is clear that the classification, in terms of human processes and to mimic thus, are not relying on any color representation of the imaging. Rather they are relying on the intensity of a single representation that is directly related to the x-ray penetrative force through the body. This value can be expressed in a single channel with an intensity degree. An obvious choice for this is the gray-scale image representation.

Since the JPG representation of the images have been made by distributing the gray-scale representation when exporting scans, taking the mean of these to produce the gray-scale image should accurately reflect the original intensity levels of the CT scan. We chose to move forward with a gray-scale representation of our images in order to remove the possibility of the network to capture noise or non significant features originating from the color representation.

Each image contains a text that describes various parameters of the scan itself such as zoom factor, slice length, slice number, scan location, etc. Initial experiments of using trained models and comparing results from images with text and the text blacked out suggested that the text are not bias towards a specific classification, but that they do add noise to the image which requires complexity for the network to process properly. The processes of deducting the text to noise and transforming it out of the resulting feature maps are not guarantied by the network at any point. Although, the performance and validation are unaffected, the stability of the network could still be affected.

Therefore we chose to remove the text by center cropping the image at the ingest of the neural network. But the text size varies from image to image based on the scanner used and the hospital providing the scan. Hence a large crop is needed which, on certain images, crops out parts of the outer body (skin, ribs, thorax, etc.). But these parts are deemed non contributing to the classification of the renal tumor by doctors and radiologists, hence why we accepted a larger crop in the final iteration of the pre-processing exploration.

The tumor is then isolated from large noise features and remain within the same constrains as explained in Sect. 2.2 in relation to scan parameters. This allows us to remove the reliance on the network to perform data transformations without any insurance of said transformations occurring and without any reliable way to check occurrences of transformations.

Finally the image dimensions went from 512×512 resized to 224×224 at ingest, to 380×380 from the crop alone without any resizing at ingest.

3.2 Improved Network Reduction

Because of the reduction of noise and non classification specific features the network requires less complexity to represent transformations that remove noise or creates the correct representation in relation to the truth labels of the data. Furthermore, as we handle the image color transformations to gray-scale manually, we can reduce the network complexity and the amount of noise and non classification specific features the network could extract within the color spectrum of the data.

Although, the initial cost of performing the exploratory data analysis in terms of time is costly when neural networks can perform the similar transformations implicitly, we are not insured that these transformations will be performed or represented as expected by the network. An obvious side effect is a more unstable network as the feature set might not be aligned in the intended way with the truth labels, but the big concern is the misalignment of the expected representation of the output in relation to the truth labeling. If the representation of the feature set is not understood then the performance of the network is not evaluated in the expected context. Therefore, an understanding throughout the life cycle of the network is critical to obtain (Fig. 2).

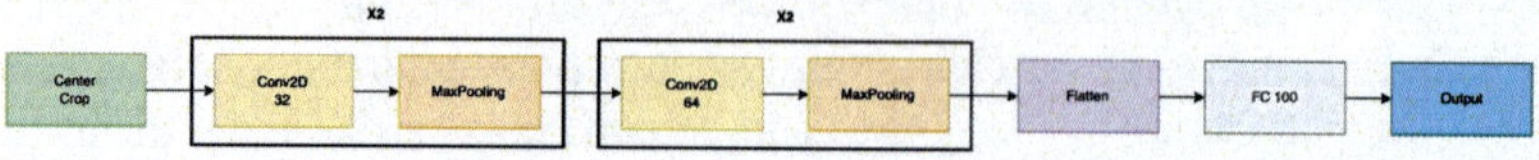

Fig. 2. The improved network. Notice the reduction in complexity of its convolutional block.

But because of the inherent problems of explaining the internal representations of deep neural networks [12] (not hints as to what happens but actual explanations that precisely describes the transformations and exact representations) we acknowledge that the understanding of transformations and representations inside the network is out of reach, hence is why we rely on the exploratory data analysis to gain insights into the data and labeling. This knowledge provides the opportunity to represent data and labels in a way that constrains the amount of noncontributing or unnecessary transformations for the given classification at hand, without relying completely on implicit processes and chance.

3.3 Improved Results

We observed an increase in network stability and performance after the network architecture and image pre-processing rework. Where our previous network plateaued at around 10 epochs, the new network architecture only needed 5 epochs of training. Additionally the training time per epoch were reduced from 9 min to 2 min, mostly from the great reduction in complexity in the model. Overall the trainable parameters in the model was reduced from 55 million to 2.887 million. By reducing the compute of the network we have gained multiple benefits in terms of clinical implementation. Currently, the use of external services to do diagnosis and process patient information is problematic due to security concerns and data anonymity, especially in the European Union [9]. But large complex deep neural networks require compute intensive specialist hardware that are not feasible to implement locally. Reducing the complexity this aggressively allows us to implement the network directly on local machines where the data leaves the machine. Furthermore we also insure that the runtime of the predictions are significantly reduced when a diagnosis requires the processing of 30–50 pictures at the time. We report that the reduction in both network and imagery complexity have a positive effect on the network performance and enables the network to pick up more significant features than our baseline network.

We observed an increase in accuracy from 93.3% to 98.64% in the test set with a per epoch validation set accuracy of 99.06%. Our external validation set showed an accuracy equivalent of our previous work going from 90.4% to 90.37%. It is clear from the test set performance increase that we have captured more significant features and less noise from the data, by reducing the representational complexity in the imagery. We argue that by manually performing meaningful data transformations before ingest we have reduced the possibility of the network to represent the data in a number unintended ways. This is also confirmed by the reduction in total training time. The network requires less training to achieve the desired representation, and thus output, while maintaining the equivalent performance of the external validation set. But the equivalence, and not increase, in the external validation set also shows that some variability in the imaging methods is being captured in the original data set. Variability in the imaging could be from different operators, machines, or simply imaging protocols, which is clear from the disparity of the external validation to the test set. Obtaining data from other regions of Denmark could provide a platform for exploring the differences in the original dataset with the external validation data. Knowledge of any non captured features outside the original dataset would provide an opportunity to produce a more representative dataset, to modify the data representation before ingest, and to modify the network architecture, which could lead to performance gains.

4 Conclusion

We have shown that exploratory data analysis can be important in the development of deep neural networks. By performing exploratory data analysis combined with the understanding of subject matter experts, we have been able to better understand the expected process and output of the classification of renal tumors.

Using this understanding we have transformed our data to represent the problem more accurately without relying on internal representations and implicit understandings of truth labels, which in turn have lead to reduced network complexity and increased performance.

Manually transforming the data before ingest into the network have allowed us to limit the possible representations of the network, and generate a better understanding of the internal representations in the network and how to evaluate the results in alignment with the input data.

This is especially shown in the reduced time to reach a satisfactory performance as an desired representation is reached faster. The validation of the new representation shows an observed increase in accuracy performance from 93.3% to 98.64%, without any significant loss in the external validation performance which stayed at 90.37%. We have achieved a better performing and more representative network by removing noise and non contributing features from our images, while constraining the number of unintended representations by exploring our data before ingest. Our results support the findings from Lai et al. [7] and Gupta et al. [4], while focusing on the data exploration as the main performance enhancer.

Furthermore, our network compute requirements have been significantly decreased from 55 millions trainable parameters to less that 3 millions. We have showed that although the reduction in complexity in both the network and imagery we still maintain or exceed the performance and feature capture of our baseline network. Not only have this allowed us to constrain the number of representations possible in the network, or the reduction in training time, but also greatly increased the possibility of implementation into a clinical context. With the reduced complexity, we are able to implement the prediction model onto local hardware meaning no data leaves the local machine, easily fulfilling the requirements of data security concerns.

Lastly, while our network shows great performance and is able to increase its performance we have also shown a lack of variability in our data. The external validation set showed only an equivalence in performance for our improved network. While the performance is still satisfactory and the variability is completely eliminated in a majority vote system, there is still room for improvement. Any variability might come from differences in equipment and personnel as well as imaging protocol. Obviously, collecting more data from other regions of the implementation area is critical to further improvement of the model in the future.

References

1. Chollet, F., et al.: Keras (2015)
2. Dey, S.K., Rahman, Md.M., Siddiqi, U.R., Howlader, A.: Analyzing the epidemiological outbreak of covid-19: a visual exploratory data analysis approach. J. Med. Virol. **92**(6), 632–638 (2020)
3. Fernández, A., García, S., Galar, M., Prati, R.C., Krawczyk, B., Herrera, F.: Learning from Imbalanced Data Sets, vol. 10. Springer, Cham (2018). https://doi.org/10.1007/978-3-319-98074-4
4. Gupta, R.K., Manhas, J.: Improved classification of cancerous histopathology images using color channel separation and deep learning. J. Multimed. Inf. Syst. **8**(3), 175–182 (2021)
5. He, K., Zhang, X., Ren, S., Sun, J.: Identity mappings in deep residual networks. In: Leibe, B., Matas, J., Sebe, N., Welling, M. (eds.) ECCV 2016. LNCS, vol. 9908, pp. 630–645. Springer, Cham (2016). https://doi.org/10.1007/978-3-319-46493-0_38
6. Heaton, J.: Ian Goodfellow, Yoshua Bengio, and Aaron Courville: Deep Learning, p. 526. Springer (2018)
7. Lai, L.L., et al.: Separation of color channels from conventional colonoscopy images improves deep neural network detection of polyps. J. Biomed. Opt. **26**(1), 1–9 (2021)
8. Mikolajczyk, A., Grochowski, M.: Data augmentation for improving deep learning in image classification problem. In: 2018 International Interdisciplinary PhD Workshop (IIPhDW), pp. 117–122. IEEE (2018)
9. European Parliament and Council. Regulation (EU) 2016/679 (General Data Protection Regulation)
10. Pedersen, M., Andersen, M.B., Christiansen, H., Azawi, N.H.: Classification of renal tumour using convolutional neural networks to detect oncocytoma. Eur. J. Radiol. **133**, 109343 (2020)
11. Pedersen, M., Christiansen, H., Azawi, N.H.: Efficient and precise classification of CT scannings of renal tumors using convolutional neural networks. In: Helic, D., Leitner, G., Stettinger, M., Felfernig, A., Raś, Z.W. (eds.) ISMIS 2020. LNCS (LNAI), vol. 12117, pp. 440–447. Springer, Cham (2020). https://doi.org/10.1007/978-3-030-59491-6_42
12. Rudin, C.: Stop explaining black box machine learning models for high stakes decisions and use interpretable models instead. Nat. Mach. Intell. **1**(5), 206–215 (2019)

Drug Protein Interaction Extraction Using SciBERT Based Deep Learning Model

Nada GabAllah(✉) and Ahmed Rafea

Computer Science and Engineering Department, American University in Cairo, New Cairo, Egypt
{nadaaym,rafea}@aucegypt.edu

Abstract. Information extraction from textual data is becoming more crucial with the increase of available data on the internet. Automatic extraction of information from biomedical data is very useful to researchers, saving time and effort exerted by them. Relation extraction between medical entities is one of the active research areas. In this paper we are presenting a relation extraction deep learning model based on SciBERT, to extract relations between drugs/chemicals and proteins/genes entities from PubMed literature. The model could achieve an average micro F1 score of 91.75% on the ChemProt test set.

Keywords: Relation extraction · Drug protection · Biomedical · Deep learning · SciBERT

1 Introduction

The amount of information on the internet is increasing every day. It is now the new norm of saving either public or private information. However, the data are not presented in a structured way, which makes it difficult to extract useful information from. Implicit relations are not easily discovered as well. Different research has been concerned with extraction of useful structured information from unstructured one. Information extraction can be considered under the umbrella of text understanding. While in text understanding the main objective is to represent all information that can be found in the text, information extraction focuses on the extraction of specific semantic information related to the extraction task [1]. Information extraction is used widely in extracting specific information from many documents, it is applied to scientific journals, hospital records, legal contracts, news records, etc. Applying information extraction helps reduce the human effort of going through many documents to extract answers to specific queries or relations between entities. Extracting semantic relations between entities in large texts is a very crucial task for a better understanding of data. It is applied in various applications, such as decision analysis and making, question and answer application, scenario prediction and analysis, etc.

The information held by the semantic relations between entities such as if-then relation or a part-and-whole relation give more insight about what the text can entail. The cause-effect relationship is one of the important relationships that can be extracted

K. Daimi and A. Al Sadoon (Eds.): ICR 2022, AISC 1431, pp. 157–165, 2022.
https://doi.org/10.1007/978-3-031-14054-9_16

from texts. It is particularly useful in the medical and biological domains [2]. The relation extraction system should be able to predict for a pair, if a given text contains a relation or not for that pair. It can also predict the type of relation based on an annotated training data of pairs and relations [3]. Lately, a lot of research has been conducted on extracting relations from medical textual data, especially the medical literature. Many datasets have been provided to researchers in order to find the best technique to extract relations between different medical entities. One of the tasks is to extract interactions (relations) between chemicals and genes (proteins). BioCreative VI task 5 provided ChemProt dataset [4] to the research community. Many techniques have been adopted to enhance the relation extraction task on this dataset. Deep neural networks have been applied in [5–8]. Some other used the ensemble methods between machine learning classifiers and neural networks as in [7, 9]. While attention networks caught some attention in [10–14]. Text representation models played an important role in enhancing the relation extraction task in general lately. The usage of different word embeddings techniques, and language models such as Bidirectional Encoder Representations from Transformers (BERT) [15] and [16] could achieve significantly promising results. BioCreativeVII provided another data set for detecting textual relations between drugs and chemical-proteins interactions (DrugProt)[1] from PubMed abstracts, which is considered an extension to the ChemProt data set. In this paper we are applying a relation extraction deep learning model based on SciBERT on the ChemProt data set and the DrugProt dataset, showing how a deep learning model based on SciBERT could achieve remarkable results. The rest of the paper is organized as follows, Sect. 2 presents the recent related work of relation extraction from biomedical data. Section 3 demonstrates the methodology used, Sect. 4 presents the experimental settings and results, and finally Sect. 5 concludes our work and suggests future work.

2 Related Work

The major relation extraction techniques used for biomedical data, specifically from the ChemProt data set can be categorized into deep learning techniques, ensemble technique, attention network technique, and using pre-trained language model like BERT. In this section we are going to highlight how those techniques were used and the scores they could achieve in extracting relations between chemicals and proteins.

2.1 Deep Learning Techniques

In [5] they applied a tree of LSTM with other additional features including a position feature, they could achieve F1 score of 58.53%. Convolutional Neural Networks (CNN) was applied in [6] along with word embedding and relative position embedding, which is the relative distance between the current word and the two target entities to find the relation between them in a sentence, they achieved F1 score of 68%. To overcome the over-confident of the model results from being trained on hard labelled data, a deep neural network with uncertainty and calibration is proposed in [17] and achieved F1 score of 78.83%.

2.2 Ensemble Technique

The ensemble of a support vector machine, a convolutional neural network, and a recurrent neural network is presented in [18], the output of the ensemble is combined using majority voting or stacking, F1 score of 64% could be achieved from this ensemble. Another ensemble of four neural networks consists of LSTM chains representing the sequence of words, part of speech tags, edges on the parse graph along the shortest dependency path between entities, is presented in [9] achieving F1 score of 63%.

2.3 Attention Networks

Attention layers has been used along with deep contextualized word representation and Bi-LSTM in [12] to achieve a F1 score of 65.9%. Another application of the attention networks is presented in [19] as the "Attention capsule", where a capsule is a set of neurons use activity vectors to represent instantiation parameters for a particular type of entity, it is used as a replacement for max pooling or average pooling in data aggregation. The attention capsule is used along with BERT as a language model for word embedding, they could achieve F1 score of 74.7%.

2.4 BERT-Based Models

BERT stands for Bidirectional Encoder Representation from Transformers [15], it is a language model design to pre-train deep bidirectional representations from unlabeled text through considering both the left and the right context in all layers instead of the common one directional models. The pre-trained model can be fine tuned by adding one additional output layer to serve as a model for various NLP tasks, such as name entity recognition, relation extraction, question answering, language inference, etc. The pre-trained model is trained using the BooksCorpus of 800M words [14], which is a large collection of free novel books written by unpublished authors, which contains 11,038 books (around 74M sentences and 1G words) of 16 different sub-genres (e.g., Romance, Historical, Adventure, etc.), and English Wikipedia 2500M words. The data is from general and various domains. SciBERT [20] is a pre-trained model based on BERT, yet trained with more specific scientific corpus. It is trained with a random sample of 1.14 million papers from Semantic Scholar with the following distribution, 18% from computer science, 82% from the general biomedical domains. The corpus consists of full text of the papers, not only the abstracts. The total token size of the corpus is 3.17 billion tokens. The sentences are split using Scispacy [21] which is the scientific version of spacy optimized for scientific text.

3 Methodology

In this section we are explaining the architecture of a relation extraction SciBERT-based deep learning model, and how it performs on ChemProt test set when trained with ChemProt training data set and a combination of ChemProt and DrugProt datasets.

3.1 ChemProt Dataset

Biocreative VI ChemProt dataset, which consists of abstracts of biomedical papers collected from PubMed. The data is labelled with chemical and genes entities and 9 possible groups of relations between them. The total number of relations is 22 relation. Table 1 shows the data distribution as training, development and test sets. The abstracts records are provided along with the entities location in the abstract and their names. The relations between entities in each abstract are provided as labels. The sentences records represent the sentences including two entities and a relation, any sentence that does not include a relation between two entities is dropped.

Table 1. ChemProt data distribution

	Training	Development	Test
Abstracts records	1020	612	800
Sentences records	4170	2428	3470

3.2 DrugProt Dataset

DrugProt data set is devised in the same manner of ChemProt, provided abstracts of PubMed abstracts along with manually annotated entities and relations between each two entities. The number of relations is 13 (included in the relations on the ChemProt dataset) and unlike the ChemProt data set they are not grouped. Table 2 shows the distribution of data as training, and development sets.

Table 2. DrugProt data distribution

	Training	Development
Abstracts records	3500	750
Sentences records	17275	3762

3.3 Pre-processing

- Load the tokenizer from the SciBERT model, the scibert-base-uncased pretrained SciBERT model is used.
- Reading provided training and test data files.
- Parse the data to separate the sentence and the relational statement and save them in data frames.
- Give ids to the relations.
- Tokenize the train and test data using the loaded tokenizer.
- Pad the sequence length of each sentence/label so they have the same length.
- Data is ready for training and predicting process.

3.4 Training the Model

After the data is prepared and processed it's used to train the model. The model takes a given relation statement *r*, in order to predict a relation type $t \cdot T$, where T is a set of given relations including the "NOT" relation which indicates that there is no relation between the given two entities. The model is based on the pre-trained model of SciBERT while training some of the final layers and adding some layers for the relation classification task. Each sentence is tokenized using the SciBERT tokenizer. The tokenizer first represents the words as IDs, such that each unique word is represented with a unique ID. The SciBERT tokenizer is based on the BERT tokenizer. Basically, this tokenizer not only separate tokens and give them IDs, but also do this separation based on the domain vocabulary of the SciBERT, such that it can separate unigrams, bigrams, or trigrams based on the context and the meaning of the word. For example, the word "beta 1-adrenoceptors" is identified as a single entity despite the space separating the two tokens. It also identifies the start and end of the sentence by adding special tokens indicating that. Afterwards, each token is embedded and represented as a vector of length 512.

3.5 SciBERT Base Model Architecture

- Input layer is a vector of tokenized words of a sentence, tokenized using the SciBERT tokenizer.
- Each sentence is represented as a tensor of embedded tokens, length of embedded vector is 512.
- Each tensor is encoded using two layers of bidirectional BiLSTM, each of 200 units as a Sequence-to-Sequence encoder.
- Load SciBERT pre-trained model to be the base network.
- Add a fully connected layer of 200 neurons and a ReLU activation function.
- Softmax is used as activation function, for multiclass classification.

3.6 SciBERT Fine-Tuned Model

In the fine-tuned model, the same steps explained in the base model are carried out, except that all layers in the SciBERT base model are retrained without freezing any layer.

Figure 1 shows an abstract architecture for the model based on SciBERT.

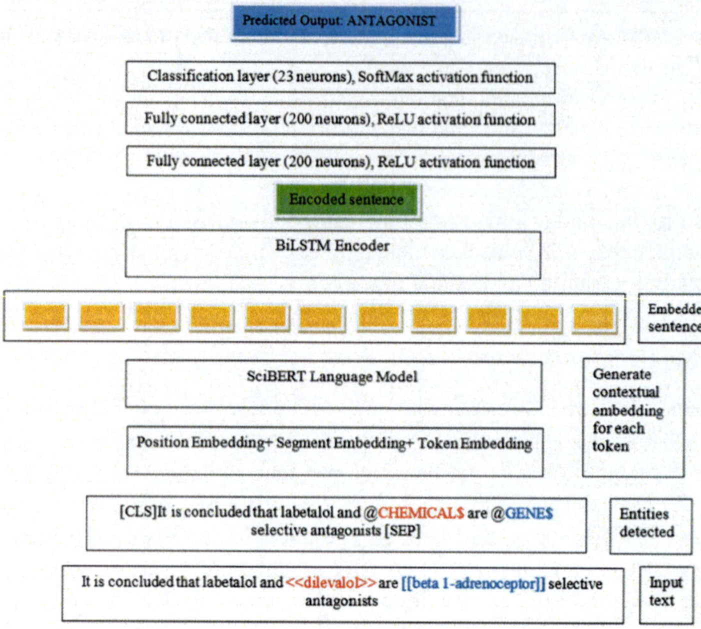

Fig. 1. Model architecture based on SciBERT

4 Experiments

In this section the experimental settings are presented to train a SciBERT based deep learning model once with ChemProt Data and once with combined training and development data from ChemProt and DrugProt and test the model on the test set of the ChemProt data set. Table 3 shows the combined training data statistic, where the training sentence records is about 5 times the training records used for the ChemProt Data. The following steps are taken for training the model on both data. Average Micro F1 score is used to evaluate the model.

Table 3. Combined data distribution

	Training	Development	Test
Abstracts records	4520	1362	800
Sentences records	21445	6190	3470

4.1 Training Setting for SciBERT Base Model

– Freeze most of the SciBERT pretrained model layers and train the types of the following layers:

- classifier
- pooler
- encoder.layer.11
- classification_layer
- blanks_linear
- lm_linear

– loss function: crossentropy, optimizer bert_adam
– Number of epochs is 75
– Learning rate 0.001

4.2 Training Setting for SciBERT Fine-Tuned Model

– Load the SciBERT pretrained model layers and train all layers
– loss function: crossentropy, optimizer bert_adam
– Number of epochs is 75
– Learning rate 0.00003

4.3 Training Setting for SciBERT Fine-Tuned Model with Extra Fully Connected Layers

– Load the SciBERT pretrained model layers and train all layers
– Add two fully connected layer before the classification layer each of 200 neurons
– loss function: crossentropy, optimizer bert_adam
– Number of epochs is 75
– Learning rate 0.00003

4.4 Results

The model is trained once with training data of ChemProt data set using the three settings mentioned above and applied to the test set. The best model out of the three settings is trained with the combined training data from ChemProt and DrugProt, then predict the same test set and record the performance. Table 4 shows the results of ChemProt is compared to the results mentioned in [16].

Table 4. ChemProt results

SciBERT Base micro F1	SciBERT fine-tuning micro F1	SciBERT fine-tuning, extra layer micro F1
75.32	82.67	**83.99**

Table 5 shows the results of the SciBERT fine-tuned with extra two layers model, trained with the combined ChemProt and DrugProt datasets and predicting the test set.

Table 5. ChemProt-DrugProt results

ChemProt SciBERT fine-tuning, extra layer micro F1	ChemProt-DrugProt SciBERT fine- tuning, extra layer micro F1
83.99	**91.75**

The results is compared to the model trained with the ChemProt data only. The model is trained with 20 epochs.

From the above results we can see that adding two fully connected layers to the fine-tuned SciBERT model enhanced the results by around 0.3%. Training the model with combined training data from the ChemProt and DrugProt enhanced the results by 7.75%, while training for less epochs, 20 instead of 75.

5 Conclusion and Future Work

We presented a relation extraction deeplearning model based on SciBERT. The model is trained with ChemProt training data set and predicted the test set and could achieve an average micro F1 score of 83.99% which is 0.3% more the base model presented in [16]. When training the model with a combined data from ChemProt and DrugProt, the model could achieve an average micro F1 score of 91.75% which is 7.75% more than the model trained with only ChemProt data set with only 20 epochs versus 75 epochs. We can observe that adding more fully connected layer to the model could enhance the performance of the fine-tuned SciBERT based model for extraction of relations between chemicals and protein/gene entities. The increase of the training data by about 5 times the sentence records lead to significant enhancement of the results. In our future work we are considering developing a generic model for relation extraction of biomedical entities, through training the model with different data sets including relations between different biomedical entities.

Acknowledgment. This research is under the project "Jesor", funded by the Academy of Scientific Research and Technology (ASRT).

References

1. Grishman, R.: Information extraction: techniques and challenges. In: Pazienza, M.T. (ed.) SCIE 1997. LNCS, vol. 1299, pp. 10–27. Springer, Heidelberg (1997). https://doi.org/10.1007/3-540-63438-X_2
2. Khoo, C.S.G., Chan, S., Niu, Y.: Extracting causal knowledge from a medical database using graphical patterns. In: Proceedings of the 38th Annual Meeting of the Association for Computational Linguistics, Hong Kong, pp. 336–343. Association for Computational Linguistics, October 2000

3. Shi, Y., Xiao, Y., Niu, L.: A brief survey of relation extraction based on distant supervision. In: Rodrigues, J.M.F., et al. (eds.) ICCS 2019. LNCS, vol. 11538, pp. 293–303. Springer, Cham (2019). https://doi.org/10.1007/978-3-030-22744-9_23
4. Krallinger, M., et al.: Overview of the BioCreative VI chemical-protein interaction track (2017)
5. Lim, S., Kang, J.: Chemical–gene relation extraction using recursive neural network. Database **2018** (2018)
6. Yüksel, A., Öztürk, H., Ozkirimli, E., Özgür, A.: CNN-Based Chemical-Protein Interactions Classification, p. 3
7. Peng, Y., Rios, A., Kavuluru, R., Lu, Z.: Extracting chemical–protein relations with ensembles of SVM and deep learning models. Database **2018** (2018)
8. Antunes, R., Matos, S.: Extraction of chemical–protein interactions from the literature using neural networks and narrow instance representation. Database **2019**, baz095 (2019)
9. Mehryary, F., Bjorne, J., Salakoski, T., Ginter, F.: Potent pairing: ensemble of long short-term memory networks and support vector machine for chemical-protein relation extraction. Database **2018** (2018)
10. Liu, S., et al.: Attention-Based Neural Networks for Chemical Protein Relation Extraction, p. 4
11. Zhang, Y., Guo, Z., Lu, W.: Attention Guided Graph Convolutional Networks for Relation Extraction. arXiv:1906.07510 [cs], March 2020. arXiv:1906.07510
12. Zhang, Y., Lin, H., Yang, Z., Wang, J., Sun, Y.: Chemical–protein interaction extraction via contextualized word representations and multihead attention. Database **2019**, baz054 (2019)
13. Lu, H., Li, L., He, X., Liu, Y., Zhou, A.: Extracting chemical-protein interactions from biomedical literature via granular attention based recurrent neural networks. Comput. Methods Programs Biomed. **176**, 61–68 (2019)
14. Verga, P., McCallum, A.: Predicting Chemical Protein Relations with Biaffine Relation Attention Networks, p. 3
15. Devlin, J., Chang, M.-W., Lee, K., Toutanova, K.: BERT: Pre-training of Deep Bidirectional Transformers for Language Understanding. arXiv:1810.04805 [cs], May 2019. arXiv:1810.04805
16. Beltagy, I., Lo, K., Cohan, A.: SciBERT: a pretrained language model for scientific text. In: Proceedings of the 2019 Conference on Empirical Methods in Natural Language Processing and the 9th International Joint Conference on Natural Language Processing (EMNLP-IJCNLP), Hong Kong, China, pp. 3613–3618. Association for Computational Linguistics (2019)
17. Choi, D., Lee, H.: Extracting chemical-protein interactions via calibrated deep neural network and self-training. In: Findings of the Association for Computational Linguistics: EMNLP 2020, (Online), pp. 2086–2095. Association for Computational Linguistics, November 2020
18. Peng, Y.: Chemical-protein relation extraction with ensembles of SVM, CNN, and RNN models, p. 4
19. Sun, C., Yang, Z., Wang, L., Zhang, Y., Lin, H., Wang, J.: Attention guided capsule networks for chemical-protein interaction extraction. J. Biomed. Inform. **103**, 103392 (2020)
20. SciBERT: A Pretrained Language Model for Scientific Text - ACL Anthology
21. Neumann, M., King, D., Beltagy, I., Ammar, W.: ScispaCy: fast and robust models for biomedical natural language processing. In: Proceedings of the 18th BioNLP Workshop and Shared Task, Florence, Italy, pp. 319–327. Association for Computational Linguistics, August 2019

Chemical-Gene Relation Extraction with Graph Neural Networks and BERT Encoder

Mina Esmail Zadeh Nojoo Kambar(✉), Armin Esmaeilzadeh, and Kazem Taghva

Department of Computer Science, University of Nevada Las Vegas, Las Vegas, NV 89154, USA
{esmailza,esmaeilz}@unlv.nevada.edu, kazem.taghva@unlv.edu

Abstract. Identifying named entities and their interactions from biomedical texts is essential for medical research. In this work, we modify the graph neural networks for relation extraction (RIFRE) model for biomedical text, named Bio-RIFRE that jointly extracts chemical-gene named entities and their interactions from biomedical texts. This model (Bio-RIFRE) utilizes the heterogeneous graph neural network model to strengthen the representation of biomedical text and relation extraction. As a result, Bio-RIFRE achieves 3% better F1-score on the CHEMPROT dataset than the other joint entity-relation extraction models. In addition, The results show that in the overlapping cases, and when the number of relations in a sentence increases, the model is robust and achieves a better F1-score.

Keywords: Relation extraction · BERT encoder · Graph neural networks · Biomedical text

1 Introduction

Automatic creation of knowledge-based systems from unstructured texts assists experts by avoiding time intensive equivalent manual activities [1]. Two of the critical parts of this process are the named entity recognition (NER) and relation extraction (RE) using natural language processing (NLP). The NER task identifies entities such as gene, chemicals, and diseases while the RE task discovers the relationships among these entities. The simplest form of the relation extractions are the binary relations in the form of triples *(Entity-1, Relation-type, Entity-2)* [2]. In the last decade, BioCreative (a critical assessment of text mining methods in molecular biology) has provided competition to extract annotated biomedical triples such as *(Chemical, Interaction-type, Gene)* from documents in PubMed [3,4].

Typically, each PubMed document may contain several triples. There are three different kind of triples based on their overlapping degree. First, *normal* sequence, in which its triples do not overlap on entities. Second, the *single*

K. Daimi and A. Al Sadoon (Eds.): ICR 2022, AISC 1431, pp. 166–179, 2022.
https://doi.org/10.1007/978-3-031-14054-9_17

entity overlap (SEO) includes at least one triple that has an entity in common with other triples. Third, *entity pair overlap* (EPO), which contains at least two triples precisely with the same entities but different relation groups [5,6]. EPO sequences are multi-label classification problems that are common in biomedical datasets such as BioCreative. For instance, given the text "DBDCT up-regulated the expression of Bax down-regulated the expression of Bcl-2 and significantly increased the ratio of Bax/Bcl-2" the pair Chem-GENE ("DBCT," "Bcl-2") is categorized as both CPR:3 and CPR:4 relation classes in BioCreative dataset [4].

The previous research, such as [7,8] mainly used pipeline methods for the task of NER and RE. Generally, the pipeline method composes of two phases. In the first phase, all possible pairs (Chemical, Gene) are extracted, in the second phase, a classification technique is used to find the relation. However, converting the RE problem to a classification task not only increases the complexity of classifying a massive number of pairs but also causes error propagation from the NER to RE tasks [9,10]. Additionally, there are other challenges that the pipeline method cannot handle such as the cases where one entity is a sub-string of other entities or triples overlapped cases as discussed in [11].

Joint models are proposed to alleviate the above mentioned difficulties by extracting the triples through a merged technique of NER and RE. These Joint learning methods employed neural network-based models [5,12] that automatically find features of the texts to generate a representation of the documents. As a result, they have significantly improved the triple extraction compared to models that do the feature extraction manually. However, previous joint models have difficulty in the following areas:

1. Methods that are not span-based cannot recognize the nested named entities. For example, they cannot consider "Baz/Bcl-2" and "Bcl-2" as two named entities simultaneously.
2. Techniques that isolate the relations from the documents' word vectors ignore the context of the sentence for generating the relations' representation of triples.
3. The previous methods' performance decreases as the number of triples increases in the sequences.

Our main contributions in this work are:

- The introduction of the Bio-RIFRE model, which is a modification of RIFRE [12] model for biomedical application. This model is trained with BioBert to capture biomedical context. Bio-RIFRE has also removed the gate section of the Graph Attention Neural Network (GANN) of RIFRE and utilized the original GANN [13] model. Adding GANN strengthens the contextual representation of the chemicals, genes, and their relationship.
- The evaluation of Bio-RIFRE on sequences with different numbers of triples shows that this model outperforms the previous model and offers a robust behavior in such a way that the performance does not change radically when the number of triples per sequence increases.

- The Bio-RIFRE outperforms the state-of-art joint model on the CHEMPROT (CPI) [4] datasets by achieving a total of 3% better F1 score.
- The result on the CPI dataset shows that in entities overlapping cases like Normal, SEO, and EPO sequences, Bio-RIFRE achieves 3%, 2%, and 14% better F-1 scores.
- The evaluation of this model on the new BioCreative dataset called DrugProt [14] also shows that although the number of relation classes and the dataset size are more extensive, our model is robust and effective.

2 Task Definition

In the chemical-protein interaction problem, the formulation of the joint entities relation extraction task is discovering all possible *(Chemical, Relation-type, Gene)* triples in the text. For simplicity, in the rest of the paper, we represent triples in (ch, r, g) form. Equation 1 illustrates the objective function of the joint chemical-products and gene-protein interaction task. We follow the notation and formulation technique proposed by [15].

$$\prod_{j=1}^{|D|}\left[\prod_{(ch,\ r,\ g)\in T_j} p((ch,\ r,\ g)|x_j)\right] \tag{1}$$

The training dataset has $|D|$ number of sequences, and j is a counter to iterate through the different training set sequences. T_j is the set of all triples available in the jth sequence. Equation (1) indicates the probability of finding all triples (ch, r, g) in the given tokenized sequence x_j. Our goal is to maximize the likelihood of finding all triples. By expanding Eq. (1) using chain rule (probability), we will achieve Eqs. (2) and (3).

$$\prod_{j=1}^{|D|}\left[\prod_{ch\in T_j} p(ch|x_j) \prod_{(r,\ g)\in(T_j|ch)} p((r,g)|ch,x_j)\right] \tag{2}$$

$$\prod_{j=1}^{|D|}\left[\prod_{ch\in T_j} p(ch|x_j) \prod_{r\in T_j|ch} p(g|x_j,ch,r) \prod_{r\in R\setminus T_j|ch} p(g_{\varnothing}|x_j,ch,r)\right]. \tag{3}$$

where $ch \in T_j$ denotes the chemicals within triples of the sequence j, and $r \in T_j|ch$ is the relations (interaction) conducted by chemical "ch". Also, $r \in R \setminus T_j|ch$, indicates all relations excluding those that are in triples with chemical "ch". In Eq. (3), a given chemical (ch) can either have relations with gene g, illustrated in $p(g|ch, x_j)$, or do not have relationships called null gene $g_{\varnothing}$ illustrated in $p(g_{\varnothing}|ch, x_j)$. We aim to maximize this objective function and find a chemical tagger that learns chemical entities in a sequence $p(ch|x_j)$, for those interactions (relation) led by the chemical in the sequence $p(g|ch, x_j)$, and those relations that chemical *ch*, does not lead indicated at $p(g_{\varnothing}|ch, x_j)$.

3 Model Architecture

In the following section, we outline the overall architecture of the Bio-RIFRE model and details of each layer and component. The model architecture shown in Fig. 1 is composed of three main layers: the word embedding layer, the Graph Attention Network (GAN) layer, and the final chemical and gene taggers.

The trained model will provide us the hidden relation embedding vector which we will use to classify the relationship between paired entities in a sentence.

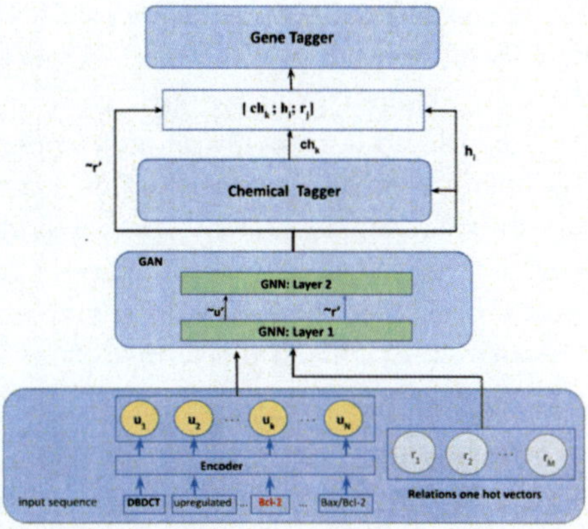

Fig. 1. An overview of Bio-RIFRE for joint entities relation extraction [12]

3.1 Word Embedding

The base layer of the model uses two different word embedding components to transform the sentence and the relations into vector representations. Given a sentence with N words, we utilize the BioBERT model [16] based on BERT encoder to create word embedding vectors. The BERT model was proposed by [17] and it employs the encoder block of the transformers architecture [18] to extract deep bidirectional representations from both the left and right contexts of words in a sentence [17,19].

The BioBERT model had been shown to outperform previous unidirectional models that its pre-trained architecture allows us to utilize it without further training. For the relation embedding, given a sentence with R relations, we initialize random one-hot vector representations to embed each relation. These relation vectors are what we intend to train in the next layers and enrich their vector representations with words embedding.

As shown in Fig. 1, the output of the embedding layer are word $[u_1, u_2, ..., u_N]$ and relation $[r_1, r_2, r_3, ..., r_M]$ tensors. Where m and n respectively indicate the number of relation classes and the sequence length. The output of the embedding layer is fed into the GAN layer to update the tensors and give a prior knowledge of potential relations to the words' and relations' representations.

3.2 Graph Attention Networks

Graph Attention Networks (GAN) was proposed by [13] to apply a self-attention mechanism to graph-structured data. Before GAN models, the Convolutions Neural Networks (CNN) [20] had been successfully utilized in various fields such as Image Processing. The success of CNNs led to an increasing interest to generalize the convolutions techniques on graph-structured data. However, these models could not be properly applied to data representations that did not have a grid-like structure, such as text data [13].

Earlier, researchers proposed Graph Neural Networks (GNN) to utilize neural networks to process structured graph data [21]. More recently, with the introduction of attention mechanisms, there is a new approach to model sequence-based data, such as words in a text, as nodes in a graph, and apply self-attention strategy to extract the relationship between nodes. In this study, we use the model proposed in [12]. Therefore, we consider two types of nodes: word nodes and relation nodes, which are connected if they participate in at least one triple. In each given GAN layer of the model, there are three steps to update the vector representation of nodes with an attention mechanism that we describe below.

First Step - Calculate Attention Weights. Given a sentence with N number of words and R number of relations, let u_i be the words and r_i be the relations in the sentence. Consider every word embedding u_i and every relation embedding r_i as nodes in a graph that are neighbors. Figure 2 shows the nodes connection.

Given word-relation pair of nodes in the graph, we calculate the attention weights, α, between each pair using the following equation [13]:

$$a_{ij} = W_a[W_q u_i : W_k r_j] \tag{4}$$

$$\alpha_{ij} = \frac{\exp(a_{ij})}{\sum_i^N \exp(a_{ij})} \tag{5}$$

in which W_a, W_q, W_k are trainable parameters in the neural network and [:] is the concatenation of two high-dimensional vectors.

Second Step - Update Vector Representations. Once we have the attention weights for each pair of word-relation nodes, we update the vector representation of each node in the graph. In this process, we take each u_i node and apply the following equation to update its vector representation considering all relation nodes and their importance to u_i. Figure 3 illustrates an example for the first word node $i = 1$ updating in GAN.

$$u_i' = u_i + \sum_j^M \alpha_{ij} W_r r_j \tag{6}$$

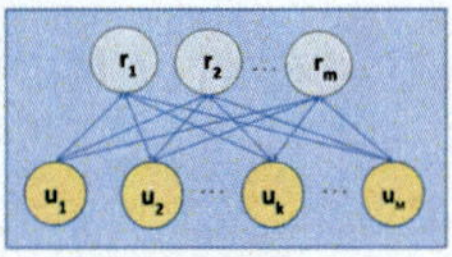

Fig. 2. GNN nodes connections

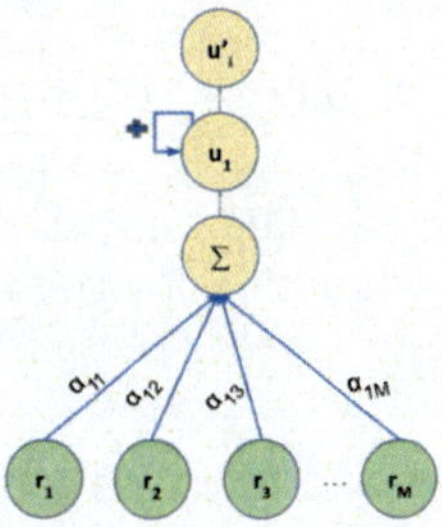

Fig. 3. A schema of how word and relation nodes are getting updated in GAN.

We perform the same calculation to update each r_i node, considering their attention to all the other u_i nodes:

$$r_i' = r_i + \sum_{j}^{N} \alpha_{ij} W_r u_j \tag{7}$$

Third Step. In the architecture proposed by [12], the third step uses a gate mechanism instead of the activation function originally described in [13]. However, we didn't find any statistically significant difference in results by using the gate mechanism, and therefore, the original activation function is used.

3.3 Relation Extraction and Tagging

After updating the word and relation representations at the last GNN layer, we use the CasRel framework from [15] to discover all chemical and gene candidate entities in a given sequence. The model consists of two cascade processes namely a Chemical and Gene tagger.

Chemical Tagger. We use the updated u_i' embeddings from the last layer of the GAN network as input to the Chemical tagger. This tagger is composed of two binary classifiers to detect the first and last word positions of the Chemical's Named Entities in a given input sentence.

$$p_i^{start_{ch}} = \sigma(W_{start} u_i' + b_{start}) \tag{8}$$

$$p_i^{end_{ch}} = \sigma(W_{end} u_i' + b_{end}) \tag{9}$$

Firstly, based on Eqs. (8) and (9), for each token of the input, the probability of being a named entity is calculated. $p_i^{start_{ch}}$ demonstrated the probability of the i-th token in the sentence to be the starting position of the chemical, and $p_i^{end_{ch}}$

is the probability of the i-th token to be the end position of the chemical. The W_{start}, W_{end}, b_{start} and b_{end} are trainable parameters and σ is the activation function [15]. The objective of the chemical tagger is to minimize the following likelihood function for the binary classifier:

$$p_{\theta}(ch|x) = \prod_{t \in \{start_{ch},\ end_{ch}\}} \prod_{i=1}^{N} (p_i^t)^{I\{y_i^t=1\}} (1 - p_i^t)^{I\{y_i^t=0\}} \tag{10}$$

where θ is parameter set of the chemical tagger, for a given sentence x, Eq. (10) calculates the probability of each word for being a chemical component, and t defines the start or end tags as $y_i^{start_{ch}}$ or $y_i^{end_{ch}}$, $I\{y_i^t = 1\}$ if the binary classifier tag is true and 0 otherwise.

We concatenate the output of the GAN layer for word nodes as h and relations nodes as r vectors with the output of the chemical tagger as ch and feed them into the tanh activation function to create the w'_{ijk} embedding vector as the input to the Gene tagger binary classifier to detect the start and end positions of Gene named entity in the sentence with their associated relations to a chemical named entity. Equation (11) shows how the input of gene tagger is created. The high-dimensional vector w'_{ijk} contains information about the chemical named entities of the sentence, and the potential relations that chemical and gene can conduct.

$$w'_{ijk} = \tanh(W_h[ch_k; r_j; h_i] + b_h) \tag{11}$$

Gene Tagger. The gene tagger finds a list of possible gene candidates for a given chemical named entity by considering all relations in the sentence iteratively. Equations (12) and (13) calculate the probability of i-th position to be the start or the end of the genes' span. W_{start}, W_{end}, b_{start}, b_{end} are trainable parameters.

$$p_i^{start_g} = \sigma(W_{start} w'_{ijk} + b_{start}) \tag{12}$$

$$p_i^{end_g} = \sigma(W_{end} w'_{ijk} + b_{end}) \tag{13}$$

The likelihood function of the gene binary classifiers is similar to the chemical tagger describes earlier with the same definitions in the chemical tagger subsection.

$$p_{\theta}(g|x, ch, r) = \prod_{t \in start_s, end_s} \prod_{i=1}^{L} (p_i^t)^{I\{y_i^t=1\}} (1 - p_i^t)^{I\{y_i^t=0\}} \tag{14}$$

Finally, the loss function for the entire model can be defined using the method described in [12] by combining the likelihood functions of the chemical and gene taggers. It is equal to taking log from Eq. (3):

$$\begin{aligned} L &= \log \prod_{(ch,r,g)\in T} p((ch,r,g)|x) \\ &= \sum_{ch\in T_j} \log p_{\boldsymbol{\theta}_{ch}}(ch|x) + \sum_{r\in T_j|ch} \log p_{\boldsymbol{\theta}_g}(g|x,ch,r) \\ &\quad + \sum_{r\in R\setminus T_j|ch} \log p_{\boldsymbol{\theta}_0}(g_{\emptyset}|x,ch,r) \end{aligned} \tag{15}$$

4 Experiment

4.1 Dataset

We assess Bio-RIFRE on two public CHEMPROT(CPI) [4] and DrugProt [14] datasets. Both datasets are from BioCreative VI track 5 and VII track 1, challenges. The goal of the datasets is to explore the chemical-genes/proteins interactions. The datasets are supervised and manually annotated to investigate the extraction of chemical-protein entity relation from PubMed abstracts. CPI's gold standard dataset has 2,420 abstract texts with five relation classes named CPR 3, CPR 4, CPR 5, CPR 6, and CPR 9. Two main groups of entities, called gene and chemical, have a total number of 30,339 and 31,831. DrugProt dataset has been recently published (2021). It analyzes 5,000 PubMed abstracts with thirteen different relation classes named INDIRECT DOWNREGULATOR, INDIRECT-UPREGULATOR, DIRECT-REGULATOR, ACTIVATOR, INHIBITOR, AGONIST, AGONIST-ACTIVATOR, AGONIST-INHIBITOR, ANTAGONIST, PRODUCT-OF, SUBSTRATE, SUBSTRATE_PRODUCT-OF, PART-OF. The number of Gene and chemical entities are 61,775 and 65,561. Table 1 illustrates the statistics of both datasets.

4.2 Evaluation Metrics and Hyperparameters

For the task of joint named entities relation extraction in a biomedical context, the model should correctly predict the chemical-gene span's start and end word positions. Therefore, a substring is not considered a valid named entity. Furthermore, it should also indicate Chemical-gene relations correctly. We use Precision(P), Recall(R), and Micro F1-score to evaluate the model.

Table 1. BioCreative VI and VII datasets statistics [22]

Dataset	Set	# Abstracts	# Relations	# Entities	
				Gene	Chemical
CHEMPROT	Training	1020	4157	12752	13017
	Development	800	2416	7568	8004
	Test	600	3458	10019	10810
DrugProt	Training	3500	17274	43255	46274
	Development	750	3761	9005	9853
	Test	750	3491	9515	9434

Based on our experiment on different pre-trained models we realized that the BioBert model [16], which is pre-trained on PubMed abstract datasets, is the best match for our purpose.

We use BioBert-cased pre-trained in Pytorch with the maximum token size of 512 in the embedding layer. Therefore the maximum sequence size is 512, and only triples that their chemical-genes entities are defined in the length of 512 are considered. It denotes the model drops all inter sequence triples. We use Stochastical Gradient Descent (SGD) for the optimizer with early stopping set to 20, which helps the model avoid overfitting. The learning rate is 0.1; the batch size was set to 10.

4.3 Baselines

We compare Bio-RIFRE with six following baseline models that have evaluated their joint methods on the CPI dataset. All the numbers are extracted from [9] and [23] papers which are the most recent studies in this field.

- **Att-BiLSTM-CRF+ELMO** [24] is attention-based. It uses CNN to extract character-level features and pretrained ELMO model in the embedding layer. Then, all collected features are concatenated and fed into two BiLSTM networks.
- **Dygiepp** [25] consists of two main layers on top of the word embedding layer. Mention recognition and relation extraction layers. This research utilizes CRF to calculate scores for Microorganism entities and their relationship.
- **SpanMB Bert** [9] proposed a novel span-based framework that fine-tuned BERT to get the contextual embeddings and then calculate span scores to classify the entities and relation types.
- **MRC4BioER** [23] utilizes BERT to convert the joint named entities relation extraction into a Machine Reading Comprehension (MRC) task and defines the sentence as Context, the relations as target Query, and the entity spans as Answer. In addition, this study provides a tagging algorithm that covers the overlapping problem by iteratively considering each span pairs for different relation classes.

- **MRC4BioER (Zheng's tagging)** the MRC4BioER model variation that utilizes Zheng's tagging [26] schema.
- **MRCBioER (Lou's tagging)** the MRC4BioER model variation that employs Lou's tagging [24] schema.

4.4 Result

Table 2 illustrates the results of models on the CPI dataset. The result indicates that using BERT in the embedding section has made a significant improvement. The SpanMB Bert model has the state-of-art with 0.88, F1-score for the NER task. The best performance between baseline models for the RE task is MRC4BioER, which achieves a 0.66 F1-score. The result shows that although Bio-RIFRE on NER task performance is not better than the SpanMB Bert model, Bio-RIFRE with a 0.69 F1-score outperforms all baseline models for RE task. This fact indicates that if Bio-RIFRE predicts chemical gene spans correctly, it will classify their relation more accurately than other baseline models.

Table 2. Result of different methods on the CPI dataset, the states-of-art are in bold format

Model	NER			RE		
	F1	R	P	F1	R	P
Att-BiLSTM-CRF+ELMo	0.811	0.798	0.825	0.551	0.512	0.595
Dygiepp	0.887	0.876	0.897	0.629	0.605	0.654
SpanMB Bert	**0.888**	**0.883**	**0.893**	0.646	0.615	0.680
MRC4BioER (Zheng's tagging)	-	-	-	0.615	0.539	0.717
MRC4BioER (Lou's tagging)	-	-	-	0.624	0.556	0.711
MRC4BioER	-	-	-	0.660	0.617	0.70
Bio_RIFRE	0.870	0.851	0.860	**0.690**	**0.70**	**0.681**

5 Discussion

We compare baseline models that provide results in term of some of their strength to handle the sequences with overlapped chemical genes named entities and sequences with different numbers of triples per sequence. Finally, we indicate that Bio-RIFRE keeps its robustness even for the datasets with more relation classes by evaluating it on the DrugProt dataset. Table 3 shows the result.

5.1 Chemical-Gene Overlapping

To compare Bio-RIFRE with some of the baseline models based on the various types of sequences, we evaluate the model separately on Normal, SEO, and

EPO sequences. MRCBioER variation models are the only baseline models that provide the result on different sequences types. Figure 5 illustrates the F1-score of the Bio-RIFRE model and three MRCBioER models. It denotes that in Normal, SEO, and EPO sequences, Bio-RIFRE increased F1-score respectively, 3% and 2% and 14%. The significant improvement for EPO sequences shows that the model works well for the multi-labeling task that assigns different relation classes to the triples with the same chemical-gene named entities.

5.2 Different Numbers of Triples per Sequence

To compare Bio-RIFRE with some of the baseline models in terms of robustness, we evaluate the model on a CPI test set with a different number of triples per sequence. For example, $N = 3$ just evaluates the model for sequences with three triples. Figure 5 illustrates the results, showing that the Bio-RIFRE model is robust when triples per sequence increase because in this trend the model's F1-score does not change significantly. Furthermore, when the number of triples in sequences is more than five, the Bio-RIFRE can figure out entities and their relationship better than other baseline models.

5.3 More Relation Classes

Table 3 indicated the result of the Bio-RIFRE model on the DrugProt dataset. This dataset is new, and there is not enough research available for comparison. However, the result shows that the Bio-RIFRE model works well even on the DrugProt dataset with thirteen different relation classes. Additionally, when the number of triples per sequence increases, the model performance does not alter significantly (Fig. 4).

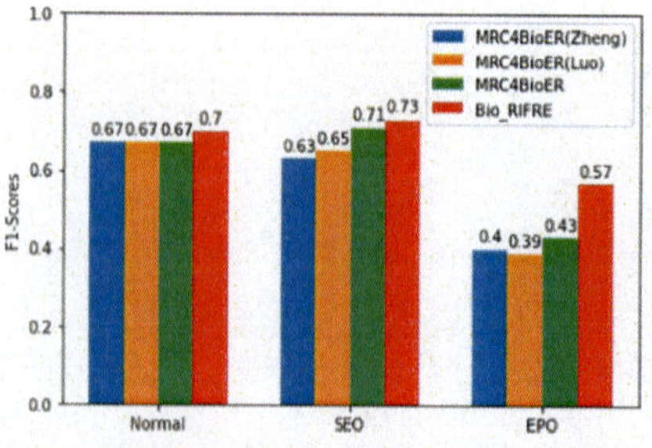

Fig. 4. F1-score of relation extraction task on Normal, SEO, and EPO sequences.

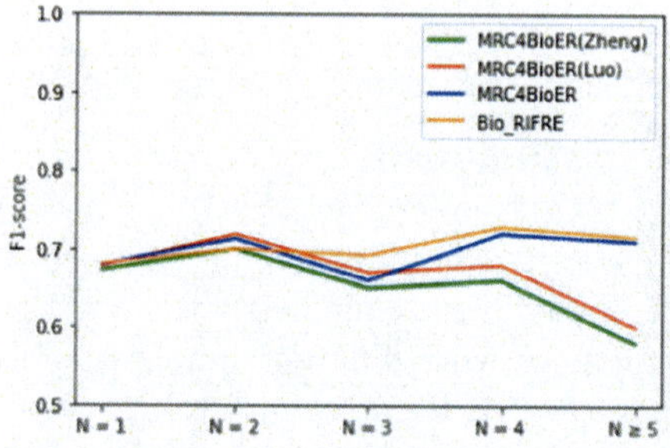

Fig. 5. F1-score of extracting different numbers of triples (N) from sequences.

Table 3. Performance of Bio-RIFRE on DrugProt with different number of triples in a sequence [22]

Number of triples	F1	R	P
N = 1	0.727	0.811	0.6595
N = 2	0.716	0.758	0.752
N = 3	0.7163	0.701	0.732
N = 4	0.7281	0.6985	0.7602
N ≥ 5	0.7144	0.6624	0.7752

6 Conclusion and Feature Work

This paper has investigated the feasibility of applying graph neural networks for the joint named entities relation extraction task in the biomedical domain. The result shows that the model outperforms the previous models on the CPI dataset and is robust when the number of relations per sentence or the number of relation classes increases. However, this model only detects the sentence-level relations and drops all those beyond a particular sentence. Therefore, we will customize the model to extract the relations at the document level in the feature.

Acknowledgment. This research is based upon work funded by the National Science Foundation under Grant No. 1625677.

References

1. Kambar, M.E.Z.N., Nahed, P., Cacho, J.R.F., Lee, G., Cummings, J., Taghva, K.: Clinical text classification of Alzheimer's drugs' mechanism of action. In: Yang, X.-S., Sherratt, S., Dey, N., Joshi, A. (eds.) Proceedings of Sixth International Congress on Information and Communication Technology. LNNS, vol. 235, pp. 513–521. Springer, Singapore (2022). https://doi.org/10.1007/978-981-16-2377-6_48
2. Zhao, S., Su, C., Lu, Z., Wang, F.: Recent advances in biomedical literature mining. Brief. Bioinform. **22**(3), bbaa057 (2020). https://doi.org/10.1093/bib/bbaa057
3. Krallinger, M., et al.: The CHEMDNER corpus of chemicals and drugs and its annotation principles. J. Cheminform. **7**(1), 1–17 (2015)
4. Krallinger, M., et al.: Overview of the BioCreative VI chemical-protein interaction track. In: Proceedings of the Sixth BioCreative Challenge Evaluation Workshop, vol. 1, pp. 141–146 (2017)
5. Zeng, X., Zeng, D., He, S., Liu, K., Zhao, J.: Extracting relational facts by an end-to-end neural model with copy mechanism. In: Proceedings of the 56th Annual Meeting of the Association for Computational Linguistics (Volume 1: Long Papers), pp. 506–514 (2018)
6. Kambar, M.E.Z.N., Esmaeilzadeh, A., Heidari, M.: A survey on deep learning techniques for joint named entities and relation extraction. In: 2022 IEEE World AI IoT Congress (AIIoT) (IEEE AIIOT 2022), Virtual, USA, June 2022

7. Warikoo, N., Chang, Y.-C., Hsu, W.-L.: LPTK: a linguistic pattern-aware dependency tree kernel approach for the BioCreative VI CHEMPROT task. Database **2018**, bay108 (2018). https://doi.org/10.1093/database/bay108
8. Lung, P.-Y., He, Z., Zhao, T., Yu, D., Zhang, J.: Extracting chemical-protein interactions from literature using sentence structure analysis and feature engineering. Database **2019** (2019)
9. Zuo, M., Zhang, Y.: A span-based joint model for extracting entities and relations of bacteria biotopes. Bioinformatics **38**(1), 220–227 (2021)
10. Zhang, Q., Liu, C., Chi, Y., Xie, X., Hua, X.: A multi-task learning framework for extracting bacteria biotope information. In: Proceedings of the 5th Workshop on BioNLP Open Shared Tasks, pp. 105–109 (2019)
11. Xiao, S., Song, M., et al.: A text-generated method to joint extraction of entities and relations. Appl. Sci. **9**(18), 3795 (2019)
12. Zhao, K., Xu, H., Cheng, Y., Li, X., Gao, K.: Representation iterative fusion based on heterogeneous graph neural network for joint entity and relation extraction. Knowl.-Based Syst. **219**, 106888 (2021)
13. Veličković, P., Cucurull, G., Casanova, A., Romero, A., Liò, P., Bengio, Y.: Graph attention networks. In: International Conference on Learning Representations (2018, accepted as poster). https://openreview.net/forum?id=rJXMpikCZ
14. Miranda, A., Mehryary, F., Luoma, J., Pyysalo, S., Valencia, A., Krallinger, M.: Overview of DrugProt BioCreative VII track: quality evaluation and large scale text mining of drug-gene/protein relations. In: Proceedings of the Seventh BioCreative Challenge Evaluation Workshop (2021)
15. Wei, Z., Su, J., Wang, Y., Tian, Y., Chang, Y.: A novel cascade binary tagging framework for relational triple extraction. In: Proceedings of the 58th Annual Meeting of the Association for Computational Linguistics, pp. 1476–1488 (2020)
16. Lee, J., et al.: BioBERT: a pre-trained biomedical language representation model for biomedical text mining. Bioinformatics **36**(4), 1234–1240 (2019). https://doi.org/10.1093/bioinformatics/btz682
17. Devlin, J., Chang, M.-W., Lee, K., Toutanova, K.: BERT: pre-training of deep bidirectional transformers for language understanding. arXiv preprint arXiv:1810.04805 (2018)
18. Vaswani, A.: Attention is all you need. In: Advances in Neural Information Processing Systems, vol. 30 (2017)
19. Esmaeilzadeh, A., Taghva, K.: Text classification using Neural Network Language Model (NNLM) and BERT: an empirical comparison. In: Arai, K. (ed.) IntelliSys 2021. LNNS, vol. 296, pp. 175–189. Springer, Cham (2022). https://doi.org/10.1007/978-3-030-82199-9_12
20. LeCun, Y., Bottou, L., Bengio, Y., Haffner, P.: Gradient-based learning applied to document recognition. Proc. IEEE **86**(11), 2278–2324 (1998)
21. Malekzadeh, M., Hajibabaee, P., Heidari, M., Zad, S., Uzuner, O., Jones, J.H.: Review of graph neural network in text classification. In: 2021 IEEE 12th Annual Ubiquitous Computing, Electronics Mobile Communication Conference (UEMCON), pp. 0084–0091 (2021)
22. Peng, Y., Rios, A., Kavuluru, R., Lu, Z.: Extracting chemical-protein relations with ensembles of SVM and deep learning models. Database **2018**, bay073 (2018). https://doi.org/10.1093/database/bay073
23. Sun, C., Yang, Z., Wang, L., Zhang, Y., Lin, H., Wang, J.: MRC4BioER: joint extraction of biomedical entities and relations in the machine reading comprehension framework. J. Biomed. Inf. **125**, 103956 (2022)

24. Luo, L., Yang, Z., Cao, M., Wang, L., Zhang, Y., Lin, H.: A neural network-based joint learning approach for biomedical entity and relation extraction from biomedical literature. J. Biomed. Inf. **103**, 103384 (2020)
25. Zhang, Q., Liu, C., Chi, Y., Xie, X., Hua, X.: A multi-task learning framework for extracting bacteria biotope information. In: BioNLP-OST@EMNLP-IJNCLP 2019 - Proceedings of the 5th Workshop on BioNLP Open Shared Tasks, pp. 105–109 (2019)
26. Zheng, S., Wang, F., Bao, H., Hao, Y., Zhou, P., Xu, B.: Joint extraction of entities and relations based on a novel tagging scheme. arXiv preprint arXiv:1706.05075 (2017)

Building Classes for Sentiment of Social Media Content Using WU Semantic Measure

Ahmad Kayed(✉) and Maha Ahmed Saidi

Faculty of Commuting and Information Technology, Sohar University, Sohar, Oman
akayed@su.edu.om, drkayed@ymail.com, maha.saidi@badailtech.com

Abstract. Sentiment classification or opinion mining is conducted to extract the core data representing opinions, and emotions. Motivated by the role of social media on appointing the dimension of the discussions, a solution is proposed to classify users' sentiments and define the most common topics deliberated by the users in Twitter. The proposed technique classifies user's sentiments by applying semantic measure to build classifications (classes) from user tweets. The classifications are alternated according to the study domain. This research has picked International Women's Day as the study domain because of the availability of historical data and the renewability of the topic. The proposed technique is building the classes that define the topics of interest. WuP (Wu and Palmer) measure is used to compute how much the tweets' words are similar to the classes' concepts. In the topic domain "International Women's Day", 2000 tweets have been used to build the four classes (Activity, Women role, Time, and Surroundings).

Keywords: Semantic measures · Sentiment analysis · Similarity measure · Social media · Opinion mining

1 Introduction

The significance of processing data is increasing with the expansion of big data. Every calculation involving the human beings is involving data as well. Therefore, processing, mining and classifying unstructured data to retrieve structured data is critical. From the general concept of data, text mining is used to collect and derive information with high quality from a text. The Human can classify the data or the information they capture from a given text into classes according to the understanding of the concept. The challenge is in large amount of substantial data that the system retrieves from the users, since it has different ambiguous sentiments. Sentiments are claims about a topic when the user define his opinion. Sentiments are used to present the emotions or opinions regarding a specific phenomenon or topic. Classification is the act of dividing things into groups according to their type.

Sentiment classification is used to transform unstructured sentiments into structured sentiments by classifying the sentiments into defined classes. There are variety of methodologies to classify the sentiments of the users, this paper proposes a way to calculate the relatedness between the text using semantic measurements. In this paper,

K. Daimi and A. Al Sadoon (Eds.): ICR 2022, AISC 1431, pp. 180–189, 2022.
https://doi.org/10.1007/978-3-031-14054-9_18

Wu and Palmer [1] semantic measure is used for sentiment classification. This paper classifies the data retrieved from the users in the social media semantically. The paper will build open classes for the topic of interest by the users. The main contribution of this paper is to build these classes (clusters) where tweets or text can be classified under theses cluster to find out the most and least topic of interest. The main objective of this paper is to semantically classify social media, users' unstructured sentiments into structured open classes according to the domain of the study in order to obtain the most interested topics of the domain.

The paper is organized as follows: section two gives background on ontology, semantic, calcification and social media. Section three presents experiment to show how to build these classes. Section four discusses the outcomes and section five concludes the paper.

2 Background Information and Related Work

2.1 Ontology and Semantic Measure

An ontology corresponds the concepts and their relationships, which can exist for an agent or a group of agents in an environment. An ontology can define specification of conceptualization. Ontology is used to enable sharing knowledge in a specific domain. For instance, when using ontology in Artificial Intelligence it can answer questions using the relationship of the concepts. Moreover, in knowledge-based system whenever an ontology exists reflect on the knowledge existence. Where the agents can retrieve the concepts, properties and relationships from the ontology and act according to that [2].

Knowledge-based measures of word-to-word semantic similarity uses information derived from semantic network to identify to which degree two words are similar [2]. Most effective semantic results are retrieved from six knowledge-based measure classified into three family groups according to their theoretical principals. First family group is Path Length Family such as Wu and Palmer Measure and Leacock & Chodorow Measure. Second family group is Information Content Family as Resnik Measure and LIN Measure. Last family is Semantic Relatedness Family for instance LESK Measure and Hirst & St-Onge Measure.

2.2 Ontology and Semantic Measure

Using sematic and calcification have used recently in many applications. Fan et al. have built a model to detect and classify toxicity in social media from user-generated content using the Bidirectional Encoder Representations from Transformers (BERT) [3]. Zhu et al. have proposed a new neural microblog sentiment classification method which learns informative representations of microblog posts by exploiting both a user's contextual information and his/her historical state information [4]. While Wu et al. have used semantic analysis to design a smart city evaluation system. They defined a list of keywords for automated information scraping; then they used semantic analysis to update the City Intelligence Quotient [5].

Sentiment classification describes opinions of the users using the context of the sentence [6]. Sentiment classification is usually applied on the document level to retrieve the overall positive or negative sentiment of the tweet. Using Sentiment classification any unstructured data can be transformed into structured data about product or phenomena. Business administration uses sentiment classification to develop their products and services according to the customers' feedback. That is why sentiment classification is highly used specially on social media to get the users opinions. An example of such a lexicon that has been widely used in the social media domain for sentiment classification is the Linguistic Inquiry and Word Count (LIWC, pronounced "Luke") [7]. Working on sentence level increase the validity of the retrieved sentiments. Therefore, this research works on the tweet level rather than group of tweets or an overall domain.

2.3 Social Media Sentiment Classification

Most of the studies have used Twitter because it is considered as an official social media site where people express their opinions via twitting their sentiments in addition it is sometimes called the news media [8]. Many literatures have been done to explain some techniques used to extract user opinions regarding either a topic or product. Twitter is a rich data source as a micro-blogging website where exchanging opinion and feelings is available and highly used by the users [9].

Kontopoulos et al. [9] have proposed a technique using language based processing of the tweet for studying the opinion of the users by either agree, disagree or neutral regarding a specific topic in live time tweets. Furthermore, Niranjan et al. [10] have proposed a methodology in form of web application to visualize user sentiments using a specific keyword or a hashtag. Tagliarino et al. [11] have used a methodology, which does not rely on a dictionary or lexicon of words to analyze the data perform. However, it uses a word-by-word analysis. Then they have applied benchmarking to the tweets using text-summarization techniques like term frequency–inverse document frequency (TF-IDF). Habtegebriel et al. [12] established another study of Twitter sentiment classification to tourism sector, the main aim of this study is to classify users' opinion regarding hotels and hotel chains by giving positive, negative or neutral feedback. They have used live time messages to retrieve exact live time data. They have applied unsupervised machine learning during the experiment.

3 Experiment (Building the Classes)

Since the main objective of this paper is to semantically classify social media, users' unstructured sentiments into structured open classes according to the domain of the study in order to obtain the most interested topics of the domain. This paper will show how to build the classes then use these classes in classifying the tweets.

The main steps of Building the classes are: Dataset collection (tweets gathering), Concept extraction, Stopping words removal, Applying Semantic measure, Building the classes, and finally Renaming the classes as in Fig. 1.

3.1 Dataset Collection

It is crucial to build the classes for the experiment from real data gathered from users' tweets; therefore, a domain for the study was defined. The domain of the study was

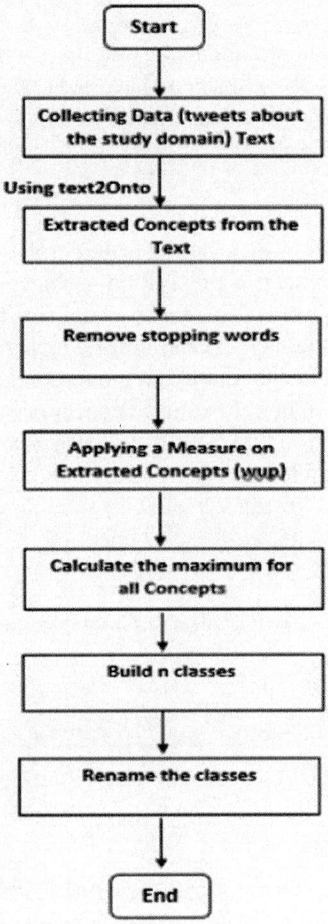

Fig. 1. Flowchart of building classes

selected based on some important criteria. First, the domain need to be well known and can be represented as a hashtag. Second, datasets are available on the real time and as historical data. Thus, we have chosen International Women's Day as it is a yearly occasion. Our collecting data approach was focusing on retrieving description of the data across large number of participants. We have applied the quantitative approach in collecting the data to get the real understanding of the domain (International Women's Day) by the users. Twenty thousand tweets were gathered using International Women's Day hashtag. The data has been collected by the second author's account on Tweeter during preparing her master thesis in the year 2019.

3.2 Concept Extraction

After collecting the tweets, the next step is extracting the concepts. For this process Text2Onto tool was used. Text2Onto represent the learning knowledge model at the meta-level in the form of instantiated modeling primitives within a so-called Probabilistic Ontology Model (POM) [13]. 36500 concepts have been extracted using Entropy concept extraction algorithm from corpus International Women's Day.

3.3 Stopping Words Removal

After concepts being successfully extracted from the corpus, notably the results comprise variety of meaningless words such as preposition, technical words, pronouns, and verb to be or to have and linking words. Thereupon, those words need to be excluded from the results to insure correct findings concentrating on main concepts from the sentences. Thus, a method has been applied to remove all the stopping words. After implementing stopping words algorithm number of extracted concepts was decreased by 17.9% (i.e. reduced by 6561 from 36500 to 29,939). In accordance to removing stopping words, only 29,939 concepts were left for the experiment. Table 1 is only a sample of forty-four concepts. The next phase is applying semantic measure on the resulted concepts to find the most related concepts and the least related once.

Table 1. Extracted concepts sample (dataset)

No	Concept	No	Concept	No	Concept	No	Concept
1	Tear	12	Ending	23	Timing	34	Industry
2	Food	13	Chain	24	Map	35	Ticket
3	Woman	14	Chef	25	Showcase	36	Friend
4	Architect	15	Role model	26	Fun	37	Restaurateur
5	Day	16	Cook	27	Experience	38	Business
6	Date	17	Environment	28	Change	39	Innovation
7	Location	18	Smile	29	World	40	Work
8	Example	19	Board	30	Mom	41	Voucher
9	Tribute	20	Moment	31	Right	42	Movement
10	World	21	End	32	Click	43	Month
11	Slogan	22	Man	33	Activism	44	Science

3.4 Apply Semantic Measure

Semantic similarity measure calculates the similarity between two words. To calculate the similarity measure there is two approaches either knowledge-based measure or corpus-based measure [14]. According to Khaja et al. [15] WuP (Wu and Palmer) measure was the most fit measure to extract words relatedness in health and food field. Accordingly, this paper has applied Wu and Palmer Measure in this experiment. Wu and Palmer Measure provides a scale of 0.0 to 1.0 of coverage similarity to a concept. The

Table 2 illustrates the results of applying WuP measure using WordNet Similarity for Java (WS4J) tool on all the extracted concepts for the entire dataset results. WS4J is online tool to compute semantic similarity using WuP.

Table 2. Extracted concepts sample (dataset)

	Tear /VB	Food /NN	Woman /NN	Architect /NN	Day /NN	Date /NN	Location /NN	Example /NN
Tear /VB	1	–	–	–	–	–	–	–
Food /NN	–	1	0.4615	0.4615	0.4615	0.8	0.5455	0.8
Woman /NN	–	0.4615	1	0.8	0.7619	0.7619	0.5333	0.4286
Architect /NN	–	0.4615	0.8	1	0.7619	0.7619	0.5333	0.2857
Day /NN	–	0.4615	0.7619	0.7619	1	0.9231	0.5	0.4615
Date /NN	–	0.8	0.7619	0.7619	0.9231	1	0.5	0.4615
Location /NN	–	0.5455	0.5333	0.5333	0.5	0.5	1	0.6667
Example /NN	–	0.8	0.4286	0.2857	0.4615	0.4615	0.6667	1

As previously mentioned, for extreme comprehensive coverage Wup similarity measure provides the result equals 1, for partial coverage the result will vary between 0.1 to 0.9 and for extreme incomplete coverage the result will be either 0 or (−). As shown in Table 2 between tear concept in first column and tear concept in first row in which both have extreme comprehensive coverage. Whereas, tear and other concepts like food, woman, architect, day, date, location and example had extreme incomplete coverage which proves the insignificance between them. There were 1543 concepts had extreme incomplete coverage which means they do not have any relation with the other concepts. For this reason, those 1543 concepts were excluded from the dataset results. The concepts: "end, commodity, home demonstrate, world, map, etc." are example of the result of extreme comprehensive coverage between two concepts.

3.5 Build the Classes

After extracting the similarity measure values of all dataset, the maximum similarity measure values between the concepts was used to build the classes. The methodology used in this research is based on first building abstract classes containing only the class name stored as class one, class two, class three, etc. Then, for each concept, the similarity of that concepts with each other concepts (peer-concepts) were sorted according to their similarity measure values. The peer-concepts with maximum similarity measure were in the top for each concept.

The peer-concepts with similarity values below 50% were excluded from the results since they are unrelated to the topic and their similarity is classified as weak similarity. The number of similarity-calculations among the concepts after removing unrelated concepts were 12,579 stored in a text file. After completing this step, only centered concepts were stored. Centered concepts are defined upon their appearance or repetition in the file after removing the unrelated concepts. Using this way, the first centered concept was the word "Example" with 250 times appeared in the calculations.

To avoid noisy and repeated data, any concept stored in a class will be removed from the similarity measure text file with all concepts which has similarity values above or equal 50%. Thus, only four hundred concepts with maximum similarity are reaming to be included in the class- building process. For instance, the concept "Example" has 250 related-concepts. For that, removing all other peer-similarity, such as "Example-idea" and "Idea" with other concepts from the file, will result ending with 400 peer-concepts. For the concept "Example" we end with only 14 unique-concepts with peer-similarity above or equal 50% out of the 250 related-concepts. Accordingly, on repeating the process of building the classes the concepts stored in any of the classes deleted from the text. The second centered concept was woman with 230 times of occurrences. Henceforth the third centered concept was day with forty occurrences and the forth was environment with twenty occurrences. Table 3 shows the classes built in the experiment.

Table 3. Build classes

Class 1	Class 2	Class 3	Class 4
Example	Woman	Day	Environment
Idea	Blogger	Date	Situation
Event	Friend	Moment	Showcase
Reality	Man	Bit	Inclusion
Experience	Architect	Year	Life
Talent	Actor	Reservoir	Opportunity
Science	Finalist	Month	Way
Right	Artisan	Today	Equality
Production	Educator	Drink	Voice
Activism	Voucher	People	Timing
Market	Cook	Part	Majority

3.6 Rename the Classes

Four classes were built with 400 concepts related to the topic. The reason behind this is in that 7680 concepts left after filtering the noisy. The system could build only four classes. As a result, of classifying the concept into four main majors the fields of discussion for the study topic were highlighted. Thereupon, an expert (human) has renamed the generated classes to get meaningful titles for each group of concepts (Class) as shown in Table 4.

Table 4. Sample of data in defined classes

Activities	Woman role	Time	Surroundings
Example	Woman	Day	Environment
Idea	Blogger	Date	Situation
Event	Friend	Moment	Showcase
Reality	Man	Bit	Inclusion
Experience	Architect	Year	Life
Talent	Actor	Reservoir	Opportunity
Science	Finalist	Month	Way
Right	Artisan	Today	Equality
Production	Educator	Drink	Voice
Activism	Voucher	People	Timing
Market	Cook	Part	Majority

4 Discussion of Findings

The experiment main aim is building the classes and then later is to classify the tweets into the defined classes. The final output of the system represents an overview of the most popular topic discussed in the study domain also the least discussed topic of interest. The system has generated four classes covering activities, woman role, time and surrounding as the highlighted topics in women international day domain. However, the system has classified the tweets datasets into those classes. There are total of four hundred tweets, which contains 10,350 words implemented by the system. The number of tweets classified into the activities class was 88 tweet. The woman role class has 168 tweets. In addition, 120 tweets have conversed about time class. However, the surrounding class had the least number of tweets with 16 tweets in the overall dataset. Therefore, to conclude the results has been a strong evidence on presenting users' sentiments towards women international day, where 43% of the tweets has discussed the women role. However only 4% of the tweets has discussed the surroundings class and this Cleary shows their interest is highly related to woman role at the first place, then time, activities and the least topic is surroundings.

5 Conclusion

Social media has become a platform for news media, one of the most famous social media site is Twitter. Where users tweet their opinion, emotions and sentiments through the application. Thereupon, each tweet can be related to one or more fields whenever it has a hashtag or mention. As a result, many companies rely in Twitter to collect feedback for their services or products. By classifying the sentiment of the users, companies can understand their thoughts. Therefore, this research has proposed a solution for sentiment classification. This technique relies on semantic measures where the data became semantically related to each other. The research has used text2Onto tool to extract concepts from datasets and then calculate the semantic measure Wup to point to the most related concepts. The proposed solution is building the classes using the most common concepts in the corpus. The results were constructing four classes, activities, woman role, time and surroundings.

References

1. Wu, Z., Palmer, M.: Verb semantics and lexical selection. In: Proceedings of the Annual Meeting of the Association for Computational Linguistics (1994)
2. Richardson, R., Smeaton, A., Murphy, J.: Using WordNet as a knowledge base for measuring semantic similarity between words (1994)
3. Fan, H., et al.: Social media toxicity classification using deep learning: real-world application UK Brexit. Electronics **10**(11), 1332 (2021)
4. Zhu, X., et al.: Exploring user historical semantic and sentiment preference for microblog sentiment classification. Neurocomputing **464**, 141–150 (2021)
5. Wu, Z., Li, X., Zhou, X., Yang, T., Lu, R.: City Intelligence quotient evaluation system using crowdsourced social media data: a case study of the Yangtze river delta region, China. ISPRS Int. J. Geo-Inf. **10**(10), 702 (2021)
6. Wilson, T., Wiebe, J., Hoffmann, P.: Recognizing contextual polarity: an exploration of features for phrase-level sentiment analysis. Comput. Linguist. **35**(3), 399–433 (2009)
7. Pennebaker, J.W., Boyd, R.L., Jordan, K., Blackburn, K.: The development and psychometric properties of LIWC 2015 (2015)
8. Kwak, H., Lee, C., Park, H., Moon, S.: What is Twitter a social network or news media. In: Proceedings of the 19th International World Wide Web (WWW) Conference, pp. 26–30 (2010)
9. Kontopoulos, E., Berberidis, C., Dergiades, T., Bassiliades, N.: Ontology-based sentiment analysis of Twitter posts. Expert Syst. Appl. **40**(10), 4065–4074 (2013)
10. Niranjan, A., Nutan, D.H., Nitish, A., Shenoy, P.D., Venugopal, K.R.: ERCR TV: ensemble of random committee and random tree for efficient anomaly classification using voting. In: 2018 3rd International Conference for Convergence in Technology (I2CT), pp. 1–5. IEEE (2018)
11. Tagliarino, N.K., Bununu, Y.A., Micheal, M.O., De Maria, M., Olusanmi, A.: Compensation for expropriated community farmland in Nigeria: an in-depth analysis of the laws and practices related to land expropriation for the Lekki free trade zone in Lagos. Land **7**(1), 23 (2018)
12. Habtegebriel, H., Edward, D., Wawire, M., Sila, D., Seifu, E.: Effect of operating parameters on the surface and physico-chemical properties of spray-dried camel milk powders. Food Bioprod. Process. **112**, 137–149 (2018)

13. Cimiano, P., Völker, J.: Text2Onto. In: Montoyo, A., Muńoz, R., Métais, E. (eds.) NLDB 2005. LNCS, vol. 3513, pp. 227–238. Springer, Heidelberg (2005). https://doi.org/10.1007/11428817_21
14. Mihalcea, R., Corley, C., Strapparava, C.: Corpus-based and knowledge-based measures of text semantic similarity. In: AAAI, vol. 6, pp. 775–780 (2006)
15. Khaja, H.I., Abate, M., Zheng, W., Abbasi, A., Adjeroh, D.: Evaluating semantic similarity for adverse drug event narratives. In: Thomson, R., Dancy, C., Hyder, A., Bisgin, H. (eds.) SBP-BRiMS 2018. LNCS, vol. 10899, pp. 292–299. Springer, Cham (2018). https://doi.org/10.1007/978-3-319-93372-6_33

Using the *Strings* Metadata to Detect the Source Language of the Binary

Ashish Adhikari and Prasad A. Kulkarni(✉)

EECS, University of Kansas, Lawrence, USA
{adhikariashish2,prasadk}@ku.edu

Abstract. We explore the question of determining the source language of program binaries. Programs compiled from different source languages are susceptible to different classes of software attacks. Therefore, knowing the source language can help the end-users assess the security risk of the binary software and allow human experts and automated binary analysis tools focus their efforts to adequately protect the software from the appropriate classes of attacks. Previous works in the related area of program provenance use complex analysis over the binary code to determine the compiler and flags used to generate the binary, but do not attempt to identify the source language of the binary. In this work we develop a simple approach that only uses the *strings* exposed by the binary to reliably determine the source language without requiring analysis of the underlying binary code, even when the binary is *stripped*. Our technique employs different machine-learning based classifiers over this simple program meta-data to accurately determine the source language over a large real-world benchmark set and 6 programming languages. We find that our simple approach can achieve an accuracy of over 98% to determine the source language over a large real-world benchmark set in all stripped and unstripped binary configurations.

Keywords: Binary · Classification · Source language · Software attack · Stripped

1 Introduction

Different high-level programming languages have differing properties, strengths and weaknesses with regards to security, robustness, resilience, and performance of the resulting binary software. Binaries from different source languages are susceptible to distinct classes of security vulnerabilities and exploits. Therefore, knowledge of the source language can provide much useful information to the customers and end-users of binary software. This knowledge can also inform security experts and automated binary analysis tools on how to best audit, protect and harden the binary against potential security relevant bugs and attacks.

Yet, to our knowledge, there is no current approach that attempts to determine the source language of the binary. Related techniques have been developed that can identify the compiler suite used to build the binary program. These techniques may use customized signature files [16] or employ complex analysis over the binary code [27] to

K. Daimi and A. Al Sadoon (Eds.): ICR 2022, AISC 1431, pp. 190–200, 2022.
https://doi.org/10.1007/978-3-031-14054-9_19

determine the source compiler. Techniques employing signatures need a specific code pattern for each compiler. Many compiler frameworks, including GCC [15] and LLVM [29], provide frontends for multiple source languages and it is unclear if techniques to identify the source compiler can be directly used to also determine the source language.

In this work we explore this important issue of identifying the source language for software binaries. We found that a simple approach that only uses easily extracted binary meta-data and does not require complex analysis of the binary code to search for patterns is sufficient in most cases to identify the source language.

Many programs have external dependencies on library functions that are resolved at run-time. The binary needs to hold this information for the runtime system. This information along with other language and compiler specific metadata is encoded as *strings* in the binary, and is present even when the binary is *stripped* of all symbol information. Simple OS tools can extract this information from the binary. Our technique uses these extracted string identifiers (using the Linux 'strings' tool) and encodes the relevant information as a vector. This vector is then fed into machine-learning (ML) based classification algorithms.

We use three ML classification algorithms: Multinomial Naive Bayes, Random Forest Classifier, and the Bernoulli Classifier for this work. Our experiments use hundreds of open-source binaries generated from six source languages and multiple compilers. We experimented with binaries generated with embedded symbol information and those that were stripped of all (unneeded) symbol and metadata information. We found that the best ML models can identify the source language of the binary with an accuracy of over 98% in most cases.

Thus, our objective in this work is to explore and develop techniques to identify the source language of any given binary software. We find that simple ML based techniques that only study the binary meta-data, and do not analyze the binary code, are sufficient in most cases to identify the source language, even for stripped binaries. We make the following contributions in this work.

1. To our knowledge, this is the first work that attempts to develop generalized techniques to reliably recover the source language information from binaries.
2. We develop several machine-learning based models to resolve this challenge and evaluate and compare their performance.
3. We compile a comprehensive benchmark set comprising hundreds of opensource programs over six source languages (C, C++, Fortran, Swift, Rust and Go) and multiple compilers for this work.

The rest of this paper is organized as follows. We present background on the security properties of our selected languages in Sect. 2. We describe our approach using ML based classification models to determine source language information from binaries in Sect. 3. We describe our experimental setup, benchmarks, experiments and results in Sect. 4. We present related work in Sect. 5. Finally conclusions and future work are presented in Sect. 6.

2 Background

Our primary goal in this work is to develop techniques to identify the source language of binary software. Several academic [3] and industry [22, 34, 36] studies report that binaries generated from different programming languages expose the end-users to different kinds and levels of security threats. For instance, one study found that programs written in the 'C' language account for the highest fraction of open-source security vulnerabilities [36]. Another study reports that while CWE-400[1], CWE-125[2], and CWE-20[3] are the most common errors in C programs, CWE-119[4] dominates C++ program errors, while CWE-400 is most common in Go programs. We also know that while buffer overflow errors (CWE-119) are common in C/C++ programs [36], these errors are not possible in memory-safe languages, like Rust and Go. Thus, knowledge of the source language can prove immensely useful for manual and automated efforts to develop the most effective strategy to secure binary software.

For this work we experiment with six popular *compiled* programming language binaries according to the TIOBE language index[5] that also have a large open-source code base. The compiled languages we selected (along with their most recent TIOBE index) are: C (ranked #2), C++ (ranked #4), Go (ranked #13), Swift (ranked #14), Rust (ranked #28), and Fortran (ranked #31). All these six are compiled languages that generate native binary executables. In the remainder of this section we describe important security relevant properties about these six languages used in this work.

C: 'C' is a low level programming language popular in computer and embedded systems applications. It can achieve high performance and is widely supported. However, memory unsafe languages, like C and C++, score poorly for security and safety [13]. These languages do not natively guaranty memory or type safety. Memory management is the responsibility of the programmer [23]. It does not support *exceptions* so programs may unintentionally ignore critical errors [37] (chapter 11 Error Handling). Secure libraries have been recently made available that can, for instance, replace vulnerable functions like `strcpy` with more secure variants, like `strncpy` and `strcpy_s`.

C++: C++ is an object oriented extension to the 'C' language that supports encapsulation, abstraction, inheritance and polymorphism. C++ suffers from many of the same security properties and challenges as C. C++ too does not impose memory safety and there is no garbage collector in typical implementations [11]. C++ is also not type safe, and the misuse of casts and unions can lead to type and memory violations. Safer APIs are also available for use in C++ programs.

Fortran: FORTRAN is popular in the domain of high-performance scientific and numeric computing. Buffer overflows are relatively harder to strings have defined length and arrays statically specify upper and lower bounds that a compiler can check for errors. However, Fortran cannot resolve invalid memory access at run-time. There is greater type safety in Fortran, and is typically considered safer as compared to C/C++ [19].

Swift: Swift is a general-purpose, powerful and popular compiled language developed by Apple Inc. as a replacement to 'Objective-C'. When 'pure' Swift is used, overflows and underflows cause a runtime trap. But interaction of Swift code with C-style pointers

Table 1. Summary and comparison of the safety properties of the programming languages employed in this work

Source language	Memory safety	Type safety	Thread safety	Availability safe APIs	Overall security
C	X	X	Y	Y	Low
C++	X	X	Y	Y	Low
Fortran	Some	X	Y	Y	Medium
Swift	Some	Some	Y	Y	Medium
Go	Y	Y	Y	Y	High
Rust	Y	Y	Y	Y	High

is permitted, and could be unsafe. Swift provides more secure library functions. Memory management is automatic. While there is no garbage collection, ARC (or Automatic Reference Counting) is used to manage memory. Swift is generally safe, but the possibility of interaction with C code can introduce hazards. Swift also suffers from insecure cryptography.

Go: Go is a compiled programming language designed at Google. This is a fairly new language that is gaining popularity in recent years. 'Go' is memory and type-safe. Bounds checking is automatic and pointer arithmetic is not permitted. Memory safety is ensured by a built-in garbage collector. However, Go programs can have data races that could be exploited to cause memory corruption. Safe API functions are available. The Go language aims to achieve both program safety and high performance.

Rust: Rust is a relatively new, open-source, statically typed programming language designed for performance and safety. Both type safety and memory management are supported by the language. Rust can guarantee memory safety by using a borrow checker to validate references. Rust is also a type safe language. It enforces thread safety of all code and data. Rust does not use *null*, so accidental null dereference errors are avoided. Safe APIs are available for programming in Rust. A Rust program is safe against data races, unlike Go.

Table 1 summarizes the safety properties of the six chosen programming languages. Among the programming languages chosen for this study, we categorize C and C++ as low-security languages, Fortran and Swift as moderately secure, and the newer Go and Rust as highly secure languages.

3 Source Language Classification Model

In this section we explain our machine-learning (ML) based approach for determining the source programming language for a given binary executable.

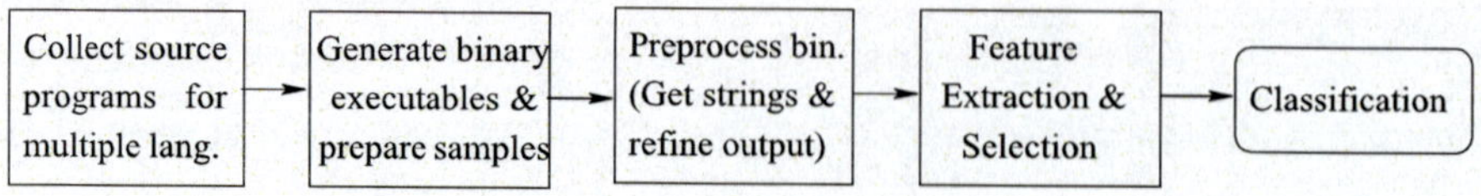

Fig. 1. Phases in our algorithm to identify the source language for binaries

We can organize our approach in the following steps or phases: (a) Collect a large dataset of binary executables for each chosen source language, (b) Extract metadata information from the binary using the available *strings* information, select and extract relevant features, and (c) Develop and explore machine-learning based classification algorithms for experimentation. These steps are illustrated in Fig. 1 and explained in more detail in the remainder of this section.

3.1 Gathering Binary Executables

We collect a large and diverse benchmark set for experimentation. We use the open-source project repository, Github to find representative programs for each of our six selected programming languages. We compile a comprehensive set of 120 benchmark programs for each of these 6 languages for experimentation.

All the open-source projects used in this work were distributed as sourcecode files, with scripts to build them into binary executables included in many cases. The choice of the compilation framework can not only affect the generated binary code, but also the binary meta-data. To study the effect of the compilation framework on the ability of ML models to correctly identify the source language, we employ multiple compilers for our C, C++ and Fortran language programs. For C and C++ we use three compiler frameworks: the GNU Compiler, Clang and ICC (Intel C++ Compiler) compilation frameworks. We use two compilers for building Fortran binaries: GNU Fortran and Intel Fortran compilers.

The older C, C++, and Fortran programming languages have a highly diverse compiler ecosystem. In contrast, a single reference compiler is usually used to build programs written in the three newer programming languages in our set, Swift, Go and Rust. We use the reference 'Swift' [30] compiler, the default 'Go' [9, 14] compiler, and the standard 'rustc' [28] compiler for building the Swift, Go and Rust programs, respectively. In the future, we will also experiment with alternative compiler frameworks for these languages.

Thus, in this phase, we gathered all the benchmark programs, generated or updated the build scripts, installed the compiler frameworks, and then built the executables for each configuration. The binaries were built with compiler optimizations switched on and the binaries were optionally stripped of all symbol information. All our programs were built for the x86-64 instruction set architecture running the Ubuntu Linux version 20.04 LTS.

3.2 Extract Meta-data Information

We use the meta-data information extracted by the Unix *strings* tools from each (stripped) binary program. The *strings* tool outputs all printable character sequences in the binary that are at least 4 characters long (and are followed by an unprintable character). We process the raw *strings* output to remove strings that are not directly useful for our task.

In this processing step, we manually identify 'string' sequences that seem useful to identify the source language. For instance, strings describing the compiler, libraries (like libstdc++.so, GLIBC, etc.), number of libraries were deemed useful. We use a simple regular expression combined with string manipulation to process the raw strings data. This extracted information is then represented in a vector form to input to our machine learning models.

3.3 Machine-Learning Based Classification

There are multiple machine-learning based classification models that could be used for this work [7]. We arbitrarily choose the following 3 popular classification algorithms for this study. The first, called Multinomial Naive Bayes classifier, is suitable for classification with discrete features of strings. Since our feature set includes the frequency of certain strings that appear in the binary, this classification scheme seems useful. The second model we use is called the Random Forest classifier. This model uses several decision tree classifiers on various subsamples of the datasets and improves its accuracy by using averaging and control over-fitting. The third classification model we use is the popular Bernoulli model. Each of these ML models need to be *trained* first to build the classifier *models*, which can then be tested for accuracy in detecting the source language of the binary. For our experiments in this work, we select 20% of our feature sets as test cases, and use the remaining 80% of the sets to train the model.

4 Experimental Results

In this section we present results of our experiments that use the trained ML models to identify the source language of binary executables. We configure three different datasets. The first dataset uses binaries that are unstripped. Unstripped binaries may embed more useful 'strings' information. Our second dataset uses only the stripped binaries. Finally, a more diverse third dataset combines binaries from both the stripped and unstripped categories in equal proportions.

As mentioned earlier, multiple compilers are used to build binaries for the C, C++ and Fortran programs. In these cases, we include an equal number of programs from each compiler in our dataset for that source language. For instance, the dataset for the C source language contains an equal number (one-third) of binaries built by the GNU GCC, Intel ICC and Clang compiler frameworks. Each compiler may use different libraries and embed different metadata strings in the binary. A more diverse dataset should improve the robustness of the machine learning models when encountering the test binaries.

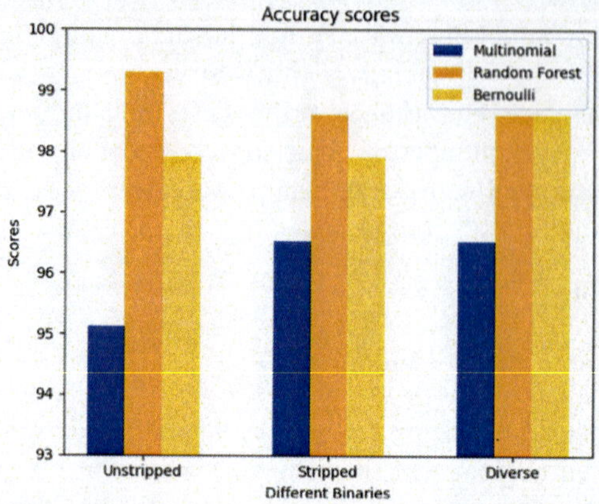

Fig. 2. Accuracy of our ML models on different datasets

Figure 2 shows the overall results of our experiments with the 3 selected classification models. Thus, we find that the best ML models achieve an accuracy of up to 99.3% when identifying the source language using the unstripped dataset. The best models achieve an overall accuracy of 98.61% when using the stripped and diverse datasets.

The results show that the Multinomial Naive Bayes algorithm achieves the poorest accuracy among all our models. While the other two ML models perform better, the Random Forest classifier achieves accuracy that is marginally higher than the Bernoulli classifier in the *stripped* and *unstripped* configurations.

Figures 3, 4, and 5 show further details about cases when the ML models fail to detect the correct source language for a binary in the *unstripped*, *stripped* and *diverse* experimental configurations, respectively. These figures employ a matrix representation, where the X-and Y-axis refer to the programming languages C, C++, Go, Rust, Fortran and Swift, respectively.

The numerals along the diagonal show the number of programs that are correctly identified, in each case. Thus, Fig. 3(a) shows that there are 28 C binaries, 22 C++ binaries, 22 Go binaries, 21 Rust binaries, 25 Fortran binaries, and 19 Swift binaries that are correctly identified by the Multinomial Naive Bayes algorithm in the *unstripped* benchmark configuration. Likewise, there are 4 C++ binaries that are misclassified as C binaries, and 2 C++ binaries that are misclassified as Fortran binaries in this same configuration.

Overall, we find that most of the misclassifications occur due to C++ binaries identified as C programs. Also, as expected, the *unstripped* and *diverse* datasets achieve accurate classification due to the availability of more useful meta-data information. However, it was surprising to find that the models achieve high accuracy even in the *stripped* configuration. Thus, our findings indicate that distinctive features are retained in the binary meta-data even after it is stripped of all symbol information (that is not needed at run-time), which allows these ML models to accurately detect the source language even for stripped binaries.

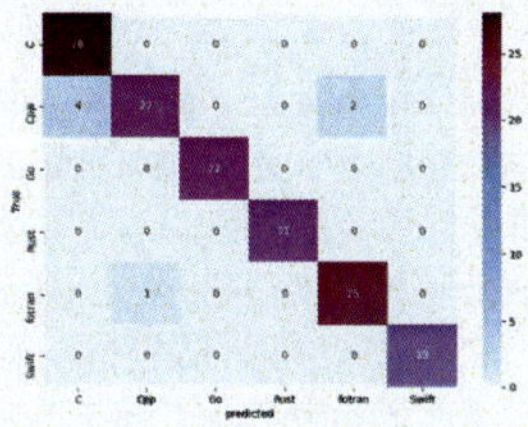

(a) Multinomial

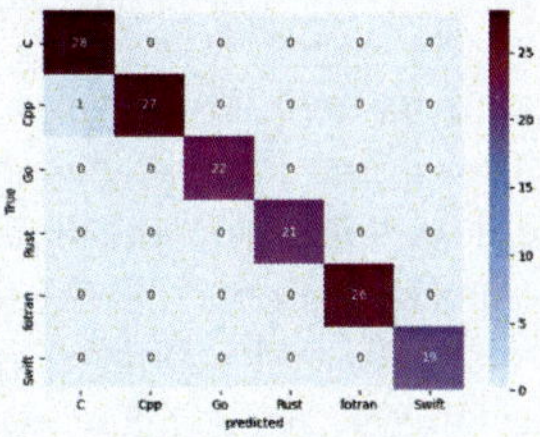

(b) Random Forest

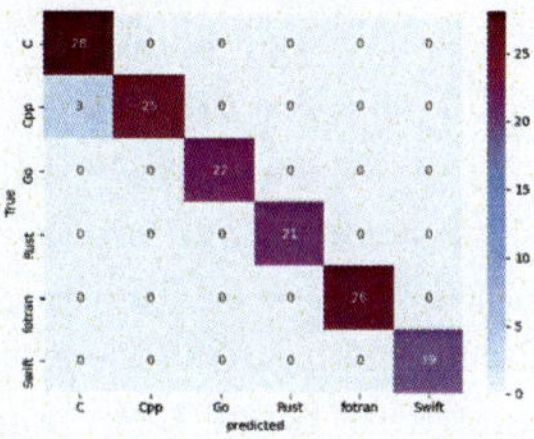

(c) Bernoulli

Fig. 3. In an unstrippped dataset

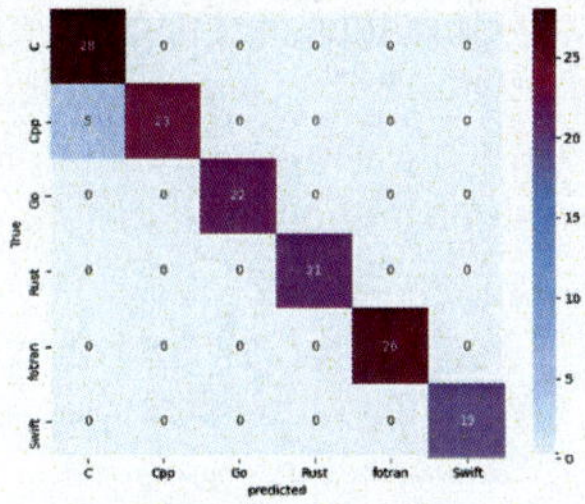

(a) Multinomial

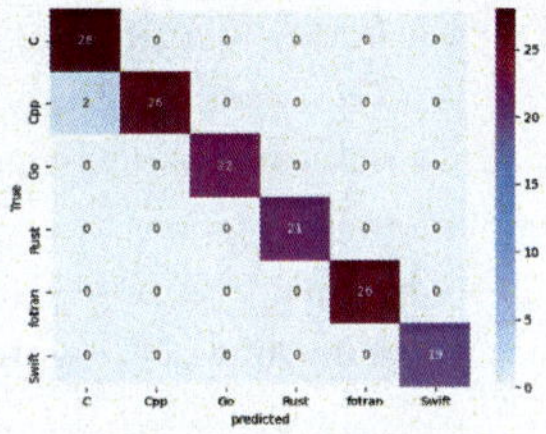

(b) Random Forest

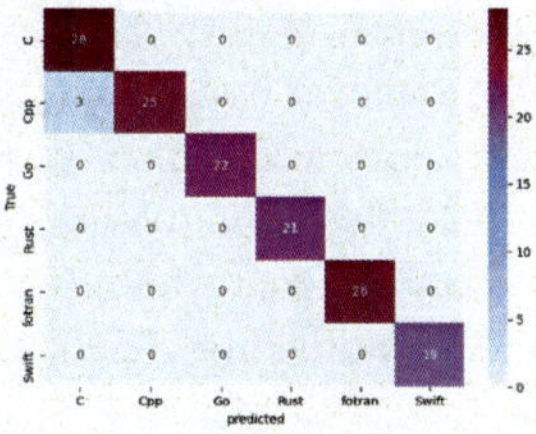

(c) Bernoulli

Fig. 4. In a strippped dataset

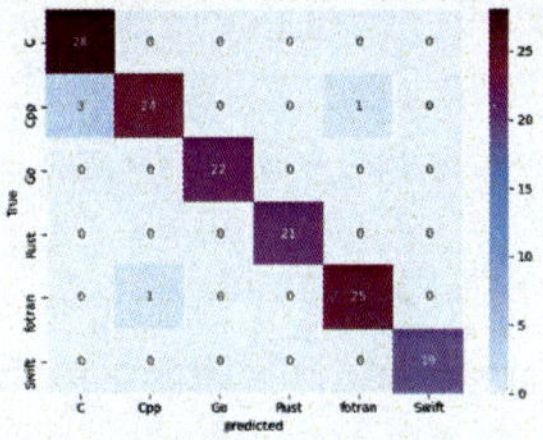

(a) Multinomial

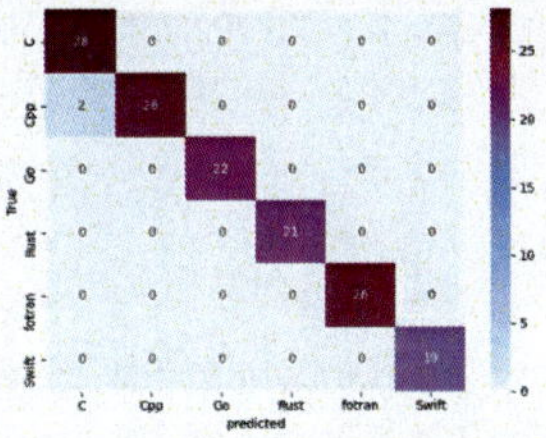

(b) Random Forest

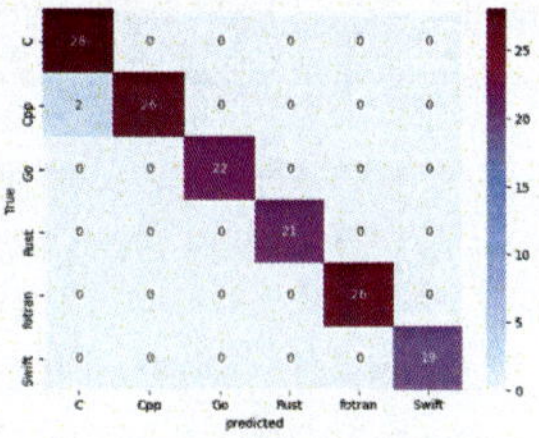

(c) Bernoulli

Fig. 5. In a diverse dataset

5 Related Works

In this section we discuss prominent research in areas that are related to this work. While there is limited research to identify the source programming language from a given binary, there is much prior research work in the related areas of compiler provenance and code authorship identification.

Research in program or compiler provenance attempts to identify the compiler tool-chain and/or optimization levels used to generate a binary program. These methods take a signature-matching or a machine-learning based approach. Signature matching methods search the binary against a set of code signatures manually generated by experts to identify the compiler used. PEiD [4] and IDA Pro [17] are examples of tools that use this signature-based method. This method relies on expert knowledge and can be easily confused by small differences in signatures. The other strategy employs ML based models to capture compiler-specific patterns from the binary code [1, 6, 24, 27, 33]. These patterns include instruction sequences or idioms [27], instruction type and frequency [5], and subgraphs from the program's CFG [25]. All these approaches require looking and deciphering properties about the binary code. Our work has a different goal and does not rely on parsing the binary code.

The topic of identifying the author of a given binary software is also related to our work [1, 2, 20, 21, 26]. This problem, called code authorship attribution, aims to categorize the authors of malware. This categorization along with information about the tools and techniques used by a set of malware that is written by the same author can help determine how the malware can spread and evolve and help in cyber-crime investigations. Most of these approaches also employ ML based methods to model various aspects of the binary code and control-flow to accurately predict the binary code authors or if different software are written by the same author.

Machine-learning based approaches are also popular is other binary analysis problems, including the detection of a virus in binary software [31], code clone detection to find the same source code in binaries compiled for different architectures [39], detection of malicious software [8, 10, 18], function recognition [35] and similarity [12] in binaries, and many others [38]. We too use a machine-learning based approach for this work.

Finally, Tian et al. proposed a classification system of identifying trojan and virus families based on printable strings [32]. We too employ the *strings* available in program binaries in this work to identify the source language of binaries.

6 Conclusions and Future Work

In this paper we explore the issue of identifying the source programming language for any given binary software. We build an experimental framework that we populate with binaries from 6 different source languages and compiled using multiple different compilers. We found that our simple machine-learning based approach that only considers the *strings* exposed by the binary and does not analyze the binary code is sufficient to accurately identify the source language, even for binaries that are optimized and stripped of all symbol information.

In the future, we will study if this approach continues to work with more programming languages. We will also experiment with binaries that may contain complex code that is obfuscated, hand-written and constructed using multiple different languages. Finally, we will explore the performance and accuracy of other ML models, including ensemble ML to further improve results.

References

1. Alrabaee, S., et al.: Compiler provenance attribution. In: Alrabaee, S., et al. (eds.) Binary Code Fingerprinting for Cybersecurity. ADIS, vol. 78, pp. 45–78. Springer, Cham (2020). https://doi.org/10.1007/978-3-030-34238-8_3

2. Alrabaee, S., Wang, L., Debbabi, M.: BinGold: towards robust binary analysis by extracting the semantics of binary code as semantic flow graphs (SFGs). Digit. Investig. **18**, S11–S22 (2016)
3. Antal, G., Mosolygó, B., Vándor, N., Hegedűs, P.: A data-mining based study of security vulnerability types and their mitigation in different languages. In: Gervasi, O., et al. (eds.) ICCSA 2020. LNCS, vol. 12252, pp. 1019–1034. Springer, Cham (2020). https://doi.org/10.1007/978-3-030-58811-3_72
4. Arghire, G.: Detect packers, cryptors and compilers bundled with PE executables with the help of this reliable piece of software that boasts a high detection rate (2017). https://www.softpedia.com/get/Programming/Packers-Crypters-Protectors/PEiD-updated.shtml
5. Austin, T.H., Filiol, E., Josse, S., Stamp, M.: Exploring hidden Markov models for virus analysis: a semantic approach. In: 2013 46th Hawaii International Conference on System Sciences, pp. 5039–5048 (2013)
6. Benoit, T., Marion, J.Y., Bardin, S.: Binary level toolchain provenance identification with graph neural networks. In: 2021 IEEE International Conference on Software Analysis, Evolution and Reengineering (SANER), pp. 131–141 (2021)
7. Bonaccorso, G.: Machine Learning Algorithms: A Reference Guide to Popular Algorithms for Data Science and Machine Learning. Packt Publishing (2017)
8. Coogan, K., Debray, S., Kaochar, T., Townsend, G.: Automatic static unpacking of malware binaries. In: 2009 16th Working Conference on Reverse Engineering, pp. 167–176. IEEE (2009)
9. Cox, R., Griesemer, R., Pike, R., Taylor, I.L., Thompson, K.: The Go programming language and environment. Commun. ACM **65**(5), 70–78 (2022)
10. Dai, J., Guha, R.K., Lee, J.: Efficient virus detection using dynamic instruction sequences. J. Comput. **4**(5), 405–414 (2009)
11. Edelson, D.R.: A mark-and-sweep collector C++. In: Proceedings of the 19th ACM SIGPLAN-SIGACT Symposium on Principles of Programming Languages, pp. 51–58. ACM (1992)
12. Eschweiler, S., Yakdan, K., Gerhards-Padilla, E.: discovRE: efficient cross-architecture identification of bugs in binary code. In: NDSS (2016)
13. Gaynow, A.: What science can tell us about C and C++'s security, 27 May 2020. https://alexgaynor.net/2020/may/27/science-on-memory-unsafety-and-security/
14. Go Team: "Download and Install Go" (2022). https://go.dev/doc/install
15. Griffith, A.: GCC: The Complete Reference, 1st edn. McGraw-Hill Inc., New York (2002)
16. Hex-Rays: IDA F.L.I.R.T. Technology: In-Depth (2022). https://hex-rays.com/products/ida/tech/flirt/in_depth/
17. IDA Pro: Hex-rays IDA pro disassembler and debugger (2017). https://hex-rays.com/
18. Islam, R., Tian, R., Batten, L., Versteeg, S.: Classification of malware based on string and function feature selection. In: 2010 Second Cybercrime and Trustworthy Computing Workshop, pp. 9–17 (2010)
19. ISO/IEC JTC 1/SC22: Fortran Language Vulnerabilities (2022). http://www.open-std.org/jtc1/sc22/wg23/docs/documents
20. Kalgutkar, V., Kaur, R., Gonzalez, H., Stakhanova, N., Matyukhina, A.: Code authorship attribution: methods and challenges. ACM Comput. Surv. **52**(1), 1–36 (2019)
21. Layton, R., Azab, A.: Authorship analysis of the Zeus botnet source code. In: 2014 Fifth Cybercrime and Trustworthy Computing Conference, pp. 38–43. IEEE (2014)
22. Lupsan, H.: Security vulnerability classes in popular programming languages (2021). https://versprite.com/blog/security-research/security-vulnerability-classes-in-popular-programming-languages/
23. Myers, N.C.: Memory Management in C++, pp. 363–374. SIGS Publications, Inc., Thousand Oaks (1996)

24. Pizzolotto, D., Inoue, K.: Identifying compiler and optimization level in binary code from multiple architectures. IEEE Access **9**, 163461–163475 (2021)
25. Rosenblum, N., Miller, B.P., Zhu, X.: Recovering the toolchain provenance of binary code. In: Proceedings of the 2011 International Symposium on Software Testing and Analysis, pp. 100–110. ACM (2011)
26. Rosenblum, N., Zhu, X., Miller, B.P.: Who wrote this code? identifying the authors of program binaries. In: Atluri, V., Diaz, C. (eds.) ESORICS 2011. LNCS, vol. 6879, pp. 172–189. Springer, Heidelberg (2011). https://doi.org/10.1007/978-3-642-23822-2_10
27. Rosenblum, N.E., Miller, B.P., Zhu, X.: Extracting compiler provenance from program binaries. In: Proceedings of the 9th ACM SIGPLAN-SIGSOFT Workshop on Program Analysis for Software Tools and Engineering, pp. 21–28. ACM (2010)
28. Rust Team: Guide to Rustc development (2022). https://www.swift.org/swift-compiler/
29. Sarda, S., Pandey, M.: LLVM Essentials. Packt Publishing (2015)
30. Swift Team: Swift Compiler (2022). https://www.swift.org/swift-compiler/
31. Tesauro, G.J., Kephart, J.O., Sorkin, G.B.: Neural networks for computer virus recognition. IEEE Expert **11**(4), 5–6 (1996)
32. Tian, R., Batten, L., Islam, M.R., Versteeg, S.: An automated classification system based on the strings of Trojan and virus families, pp. 23–30, November 2009
33. Tian, Z., Huang, Y., Xie, B., Chen, Y., Chen, L., Wu, D.: Fine-grained compiler identification with sequence-oriented neural modeling. IEEE Access **9**, 49160–49175 (2021)
34. Tung, L.: Programming language security: These are the worst bugs for each top language (2020). https://www.zdnet.com/article/programming-language-security-these-are-the-worst-bugs-for-each-top-language/
35. Wang, S., Wang, P., Wu, D.: Semantics-aware machine learning for function recognition in binary code. In: 2017 IEEE International Conference on Software Maintenance and Evolution (ICSME) (2017)
36. WhiteSource: What are the most secure programming languages? (2021). https://www.whitesourcesoftware.com/most-secure-programming-languages/
37. Wikibooks: C programming (2017). https://en.wikibooks.org/wiki/C_Programming
38. Xue, H., Sun, S., Venkataramani, G., Lan, T.: Machine learning-based analysis of program binaries: a comprehensive study. IEEE Access **7**, 65889–65912 (2019)
39. Zeng, J., Fu, Y., Miller, K.A., Lin, Z., Zhang, X., Xu, D.: Obfuscation resilient binary code reuse through trace-oriented programming. In: Proceedings of the 2013 ACM SIGSAC Conference on Computer & Communications Security, pp. 487–498 (2013)

Expanding Queries with Maximum Likelihood Estimators and Language Models

Christos Karras[1](✉), Aristeidis Karras[1], Leonidas Theodorakopoulos[2], Ioanna Giannoukou[2], and Spyros Sioutas[1]

[1] Computer Engineering and Informatics Department, University of Patras, 26504 Patras, Greece
{c.karras,akarras,sioutas}@ceid.upatras.gr

[2] Department of Management Science and Technology, University of Patras, 26334 Patras, Greece
{theodleo,igian}@upatras.gr

Abstract. The employment of various language modelling techniques in the area of information retrieval is gaining wide adoption in the state of the art methods. The precision of the language model enables the solution of the issue of information retrieval in a huge corpus of texts. To accomplish this, these techniques begin by estimating a probabilistic linguistic model for each article in the collection that is capable of generating a ranking of relevant texts in response to a query. One of the difficulties that this family of methods faces is a shortage of data. As a result, smoothing methods capable of changing the maximum likelihood estimator are required to account for the imprecision created. This paper highlights its use surpasses established approaches, such as tf-idf, for creating rankings of documents sorted by relevance. Finally, we examine various ideas related to query expansion by utilizing such methods.

Keywords: Expansion of queries · Language models · Cosine similarity · Maximum likelihood estimators · Decision making · Deep learning

1 Introduction

Throughout the years, query expansion strategies have been presented as a way to address the issue of term mismatches between a query and the documents it refers to. Typically, two kinds of query expansion technique families exist: local (based on Pseudo, Relevance, Indirect Feedback) and global (based on the creation and usage of a dictionary) [1]. This paper is focusing on the first category. Due to the difficulties of obtaining user input, only the first documents retrieved will be deemed significant. Pseudo-relevant documents are scanned for potential candidate phrases that may aid in expanding the query [2].

K. Daimi and A. Al Sadoon (Eds.): ICR 2022, AISC 1431, pp. 201–213, 2022.
https://doi.org/10.1007/978-3-031-14054-9_20

This strategy has been expanded upon inside the framework of the Language Model idea [3]. Statistical language models are frequently employed in information retrieval because they have a strong theoretical foundation and perform well empirically. The Robertson and Sparck Jones model [4] and the Croft and Harper model [5] are two well-known probabilistic techniques for information retrieval at the state of the art. Both approaches evaluate the likelihood that each page is relevant to a given query. Clearly, the two primary issues are related to accurately predicting both the query and document models. By predicting the factored form of the distribution $P(q, D)$, a Language Model determines the relevance of a document d to a query q [6].

The construction of a fine-tuned Language model must necessarily make use of smoothing models when one or more terms do not appear in a document. In the latter case, the maximum likelihood estimator would produce a probability equal to zero, invalidating the creation of the model itself [7,8]. Another notion that is advantageous for widening the query and is extensively employed throughout the paper is that of *Word Embeddings*. The latter is gained via the usage of Language models, or more specifically through the co-occurrence of the words made accessible. This technique is predicated on the ability to map each word into a vector of real numbers contained inside a vector space. The goal is to be able to compare their distances in order to determine their similarity. If two words are similar, they are categorized as synonyms.

The remainder of the paper is organized as follows. In Sect. 3, the objectives of the paper will be introduced followed by a brief overview of the problem definition. Section 4, describes the implementation of the system in both theory and application level while Sect. 5 highlights the experimental results and their findings. Finally, the conclusions and future directions of this work are presented in Sect. 6.

2 Related Work

Information retrieval is a rapidly growing field inextricably linked with deep learning methods. Machine Learning models as in [9] are the foundation for extracting knowledge as well as events and patterns. Markov Chain Monte Carlo (MCMC) methods are on their turn employed in the knowledge representation field as they are stochastic processes that check the underlying distributions within a set of data [10,11]. Additionally, heuristics are often utilized in gaining useful insights from complex geometric objects so as to extract features or information [12]. Smart IoT infrastructures as in [13] utilize innovative methods and emerging technologies for event detection purposes as well as for knowledge extraction in the field of smart agriculture supply chain.

3 Problem Definition

Language models have a wide range of applications, including voice recognition, spelling correction, grammar correction, and machine translation. All of these applications are tasked with the responsibility of assigning a probability to a sequence of words based on their frequency of occurrence in one or more texts. As briefly described in the introductory section, the goal of the following paper is to prove the existence of another technique capable of extending a query that takes use of the idea of language model, especially an emphn-grams model. To accomplish this purpose, the mismatch between the words in the query and the terms in a corpus of documents must be resolved. The likelihood of creating a new q query given an estimate of the Language Model for an D document can only be determined by ranking relevant documents. When dealing with a big corpus of documents, creating n Language models with n equal to the number of documents proves to be a computationally difficult procedure.

This research paper utilizes a beneficial strategy to build a preliminary rating of documents sorted by relevance for a given query q. The *tf-idf* recovery model is being used in accordance with word weighting, which is extensively employed in informational retrieval area, leading to sufficient results. The inclusion of the *LM* and other semantic analysis approaches enabled us to surpass the *tf-idf* baseline, producing a ranking of texts, more relevant to a given query q [14].

4 Methodology

It should be emphasised that the ranking is generated using the weight vectors of the *tf-idf* technique utilising the well-known *cosine similarity* measure between the weight vectors. To meet the specified aim, the location of the relevant target document, that is, the document for which the user is seeking, was tracked. This was made feasible by selecting a query from the available ones that was similar to the title of this document. The score supplied to the target document will serve as the minimal *threshold* for constructing the new document ranking. This step is critical since specifying a higher threshold would result in the target document being omitted from future computations.

By lowering the threshold, however, documents that constitute noise will be considered. The *LMs* for each document will be generated based on this ranking, yielding n *LMs*, with n equal to the number of relevant documents based on the query keywords. It should be noted that this step was performed using the *skip-gram idea*, with step s equal to two. Each LM may be created only after using one of the available smoothing procedures. To avoid a linguistic model giving 0 probability to an unseen event, i.e. when a word in the query is not included in an LM, we should remove some probability mass from certain more common events and apply it to occurrences we have not seen before.

Smoothing may be accomplished in a number of ways, including Laplace (add-one) smoothing, Linear Interpolation smoothing [15], add-k smoothing [16], back-off smoothing [16], and Kneser-Ney smoothing [17]. Among them, the proposed method evaluates the usage of the first two smoothing approaches, each of which produces results that are effective in accomplishing the ultimate aim. The strength of the algorithm is in its ability to determine the optimal ranking of relevant pages using the initial query, iteratively, as s evolves.

This variation leads to the generation of several LMs, each with step s, with $s = \{2, 3, \ldots, 10\}$. At each iteration, a new ranking of documents will be generated, thanks to the calculation of the Maximum Likelihood Estimation *MLE*, between the query q and each document d as shown in (1).

$$P(q|d) \approx P(q|M_d) \approx \prod_i^n P(w_i|w_{i-1}) \approx \frac{count(w_i, w_{i-1})}{\sum_{j=1}^n count(w_j, w_{i-1})} = \frac{count(w_i, w_{i-1})}{count(w_{i-1})} \tag{1}$$

After sorting all nine ranks, the one with the target document in the highest position, near to the top, will be selected. Additionally, this will allow for the determination of the λ parameters used in the interpolation smoothing process. By concentrating on the latter approach, it became important to execute the notion given by [7] about linear interpolation computation. Rather of adding one to the probability calculation, as the smoothing of Laplace does see Eq. (2), linear interpolation iteratively calculates the MLE of order two (*bi-grams*) see Eq. (3), all the way down to zero (*zero-grams*) see Eq. (4).

$$P(w_i|w_{i-1}) = \frac{count(w_{i-1}) + 1}{count(w_{i-1}) + |V|} \tag{2}$$

$$P(w_i|w_{i-1}) = \lambda P(q|M_d) + (1 - \lambda)P(q|M_c) \tag{3}$$

$$P(w_i) = \lambda \frac{1}{|V|} + (1 - \lambda)P(w_i) \tag{4}$$

where:

- $\sum_i \lambda_i = 1$
- M_d: represents the language model of the single document;
- M_c: represents the language model of the entire collection of documents;
- $|V|$: represents the number of unique words within the corpus of documents.

It is usually prudent to note that, similar to the iterative process of steps s, both λ parameters follow the same logic. The aim is to give both values a range of integers $\lambda = \{0.1, 0.2, \ldots, 1\}$. The amount of *perplexity* between the query word set $W = \{w_1, w_2, \ldots, w_N\}$ and the language model of the target page included in the ranking of relevant texts supplied by the tf-idf model will be computed in both smoothing procedures [18]. The calculation is shown in Eq. 5.

$$pp(W) = \sqrt[N]{\prod_{i=1}^N \frac{1}{P(w_i|w_{i-1})}} \tag{5}$$

After achieving the optimal ranking, the next step is to construct a *term-term matrix* [18], in which the terms include both those from the query and those from the language model of the whole collection of relevant texts included in the ranking. The co-occurrences of all words will be given in this matrix. On this sort of matrix, the computation of *Positive Pointwise Mutual Information (PPMI)* is feasible. PPMI is based on the assumption that the easiest method to assess the relationship between two words is to determine how much more often the two words occur in our corpus than we would have expected them to occur randomly. This metric is derived from the conventional PMI, which is a measure of the frequency of two occurrences, x and y, in comparison to what we would anticipate if they were independent (see Eq. 6).

$$pmi(x,y) = \log_2 \frac{P(x,y)}{P(x)P(y)} \tag{6}$$

The ratio indicates how much more often the two terms appear than we would predict by chance. Positive, negative, or infinite PMI values are all possible.Negative values, which indicate that occurrences occur less often than we would anticipate by chance, are notoriously untrustworthy when dealing with documents that include few words, as we do here. To resolve this issue, the PPMI is calculated, which substitutes negative values with zero as shown in Eq. 7.

$$PPMI(x,y) = \max(\log_2 \frac{P(x,y)}{P(x)P(y)}, 0) \tag{7}$$

However, why is the PPMI computation used? This is advantageous for calculating the similarity of words, i.e. their synonymy, for searching for paraphrases, for tracking the change in meaning of words, and for automatically discovering the meanings of words in various datasets. The cosine similarity is performed on the first 10 word vectors with the greatest positive PPMI values to determine the most comparable terms to those in the query. By the end of the inquiry, each token will have a maximum of 10 expansion terms. As a result, we can immediately understand how query expansion may be accomplished. Moving on, there is one more issue to resolve before we can compute the similarity of the cosine: the *high dimensionality* of the matrix.

To achieve a high degree of similarity while maintaining a low computing cost, another idea has been implemented which is the *Singular Value Decomposition (SVD)* presented the notion of using SVD on a term-term matrix [19]. By switching from sparse to dense vectors, it is possible to do more accurate similarity comparisons. The SVD algorithm allows for the decomposition of the term-term matrix (A), with dimensions txd, into three matrices [20] as shown in Eq. 8.

$$A = USV^T \tag{8}$$

where:

- U: matrix of dimension txm where the columns represent the left singular vectors of matrix A;
- S: diagonal matrix of dimension mxm, containing the singular values of matrix A;
- V^T: transposed matrix, of dimensions mxd, where the columns represent the right singular vectors of matrix A.

By multiplying the matrix U by the matrix S, a new matrix $\mathcal{D}$ of form as in 9, of dimension txm, is formed containing all the terms that will be compared via cosine similarity with the query terms contained in the matrix *mathcalT* as shown in Eq. 10 given by the product of S and V^T.

$$\mathcal{D} = U \times S \tag{9}$$

$$\mathcal{T} = S \times V^T \tag{10}$$

With all potential terms readily accessible for inclusion in the query tokens, we can now produce all conceivable queries. The number of queries generated is dependent on the number of words in the first query and any words received via the cosine similarity computation. With a maximum of ten words per token, the total number of produced queries is equal to the product of the number of possible pairings of terms and the number of possible pairs of terms as in 11.

$$\#Queries = \prod_{i}^{q}(\#sim\_words_i) \tag{11}$$

where i denotes a single word in the query and q denotes the total number of words in the initial question. As new inquiries, they will follow the same method as the original query, i.e., new LMs will be generated, along with new rankings of documents that include the target document in the first locations. Finally, the best query, or queries, will be chosen based on the level of perplexity reached.

5 Experimental Results

The dataset used for the experiments is the famous *Recipes1M+* [21], a collection created by MIT, consisting of more than one million culinary recipes. Of all these recipes, only a subset of 51235 documents of it was used due to their informative content which best fits the purpose of this paper. According to the information about the line distributions for each recipe, the instruction field has a greater number than the ingredients field. To optimise our search performance, we used the 'instructions' field (Fig. 1). The first ranking of significant papers produced by the tf-idf algorithm was reviewed using two distinct methods that were most closely related to the notion described in [22].

To be more precise, each category in a recipe is treated as a distinct item connected with a document. Both techniques depend on the ability to match relevant documents' categories to the category of the target document. Because the categories are not included in the dataset, the two suggested methodologies focus on "extracting" them straight from the web. The first solution makes use of an API called *Scrape Schema Recipe*, which scrapes the correct category using the link to the recipe website included in the dataset. Unfortunately, not all connections remain active, and hence the ranking is determined using three distinct methods:

1. **Overestimated**: consider the uncategorized document as good.
2. **Underestimated**: considers the uncategorized document not good.
3. **Discarded**: Discard the uncategorized document from the evaluation.

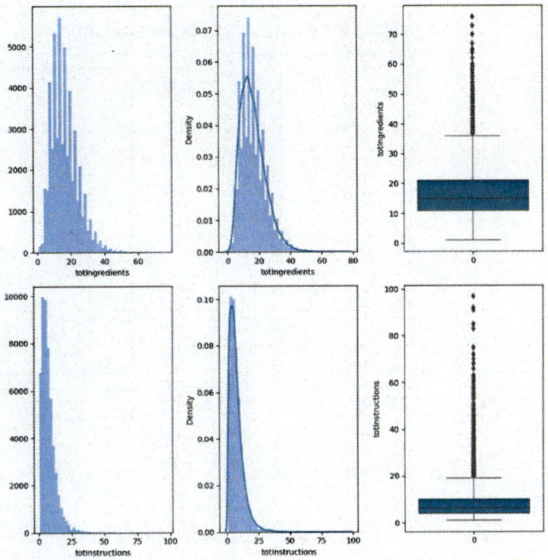

Fig. 1. Distributions of lines per ingredients and instructions.

As for the second method, this makes use of the *USDA* API, a library that has the task of taking every single ingredient of the recipe and fetching the corresponding category from a large database belonging to the United States Department of Agriculture. Compared to the first approach, the recipes that did not have a category are only four recipes. It is worth mentioning that both approaches are computationally expensive as the extraction of all categories took about two days.

In addition to all these evaluations, we decided to create a last one derived from a mixed approach (Scrape + USDA). Taking five random queries, the evaluations of the corresponding rankings are those reported in Table 1. As you can see, the mixed approach is the one that, in terms of average precision, manages to achieve the best evaluation. The performances, in terms of precision, recall and

Table 1. Average Precision on each query for each method.

Scrape schema recipe					
Queries	Overestimate	Underestimate	Discarded	USDA	Mixed (Scrape+USDA)
1	0.7562	0.3734	0.5962	0.9823	0.9953
2	0.9402	0.6792	0.9064	0.9974	0.9989
3	0.7542	0.2761	0.5429	0.9782	0.9986
4	0.8958	0.5334	0.8447	0.9528	0.9872
5	0.8346	0.5044	0.7558	0.9860	0.9948
Average	0.8379	0.4736	0.7290	0.9755	**0.99487**

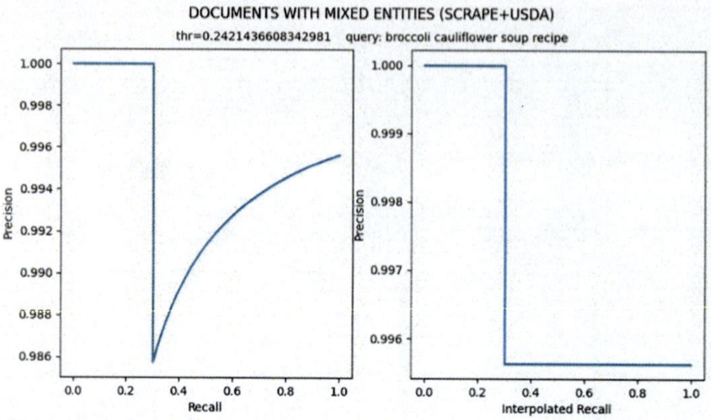

Fig. 2. Performance in terms of Precion, Recall and Interpolated Recall of mixed approach (Scrape+USDA)

interpolated recall, shown in (Fig. 2), demonstrating that the mixed approach is the best. Moving on to the evaluation of the new queries generated, a visual comparison, based on a PCA, was used between the ranking generated by the tf-idf method and each new query produced by the proposed method (Figs. 3, 4, 5, 6, 7).

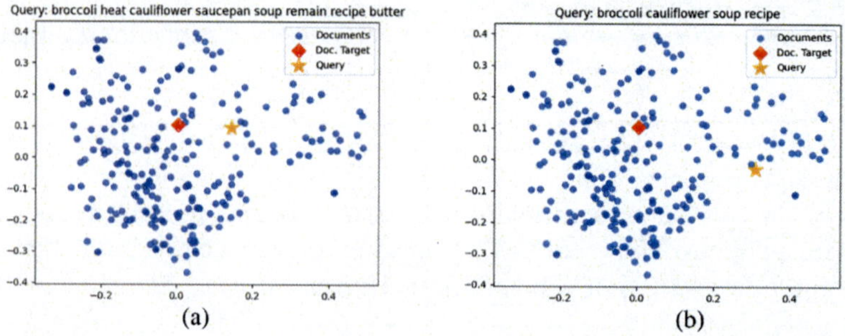

Fig. 3. Query (a) broccoli heat cauliflower saucepan soup remain recipe butter (b) broccoli cauliflower soup recipe

The goal is to find a query whose distance from the target document is less than all other distances produced by the remaining queries. As we can see, compared to the position of the original query, a query with a smaller distance has always been found. For each new query generated, the perplexity is calculated as the skip-grams step varies, with the language model of the target document. After various tests, with a higher number of queries, it can be stated that the skip-gram step and the perplexity are two inversely proportional measures, that is, as the step s increases, the perplexity p decreases. The same behavior occurs

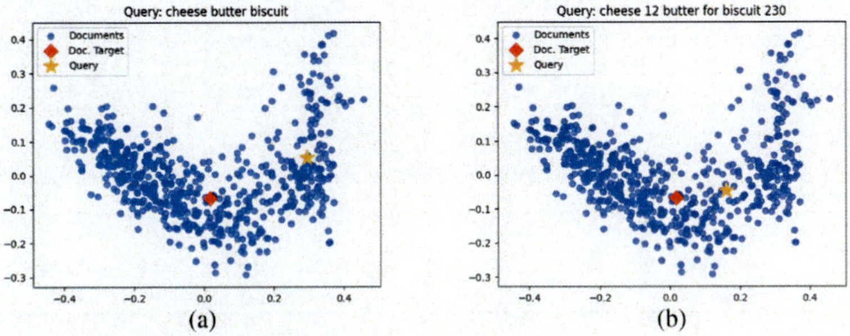

Fig. 4. Query (a) cheese butter biscuit (b) cheese 12 buffer for biscuit 230

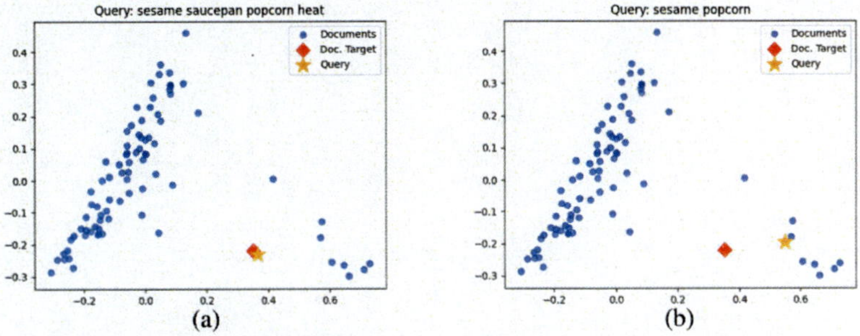

Fig. 5. Query (a) sesame saucepan popcorn heat (b) sesame popcorn

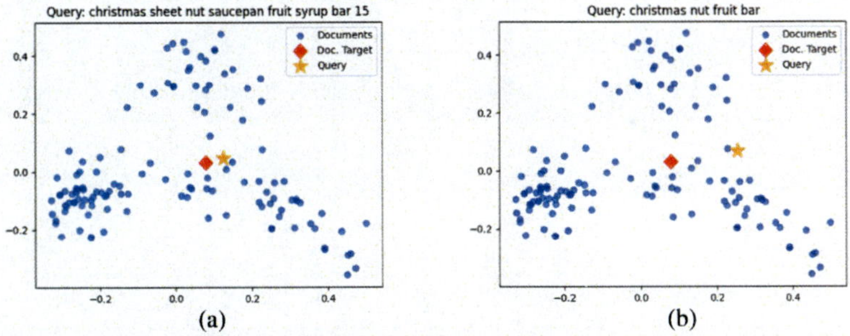

Fig. 6. Query (a) Christmas sheet nut saucepan fruit syrup bar 15 (b) Christmas nut fruit bar

with the λ_1 and λ_2 parameters present in the interpolated smoothing. When λ_1 is less than λ_2, perplexity always tends to decrease (Fig. 8). For the evaluation of the system four distinct libraries capable of tokenizing documents and queries were utilized: **Spacy**, **Gensim**, **Nltk**, and **Keras**. Each of them generates results that vary in terms of perplexity, the number of queries produced, calculation time (Table 3), and ranking (Table 2). As shown by the results, each strategy offers

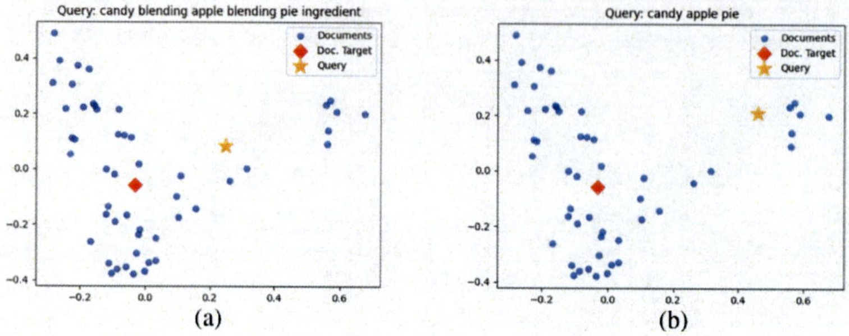

Fig. 7. Query (a) candy blending apple blending pie ingredient (b) candy apple pie

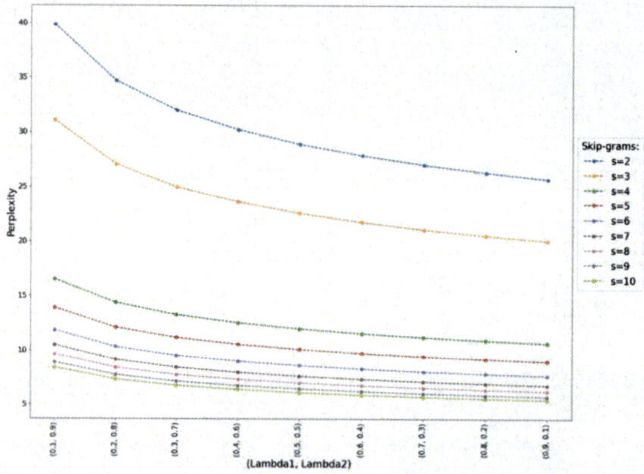

Fig. 8. Variation of the perplexity value based on the change of the step s and of the λ_1 and λ_2 values of interpolated smoothing.

Table 2. Target document position in the ranking of relevant documents. (T: *tf-idf*, P: *Proposed*)

Method	1		2		3		4		5	
	T	P	T	P	T	P	T	P	T	P
Keras	229	0	627	0	86	0	129	0	56	0
Nltk	229	0	627	0	86	0	129	0	55	0
Spacy	223	0	651	0	85	0	144	0	79	0
Gensim	241	0	656	37	88	0	117	0	42	0

distinct advantages. What each strategy has in common is that the target page is ranked first.

Looking at the results obtained with an additional five queries Table 4, for a total of ten queries, we can see that the best results come from Gensim. This is therefore able to find a greater number of queries that have less perplexity

Table 3. Performance in terms of number of queries (#Queries) and computation time.

Method	#Queries	Time
Keras	15.500	***Low***
Nltk	15.500	***Low***
Spacy	20.400	*High*
Gensim	**22.090**	*Medium*

Table 4. Euclidean Distance (D) between a query and the target document at a specific perplexity (P).

Queries	Keras		Nltk		Spacy		Gensim	
	D	P	D	P	D	P	D	P
1	0.15	16.42	0.15	16.58	0.11	34.87	0.13	90.16
2	227	17.91	0.11	22.37	0.21	11.56	0.15	53.44
3	0.03	05.42	0.022	05.41	0.07	05.15	0.01	05.03
4	0.04	12.39	0.05	12.45	0.09	12.44	0.01	10.83
5	0.35	23.04	0.31	23.22	0.43	42.25	0.27	10.36
6	0.24	06.39	0.22	06.39	0.24	03.93	0.21	04.02
7	0.13	1429.33	0.12	1521.33	0.24	06.03	0.12	03.43
8	0.38	13.87	0.39	13.81	0.46	13.65	0.27	08.11
9	0.57	05.31	0.56	05.31	0.61	04.76	0.41	03.92
10	0.01	04.27	0.01	04.29	0.06	05.12	0.01	04.28

with the target document than the other methods. To verify the veracity of the results, the Euclidean distance between the new query and the target document was calculated. As we can observe, a smaller distance implies a lower perplexity between the query and the target document. As for the other systems, Keras and Nltk obtain similar results, unlike the latter producing queries with the highest perplexity. As for Spacy, this produces queries with the greatest distance from the target document and in fact, comparing with the results obtained with Gensim, we can see that as the distance increases, the perplexity of each specific queries generated by Spacy also increases.

6 Conclusions and Future Work

In conclusion, it can be said that new queries are generated appropriately and that Gensim is the system that achieves the best performance. However, other things need improvement, such as defining a way for establishing a suitable threshold for creating each ranking of relevant documents. Throughout the research, the thresholds supplied by the sklearn library's precision recall curve function were considered. Regrettably, not all of them had a sufficient score to examine the target document. As a result, it was decided to take into account the initial threshold, referred to as the weight supplied to the target document using the cosine similarity approach.

This paper could be extended in various ways. Future directions of this work include improvements in search performance, where an ad hoc barrier can be established to prevent the ranking of relevant documents from including all of the collection of documents. Another enhancement is the decrease of the term matrix (with stochastic gradient descent). Concerning the usage of the various parsers, it would be interesting to design a hybrid system capable of producing a large number of questions in a short period of time. Moreover, it would be interesting to provide a mechanism capable of extending the initial query with words from a vocabulary such as Wordnet.

References

1. Cummins, R., O'Riordan, C.: Evolving co-occurrence based query expansion schemes in information retrieval using genetic programming. In: AICS 2005, p. 137 (2005)
2. Lafferty, J., Zhai, C.: Document language models, query models, and risk minimization for information retrieval. In: Proceedings of the 24th Annual International ACM SIGIR Conference on Research and Development in Information Retrieval, SIGIR 2001, pp. 111–119. ACM, New York (2001)
3. Ponte, J.M., Croft, W.B.: A language modeling approach to information retrieval. In: Proceedings of the 21st Annual International ACM SIGIR Conference on Research and Development in Information Retrieval, SIGIR 1998, pp. 275–281. Association for Computing Machinery, New York (1998)
4. Robertson, S.E., Jones, K.S.: Relevance weighting of search terms. J. Am. Soc. Inf. Sci. **27**(3), 129–146 (1976)
5. Croft, W.B., Harper, D.J.: Using probabilistic models of document retrieval without relevance information. J. Doc. (1979)
6. Zaragoza, H., Hiemstra, D., Tipping, M.: Bayesian extension to the language model for ad hoc information retrieval. In: Proceedings of the 26th Annual International ACM SIGIR Conference on Research and Development in Information Retrieval, SIGIR 2003, pp. 4–9. Association for Computing Machinery, New York (2003)
7. Gutkin, A.: Log-linear interpolation of language models. Mémoire de DEA, University of Cambridge (2000)
8. Chen, S.F., Goodman, J.: An empirical study of smoothing techniques for language modeling. Comput. Speech Lang. **13**(4), 359–394 (1999)
9. Karras, C., Karras, A., Sioutas, S.: Pattern recognition and event detection on IoT data-streams. arXiv preprint arXiv:2203.01114 (2022)
10. Karras, C., Karras, A., Avlonitis, M., Sioutas, S.: An overview of MCMC methods: from theory to applications. In: Maglogiannis, I., Iliadis, L., Macintyre, J., Cortez, P. (eds.) AIAI 2022. IFIPAICT, pp. 319–332. Springer, Cham (2022). https://doi.org/10.1007/978-3-031-08341-9_26

11. Karras, C., Karras, A., Avlonitis, M., Giannoukou, I., Sioutas, S.: Maximum likelihood estimators on MCMC sampling algorithms for decision making. In: Maglogiannis, I., Iliadis, L., Macintyre, J., Cortez, P. (eds.) AIAI 2022. IFIPAICT, pp. 345–356. Springer, Cham (2022). https://doi.org/10.1007/978-3-031-08341-9_28
12. Karras, C., Karras, A.: DBSOP: an efficient heuristic for speedy MCMC sampling on polytopes. arXiv preprint arXiv:2203.10916 (2022)
13. Karras, A., Karras, C., Drakopoulos, G., Tsolis, D., Mylonas, P., Sioutas, S.: SAF: a peer to peer IoT LoRa system for smart supply chain in agriculture. In: Maglogiannis, I., Iliadis, L., Macintyre, J., Cortez, P. (eds.) AIAI 2022. IFIPAICT, pp. 41–50. Springer, Cham (2022). https://doi.org/10.1007/978-3-031-08337-2_4
14. Lavrenko, V., Croft, W.B.: Relevance models in information retrieval. In: Croft, W.B., Lafferty, J. (eds.) Language Modeling for Information Retrieval. INRE, pp. 11–56. Springer, Dordrecht (2003). https://doi.org/10.1007/978-94-017-0171-6_2
15. Blu, T., Thevenaz, P., Unser, M.: Linear interpolation revitalized. IEEE Trans. Image Process. **13**(5), 710–719 (2004)
16. Falahatgar, M., Ohannessian, M.I., Orlitsky, A.: Near-optimal smoothing of structured conditional probability matrices. In: Advances in Neural Information Processing Systems, vol. 29 (2016)
17. Song, M., Yoo, C.D.: Multimodal representation: Kneser-ney smoothing/skip-gram based neural language model. In: 2016 IEEE International Conference on Image Processing (ICIP), pp. 2281–2285. IEEE (2016)
18. Jurafsky, D., Martin, J.H.: Speech and Language Processing: An Introduction to Natural Language Processing, Computational Linguistics, and Speech Recognition, vol. 3 (2008)
19. Schütze, H.: Dimensions of meaning. In: Proceedings of the 1992 ACM/IEEE Conference on Supercomputing, Supercomputing 1992, pp. 787–796. IEEE Computer Society Press, Washington (1992)
20. Deerwester, S., Dumais, S.T., Furnas, G.W., Landauer, T.K., Harshman, R.: Indexing by latent semantic analysis. J. Am. Soc. Inf. Sci. **41**, 391–407 (1990)
21. Marin, J., et al.: Recipe1M+: a dataset for learning cross-modal embeddings for cooking recipes and food images. IEEE Trans. Pattern Anal. Mach. Intell. **43**, 187–203 (2019)
22. Parvez, M.R., Chakraborty, S., Ray, B., Chang, K.W.: Building language models for text with named entities. arXiv preprint arXiv:1805.04836 (2018)

Grouping Test Results with the Common Root Cause Using String Similarity Algorithms

Vladimir T. Kramar[1](✉), Jukka K. Nurminen[1], and Tatu Aalto[2]

[1] University of Helsinki, Helsinki, Finland
{vladimir.kramar,jukka.k.nurminen}@helsinki.fi
[2] F-Secure, Helsinki, Finland
tatu.aalto@withsecure.com

Abstract. This paper presents an innovative concept of test log categorization that demonstrates how five different string similarity algorithms such as Pythons built-in diff library, Jaccard index, Jaro-Winkler distance, cosine similarity and Levenshtein ratio are applied on test logs from pytest - one of the popular assertion-based test frameworks. In order to minimize manual, error-prone work for software engineers of analyzing multiple test runs daily, these test logs are grouped into the following three distinctive categories; C1 - has similar failures in the same test, C2 - has a similar failure in two different tests and C3 - has a different failure in two same tests for easier root-cause analysis and fixes. The presented work demonstrates how efficient the string similarity algorithms can be.

Keywords: String similarity · Pytest · Testing · Software logs · Test logs · Machine learning

1 Introduction

In software development, the utilization of software logs that are generated during a run-time, usually on a system level, is not a novel concept and has been researched plenty. Software logs and information within them can be used but are not limited to such tasks as anomaly detection, health monitoring of a soft- ware system or many other applications [1]. Additionally, many commercial log analysis companies have been successful in providing different insights to their customers with logs such as Splunk or Sematext Logs [2, 3].

A fundamental question that almost all of the log analysis processes try to answer is: "How to turn unstructured log data into structured data?". Many studies propose different ways of turning unstructured log messages into structured ones. For example, Drain or Spell algorithms for log parsing are applicable [4, 5]. Alternatively, bolstering these and other different log parsing algorithms data science methods are applied. Statistical methods like Conformal Prediction or even applying deep learning methods are utilized [6, 7].

Among the studies regarding the utilization of software logs, studies focusing on utilizing test logs have not been found. The reason for that might be because the software

K. Daimi and A. Al Sadoon (Eds.): ICR 2022, AISC 1431, pp. 214–224, 2022.
https://doi.org/10.1007/978-3-031-14054-9_21

log analyses and log parsing focus mostly on their preventative nature, where failure is identified before it happens. The approach proposed in this paper focuses on achieving a time-saving solution to process the logs indicating a failure. That is expected to support software development where tests play an important role.

Continuous integration is a software development practice that relies on frequent commits and automated tests [8]. Modern software companies and open source projects utilize continuous integration in their software development pipeline [9]. Tests are essential practices of continuous integration. The tests produce logs in the same way as the software produce logs. Among these tests can be small unit tests or advanced end-to-end tests consisting of multiple smaller tests.

In this paper, we propose a concept and implementation of the introduced concept that categorizes failures that emerge in the pytest testing framework test logs into three categories. This is achieved by applying string similarity algorithms like Pythons built-in diff library, Jaccard index, Jaro-Winkler distance, cosine similarity and Levenshtein ratio on two tests logs that contain the test log and the failure within it [10–14].

Lastly, this paper presents the results of this approach on the test logs that were generated from the software that is being used in the production environment. Five different algorithms are applied to two different from each other data sets to validate the approach described above. Results show the great potential of this approach with this limited data set but have a shortcoming of mixing up the categories if the failures within the test logs are similar to each other. Nevertheless, even with such results the information that this approach provides warrants further development and shows promise.

The rest of the text is structured as follows. The Methodology section gives an overview of the problem and the proposed concept to solve the problem. In the Concept section, the main concept is presented along with the detailed groups and subgroups. In the Implementation section, a walk-through of the implementation of the concept is presented, including test log pre-processing and data set description. In the Results section, the findings from two different data sets are presented. In the Discussion section, some thoughts are given regarding the findings of this paper, including the benefits and drawbacks of this approach and the future perspective is introduced. Finally, the summarizing remarks are given in the Conclusion section.

2 Methodology

The work presented in this paper was performed as applied research in collabo- ration with the team of software developers from WithSecure [15]. WithSecure is a cyber-security software company that develops virus protection software.

As a real-world challenge, on a daily basis, software engineers face analyzing manifolds of failed tests. Sophisticated tools already aggregate the failing tests by the count and present the data in a convenient way for analysis. While a software engineer can fix the failing test with the most failures, this leaves other tests that are caused by the same failure potentially undetected and are left there to be discovered after the tests are rerun. In order to avoid this, a software engineer has left with grouping the tests that fail in the same way by hand. This task takes time and is easily error-prone, especially since the software logs come in all shapes and forms.

In order to avoid the error-prone manual work of grouping the test logs, this paper proposes and demonstrates the implementation of a concept of test log categorization utilizing string similarity algorithms. The analyzed algorithms are Python library diff, Jaro-Winkler distance, Jaccard score, cosine similarity and Levenshtein ratio.

In collaboration with WithSecure software engineers, it has been decided to categories the logs into three distinctive categories. Those categories are the following:

- Category 1: Similar failure within two same tests.
- Category 2: Similar failure within two different tests.
- Category 3: Different failure within two same tests.

Using such categorization, software developers can focus on fixing errors be- longing to one category only, which essentially saves resources and improves the quality of software testing processes. Test logs that were the input for the experiments were produced by pytest Python-based framework [16]. The generated test logs are a part of the production version of WithSecure software.

3 Concept

As a starting point, three categories of test logs are identified. In order to achieve a clear distinction between the categories, the similarity score from different string similarity algorithms was used as a measure. Similarity scores consist of two values. The first is an overall similarity score between the two tests. The score is calculated by comparing two test runs in their entirety with each other. The second is the failure similarity if the failure exists in the test run. This is calculated by comparing two failures from the tests in question with each other. Based on those metrics, categories and subcategories may be described as follows:

- Category 1 (C1) - Same failure, same test: Similarity score is high between a failing test in a test run and the same failing test in a different test run if the reason for failure is similar.

    - Category 1.1 (C1.1) - Same failure: Similarity score is high between the same failures in different test runs.

- Category 2 (C2) - Same failure, different test: Similarity score is high be- tween two different tests in different test runs that fail in a similar fashion. Additionally, it is lower than Category 1.

    - Category 2.1 (C2.1) - Same failure: Similarity score is high between the same failures in different test runs.

- Category 3 (C3) - Different failure, same test: Similarity score is low between two same tests in different test runs if the failure is different. Additionally, it is lower than in Category 2 and Category 3

- Category 3.1 (C3.1) - Different failure: Similarity score is low between two failures if the failure is different within the same test in different test runs.

Let us denote Categories 1, 2, and 3 as $C1$, $C2$ and $C3$ and subcategories 1.1, 2.1, and 3.1 as $C1.1$, $C2.1$ and $C3.1$. The relationship between the similarity scores of those categories can be summarized in Eq. 1 as such:

$$(C1 > C2 > C3) \land (C1.1 > C2.1 > C3.1) \tag{1}$$

4 Implementation

4.1 Data Description

Two data sets containing logs that represent typical software errors were pre- pared from the development logs and analyzed in this work. The first data set contained sixteen different log files. In every of those log files were several individual tests. Four of those log files were the result of the passed tests. Twelve of those were the results of the failed test runs. The second data set contained twelve different log files. Three of those log files were the result of the passed tests. Nine of those were the results of the failed test runs.

Both data sets have contained one failure per test, as this covers 99% of cases of failures in the production environment. All of the failures presented in those logs were artificially created, meaning that the test runs were intentionally meant to fail in a certain place and in a certain way. Nevertheless, they were developed to mimic the real-life scenarios from the actual test logs.

4.2 Test Log Prepossessing

Pytest test log files contain multiple tests. Every test starts with the "setup" keyword being present in the log message, and each test ends with a "teardown" keyword present in the log message. The keywords are used at later stages to extract different tests from test logs consisting of multiple tests. Additionally, each individual line within the test follows also a pattern. This pattern consists of a timestamp in a format of year-month-day hour-minute-second, millisecond. Secondly, a level of debugging that can take values such as "[INFO]", "[DEBUG]" or in a case of a failure present within a test – "[CRITICAL]". Lastly, the actual log message that has previously mentioned keywords like "call" and "teardown". Table 1 shows examples from multiple different test logs that are used in this paper. These logs are not in order and are there just to illustrate better what has been described above. Due to the sensitive nature of text and privacy concerns, some parts of the log message have been transformed into log messages.

Given the reasons above, one can transform each line in the unstructured log files into a structured format such as a pandas data frame for deeper analysis. These lines can be parsed into three columns. Those columns are the date and a timestamp, the logging level, and the log message itself. Line by line the log entries are then parsed using a built-in function of Python ".split()" utilizing "["and"]" characters into the structured data frame.

Additionally, as noted before, each test long may contain multiple tests. Using the freshly created data frame that contains processed test logs, these test logs need to be separated into smaller tests. That is done by utilizing "setup" and "teardown" keywords found in the log message. These keywords denote the start and end of an individual test. Splitting is done by selecting all rows between log lines that contain the above-mentioned keywords and extracting the test name from the line that contains "setup" keywords. The selected lines are considered as separate data frames and placed into a separate array. The actions described lead to an array full of data frames that are considered to be individual test runs within different test runs.

As the last step in the pre-processing phase, manual categorization takes place. This manual categorization is only done to validate the effectiveness of different string similarity algorithms and validation of the hypotheses presented in the Concept part. Manual categorization is achieved in two steps with the utilization of descriptive names of the logs.

The first step is the permutation of two, created from the array of data frames originated from the previous steps of the pre-processing phase. The permutation simplifies the comparison and access to the two individual tests.

The categorization is achieved by iterating over permutations of individual tests and utilizing the name of a test log to which an individual test belongs to, to assign that individual test to a category based on the rules described in the "Concept" part of the paper.

The outcome above-mentioned steps of pre-processing lead to an array of tuples. Each item of two items from the tuple is an individual test from a bigger test run log that now belongs to one of the categories or none. Table 2 shows an example of one of the items from a random tuple. Column "log name" tells to which test log does a test in question belong to, column "timestamp" is the extracted timestamp, column "level" describes the level of debugging, column "log message" contains the log message, column "testname" tells the name of the test that was extracted and lastly column "category" contains the category to which this test log name and test name belong to.

4.3 String Similarity Algorithms

String similarity algorithms accept two strings and return a score between 0 and 1, on how similar these two strings are. 0 means that strings are not similar at all and 1 means that strings are identical. Additionally, if a failure is present in both of items of the tuple then the lines that correspond to the failure and their similarity are calculated separately. The algorithms were chosen based on the group that they belong to and the ease of access to them via popular Python external python packages or built-in (Table 3).

Table 1. Example of pytest logs

testlog
2022-01-27 11:31:38,285 [DEBUG] *log message*
2022-01-27 11:31:38,285 [DEBUG] setup: *log message*::test 01
2022-01-27 11:31:38,300 [DEBUG] call: *log message*::test 01
2022-02-11 15:45:01,618 [CRITICAL] *failure stack trace*
2022-01-27 11:31:41,941 [DEBUG] teardown: *log message*::test 01

Table 2. Example data frame after log prepossessing

log name	time stamp	level	log message	test name	category
pass 1	*timestamp*	debug	*log message*	test 01	no failure
fail same error 1	*timestamp*	critical	*log message*	test 01	C1
fail diff error 3	*timestamp*	info	*log message*	test 99	C3
fail diff test 1	*timestamp*	info	*log message*	test 02	C2

Table 3. Algorithms

Name	Type
Similarity ratio	Sequence-based algorithm
Jaro-Winkler distance	Edit distance-based algorithm
Levensthein ratio	Edit distance-based algorithm
Jaccard index	Token-based algorithm
Cosine similarity	Fuzzy matching algorithm-

5 Results

Results were analyzed by plotting the score similarities calculated by similarity algorithms on an x and y-axis. Where an overall test similarity is plotted on an x-axis and failure similarity is plotted on a y-axis. Ideally, plotting these values would form distinct three groups where each group is a representation of categories described in the Concept section. The best performing algorithm is chosen by applying the following metrics:

Question 1 (Q1) - Are the three categories identifiable?
Question 2 (Q2) - Does the Eq. 1 hold, e.g., are the categories in the correct order?
Question 3 (Q3) - What is the mean distance between the center of each category?

For Q1, if the categories are easily identifiable and can be grouped without any doubt, then it is considered a positive in terms of this research paper for an algorithm in question. For Q2, if the algorithm scored the groups in an order that was specified in Eq. 1 then it is considered positive in terms of this research paper for an algorithm in question. For Q3, the higher the mean distance be- tween clusters of categories, the better it is. This means that the clusters are further apart in a significant matter, and the difference between categories is more significant.

5.1 Data Set 1 Results

Figure 1 depicts all of the five algorithms applied to the first data set. Table 4 answers each question specified above for each of the algorithms.

Table 4. Data set 1 results

	Sm ratio	cos similarity	Jaccard index	Jaro-Winkler	Levenshtein ratio
Q1	No	Yes	No	Yes	Yes
Q2	No	No	No	No	No
Q3	0.5272	0.5260	0.0807	0.1433	0.3606

5.2 Data Set 2 Results

Figure 2 depicts all of the five algorithms applied to the second data set. Table 5 answers each question specified above for each of the algorithms.

Table 5. Data set 2 results

	Sm ratio	cos similarity	Jaccard index	Jaro-Winkler	Levenshtein ratio
Q1	Yes	Yes	No	No	Yes
Q2	No	Yes	No	No	Yes
Q3	0.3761	0.1135	0.0833	0.1051	0.2014

6 Discussion

In the first tested data set, three out of five algorithms formed three distinct groups, with the “Eq. 1” not holding for any of the algorithms. The biggest difference in the groups was achieved by the Levenshtein index and the cosine similarity algorithms.

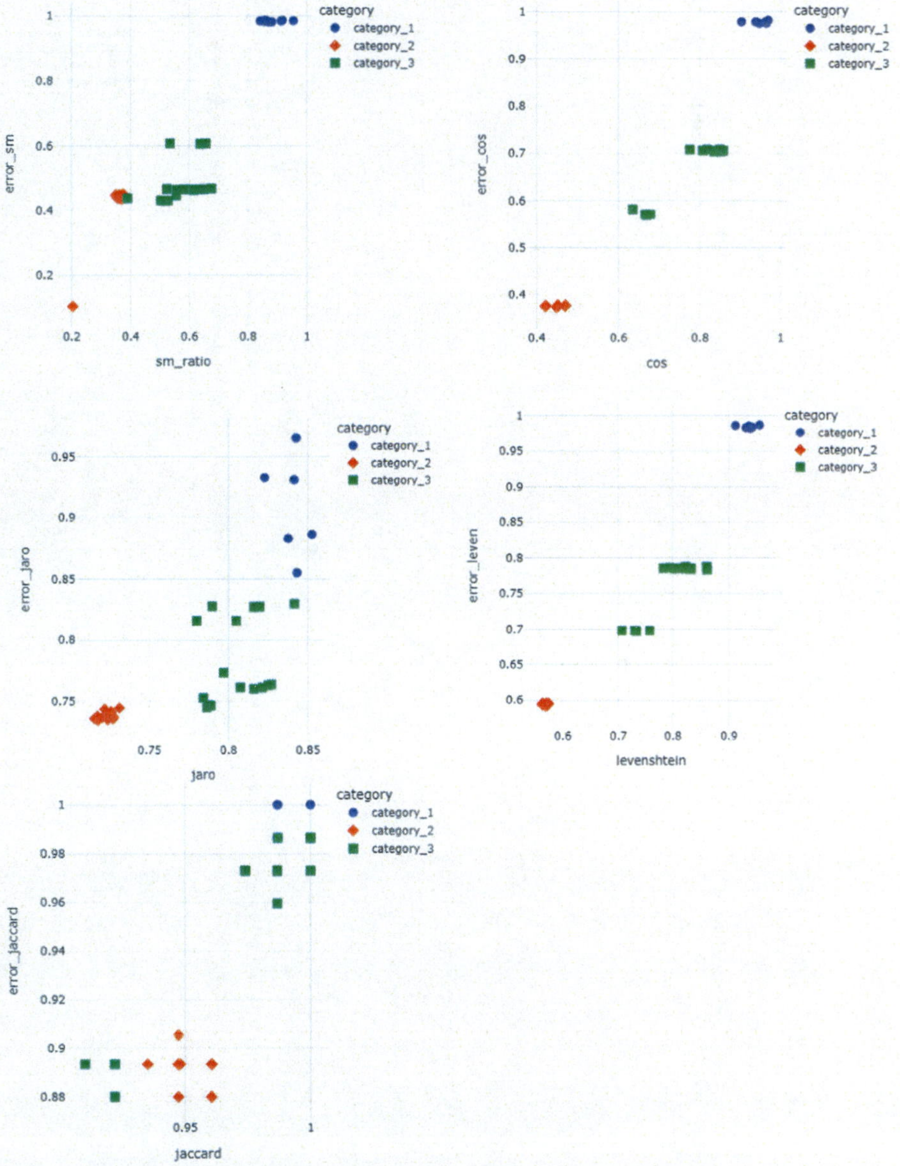

Fig. 1. Data set 1. Five algorithms. Starting from the top left: **similarity ratio**, **cosine similarity**, **Jaccard index**, **Jaro-Winkler distance** and **Levenshtein ratio**

Upon closer examination of the data set test logs, it be- came apparent that the failure that was happening in all the instances of the second category and the third category was way too similar to the one in the first category instances. This caused the misalignment of the categories and has been identified as the biggest shortcoming of this approach. The second data set excluded such a situation as the data was formed to make sure to contain

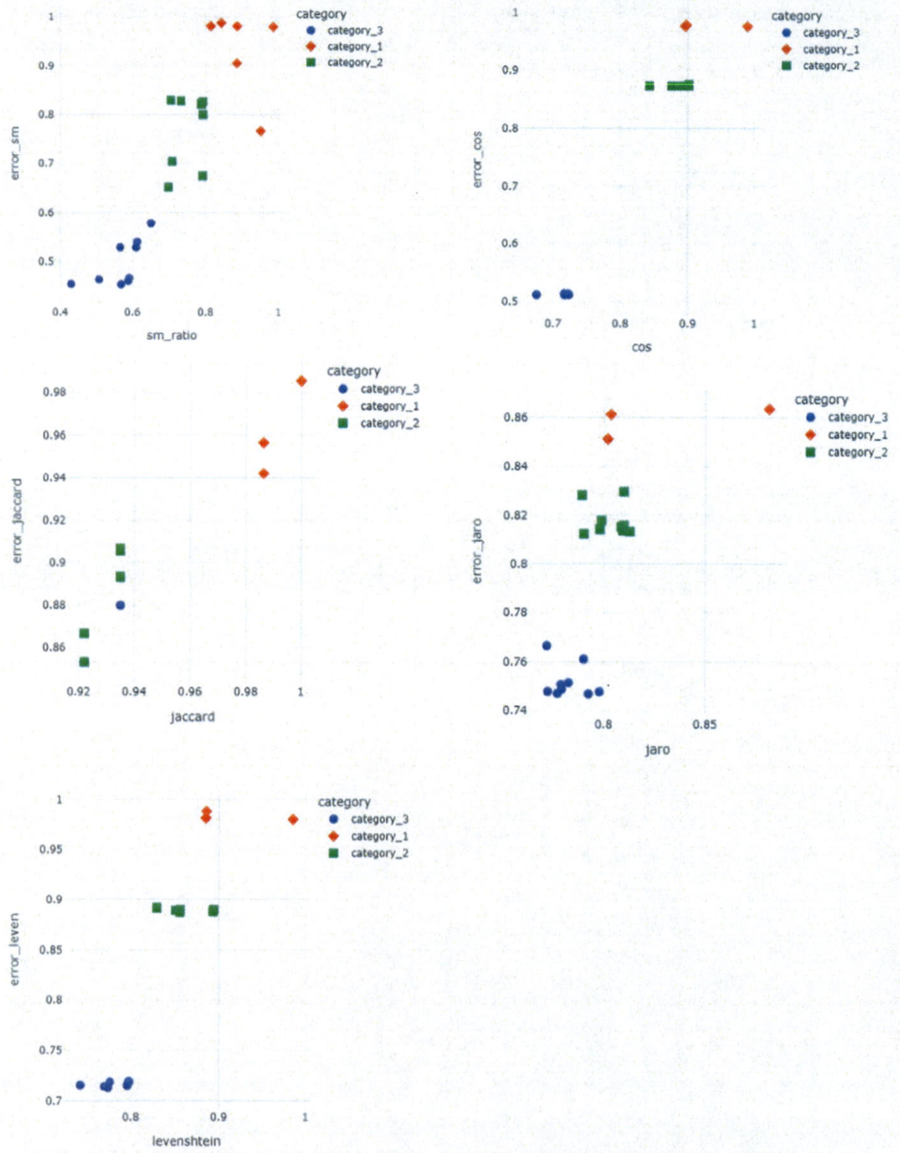

Fig. 2. Data set 2. Five algorithms. Starting from the top left: **similarity ratio**, **cosine similarity**, **Jaccard index**, **Jaro-Winkler distance** and **Levenshtein ratio**

different enough failures. With clear enough failures in the second data set, categories align correctly and Eq. 1 holds. Similarly, to the first data set, the best performing algorithms were the cosine similarity and the Levenshtein index.

Even though the Eq. 1 did not hold for the first data set, even with the three distinctive groups being separate enough and grouped together, it brings an explicit value to a software engineer. The goal of all the three approaches is to find groups of failures and tests that are akin to each other, and this approach accomplishes exactly that. From a point of view of a software engineer, the most interesting result is the clusters, which imply the similarity between the failures. This in return could indicate that fixing the failure that is dominant in a specific cluster would cause other tests in the cluster to be fixed as well.

Both the concept and the implementation were presented to WithSecure and validated by the software engineers of the company. This approach, though, needs to be even further validated with real test log data from software that is deployed in production, has more complex failures in the logs and lastly tests and different amounts of instances in each category. These three points will be the next undertaking of the team. The current hypothesis is that manual categorization will not always be available, especially in the production environment. Therefore, the application of machine learning, e.g., clustering algorithms, may be applied to form the three categories.

7 Conclusion

Both the concept and the implementation were presented to F-Secure and vali- dated by the software engineers of the company. This approach, though, needs to be even further validated with more sophisticated data that has more complex failures of the tests and different amounts of instances in each category. These three points will be the next undertaking of the team. The current hypothesis is that manual categorization will not always be available, especially in the production environment. Therefore, the application of machine learning, e.g., clustering algorithms, may be applied to form the three categories.

Out of five different algorithms, the best performing on both data sets were the Levenshtein index and the cosine similarity. The presented approach was found to be useful, warranting further research and development of the approach. The next steps are to investigate the applicability of the approach to more com- plex failures, different counts of failures and deployment of a tool utilizing the presented concept to the production environment as part of the continuous integration pipeline. Yet the other next step in the development of the presented concept is the application of machine learning clustering algorithms to automate the data processing.

Acknowledgements. This work was funded by local authorities ("Business Finland") under grant agreement ITEA-2019-18022-IVVES of ITEA3 programme [17]. The authors would like to express gratitude to Alexei Vyskubov and Matvej Pashkovskiy from F-Secure for the discussions and their insightful input that lead to the findings of this paper.

References

1. Uspenskij, M.B.: Log mining and knowledge-based models in data storage systems diagnostics. In: E3S Web of Conferences, vol. 140, p. 03006 (2019)
2. Splunk—Turn Data Into Doing. https://www.splunk.com/
3. Sematext Logs—Cloud Log Management Service—Hosted ELK. https://sematext.com/logsene/
4. He, P., Zhu, J., Zheng, Z., Lyu, M.R.: Drain: an online log parsing approach with fixed depth tree. In: 2017 IEEE International Conference on Web Services (ICWS), pp. 33–40. IEEE (2017)
5. Du, M., Li, F.: Spell: online streaming parsing of large unstructured system logs. In: IEEE Transactions on Knowledge and Data Engineering, vol. 31, no. 11, pp. 2213–2227 (2019). https://ieeexplore.ieee.org/document/8489912/
6. Ren, Y., et al.: System log detection model based on conformal prediction. Electronics **9**(2), 232 (2020)
7. Du, M., Li, F., Zheng, G., Srikumar, V.: DeepLog. In: Proceedings of the 2017 ACM SIGSAC Conference on Computer and Communications Security, New York, NY, USA, pp. 1285–1298. ACM (2017)
8. Continuous Integration. https://martinfowler.com/articles/continuousIntegration.html
9. Durieux, T., Abreu, R., Monperrus, M., Bissyand´e, T.F., Cruz, L.: An analysis of 35+ million jobs of Travis CI; an analysis of 35+ million jobs of Travis CI. In: 2019 IEEE International Conference on Software Maintenance and Evolution (ICSME) (2019). https://travis-ci.org
10. difflib - Helpers for computing deltas (2022). https://docs.python.org/3/library/difflib.html
11. Cohen, W.W., Ravikumar, P., Fienberg, S.: A comparison of string metrics for matching names and records (2003)
12. Jaccard, P.: The distribution of the flora in the alpine zone.1. New Phytol. **11**(2), 37–50 (1912)
13. Han, J., Kamber, M., Pei, J.: Getting to know your data. In: Data Mining, pp. 39–82. Elsevier (2012). https://linkinghub.elsevier.com/retrieve/pii/B9780123814791000022
14. Levenshtein, V.I., et al.: Binary codes capable of correcting deletions, insertions, and reversals. In: Soviet Physics doklady, vol. 10, no. 8, pp. 707–710 (1966)
15. Home—WithSecure™. https://www.withsecure.com/en/home
16. pytest: helps you write better programs—pytest documentation. https://docs.pytest.org/en/7.0.x/
17. Home - Ivves. https://ivves.eu/

Download Speed Optimization in P2P Networks Using Decision Making and Adaptive Learning

Aristeidis Karras[1(✉)], Christos Karras[1], Konstantinos C. Giotopoulos[2], Ioanna Giannoukou[2], Dimitrios Tsolis[3], and Spyros Sioutas[1]

[1] Computer Engineering and Informatics Department, University of Patras, Patras, Greece
{akarras,c.karras,sioutas}@ceid.upatras.gr

[2] Department of Management Science and Technology, University of Patras, Patras, Greece
{kgiotop,igian}@upatras.gr

[3] Department of History and Archaeology, University of Patras, Patras, Greece
dtsolis@upatras.gr

Abstract. Pure peer-to-peer networks serve to secure information in a decentralized, distributed topology. The multi-armed bandit (MAB) problem formulation proves to be a useful tool for analyzing the problem of optimizing new peer connections. In this paper, we outline the new peer scenario described as a reinforcement learning problem with MABs in order to identify the fastest peer to download from during the connection process. The MAB problem involves k slot machines which are also called one-armed bandits and pay out reward values according to an internal distribution, of which the agent is not aware. The aim is to choose a strategy to learn which arms pay out the most in order to maximize total reward over a set number of rounds. Results indicate that UCB and ε-first performed the best at selecting the optimal peer in each of our test scenarios. Contrariwise, SoftMax and ε-greedy unperformed.

Keywords: P2P networks · Reinforcement learning · Decision making · Intelligent agents · Adaptive learning · Multi-armed bandit · Strategies

1 Introduction

Peer-to-peer (P2P) computer networks provide an environment for content distribution in which the integrity of the system is not endangered by the loss of a single, centralised node. Based on [1], true p2p systems require peers to be directly accessible (without intermediary entities) and the network state or quality of service to be retained in the event that a peer is withdrawn from the network for any reason. The prerequisites for peer-to-peer networks differ per application domain. However, new peers that connect to the server for the

K. Daimi and A. Al Sadoon (Eds.): ICR 2022, AISC 1431, pp. 225–238, 2022.
https://doi.org/10.1007/978-3-031-14054-9_22

first time have no knowledge of the network status. As a result, new peers cannot be held responsible for preserving the network state and content if existing nodes disconnect. It is critical that this new peer receives relevant data as soon as feasible in order to meet both the needs of a real p2p ecosystem and any required quality of service standards. With the extra volatility of a dynamic network configuration, the velocity at which a new peer may be brought up to speed becomes significantly more important. P2P systems may also be seen as streaming applications where event detection techniques can be used to find a new peer in the network [2] while MCMC methods [5,6] and heuristics as in [3] can be used to discover the fastest peer to download from.

For example, consider the case of a p2p network wherein a new peer joins with the intent to be brought up to speed with the rest of the network as soon as feasible (i.e. download all the data in the network from other peers). However, the new peer does not have prior knowledge for the network speeds of its seeds, only just how much data it receives over time when it chooses a peer and receives data from them in one (or more) time step(s). The reward is the average number of bytes received across the number of time steps spent on that action. At this point, it is assumed that data packets are UDP datagrams.

Time steps should not be confused with steps (or rounds) in the algorithm. Multiple time steps can happen during a single round, as a step is when the agent makes a decision for a given number of time steps. Rounds and steps are used interchangeably within the paper. The agent should aim to choose the peer that is transmitting the fastest. However, consider that network speeds may change, and the optimal seed to leech from will not always be the best. This is named as a restless scenario. We simulate these dynamics by assigning each peer a set of possible states, as well as a transition matrix of probabilities to transit from one state to another at every time step. In this case, every peer is running its own Markov process in the background, irrespective of the action by the agent.

This case can be solved with a multi-armed bandit (MAB) approach where each peer is considered as an arm in the MAB algorithm. The agent will choose to pull an arm and receive reward for a certain number of time steps. During every time step, the network dynamics shift, and each arm may transit to an other one of its states (regardless of if it was the arm selected or not). Naturally, this creates greater variance in average reward payout, which serves to simulate the noise present in real-world network systems.

Previous works [4,7,8] investigate p2p networks where the peers communicate or compete with one another. However, in our case we assume no information about peers is initially present on the hardware of the new peer, and that transmitting this information ahead of the vital data packets should not be a priority. Therefore, the trial-and-error methodology of MAB agents fits the learning requirements under these constrained conditions. Various algorithms are considered to solve the MAB problem, and a few are selected and implemented in order to evaluate their efficiency against this problem.

The remainder of the paper is organized as follows. In Sect. 2 related work in the field of multi-armed bandits is surveyed and covered in order to compare our work with solutions to similar problems and verify the validity of our results. Section 3 describes the methodology in both theory and application level while Sect. 4 highlights the experimental results and their findings. A brief discussion takes place in 5 and finally, the conclusions and future directions of this work are presented in Sect. 6.

2 Related Work

Multi-armed bandits (MABs) serve as a useful abstraction for optimization problems that require decision making with reward outcomes that are initially unknown. In [9], secondary user nodes pick a single channel without knowing its quality or availability in cognitive radio networks utilizing a MAB strategy. The authors employ an upper confidence bound (UCB) algorithm named QoS-UCB. Extending the bandit model makes wireless network selection more flexible, maximizing end-user perceived quality [10]. In this formulation, the agent may perform two tasks: measure or utilise. Measuring simply permits assessment while utilising adds exploitation. Measuring is faster than utilising, which might require many stages. The payout distributions are determined by the algorithm selection. Aggressive algorithms like poker have little regret but high variability, making them less dependable [10] while more efficient methods are shown in [11].

In [4], strategies are provided for coordinating numerous MABs agents and learning stochastic network conditions. The agent transmits instead of receiving in their problem formulation. While outbound transmission speed or success may be measurable, reception rate is not. The final receiver may not have the resources to unpack transmission bundles in time, causing congestion. In [12], scheduling algorithms for MAB problems in wireless networks are presented. ε-greedy, an algorithm that balances exploration and exploitation, has flaws in its pure randomness and does not take confidence intervals into consideration. UCB uses this and gradually reduces exploration. There is a distinguish between single and multi-player multi-armed bandits (SMAB and MMAB). SMAB is used in single-peer leeching and centralised network methods while MMAB typically compromises independence for synchronisation overheads.

The study in [13] investigates how k players cooperate to locate an ε-optimal arm in an MAB environment and find communication only once players learn $\sqrt{k}$ times quicker than a single player. This strategy may be handy if network peers vary or service quality varies. Little effort has been put towards adapting bandit algorithms to p2p network contexts [7]. This paper implements the ε-greedy stochastic algorithm in a p2p network, scaling with network size, obtaining a linear speedup in terms of the number of peers, and retaining the asymptotic behaviour of the standalone version. In p2p networks, competition is unavoidable, particularly when peers attempt to stay up to date. Unpredictable competition makes management tough. Hence, distributed clustering scenarios are utilized for overcoming MAB difficulties in p2p networks [14]. All peers solve the same issue in one setting, whereas a cluster of peers solves the same problem within its cluster. This achieves an ideal regret rate, defined as the difference between the optimal reward total and the collected rewards.

In [8], an online learning strategy based on an MAB architecture is designed to handle peer rivalry and delayed feedback. The work in [15] optimises data rate transfers and minimises power consumption in wireless p2p networks. Similar constraints are common when examining graphical processing units (GPUs), as in [16]. MAB problems are also highlighted in [17], where the integration of MAB problems with recommendation systems is presented.

3 Methodology

In this section, we present a brief summary of each algorithm investigated, as well as our methodology for creating test cases and evaluating the performance of the algorithms on the new peer update task using a limited number of hyper-parameters.

3.1 Employed Algorithms

The most common algorithm utilized to multi-armed bandit (MAB) problems is named ε-greedy. In ε-greedy a single hyperparameter ε is taken which indicates the probability of exploration (i.e., choosing a random arm from the possible selections), with $1-\varepsilon$ being the probability of choosing the optimal arm based on the average rewards so far. ε-greedy is utilized as well as some of its variants in this paper.

Initially, ε-first is an ε-greedy strategy in which only exploration is done for the initial $T\varepsilon$ rounds, and pure exploitation occurs during the remaining rounds. The number of rounds (also called steps) is defined as T per run [18]. This forces exploration meaning peak rewards will be delayed, but broader experience is gained as a trade-off. Additionally, ε-decreasing is one more ε-greedy variant whereabouts the initial ε value ε_0 is decreased over the number of rounds completed. In particular, the probability of exploration at a given time t is defined as

$$\varepsilon_t = \min\left\{1, \frac{\varepsilon_0}{t}\right\} \text{ where } \varepsilon > 0 \tag{1}$$

The values for ε_0 are typically not on the interval $[0,1]$, instead values like 1.0, 5.0, and 10.0 are used [18].

The SoftMax method (also called Boltzmann Exploration) performs action decisions based on *probability matching* methods [18]. Each arm a of k arms holds an associated probability

$$p_a = e^{Q_a/\tau} / \sum_{a'} e^{Q_{a'}/\tau} \tag{2}$$

where Q_a is the estimated action value associated with action a. The hyperparameter of SoftMax is τ, called the *temperature*. It can be varied similar to ε in ε-greedy.

Another variant of SoftMax is Exp3, using the idea of Boltzmann Exploration and probability matching [18]. Each arm a of k arms has an associated probability

$$p_a(t) = (1-\gamma)\frac{w_a(t)}{\sum_{j=1}^{k} w_j(t)} + \frac{\gamma}{k} \tag{3}$$

of being pulled at time t. The single hyperparameter γ indicates the learning rate. The weights associated with each action a at time t are denoted $w_a(t)$.

In many of the previously mentioned works, UCB (Upper Confidence Bound) and slight alterations of UCB were used. Given its popularity and excellent results we hoped it would also perform well within our environment setup. Instead of selecting actions based on probabilities, UCB alters its exploration and exploitation as it gathers information about the environment. Least-taken actions are prioritized during the exploration phase, and once the estimated action values are more established, UCB exploits the action with the highest estimated reward. This action selection is derived from the following

$$A_t = argmax_a \left[Q_t(a) + C\sqrt{\log t / N_t(a)} \right] \tag{4}$$

where $Q_t(a)$ is the estimated value of action a at time t, C is a confidence value hyperparamter that controls the level of exploration, and $N_t(a)$ is the number of times action a has been selected prior to time t. The exploitation part of the equation is $Q_t(a)$, while the second half handles the level of exploration also controlled by the hyperparameter C. UCB-1 slightly alters the default algorithm by including a constant of 2 being multiplied by the $\log t$ as such,

$$A_t = argmax_a \left[Q_t(a) + C\sqrt{2\log t / N_t(a)} \right] \tag{5}$$

This is a popular point of view on the original UCB algorithm that we considered to include to see how they may differ in our implementation.

Another MAB algorithm named poker was introduced in [10] which has low regret but is unreliable due to high variance. Hence, because of these problems, time constraints, and the complexity of the pseudo-code included in the paper, we decided to not cover poker in our evaluation.

3.2 Implementation

The initial peer setup for this work is comprised from a set of 5 single-state peers we call *init*5: $PeerArm(2,1)$, $PeerArm(4,1)$, $PeerArm(6,1)$, $PeerArm(8,1)$, $PeerArm(10,1)$. This simple layout removes the simulated dynamism of multi-state peers, but provides a descent baseline evaluation for each algorithm.

For the automation of the creation of multiple peers, we introduce Algorithm 1 which takes as input a number of peers to generate, and three distributions (with their associated hyperparameters) from which it samples the number

Algorithm 1. produce_peers

Require: number of peers n, the distribution for state counts $\mathbb{S}$ and its parameters s_p, the distribution for means $\mathbb{M}$ and its parameters m_p, and the distribution for standard deviations $\mathbb{D}$ and its parameters d_p
Ensure: An array of $PeerArm$ objects $\boldsymbol{\Phi}$

Initialize $\boldsymbol{\Phi}$ as an empty array
for p = 0 **to** n **do**
  $n_s \sim \mathbb{S}(s_p)$
  if $n_s < 1$ **then**
    $n_s = 1$
  end if
  Initialize Π as an empty array of means
  Initialize Σ as an empty array of standard deviations
  for p = 0 **to** n_s **do**
    $\pi \sim \mathbb{M}(m_p)$
    $\sigma \sim \mathbb{D}(d_p)$
    Append π to Π
    Append σ to Σ
  end for
  Initialize T as an empty $n_s \times n_s$ transition matrix
  for i = 0 **to** n_s **do**
    Sample n_s values $\rho_i \sim Uniform(0, 1)$
    Set each $T_{i,j}$ to $\frac{\rho_{i,j}}{\sum_j \rho_i}$ $\forall j \in [0, n_s)$
  end for
  $\phi = PeerArm(\Pi, \Sigma, T)$
  Append ϕ to $\boldsymbol{\Phi}$
end for
Return $\boldsymbol{\Phi}$

of states a peer will have, and the mean and standard deviation for each state reward. Each state requires a mean and standard deviation because rewards are generated utilizing a normal distribution.

The generate function $prod10$ set of peers utilizes Algorithm 1 to produce 10 peers using the specification below, each of which is more realistic in their transmission speed (reward) variance than $init5$. Respectively we perform the same task for 20 peers, labelled $prod20$.

- $prod10 = produce\_peers(10,$
- $np.random.poisson, dict(lam = 5.0),$
- $np.random.normal, dict(loc = 10.0, scale = 1.5),$
- $np.random.normal, dict(loc = 0.5, scale = 0.1))$

The algorithms outlined in Sect. 3.1 are implemented in *Python* 3.9 language and evaluated using a *PyCharm* Jupyter Notebook. Each algorithm utilizes a generic *BanditEnv* environment in order to execute actions and resets the environment after each execution. The estimates of the action value are computed by using a sample-average estimate of action value, with an initial estimate of 0 for each peer. This method does not exploit the stochastic state-changing Markov process in each peer, as the agent would have to learn the transition matrix for each peer as well. In the purpose of conserving time and preserving room for future study, this work uses the sample-average estimation approach. By default, the MAB algorithms will take an action for 1 time step, but we have added functionality such that it is possible to take more than 1 action, and the end reward for that step is simply the average of rewards received by taking that action for that many time steps. Bear in mind that the state of peer transitions will remain to be active for each time step. Therefore, the agent cannot lock the network state by taking an action for several time steps.

4 Experimental Results

Each algorithm completes 100 runs, with a fixed number of n steps. In this experiments we test for $n = 1$ and $n = 20$. The number of steps relates to how long the peer will be receiving data from its peers. This number is varied in order to visualize the algorithmic performance in the short and long-term.

The average reward for each step is averaged across 100 runs, and each of these averages is plotted across the number of steps. In the following subsection, we present plots created by *matplotlib* library and *seaborn* package containing visually definitive evaluations of each algorithm in our test environment. Our experiment results do not include UCB-1.

Due to the similarities to UCB, UCB-1 produces almost identical results. This was not unexpected, and it was excluded in order to simplify the comparisons with the other algorithms. We also decided to drop ε-decreasing, as its poor performance produced nothing of note.

4.1 Evaluation

Figure 1 shows the general performance of each algorithm when it comes to the set of static peers, *init*5.

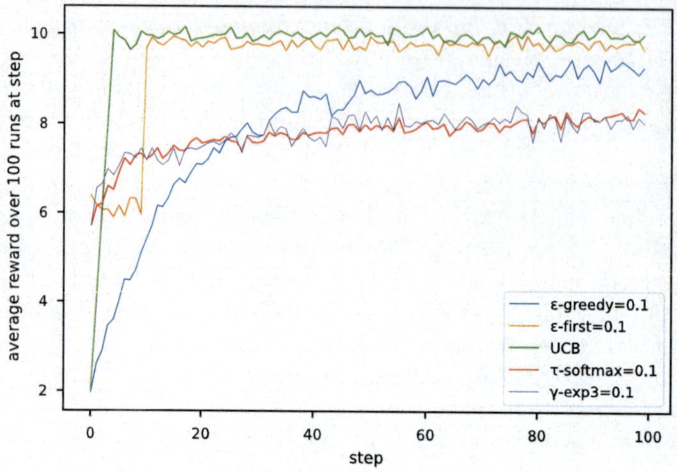

Fig. 1. Average reward over time for each algorithm over 100 steps using the *init*5 peers with 1 time step per action.

The aforementioned papers, seem to agree that ε, τ, and γ values should be around 0.1. However, we decided to see if stronger exploitation would benefit the learning curve. We noticed that lowering the C hyperparameter of UCB did not improve its already strong performance at $C = 1$, so we increased it instead.

Figure 2 uses the *init*5 peers with C value of UCB set to 15, and all other algorithm hyperparameters set to 0.01.

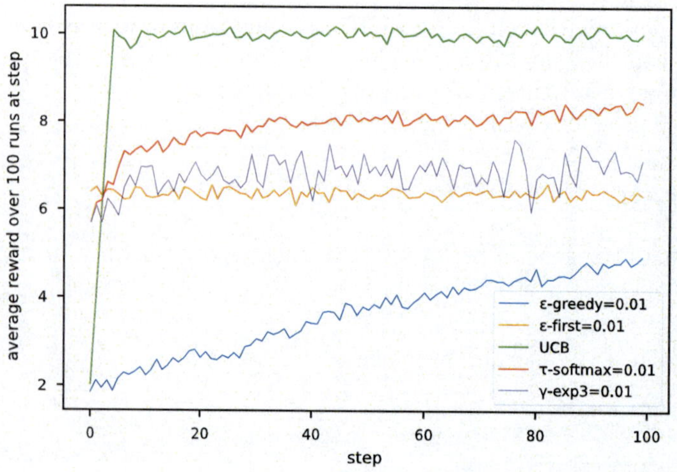

Fig. 2. Average reward over time for each algorithm over 100 steps using the *init*5 peers with 1 time step per action. Different hyperparameters are noted. UCB uses $C = 15$ as opposed to $C = 1$.

Figure 3 uses the dynamic *prod*10 peer set. Exp3 seems to peak higher than SoftMax compared to Fig. 1, but then they are almost identical. The other algorithms have similar performance, although it seems that the dominance of UCB suffers only slightly in stochastic scenarios.

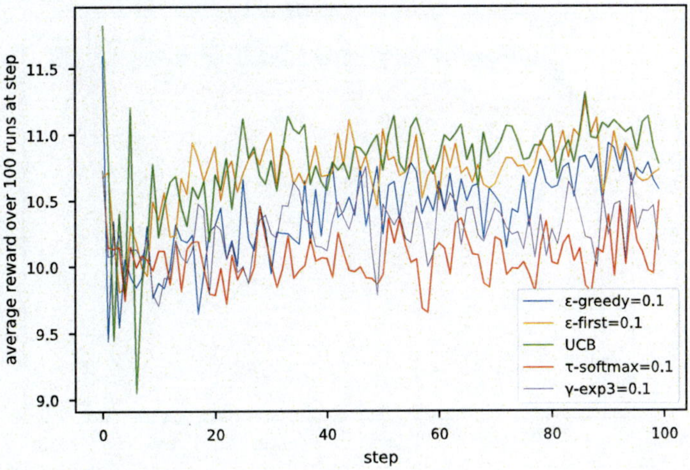

Fig. 3. Average reward over time for each algorithm over 100 steps using *prod*10 peers with 1 time step per action.

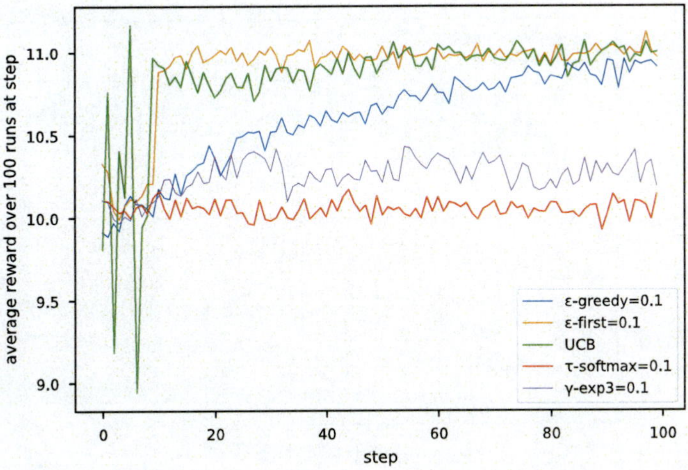

Fig. 4. Average reward over time for each algorithm over 100 steps using *prod*10 peers with 20 time steps per action.

Increasing the time steps to 20 (the amount of time steps the agent will dedicate to a particular peer) shows a slight reduction in the variance of SoftMax and Exp3 in Fig. 4. However, it is also noteworthy that the overall average reward peaks higher for each algorithm, compared to Fig. 3, with 1 time step per action.

Based on the results in Fig. 1, we wanted to find out if SoftMax would ever overtake ε-greedy. In Fig. 5 we see that SoftMax eventually stabilizes with lower variance but it is still lower than ε-greedy.

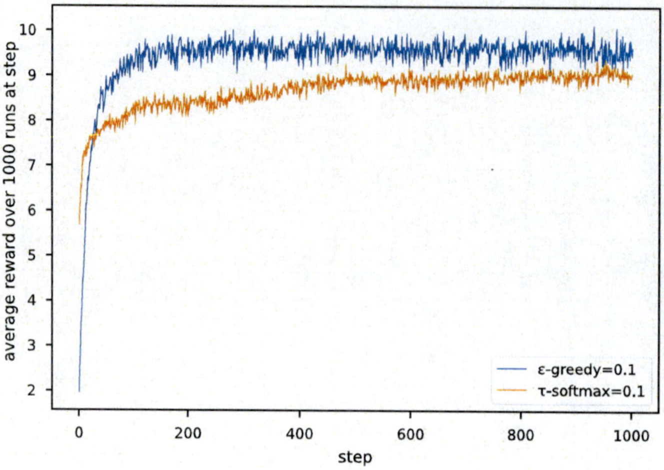

Fig. 5. Average reward over time for ε-greedy and SoftMax over 1000 steps using *init*5 peers with 1 time step per action.

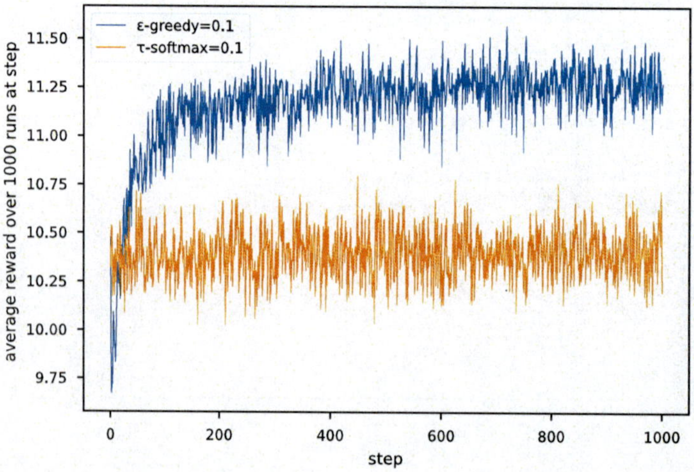

Fig. 6. Average reward over time for ε-greedy and SoftMax over 1000 steps using *prod*10 peers with 1 time step per action.

However, Fig. 6 shows that this is not the case for the more dynamic *prod*10 peers. Even after only 1000 steps, it is clear that SoftMax is not rising above ε-greedy while on *init*5 its performance was significantly higher.

As we have seen, ε-first is capable of competing with UCB in optimal peer selection. In Fig. 7, we show that extending the exploration proportion for more peers does not present noticeable improvements. We can therefore say that $\varepsilon = 0.1$ is a safe heuristic for ε-first, but also that, in this case, more peers lead to a reduction in average reward variance in the exploitation phase.

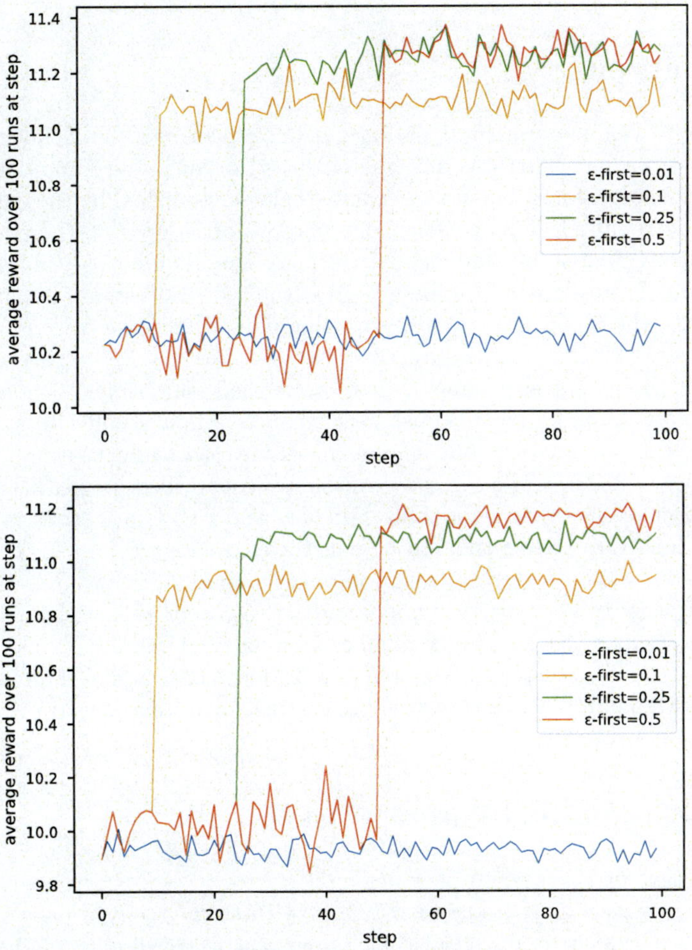

Fig. 7. Comparing average reward over time for various ε values in ε-first using 10 peers (above) and 20 peers (below) with 1 time step per action.

As seen in Fig. 7, the set with the greater number of peers, attains a higher average reward than the set with fewer peers. Note that all peers in both sets are created from the same distributions. This is due to the fact that more peers means more chances for a single peer to be significantly better than the best peer in a set of fewer peers. In Fig. 7 in the top subfigure, the plots are created using the *prod*10 function, indicating that the number of peers is 10 while in the bottom subfigure, the plots are created using the *prod*20 function indicating that the number of peers is 20. Additionally, noteworthy is the fact that ε-first=0.5 took almost 50 steps to reach a descent amount of reward and therefore the performance was the highest. This leads us to the initial observation where as other works highlighted, the value of ε-first must be within $[0.01, 0.25]$ range.

5 Discussion

According to our experimental findings, UCB performed significantly well in every test situation. This was anticipated based on our study and conclusions from comparable efforts, but we were nevertheless astonished by the small number of steps required. This performance may be attributed to the specified C value, which regulates the amount that the algorithm requires of exploration and exploitation. As anticipated, running UCB with $C = 15$ substantially altered the behaviour of the algorithm, resulting in a significant increase in the number of learning steps before reaching stability.

The methods ε-greedy and ε-first performed smoothly, although they required more steps to get a robust performance. ε-first seemed to struggle in the first ~10 learning steps, but it immediately leaped to fluctuating about the performance of UCB, while ε-greedy eventually got itself to beneath UCB.

In respect to the other algorithms, SoftMax and Exp3 have significant short-term and long-term trade-offs. As demonstrated in Figs. 5 and 6, we directly compared SoftMax to ε-greedy over a longer period of steps and varied the number of peers to get a better understanding. We were able to determine that SoftMax exceeds ε-greedy for low number of steps while as the number of steps increases, ε-greedy overtakes. This offers SoftMax some appeal if we were in a scenario with a small number of peers operating for a long period of time, but this is very improbable.

6 Conclusions and Future Work

In the context of the peer-to-peer network system presented, we were able to investigate a variety of well-known MAB algorithms (ε-greedy, ε-first, UCB and more) each of which produced distinct outcomes. To verify the validity of the results, related literature is surveyed in order to compare our work with solutions to similar problems. In terms of performance, the most robust of the group was UCB, while ε-first performed almost identically in the example with the 1 time step per action. Increasing the number of peers inside a network causes the average reward value to rise. There may be a negative relationship between the number of peers and the variance, but the data are ambiguous. This suggests that our solution may scale effectively as the number of peers in the network rises; nevertheless, this variance connection requires more investigation.

Future directions of this work include the implementation of the aforementioned poker algorithm along with additional methods explored in related works, such as a gossip-based algorithm. The outcomes of these future experiments can aid in our comprehension of the performance of more complicated and modern algorithms in contrast to these undemanding ones. Moreover, a modification of the behaviour of the environment in the hopes of simulating a peer-to-peer network that would permit various types of user communication can occur. This will qualify for a more realistic stochastic environment, which should make algorithm performance comparisons more interesting and accurate, similar to a real-world scenario where noise is present to all types of communications.

References

1. Schollmeier, R.: A definition of peer-to-peer networking for the classification of peer-to-peer architectures and applications. In: Proceedings First International Conference on Peer-to-Peer Computing, pp. 101–102. IEEE (2001)
2. Karras, C., Karras, A., Sioutas, S.: Pattern recognition and event detection on IoT data-streams. arXiv preprint arXiv:2203.01114 (2022)
3. Karras, C., Karras, A.: DBSOP: an efficient heuristic for speedy MCMC sampling on polytopes. arXiv preprint arXiv:2203.10916 (2022)
4. Avner, O., Mannor, S.: Multi-user communication networks: a coordinated multi-armed bandit approach. IEEE/ACM Trans. Netw. **27**(6), 2192–2207 (2019)
5. Karras, C., Karras, A., Avlonitis, M., Giannoukou, I., Sioutas, S.: Maximum likelihood estimators on MCMC sampling algorithms for decision making. In: Maglogiannis, I., Iliadis, L., Macintyre, J., Cortez, P. (eds.) AIAI 2022. IFIP Advances in Information and Communication Technology, vol. 652, pp. 345–356. Springer, Cham (2022). https://doi.org/10.1007/978-3-031-08341-9_28
6. Karras, C., Karras, A., Avlonitis, M., Sioutas, S.: An overview of MCMC methods: from theory to applications. In: Maglogiannis, I., Iliadis, L., Macintyre, J., Cortez, P. (eds.) AIAI 2022. IFIP Advances in Information and Communication Technology, vol. 652, pp. 319–332. Springer, Cham (2022). https://doi.org/10.1007/978-3-031-08341-9_26
7. Szorenyi, B., Busa-Fekete, R., Hegedus, I., Ormándi, R., Jelasity, M., Kégl, B.: Gossip-based distributed stochastic bandit algorithms. In: International Conference on Machine Learning, pp. 19–27. PMLR (2013)
8. Yang, M., Zhu, H., Wang, H., Koucheryavy, Y., Samouylov, K., Qian, H.: Peer to peer offloading with delayed feedback: an adversary bandit approach. In: ICASSP 2020–2020 IEEE International Conference on Acoustics, Speech and Signal Processing (ICASSP), pp. 5035–5039. IEEE (2020)
9. Modi, N., Mary, P., Moy, C.: QoS driven channel selection algorithm for cognitive radio network: multi-user multi-armed bandit approach. IEEE Trans. Cogn. Commun. Netw. **3**(1), 49–66 (2017)
10. Boldrini, S., De Nardis, L., Caso, G., Le, M.T., Fiorina, J., Di Benedetto, M.G.: muMAB: a multi-armed bandit model for wireless network selection. Algorithms **11**(2), 13 (2018)
11. Vial, D., Shakkottai, S., Srikant, R.: Robust multi-agent multi-armed bandits. In: Proceedings of the Twenty-second International Symposium on Theory, Algorithmic Foundations, and Protocol Design for Mobile Networks and Mobile Computing, pp. 161–170 (2021)

12. Li, F., Yu, D., Yang, H., Yu, J., Karl, H., Cheng, X.: Multi-armed-bandit-based spectrum scheduling algorithms in wireless networks: a survey. IEEE Wirel. Commun. **27**(1), 24–30 (2020)
13. Hillel, E., Karnin, Z.S., Koren, T., Lempel, R., Somekh, O.: Distributed exploration in multi-armed bandits. In: Advances in Neural Information Processing Systems, vol. 26 (2013)
14. Korda, N., Szorenyi, B., Li, S.: Distributed clustering of linear bandits in peer to peer networks. In: International Conference on Machine Learning, pp. 1301–1309. PMLR (2016)
15. Si, P., Yu, F.R., Ji, H., Leung, V.C.: Distributed sender scheduling for multimedia transmission in wireless mobile peer-to-peer networks. IEEE Trans. Wirel. Commun. **8**(9), 4594–4603 (2009)
16. Tasoulas, Z.G., Anagnostopoulos, I.: Improving GPU performance with a power-aware streaming multiprocessor allocation methodology. Electronics **8**(12), 1451 (2019)
17. Silva, N., Werneck, H., Silva, T., Pereira, A.C., Rocha, L.: Multi-armed bandits in recommendation systems: a survey of the state-of-the-art and future directions. Expert Syst. Appl. **197**, 116669 (2022)
18. Vermorel, J., Mohri, M.: Multi-armed Bandit Algorithms and Empirical Evaluation. In: Gama, J., Camacho, R., Brazdil, P.B., Jorge, A.M., Torgo, L. (eds.) ECML 2005. LNCS (LNAI), vol. 3720, pp. 437–448. Springer, Heidelberg (2005). https://doi.org/10.1007/11564096_42

Systematic Review for Selecting Methods of Document Clustering on Semantic Similarity of Online Laboratories Repository

Saad Hikmat Haji[1](✉), Karwan Jacksi[2], and Razwan Mohmed Salah[3]

[1] Department of Information Technology, Duhok Polytechnic University, KRA, Dahuk, Iraq
saad.hikmat91@gmail.com
[2] Department of Computer Science, University of Zakho, KRA, Zakho, Iraq
karwan.jacksi@uoz.edu.krd
[3] Department of Computer Science, University of Duhok, KRS, Dahuk, Iraq
razwan.mayi@uod.ac

Abstract. In the era of digitalization, the number of electronic text documents has been rapidly increasing on the Internet. Organizing these documents into meaningful clusters is becoming a necessity by using several methods (i.e., TF-IDF, Word Embedding) and based on documents clustering. Document clustering is the process of dynamically arranging documents into clusters such that the documents contained within a cluster are very similar to those contained inside other clusters. Due to the fact that traditional clustering algorithms do not take semantic relationships between words into account and therefore do not accurately represent the meaning of documents. Semantic information has been widely used to improve the quality of document clusters by grouping documents according to their meaning rather than their keywords. In this paper, twenty-five papers have been systematically reviewed that are published in the last seven years (from 2016 to 2022) linked to semantic similarities which are based on document clustering. Algorithms, similarity measures, tools, and evaluation methods usage have been discussed as well. As result, the survey shows that researchers used different datasets for applying semantic similarity-based clustering regarding the text similarity. Hereby, this paper proposes methods of semantic similarity approach-based clustering that can be used for short text semantic similarity included in online laboratories repository.

Keywords: Document clustering · Semantic document clustering · Semantic similarity · TF-IDF · Word embedding · Online laboratories

1 Introduction

The huge success of the Information Society and the World Wide Web has generated in a considerable rise in the volume of textual electronic information available. As a result, the research community has developed a strong interest in computer comprehension of text in order to enable the correct exploitation, administration, categorization, and retrieval of textual material [1–3].

K. Daimi and A. Al Sadoon (Eds.): ICR 2022, AISC 1431, pp. 239–252, 2022.
https://doi.org/10.1007/978-3-031-14054-9_23

Clustering is a critical technique for unsupervised learning. In this context, related items are clustered together into a single cluster during the clustering process. Accordingly, within a cluster, documents are distinct from those in neighboring clusters. In general, clustering is a strategy for grouping texts based on their content similarity. And document clustering's objective is to aid humans in finding and digesting information [4, 5].

Traditional document clustering algorithms treat the terms "words" in the documents as features; however, the semantic relationship between these terms in the texts is ignored. Certain difficulties, such as synonymy and polysemy, ambiguity, and excessive dimensionality, can be addressed by conventional procedures. As a result, a solution to the challenge of grouping document descriptions in a way that satisfies the unique requirements of document clustering is required [6, 7]. To compile documents into coherent clusters, it is critical to leverage the documents' semantic associations between terms and concepts. Semantic similarity is required in this case. The term of semantic similarity refers to a precise measure for certain pamphlets or concepts instead of a similarity that can be calculated roughly concerning reflect grammar, such as string format. Consequently, statistical methods are used for asset estimation semantic connections between language units and concepts or examples by comparing knowledge that confirms their significance or representation of life, using a numerical definition [8].

Numerous methods for document clustering have been proposed. The Term Frequency Inverse Document Frequency (TF-IDF) has been the most frequently used way of representing a corpus before applying a clustering method. Additionally, Word Embedding methods like Glove and Word2vec are used to represent words as n-dimensional vectors, clustered using a clustering algorithm such as K-Means, hierarchical agglomerative clustering (HAC), DBSCAN, or the other clustering algorithm [9, 10].

The main goal of this paper is to provide a comprehensive overview of several semantic-driven strategies for document clustering that can improve the quality and performance of the clusters created, followed by a solution to the following question: Which methods can be used for document clustering of the Online Laboratories Repository?

With the excessive supply of broadband Internet at the end of the last decade, many research groups all over the world have started the exploration of ways to support and facilitate the learning activities of students by using new possibilities. Online laboratories are fundamental for home experimentation because they are specially designed for distant learning students to acquire introductory hands-on experience and familiarize themselves with real-life phenomena. These online experiments can be found in different fields, including electronics, mechatronics, informatics, etc. [11].

The rest of this paper is organized as follows: Sect. 2 explains the fundamentals of document clustering. Section 3 reviews in detail prior recent 25 papers. Presents the results and as well as analyses in Sect. 4. The proposed methodology can be shown in Sect. 5. Section 6 concludes this paper and findings.

2 Principles of Document Clustering

This section examines document clustering and its two methodologies, conventional and semantic, significant obstacles and issues associated with document clustering. Additionally, it discusses the advantages of semantic clustering over traditional clustering.

As shown in Fig. 1, Clustering is the automated organization of text documents into numerous meaningful clusters or groupings. One cluster comprises papers with a similar subject that are distinct from those in the other cluster, which contains documents with a different subject. Two traditional methods and semantics can be used to integrate the documents [6].

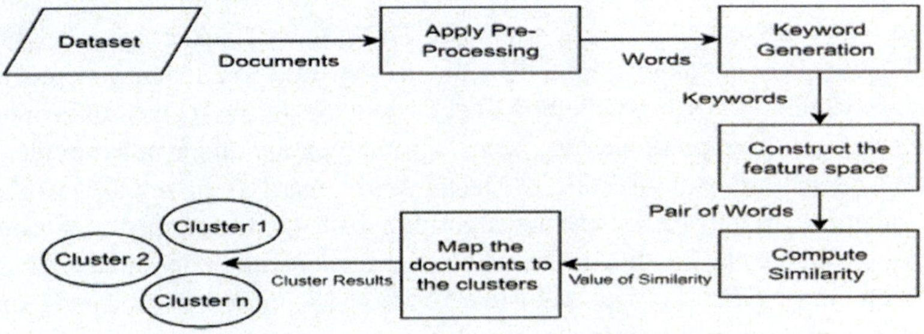

Fig. 1. Clustering documents as a typical process [6]

In general, some challenges and difficulties with document clustering can be included such as suitable documents feature for document clustering, appropriate similarities in the term-document and document-document similarities measuring calculation, proper clustering technique for effective cluster construction based on similarity results. Appropriate valuation metrics are required to evaluate the clustering's quality and adequate tools for running a clustering procedure on documents [6]. Synonymy and Polysemy, High dimensionality and Cluster labelling issues can be accounted as well [12].

The traditional model of clustering document has employed the Bag of Words (BOW) form to generate keyword phrases that identify duplicate words inside the document. The primary issue in traditional model has ignored the semantic links between words. A semantic document cluster can be used to generate a clustering of the documents since it requires rethinking of meaningful relationships, which may be unable to discriminate between two distinct groups [13].

On the other hand, semantic collection is one of the most essential strategies for document clustering. This approach focuses on the relationship between semantics, such as (words and phrases) that are considered in attempting to identify the meaning of a language element and how it is formed differently depending on the language, where significant documents are put together in one block. In contrast, non-significant documents are grouped together in another. With the result that clustering can assist in defining a cluster's topic, and sentences can be ethically connected to one another in a variety of ways [14, 15].

3 Related Work

In the current studies, researchers are focused on semantic features of clustering document to improve cluster accuracy. Therefore, authors consult external databases such as WordNet, Wikipedia, Lucene, and others. By the same token, the authors in their study have used different clustering algorithms, methods, similarity measures, datasets, and evaluation measures.

In 2016, Desai and Laxminarayana [16] Introduced a model for clustering documents that categorize texts based on their shared concepts. The suggested model begins by identifying all of the coreferences in each collection's documents. Polysemy and synonymy are addressed by capturing an appropriate understanding of the term based on its context using WordNet and Semantic similarity. The proposed clustering model is implemented on the classic4 dataset, and the results demonstrate an efficiency improvement. The suggested model's primary method to document clustering included five modules: coreference resolution, preprocessing, sense disambiguation and synonymy identification, feature selection, and bisecting K-Means. With regard to the research of Zandieh and Shakibapoor [5] they have presented algorithm to cluster texts based on meanings of the words through a new method to find semantic relationship between words based on Wordnet ontology. Then text data is clustered using the proposed method and hierarchical clustering algorithm. The steps followed as: Documents preprocessed, converted to vector space model, and then are clustered using the proposed algorithm semantically. The experimental results showed that the quality and accuracy of the proposed algorithm are more reliable than the existing hierarchical clustering algorithms. the stages of proposed algorithms are deleting numbers and punctuations, tokenizing documents and converting them to the smallest semantic unit (token), then deleting stop words, Words' stemming, and after that, representing documents in form of vector space model, creation of TF-IDF matrix, making semantic TF-IDF matrix and creating distance matrix.

Jacksi et al. [15] proposed an efficient semantic clustering strategy for the Wikipedia and IMDB movie datasets. Two clustering algorithms, HAC and K-Means, were utilized, and the findings were clarified so that they could be compared. For internal evaluation purposes, the results achieved by employing the silhouette metric can be considered the best results acquired by applying the K-Means algorithm to the 20-Newsgaroap dataset. In contrast, the lowest result was obtained by applying the HAC algorithm to the txt-Sentoken dataset. The best result was obtained for external evaluation by applying the K-Means algorithm with the purity metric to the txt-Sentoken dataset. In contrast, the worst result was obtained by applying the HAC method with the 20 Newsgroup dataset and the Adjust-rang-score metric. Additionally, the running time consumption of both algorithms was determined, with the HAC algorithm achieving the best result in all states. In addition, Mohammed et al. in their research [17] presented a semantic document clustering technique based on Glove word embeddings and the DBSCAN algorithm. Their proposed system consists of four major steps: downloading and grouping datasets, preprocessing data, applying the Glove word embedding.

In 2016, Bafna et al. [10] used TF-IDF technique, fuzzy K-means, and a hierarchical algorithm. The experiment is being conducted on a limited dataset, and cluster analysis is being performed. The experiments are tried on different real and artificial dataset such as NEWS 20, Reuters, emails, research papers on different topics. Radu et al. [18] compared the accuracy of four standard clustering methods (K-Means, Spherical K-Means, LDA, and DBSCAN) in conjunction with the Document to Vector model. They used two stemmers and a lemmatizer to preprocess the input corpus to ensure that the Doc2Vec embeddings are independent of the preprocessing strategy. The results reveal that Doc2Vec performed better in all clustering algorithms. Salih and Jacksi, [19] provided a method for grouping documents using the NLTK vocabulary based on semantic similarity. The approach begins with the definition of synopses from the IMDB and Wikipedia datasets, tokenization, and stemming. Following that, a vector space is generated using TF-IDF, and the ward's approach and K-means algorithm are used for clustering. Each algorithm can be implemented in one of three ways: without preprocessing, with preprocessing but without stemming, or with stemming. The Silhouette metric is used in conjunction with seven other measures to determine the degree of similarity between the five distinct datasets. The outcome demonstrated that for small datasets, Ward's technique outperforms K-means. Additionally, Stanchev, [20] proposed the semantic clustering approach based on a similarity graph that stores the degree of semantic association between terms, where a term can be either a word or a phrase. They validate their system experimentally using the Reuters-21578 benchmark, which has 11 362 newswire stories that are manually classified into 82 categories. They group the documents using the k-means clustering algorithm.

Hssina et al. [21] evaluated the approaches for calculating semantic similarity between text documents. The methods for estimating document similarity are critical components of document clustering. They concentrated on approaches for calculating semantic similarity using the WordNet lexical database and the VSM. And can be thought of as the descriptors and weighting retrieved from their text corpus. An experiment was done with students who created text documents to evaluate the procedures. Experiments on WordNet demonstrate that the suggested system enhances the accuracy of semantic similarity between text documents. In addition, Fatimi et al. [13] demonstrated how to use semantic web tools to cluster and review textual documents. they highlighted some of the recent works on RDF code modification and was inspired to introduce a related pipeline of semantic operations for RDF-based semantic text clustering. The most important feature is to provide an overall architecture for semantic text clustering focused on RDF data modeling. This approach incorporates many approaches to create a compelling and powerful structure capable of analyzing textual documents using machine learning techniques coupled with semantic web principles.

Stanchev, [22] discussed on how to generate a probabilistic graph using WordNet knowledge. They improved existing algorithms by tagging each word and meaning with a segment of expression. They then showed how to extend the graph using DBPedia data. They put the algorithm to the test by comparing it to an algorithm that uses the cosine similarity metric and an algorithm that only uses WordNet knowledge. The findings show that adding DBPedia information increases the stability of the Reuters-21578 benchmark while also making it more reminiscent of the algorithm. However, Banik et al. [23] developed a technique that uses a score or weight-based semantic relationship between user queries to provide a more meaningful result. This framework moderates Wikipedia-related articles derived from the Wikipedia API. By computing similarity between two papers, the similarity level between two articles is calculated based on keyword information. Based on their studying of various proposals in this regard, so the proposed system seeks to refine the findings and present state-of-the-art research. In comparison to other similarity methods, the proposed approach has the most significant Pearson correlation coefficient. In addition, Zafar et al. [24] discussed that the principle of document clustering, in conjunction with ontology, allows users to resolve the challenges associated with traditional keyword-based search. It aims to shorten search times and improve the retrieval of relevant documents. This study proposes a semantic-based document clustering technique based on the K-means clustering algorithm applied to a definition weight matrix computed using a modified TF-IDF approach. The weights are determined uniquely for the WordNet ontology features and relations. The silhouette coefficient is used to assess cluster purity.

Wang and Koopman, [25] used two classification methods in the Astro dataset to recognize clusters. In this analysis, the author constructed semantic article representation and attempted to detect articles clusters based on their semantic similarity. Two well-known clustering techniques, K-Means and a Louvain group detection algorithm, were used to generate our two OCLC-31 (K-Means) and OCLC-Louvain named clustering solutions (standing for Louvain). Al-Azzawy and Al-Rufaye, [26] described new word clusters based on specific text features, constructing a framework to cluster text words according to characteristics, such as morphological, syntactical, and semantically characteristics. Clustering is a form of Unattended Machine Learning, where it extracts terms with similar features from the Similarity Function clusters to calculate their distances. The authors relied on k-means for Clustering to calculate the distance between the sentences and cluster all words of the document. Finally, with the standard assessment methods, the authors evaluated system performance by calculating precision, Recall, and F-Measure. Blokh and Alexandrov, [27] proposed a method for grouping news data using ontology-based similarity estimates on Facebook-specific mass media news data. the objective of this article is to define an efficient algorithm for news clustering in the mass media and derive the related topic distribution. The method is divided into two stages. In the first, they preprocess news data by building a similarity matrix, which they use to evaluate the similarity of news sentences based on their sense and context. They next do clustering to determine how news could be clustered. They used official Facebook news media accounts as a data source. Experiments demonstrate that messages may be classified into semantic clusters, with each cluster representing a distinct theme. They created a distribution of topics based on the volume of news messages.

Afreen and Srinivasu, [28] combining WordNet with lexical chains to address the issues of extracting core semantic information from texts and giving appropriate descriptions to the resulting clusters. The suggested solution uses a technique that identifies the document's subject using disambiguated fundamental semantic properties derived from the document and the characteristics of a lexical chain based on WordNet. In proposed approach the main contributions are preprocessing of document which identifies the noun as a feature by performing tagging and lemmatization, performing word sense disambiguation to obtained candidate words based on the modified similarity approach and finally the generation of cluster based on lexical chains. They observed better performance of lexical chain based on the chain evaluation heuristic whose threshold is set to 50%. Jang et al. [29] provides a unique density-based clustering approach for identifying lexical similarities in word embedding spaces with varying density distributions and suggests features for dialogue acts and emotion categorization using the density-based clustering results. In addition, Lwin [30] illustrated the experimental findings of the proposed approach applying the domain Ontology which applies the semantic relationship in the extraction phase of the function and the algorithm Swarm Optimization (PSO). The performance of intracluster similarity is highly acceptable according to the result. In addition, it is discovered that the similarity between the clusters also achieves an accurate result. The suggested method provides a satisfactory outcome of the F-measure value (100 documents) on the News Group dataset.

In 2016, Rafi et al. [31] developed a method for document representation based on extracting three distinct features from a given document. This includes lexical, syntactic, and semantic characteristics. A meta-descriptor is proposed for each document based on these three characteristics: lexical, syntactic, and semantic. Moreover, Rafi et al. [32] suggested a multi-layer strategy for semantically focused document clustering. The document is divided into lexical, syntactic, and semantic layers. Each layer generates a unique matrix of document-to-document similarity using the cosine similarity metric, which is then aggregated using the weighted average method. These weights were learned via a supervised approach, and they are then used to execute clustering via Hierarchical Agglomerative clustering (HAC). When purity and F-measure are compared, the clustering result obtained by combining similarity measures is superior to that obtained by syntactic and semantic clustering. Moreover, A recent paper published by Ibrahim et al. [9] introduced a novel method for grouping documents based on textual similarities. The NLTK dictionary is used to find, identify, and stop text synopses from Wikipedia and IMDB databases. The next step is to create a vector space with TF-IDF and cluster it using k-Means technique. the outcomes depending on three different scenarios: First, there is no treatment; second, there is preprocessing without derivation; and third, there is derivative processing. More recent paper published by Singh et al. [33] developed an approach for reducing superfluous features based on word embedding Glove. The proposed method clusters phrase with similar semantic meaning using Glove. Based on semantic similarity and multidimensional scaling analysis, Shan and Du, [34] suggested a method for clustering online services. They began by calculating the semantic similarity of documents using Wordnet and then calculated the semantic distance matrix. Subsequently, they employed multidimensional scaling analysis to obtain the semantic distance vector (SDV) and then clustered the SDV using K-means clustering techniques to achieve web service clustering. Finally, Jalal and Ali, [2] developed a classification strategy for clustering research articles to streamline and automate the process of arranging and classifying scientific articles. They use simple crawler techniques to extract the contents of each cluster's theme, title, abstract, and keywords in this suggested system. The dataset is then preprocessed using the TF-IDF algorithm and cosine similarity. The experimental results indicate that it is possible to classify over 96% of articles into similar scopes.

4 Results and Discussion

The 25 selected papers have been systematically reviewed and shown in Table 1. This table summarizes the features of these papers based on methods of similarity, utilized datasets, similarity measures, clustering algorithms, and evaluation measures. In addition, the main findings of the studies were clarified. The result of a survey shows that the majority of methods make use of the TF-IDF technique or Word embedding, which are mostly used and well-known similarity metrics in authors' work. When TF-IDF and cosine are utilized, the clustering is precise and efficient.

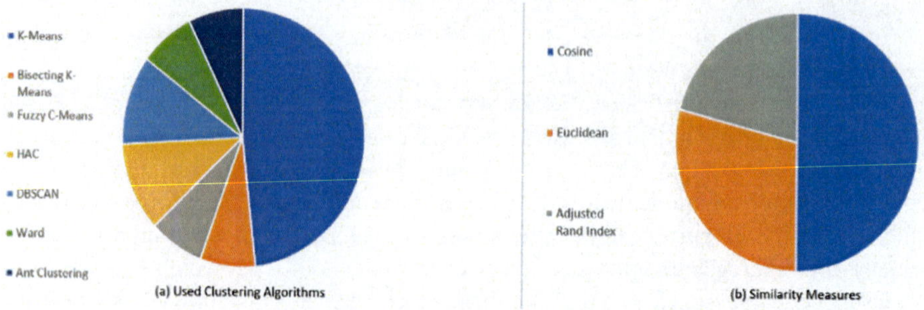

Fig. 2. (a) Used clustering algorithms (b) similarity measures.

TF-IDF technique is the most common way to display vector space documents. However, its results are extremely dimensionally challenging to achieve due to the dimensional curse of the classic clustering algorithms. Recent work embedding techniques may reduce the dimensionality of the documents and preserve semantical relations between word. Besides, the TF-IDF technique is used, which eliminates the most frequent words from the corpus and extracts only the most important ones.

Furthermore, the cosine similarity test was used by the authors to measure the similarity of documents in their works. Cosine similarity parameters outperformed other approaches to similarity. Cosine similarity is one of the most common metrics for proximity in the various recovery and clustering applications as shown in Fig. 2. Moreover, in their work on document clustering, several authors use K-means and the hierarchical clustering algorithm because it is an easy method to cluster and highly scalable as seen in Fig. 2. Nevertheless, in their works, some writers use the Jaccard and the Euclidean distance similarity scales. In finding the similarity text, the Jaccard similarity coefficient evaluates the similarity between documents and ontology, see Fig. 2.

Based on this survey study, some authors used fuzzy C-Means, Bisecting K-Means, HAC, DBSCAN and SVM in their research but fewer than K-Means. In a nutshell, Bisecting K-Means Algorithm is a variant of the K-Means algorithm. It is capable of producing partitional/hierarchical clustering. It can identify clusters of any shape or size. This algorithm is applicable. In terms of entropy estimation, it outperforms K-Means. Likewise, in the assessment of results by different authors, specific metrics such as Recall, precision, F-Score, F-Measure, purity, Rand Index, and entropy are frequently used. Accuracy and recall assessment tests are standard and popular instruments used to assess the consistency and performance of the clusters.

Finally, based on our survey, the authors noticed that the performance and accuracy of each method varies because it relies on the dataset type and the methods used for preprocessing and vectorization. Some methods got high performance and accuracy for large datasets while some performed best for the short dataset.

Table 1. Summary of reviewed papers using semantic similarity based on document clustering.

Paper	Semantic approach	Similarity measures and evaluation	Clustering algorithms/methods	Other measures	Used dataset
Singh et al. 2022 [33]	Enhanced text clustering	Precision, recall, F-measure,	Naïve bayes classifier	Glove word embedding	BBC corpus, Classic4, 20-newsgroup
Shan and Du 2021 [34]	Clustering web services	Precision, Recall, F-measure	K-Means	Wordnet	Programmable Web
Ibrahim et al. 2021 [9]	Semantic Approach based on Document Clustering	Euclidian	K-Means	TF-IDF	IMDB, Wiki, 20-Nesgroup, nltk-Reuters, txt_sentoken, nltk_brown
Jalal and Ali 2021 [2]	Clustering the research papers	Cosine Similarity, Precision, Recall	K-Means	TF-IDF	518 research papers from BEEI Journal
Jacksi et al. 2021 [15]	Clustering Movies synopses	Euclidean, Silhouette metric, purity,	HAC and K-means	TF-IDF	IMDB & WIKI
Mohammed et al. 2020 [17]	Semantic Similarity approach for Document Clustering	Cosine and Euclidean, Silhouette average, purity, accuracy, F1,	DBSCAN	Glove word embedding	Wikipedia and IMDB. nltk-Broun, 20newsgroups, txt_sentoken, and Reuters
Radu et al. 2020 [18]	Document Clustering	Cosine, Euclidean, Homogeneity,Adjusted Rand	DBSCAN, K-Means	TF-IDF Word2Vec	12 263 articles from Arxiv1
Salih and Jacksi 2020 [19]	Document Clustering based semantic approach	Silhouette Ratio, Homogeneity and, F1-Measure, Purity	K-Means and Wards	TF-IDF and Wordnet	IMDP& Wiki, nltk_reuters, txt_sentoken, 20Newsgroup
Fatimi et al. 2020 [13]	Text Clustering Semantic Approach	Cosine and Precision	K-Means, Hierarchical Clustering	TF-IDF	DBPedia
Lwin 2019 [30]	Document Clustering semantic approach	precision, recall, and F-measure	HAC	Not Mentioned	Amazon, Alibaba, BBC skysport

(*continued*)

Table 1. (*continued*)

Paper	Semantic approach	Similarity measures and evaluation	Clustering algorithms/methods	Other measures	Used dataset
Stanchev 2018 [22]	Semantic Document Clustering	Cosine, Precision, Recall, F-Measure	K-Means	Wordnet	Reuters-21578 benchmark
Banik et al. 2018 [23]	Wikipedia Documents Clustering based on semantic similarity	Cosine, F-Measure, Precision and Recall	Ant Clustering Algorithm	Wordnet	Wikipedia
Zafar et al. 2018 [24]	Semantic Document Analysis and clustering	silhouette coefficient, F-Score and purity	K-Means	TF-IDF and Wordnet	Banks Annual Reports
Zandieh and Shakibapoor 2017 [5]	Clustering Data text based on Sematic Similarity	Cosine and Euclidean, Adjusted Rand Index	Fuzzy C-Means	TF-IDF and Wordnet	20 Newsgroups
Wang and Koopman 2017 [25]	Article Clustering based on semantic approach	Cosine, F1-Score and adjusted F1- Score	Louvain Method and K-Means	Not Mentioned	Astro Dataset
Al-Azzawy and Al-Rufaye 2017 [26]	Arabic Text Clustering based	Precision, F-Measure, Recall	K-Means	TF-IDF	20 texts (10 from news and 10 short stories)
Blokh and Alexandrov 2017 [27]	News Clustering based on Semantic Approach	JCN	Not Mentioned	Wordnet	News Message from Facebook official mass Media
Afreen and Srinivasu 2017 [28]	Semantic Document Clustering Using Lexical Chains	Not Mentioned	Not Mentioned	Wordnet	30 Documents from 20Newsgroup

(*continued*)

Table 1. (*continued*)

Paper	Semantic approach	Similarity measures and evaluation	Clustering algorithms/methods	Other measures	Used dataset
Desai and Laxminarayana 2016 [16]	Semantic Based approach for Document Clustering	Cosine, Purity	Bisecting k-Means	TF-IDF for feature selection	Classic4 text document dataset
Stanchev 2016 [20]	Document Clustering based on semantic approach	Cosine, Precision and Recall	K-Means	Wordnet	Reuters - 21578
Hssina et al. 2016 [21]	Semantic Similarity evaluation for textual corpus	Euclidean distance and Cosine	K-Means and Fuzzy C-Means	TF-IDF and Vector Space Model	1224 words created from 32 text documents
Bafna et al. 2016 [10]	Document Clustering	Cosine, Entropy, F-Measure	k-means and HAC	TF-IDF for feature selection	News20, Reuters, Emails
Jang et al. 2016 [29]	Word Embedding for semantic similarity clustering	Precision, Recall, F1-Score	DBSCAN and DENCLUE	Word2vec	Korean news article
Rafi et al. 2016 [32]	Document Clustering - semantic approach	Cosine, F-Measure and Purity	HAC	TF-IDF	NEWS20
Rafi et al. 2016 [31]	Semantic in Document Clustering	Cosine, F-Measure, Purity	Candidate based clustering algorithm	TF-IDF	*News20 and Reuters21758*

5 Proposed Work

Based on the literature reviewed and its consequence, the proposed system is to cluster online educational laboratories based on semantic similarity. The process will be achieved by identifying these labs from repositories; the clustering will be performed on the description of the labs by understanding their description and clustering them accordingly. The results will be visualized and presented as an interactive webpage showing the categories of the clustered remote labs.

As mentioned above, most researchers used documents in different fields for clustering based on semantic approach; rarely can you find semantic clustering for online educational laboratories as Qona'ah et al. [11] which used traditional clustering techniques for clustering online labs based on the productivity of the laboratories, and they used different algorithms such as K-Means, K-Medoids, and model-based clustering.

So, the methodology of the proposed work will be as follows as shown in Fig. 3.

- Finding data: fining a dataset containing remote lab descriptions
- Tokenization and stemming
- Use an algorithm to generate a group of words as a vector which are TF-IDF and Word Embedding
- Cluster them using a suitable clustering algorithm like K-Means and HAC as it's suitable algorithms for short text clustering [35].
- Generating JSON: converting the result to (json) as list of nodes and links.
- Present the results: generate webpages and create relationships between the labs.

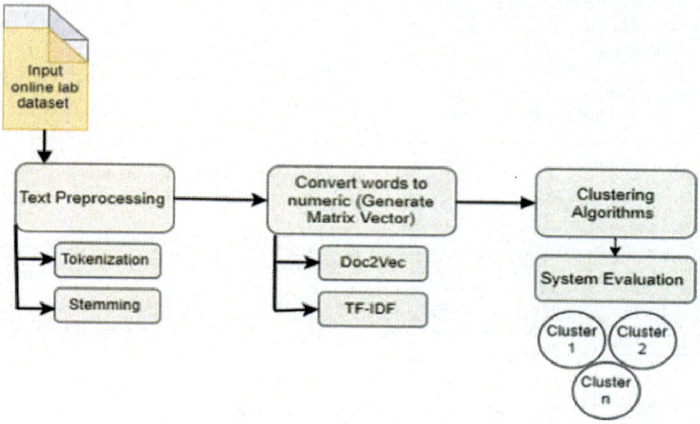

Fig. 3. Proposed system methodology

6 Conclusion

This paper provides an in-depth review of semantic text clustering. It involves a study of both conventional and novel approaches to semantic text clustering. Both methods go through several steps, including stemming, stop word elimination, tokenization, and text clustering. Therefore, clustering is accomplished through the use of clustering algorithms. In addition, the K-means algorithm is the most popular one for its improved usability. There are others that can provide closer clustering, such as bisecting K-means, Fuzzy C-mean, and Hierarchical agglomerative clustering. Furthermore, semantic-based approaches to document clustering have greater precision, results, and cluster consistency than conventional methods. Different clustering methods were compared and analyzed. Commonly, this systematic review of recent works related to Selecting Methods of Semantic Similarity based on Document Clustering allows the assessment of methods quality and identifying and guiding the methodology of future research can apply to Online Laboratories Repository.

References

1. Mehta, V.: Stamantic clustering: combining statistical and semantic features for clustering of large text datasets. Expert Syst. Appl. **174**, 9 (2021)
2. Jalal, A.A., Ali, B.H.: Text documents clustering using data mining techniques. Int. J. Electr. Comput. Eng. IJECE **11**(1), 664 (2021). https://doi.org/10.11591/ijece.v11i1.pp664-670
3. Haji, S.H., Abdulazeez, A.M., Zeebaree, D.Q., Ahmed, F.Y.H., Zebari, D.A.: The impact of different data mining classification techniques in different datasets. In: 2021 IEEE Symposium on Industrial Electronics and Applications (ISIEA), Langkawi Island, Malaysia, pp. 1–6 (2021). https://doi.org/10.1109/ISIEA51897.2021.9510006
4. Diallo, B.: Multi-view document clustering based on geometrical similarity measurement. Int. J. Mach. Learn. Cybern. **13**, 663–675 (2022). https://doi.org/10.1007/s13042-021-01295-8
5. Zandieh, P., Shakibapoor, E.: Clustering data text based on semantic. Int. J. Comput. **26**(1), 8 (2017)
6. Saiyad, N.Y., Prajapati, H.B., Dabhi, V.K.: A survey of document clustering using semantic approach, p. 8 (2016)
7. Ali, I., Melton, A.: Semantic-based text document clustering using cognitive semantic learning and graph theory. In: 2018 IEEE 12th International Conference on Semantic Computing (ICSC), Laguna Hills, CA, USA, pp. 243–247 (2018). https://doi.org/10.1109/ICSC.2018.00042
8. Polus, M.E., Abbas, T.: Intelligent text clustering based on semantics similarity, p. 7 (2020)
9. Ibrahim, R.K., Zeebaree, S.R.M., Jacksi, K., Sadeeq, M.A.M., Shukur, H.M., Alkhayyat, A.: Clustering document based semantic similarity system using TFIDF and k-mean. In: 2021 International Conference on Advanced Computer Applications (ACA), Maysan, Iraq, pp. 28–33 (2021). https://doi.org/10.1109/ACA52198.2021.9626822
10. Bafna, P., Pramod, D., Vaidya, A.: Document clustering: TF-IDF approach, p. 6 (2016)
11. Qona'ah, N., Devi, A.R., Dana, I.M.G.M.: Laboratory clustering using k-means, k-medoids, and model-based clustering. Indones. J. Appl. Stat. **3**(1), 64 (2020). https://doi.org/10.13057/ijas.v3i1.40823
12. Lakshmi, R., Baskar, S.: Efficient text document clustering with new similarity measures. Int. J. Bus. Intell. Data Min. **18**, 24 (2021)
13. Fatimi, S., El, C., Alaoui, L.: A framework for semantic text clustering. Int. J. Adv. Comput. Sci. Appl. 11(6) (2020). https://doi.org/10.14569/IJACSA.2020.0110657
14. Alian, M.: Semantic similarity for English and Arabic texts: a review, p. 29 (2020)
15. Jacksi, K., Ibrahim, R.K., Zeebaree, S.R., Zebari, R.R., Sadeeq, M.A.: Clustering documents based on semantic similarity using HAC and k-mean algorithms. In: 2020 International Conference on Advanced Science and Engineering (ICOASE), Duhok, Iraq, pp. 205–210 (2020). https://doi.org/10.1109/ICOASE51841.2020.9436570
16. Desai, S.S., Laxminarayana, J.A.: WordNet and semantic similarity based approach for document clustering. In: 2016 International Conference on Computation System and Information Technology for Sustainable Solutions (CSITSS), Bengaluru, India, pp. 312–317 (2016). https://doi.org/10.1109/CSITSS.2016.7779377
17. Mohammed, S.M., Jacksi, K., Zeebaree, S.R.M.: Glove word embedding and DBSCAN algorithms for semantic document clustering. In: 2020 International Conference on Advanced Science and Engineering (ICOASE), Duhok, Iraq, pp. 1–6 (2020). https://doi.org/10.1109/ICOASE51841.2020.9436540
18. Radu, R.-G., Radulescu, I.-M., Truica, C.-O., Apostol, E.-S., Mocanu, M.: Clustering documents using the document to vector model for dimensionality reduction. In: 2020 IEEE International Conference on Automation, Quality and Testing, Robotics (AQTR), Cluj-Napoca, Romania, pp. 1–6 (2020). https://doi.org/10.1109/AQTR49680.2020.9129967

19. Salih, N.M., Jacksi, K.: Semantic document clustering using k-means algorithm and ward's method. In: 2020 International Conference on Advanced Science and Engineering (ICOASE), Duhok, Iraq, pp. 1–6 (2020). https://doi.org/10.1109/ICOASE51841.2020.9436588
20. Stanchev, L.: Semantic document clustering using a similarity graph. In: 2016 IEEE Tenth International Conference on Semantic Computing (ICSC), Laguna Hills, CA, USA, pp. 1–8 (2016). https://doi.org/10.1109/ICSC.2016.8
21. Hssina, B., Bouikhalene, B., Merbouha, A.: Evaluation of semantic similarity using vector space model based on textual corpus. In: 2016 13th International Conference on Computer Graphics, Imaging and Visualization (CGiV), Beni Mellal, Morocco, pp. 295–300 (2016). https://doi.org/10.1109/CGiV.2016.64
22. Stanchev, L.: Semantic document clustering using information from WordNet and DBPedia. In: 2018 IEEE 12th International Conference on Semantic Computing (ICSC), Laguna Hills, CA, USA, pp. 100–107 (2018). https://doi.org/10.1109/ICSC.2018.00023
23. Banik, P., Gaikwad, S., Awate, A., Shaikh, S., Gunjgur, P., Padiya, P.: Semantic analysis of Wikipedia documents using ontology. In: 2018 IEEE International Conference on System, Computation, Automation and Networking (ICSCA), Pondicherry, pp. 1–6 (2018). https://doi.org/10.1109/ICSCAN.2018.8541162
24. Zafar, A., Awais, M., Aftab, M.A.: Ontology based document data analysis, p. 7 (2018)
25. Wang, S., Koopman, R.: Clustering articles based on semantic similarity. Scientometrics **111**(2), 1017–1031 (2017). https://doi.org/10.1007/s11192-017-2298-x
26. Al-Azzawy, D.S., Al-Rufaye, F.M.L.: Arabic words clustering by using k-means algorithm. In: 2017 Annual Conference on New Trends in Information and Communications Technology Applications (NTICT), Baghdad, Iraq, pp. 263–267 (2017). https://doi.org/10.1109/NTICT.2017.7976098
27. Blokh, I., Alexandrov, V.: News clustering based on similarity analysis. Procedia Comput. Sci. **122**, 715–719 (2017). https://doi.org/10.1016/j.procs.2017.11.428
28. Afreen, S., Srinivasu, D.B.: Semantic based document clustering using lexical chains, vol. 04, no. 01, p. 7 (2017)
29. Jang, J., Lee, Y., Lee, S., Shin, D., Kim, D., Rim, H.: A novel density-based clustering method using word embedding features for dialogue intention recognition. Cluster Comput. **19**(4), 2315–2326 (2016). https://doi.org/10.1007/s10586-016-0649-7
30. Lwin, W.: Impressive approach for documents clustering using semantics relations in feature extraction. In: 2019 the 9th International Workshop on Computer Science and Engineering (2019). https://doi.org/10.18178/wcse.2019.03.007
31. Rafi, M., Naveed, M., Arshad, W., Rafay, H.: Exploiting document level semantics in document clustering. Int. J. Adv. Comput. Sci. Appl. **7**(6) (2016). https://doi.org/10.14569/IJACSA.2016.070660
32. Rafi, M., Sharif, M.N., Arshad, W., Mohsin, S., Rafay, H.: Multi-layer semantics based document clustering. In: Proceedings of the 6th International Conference on Web Intelligence, Mining and Semantics, Nîmes France, pp. 1–4, June 2016. https://doi.org/10.1145/2912845.2912880
33. Singh, K.N., Devi, S.D., Devi, H.M., Mahanta, A.K.: A novel approach for dimension reduction using word embedding: an enhanced text classification approach. Int. J. Inf. Manag. Data Insights **2**(1), 100061 (2022).https://doi.org/10.1016/j.jjimei.2022.100061
34. Shan, C., Du, Y.: A web service clustering method based on semantic similarity and multidimensional scaling analysis. Sci. Program. **2021**, 1–12 (2021). https://doi.org/10.1155/2021/6661035
35. Han, M., Zhang, X., Yuan, X., Jiang, J., Yun, W., Gao, C.: A survey on the techniques, applications, and performance of short text semantic similarity. Concur. Comput. Pract. Exp. **33**, 17 (2021)

Hate Speech Detection in Social Media for the Kurdish Language

Ari M. Saeed[1(✉)], Aso N. Ismael[1], Danya L. Rasul[1], Rayan S. Majeed[1], and Tarik A. Rashid[2]

[1] Department of Computer Science, College of Science, University of Halabja, Halabja, Iraq
Ari.said@uoh.edu.iq

[2] Department of Computer Science and Engineering, University of Kurdistan Hewler, Erbil, Iraq
tarik.ahmed@ukh.edu.krd

Abstract. With the rapid growth of technology over the world, especially, on the internet, people enormously use social media freely to express their ideologies. Sometimes the freedom of media is caught up and the rights of others are beaten down by hate speech. Moreover, social media is an easy and vague way to desecrate people, groups, and parties since there is no any way to recognize anonymous users over social media. Testing human speech is common for English, Arabic, and Turkish languages while there is no attempt for the Kurdish language. For that reason, the Kurdish hate speech dataset is collected from comments on the Facebook application as an effort for detecting hate speech and removing them. The raw dataset consists of 6882 comments which are divided into hate and hot hate classes. Support Vector Machine (SVM), Decision Tree (DT), and Naïve Bays (NB) algorithms are implemented and compared. Based on the results, the SVM is found most excellent with the F1 measure being 0.687.

Keywords: Kurdish hate speech detection · Machine learning algorithms · Text classification

1 Introduction

Nowadays, social media is popular media for communicating with people around the world. With increasing the number of users who share their opinion and exchange their idea, the volume of information is increased massively as well. Facebook is an application that is used as a social media in almost all countries and regions. The Kurdistan region in Iraq is one of them in which people utilize Facebook freely. Kurdish people use the Kurdish language for communication through Latin and Arabic scripts for expressing and posting over Facebook. Moreover, there is not any filtration for publishing the posts. Sometimes people use hate and offensive speeches toward others. There is no doubt, that expressing online hate speech toward opposition has a massive impact by comparing with offline hate speech since more people can see it [1–3]. Based on that fact, users, groups, and parties disturb others by desecrating religion, instigating racism, devaluating freedom rights, culture, and so on. When there is not any filtration for blocking a hate

K. Daimi and A. Al Sadoon (Eds.): ICR 2022, AISC 1431, pp. 253–260, 2022.
https://doi.org/10.1007/978-3-031-14054-9_24

post in the Kurdish language by internet providers, people can publish hate speeches without caring to filter and banding their posts. Fortunately, detecting hate speech in international languages, such as English is improved and progressed while there is no attempt for the Kurdish language [4]. For those reasons, detecting hate speech for a national language, such as Kurdish has become a necessary and urgent case. In this study, a new model is created for detecting hate speech in the Kurdish language as a new effort by implementing algorithms and techniques in machine learning and data mining.

2 Motivation and Related Work

With publishing a large volume of hate speeches over social media. A new challenge in data mining techniques is raised for detecting those speeches. Hate speech detection has become a new area that researchers work on it due to its negative effect on socials life. The number of researchers that worked in this domain are few who used machine learning algorithms for the detection of hate speech [1]. For that reason, this dataset is collected from comments and called a Kurdish Hate Speech Dataset (KHSD). KHSD is available for use in some fields of data mining techniques, such as (sentiment analysis, text summarization, and text to speech). It can be utilized by other languages, such as Arabic, Persian, and Urdu since the Kurdish language uses, particularly the same alphabet. Moreover, it can be used for automatic systems in artificial intelligence (AI), such as AI assistants, automated content generation, and automated hate speech detection [4, 5]. Indonesian hate speech text was detected by using the skip-gram model and the word2vec method with Text CNN was implemented. Moreover, the imbalanced dataset was solved by using class weight, random undersampling, and oversampling. The results showed that the F-score is 93.70% [6].

SVM and Long Short Term Memory (LSTM) were utilized for detecting Italian hate speech text on Facebook applications. The ten-fold cross-validation technique was used for partitioning the dataset for training and testing data. The results showed that the effectiveness of automatic hate speech detection was more than the manual classification by using those two algorithms. The accuracy of SVM was 64.61%, which was higher than LTSM, which was 60.50. [7] compares five different text datasets for detecting racist and sexist hate speech. Moreover, different classical data mining algorithms were implemented, such as SVM, GBDT, NB, and LR while CNN with LTSM is used as deep learning classifiers. In this paper, the word-embedding, TF-IDF n-gram, and word gram are utilized [5].

3 Experimental Framework

In this section, a series of steps are implemented for generating the right model data mining fields. The steps are Data collection, Data Description, and Labeling, Preprocessing, Classification as shown in Fig. 1:

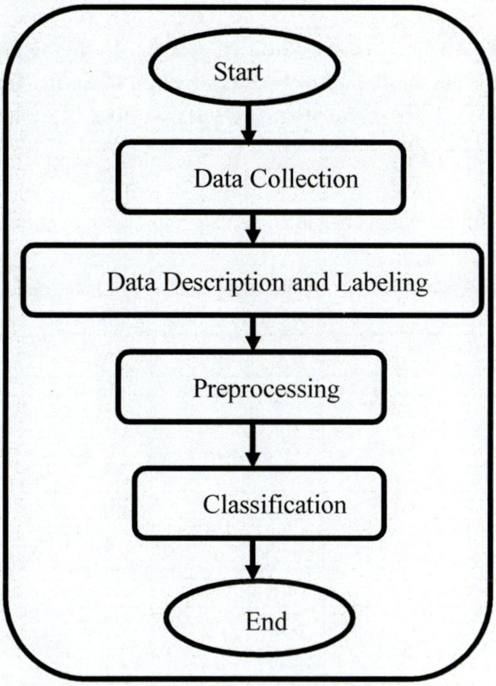

Fig. 1. Experimental framework

3.1 Data Collection

Data collection is the first step in machine learning to predict the right model and it is important to collect data from valid sources. Different challenges have been tackled in hate speech data collection on social media for some languages, such as English, Italic, Arabic, and so on. For collecting the comments of the dataset on the Facebook application, there are different types of tools that have been utilized. Facepager tool that is applied in this project for collecting comments. The comments on this dataset are collected from different TV channels, athletes, religions, politicians, doctors, ministries, and some specific pages. After installing the tool, the first step is to log into the facepager tool, then, create a new database and add a new node to insert the specified Facebook link for getting the comments. The second step is clicking on the fetch data button to get data and it can increase the page size to get more data. The third step is to export fetching data into a CSV file [8].

3.2 Data Description and Labelling

The Kurdish language is spoken by 40 million people with various dialects. The Kurdish language is not unified since the Kurdish of Syria and Turkey use the Kurmanji dialect with Latin script whilst the Sorani dialect is used in Iran and Iraq with Arabic script. In this project, the Sorani dialect is used to collect the dataset. The dataset consists of 6882 comments of users on the Facebook application. On social media, there are different types of hate speech is concerned based on categories. In this work, hate and hot hate speech are extracted from eight classes (Politic, Religion, Sport, Terrorism, Education, Race, Freedom, and Sex) [9]. The percentage and number of gathering comments are different for each class as shown in Table 1.

Table 1. Numbers and percentage ratio of eight classes

Class	Number of comments	Hate speech's numbers	Not hate speech's number	Percentage
Politic	1081	431	650	15.7%
Religion	842	415	427	12.2%
Sport	978	406	572	14.2%
Terrorism	718	459	259	10.4%
Education	760	272	488	11%
Race	862	683	179	12.5%
Freedom	693	368	325	10%
Sex	948	632	316	13.7%
Total	6882	3666	3216	100%

After reading the 6882 comments accurately one by one, then, the process of labeling comments is started by four annotators to annotate the comments manually. For annotators, it is not easy to predict users' expressions due to the comments being enigmatic and it is a big challenge to classify a comment to hate or not. In this project, the comments are classified to hate or not hate based on the meaning of sentences [5, 13].

3.3 Data Preprocessing

In this subsection, a series of preprocessing steps are applied to the dataset to be ready for use in data mining fields. The preprocessing techniques are Tokenization, Normalization, Removing Stop words, and Stemming.

a- Tokenization: is the process of splitting the comments for words by removing spaces.
b- Normalization: is used to normalize the comments by (Removing Special Characters, Punctuation, Numbers, URLs, hashtags & user mentions if it is English,

English letter, words, sentences, Arabic letter, Sentences that has no meaning) and replacing Arabic characters that are used instead of Kurdish characters since different scripts among users over social media are used without knowing its Kurdish script or Arabic script as shown in Table 2.

The comments are read one by one, if the comments don't have any meaning and are corrupted, then they are removed. For that purpose, the number of comments after preprocessing steps is decreased from 6882 to 6607 [9–11]. On the other hand, 240

Table 2. Replacing Arabic characters with Kurdish characters

NO	Arabic Characters	Example	Replaced with Kurdish Characters	Example
1.	ي	نه كه ي	ی	نه که ی
2.	ة	نية	ه	نیه
3.	ۆ	بۆ	ۆ	بۆ
4.	ێ at the end	نوێ	ێ	نو ێ
5.	ه (U+0647) at the end	باره	ە (U+06D5)	بارە
6.	ك rarely used in Kurdish	جاك	ک	جاک
7.	ھ (0+06be)	ھێز (U+06BE)	ه (U+0647)	هێز

stop words are removed to decrease noise and high dimensionality of feature space [4]. Moreover, Stemming is implemented by removing prefixes and suffixes of words to get the stem (root) of words [9].

3.4 Classification

One of the most important points to be discussed is the balanced dataset. In this study, the KHSD data set is 6882 comments that are divided into two categories hate and note hate. It can be said that the KHSD is almost balanced since the number of hate is 3669 while not hate is 3084. Another important factor is using algorithms, such as SVM, NB, and CNN. Cross-validation is used as a technique for dividing the dataset for training and testing sets. In this experiment, 9-fold is used as training for predicting the models, and 1-fold is used as testing to predict the labels. For evaluating the classifiers, four popular criteria are used for detecting hate speech in text. The following equations are used as shown below [12, 13].

$$\text{Precision} = \frac{TP}{TP + FP} \tag{1}$$

$$\text{Recall} = \frac{TP}{TP + FN} \tag{2}$$

$$\text{F1} = 2 * \frac{Recall * Precision}{Recall + Precision} \tag{3}$$

$$\text{Accuracy} = \frac{TP + TN}{TP + FP + TN + FN} \tag{4}$$

Three different classification algorithms are implemented on the KHSD dataset. The performance of each algorithm is different based on various tests. Six different tests are applied as shown below:

1. Raw Sentences (RS) are implemented without any preprocessing technique.
2. Raw Sentences are Normalized (RSN).
3. Raw Sentences are Normalized and Stop Words are removed (RSNSW).
4. Raw Sentences are Normalized and Stemmed (RSNS).
5. Raw Sentences are Normalized and Stop Words are removed and then stemmed (RSNSWS).

6. Raw Sentences are Normalized and Stemmed then Stop Words are removed (RSNSSW).

The F1 measure is used for evaluating the classification methods as the average of precision and recall as shown in Table 3.

Table 3. F1 measure for SVM, C4.5, and NV

	RS	RSN	RSNSW	RSNS	RSNSWS	RSNSSW
SVM	0.644	0.643	0.686	0.650	0.687	0.651
DT (C4.5)	0.560	0.584	0.548	0.584	0.583	0.566
NB	0.560	0.541	0.506	0.558	0.548	0.500

As shown in Table 3 the performance of the F1 measure is increased and decreased gradually based on the algorithms and tests. In SVM the F1 measure is 0.644 for RS while RSNSWS is 0.687, which means the F1 measure is increased slightly by 0.043. In DT the value of RSNS and RSN is 0.584 while in RSNSW is 0.548, which means the difference is 0.036. Moreover, RS decreased from 0.560 to 0.548 in RSNSW. In NV the F1 is 0.560 in RS while it is decreased in all other tests. In Fig. 2, the results of the experiment are different, the SVM is the best classifier for detecting hate speeches for all tests by comparing with DT and NV. The F1 for DT and NV are the same for RS while for all other tests DT is better than NV.

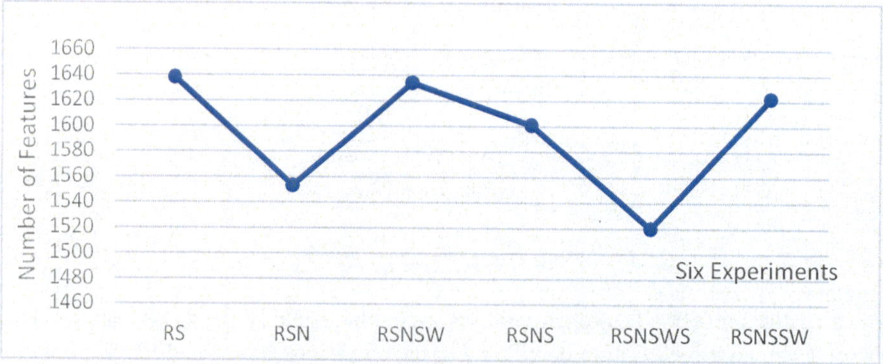

Fig. 2. F1 performance in SVM, DT, and NV for six tests

One more crucial point in this experiment is decreeing the number of features by implementing preprocessing steps as shown in Fig. 3.

As depicted in Fig. 3, six different tests are implemented. It is clear that in RSNSW, the number of features is decreased significantly since the number of features in RS is 1638 and it becomes 1520 while in RSN it is 1553. Moreover, when RSNSW is tested,

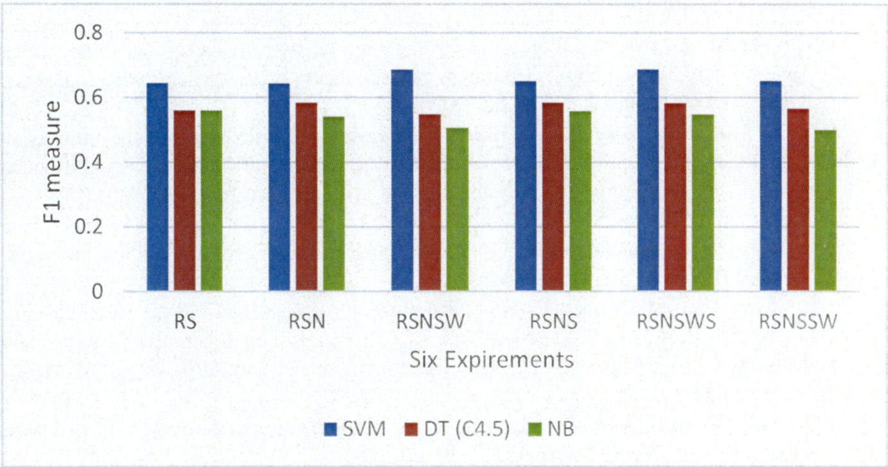

Fig. 3. Number of features for six experiments

the number of features is 1634. On the other hand, the number of features is decreased by 37 and 16 for each RSNS and RSNSSW respectively to be compared with RS.

4 Conclusion and Future Work

In this study, detecting hate speech in Kurdish text is implemented by using three different classifiers on six various tests. The results are comparable for each test and different results are considerable. The F1 score is used for evaluating the results and comparing them. Based on the results, the best result F1 score for SVM, DT, and NV is 0.687, and 0.584 0.56 respectively. In the future, the preprocessing techniques can be improved and investigated to increase the high F1 score.

References

1. Al-Hassan, A., Al-Dossari, H.: Detection of hate speech in social networks: a survey on multilingual corpus. In: 6th International Conference on Computer Science and Information Technology, vol. 10 (2019)
2. Saeed, A.M., Rashid, T.A., Mustafa, A.M., Agha, R.-R., Shamsaldin, A.S., Al-Salihi, N.K.: An evaluation of Reber stemmer with longest match stemmer technique in Kurdish Sorani text classification. Iran J. Comput. Sci. **1**(2), 99–107 (2018). https://doi.org/10.1007/s42044-018-0007-4
3. Alotaibi, A., Hasanat, M.H.A.: Racism detection in twitter using deep learning and text mining techniques for the Arabic language. In: 2020 First International Conference of Smart Systems and Emerging Technologies (SMARTTECH), pp. 161–164. IEEE (2020)
4. Rashid, T.A., Mustafa, A.M., Saeed, A.R.: Automatic Kurdish text classification using KDC 4007 dataset. In: Barolli, L., Zhang, M., Wang, X. (eds.) Advances in Internetworking, Data and Web Technologies, vol. 6, pp. 187–198. Springer, Cham (2017). https://doi.org/10.1007/978-3-319-59463-7_19

5. Istaiteh, O., Al-Omoush, R., Tedmori, S.: Racist and sexist hate speech detection: literature review. In: 2020 International Conference on Intelligent Data Science Technologies and Applications (IDSTA), pp. 95–99. IEEE (2020)
6. Alfina, I., Mulia, R., Fanany, M.I., Ekanata, Y: Hate speech detection in the Indonesian language: a dataset and preliminary study. In: 2017 International Conference on Advanced Computer Science and Information Systems (ICACSIS), pp. 233–238. IEEE (2017)
7. Del Vigna12, F., Cimino23, A., Dell'Orletta, F., Petrocchi, M., Tesconi, M.: Hate me, hate me not: hate speech detection on Facebook. In: Proceedings of the First Italian Conference on Cybersecurity (ITASEC17), pp. 86–95 (2017)
8. Nazir, M.U., et al.: Social media competitive analysis - a case study in the pizza industry of Pakistan. In: Bajwa, I., Kamareddine, F., Costa, A. (eds.) Intelligent Technologies and Applications, vol. 932, pp. 313–325. Springer, Singapore (2019). https://doi.org/10.1007/978-981-13-6052-7_27
9. Rashid, T.A., Mustafa, A.M., Saeed, A.: A robust categorization system for Kurdish Sorani text documents. Inf. Technol. J. **16**(1), 27–34 (2017)
10. Sohrabi, M.K., Hemmatian, F.: An efficient preprocessing method for supervised sentiment analysis by converting sentences to numerical vectors: a twitter case study. Multimedia Tools Appl. **78**(17), 24863–24882 (2019). https://doi.org/10.1007/s11042-019-7586-4
11. Hegazi, M.O., Al-Dossari, Y., Al-Yahy, A., Al-Sumari, A., Hilal, A.: Preprocessing Arabic text on social media. Heliyon **7**(2), e06191 (2021)
12. Mullah, N.S., Zainon, W.M.N.W.: Advances in machine learning algorithms for hate speech detection in social media: a review. IEEE Access **9**, 88364–88376 (2021). https://doi.org/10.1109/ACCESS.2021.3089515
13. Huang, Y., Wang, R., Huang, B., Wei, B., Zheng, S.L., Chen, M.: Sentiment classification of crowdsourcing participants' reviews text based on LDA topic model. IEEE Access **9**, 108131–108143 (2021)

Deep Learning Algorithm for Predicting Drug Synergy Against Cancer: Data, Drug Feature Extraction, Prediction and View (DDPV) Taxonomy

Usha Kiran Gautam[1], Tarik A. Rashid[2], Qurat Ul Ain Nizamani[3(✉)], Rashidul Mubasher[3], Nectarios Costadopoulos[3], Razwan Mohmed Salah[4], and Ahmad Alrubaie[5]

[1] Study Group Australia, Sydney, Australia
[2] University of Kurdistan Hewler, KRG, Erbil, Iraq
[3] Kent Institute Australia, Sydney, Australia
{Qurat.Nizamani,Rashidul.Mubasher, Nectarios.Costadopoulos}@kent.edu.au
[4] The University of Duhok, Duhok, Iraq
razwan.mayi@uod.ac
[5] University of New South Wales, Kensington, Australia

Abstract. The Deep learning prediction technique has become more popular day by day in the medical sector, mainly in predicting anti-cancer drug synergy. However, a deep learning algorithm has not been introduced sufficiently in predicting drug development against cancer. This paper aims to research literature based on the deep learning techniques to provide predictions about the effects of drug combinations based on the developed taxonomy. The end-users can see the type of data used, feature extraction tools, prediction techniques and visual display of the synergistic drug combinations that will help them to derive a more accurate drug synergy score for smooth anti-cancer treatment.

Keywords: Deep learning · Prediction algorithm · Anti-cancer · Taxonomy · Drug synergy

1 Introduction

Deep learning (DL) has become a core attraction for research in the medical field for cancer prediction, detection, classification, and diagnosis. It is among the best machine learning technology that provides knowledge to pathologists to make an accurate prediction from complex data [1]. This technology in anti-cancer drug synergy aims to identify the complex synergistic data for predicting the effects of the drug combination. This is usually achieved by extracting high-level data features from the patient data using classification to train the deep learning model to visualize the system to the pathologist or the pharmacologist. The importance of data, prediction, and view is sig-nificant in applying deep learning for predicting drug synergy against cancer [2].

K. Daimi and A. Al Sadoon (Eds.): ICR 2022, AISC 1431, pp. 261–269, 2022.
https://doi.org/10.1007/978-3-031-14054-9_25

By addressing the issues of the generic domain, new technology based on a novel deep learning model and drug synergy prediction against cancer has been proposed. This technology has been used in the generic domain to predict cancer disease and in the sub-domain to make novel synergistic drug predictions. But the integration of additional omics data with gene expression data is a challenge in an accurate drug response prediction [3]. Due to heterogeneity in tumor cell lines, it is tough to predict a novel drug synergy [1]. Therefore, our research will focus on a novel deep learning model that integrates multi-data to provide highly predictive drug values. Data, prediction, and view (DPV) taxonomy allow the developers to make alterations and improvements. The criteria we have used to verify the DPV taxonomy are accuracy, quality, and completeness.

Our taxonomy concentrates on the deep learning model in drug synergy prediction against cancer. Deep learning is the advanced transformation of machine learning technology to learn knowledge without prior concern [4]. It can automatically learn the nonlinear structures from the vast data sets, which helps describe the unknown relationship between the classifiers [5]. This deep learning technology is already applied in bioinformatics for extracting genomic features to predict accurately. Our contributions for this paper include providing a new solution called Data, Drug feature extraction, Drug target prediction and View (DDPV) taxonomy. Further, we discuss a method for high- level feature extraction from a public dataset. This work also highlights the key issues and challenges of predicting drug synergy against cancer.

2 Literature Review

Past prediction taxonomies and publications have focused on only two or three factors: e.g., data, view, or interaction tool. But, in the following section, we have proposed and discussed four taxonomies (DDPV) for prediction and other essential aspects of the prediction process.

Many papers have only explained one factor: data or view as the basis for classifying prediction techniques [2]. Enhanced Novel deep learning-based method-Deep synergy to reduce the challenges posed by combinatorial space. They improve the synergy score by using a chemopy and normalization strategy. This solution hence offers high accuracy synergy scores and best prediction in a cross-validation set; however, the datasets used by this work has few quantities of drugs and cancer cell lines. As a result, highlevel features may not be extracted [1]. Extended this idea by developing deep learning to predict drug response (DeepDR) algorithm to minimize the gaps between cell lines and tumors [7]. Enhanced AuDNNsynergy (Deep Neural Network Synergy model with Autoencoders) to minimize the screening problem of drug interactions. They offer a solution to the problem by using the linear unit and rectified linear unit, which has improved the quality of the estimator [9]. Enhanced deep learning-based drug-target binding affinity model (DeepDTA) to minimize the challenges in predicting drug-target affinity prediction. They offer a solution to the problem by using a dropout regularization technique to remove the overfitting problem [10]. Enhanced deep learning-based transcriptome data classification model to downgrade the cost of in silico prediction.

They develop a solution to the problem by using k-fold cross-validation and softmax regression to optimize the neuron layers. Their method provided a validation accuracy of 90.53% and an F-score of 86.38%. Finally, [6] described a deep neural network (DNN) model based on four components/stages (Data, drug feature extraction, prediction of drug-target interaction and view/display) and transformation operators (data transformation, drug feature transformation, prediction transformation and data mapping transformation.)

The DNN model with an application to anti-cancer therapy begins with collecting different types of data gathered from publicly available databases of cancer patients (example, gene expression data, cancer cell line and 2D descriptors). The feature extraction step extracts the high-level data representations and transforms them into the prediction step. The prediction technique involves training the deep neural network model and predicting the drug-target interaction to find the most effective synergy score. The view step gets the prediction transformation displayed in the devices or screen and how the physicians and patients react to the predicted drug target synergy score.

In our work, we have proposed a more accurate and complete taxonomy by including most of the prediction (DDPV) components with data, their subclasses, drug feature extraction, drug target prediction and display or view to make it more interactive for the user in a real or virtual environment.

3 Proposed DDPV Taxonomy

The proposed system was based on the taxonomy called DDPV (Data, Drug feature extraction, Prediction of drug target and view of drug combination), which was reviewed by conducting the study on both current and past deep learning-based prediction techniques for anti-cancer. We iteratively developed a taxonomy that includes essential factors for creating, validating, and evaluating a proposed system by analyzing cancer treatment therapy's prediction and deep learning network.

The inclusive criteria are based on the datasets that consist of different data types (raw, imaging and visually processed). It also includes identifying different kinds of techniques for calculating novel synergistic drug combinations. Likewise, inclusive criteria also include different tools that were used for implementing deep learning. Finally, it also talks about the results displaying devices, display location and the virtual and hardware tools.

Based on literature review, we tend to believe that to develop an effective system that can assist pathologists and medical professionals in predicting anti-cancers drug synergy, three critical points need to be considered: a. which of the most extensive available data should be used and b. how the data can be extracted and predicted, and.

c. how they can be viewed and interacted with. Hence, we determine deep learning-based anti-cancer drug synergy prediction in terms of three components: *data, prediction, and view.*

The first component that is used in the proposed DDPV taxonomy is data. It includes raw data, analyzed imaging data and visual data with various properties of dimensionality, acquisition process, underlying process, semantics, data object and whether the data were acquired publicly or paid from the database. The second component used is drug feature extraction, which includes tools and techniques to extract the dataset's relevant and high-level representations of drug characteristics. The third component is a prediction of drug-target, which analyses the visual and data samples and predicts synergistic drug interaction in anti-cancer therapy. The last component used is the view for drug combination, and involves a display used, a location where data are introduced, and the data's interface. All of these factors, their subclasses and relations are portrayed in Fig. 1.

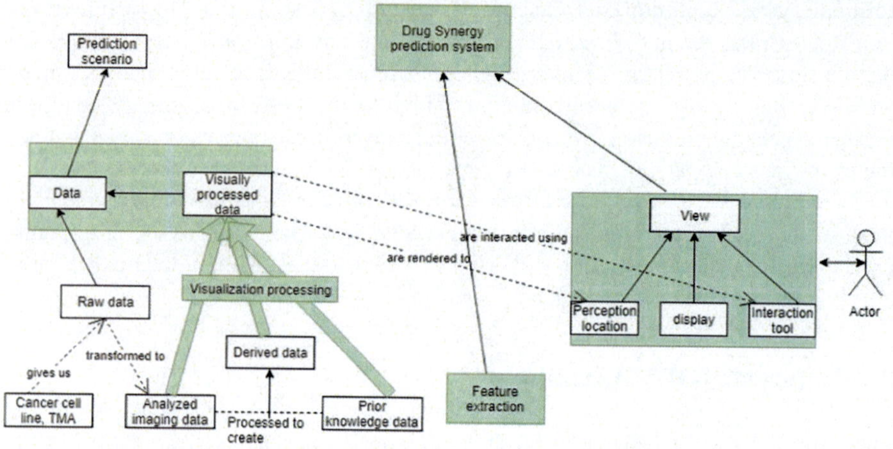

Fig. 1. The figure shows four factors of prediction taxonomy DDPV (Data, prediction and view) with their classes and subclasses, represented by solid-line arrows. Dashed line arrows represent the relationship between classes and subclasses. The component view consists of three subclasses, and the data interact with the user using interactive tools.

3.1 Description of Each Component

1) **Data.** Most of the researched publications used analyzed imaging data. Some of them have used raw imaging data, and a few have used visually processed data. The explanation of each subclass is given as: Raw Data. Many journal articles used the cancer cell line for predicting the drug synergy in cancer treatment. Analysed imaging data. The majority of the publications have used analysed imaging data which can be used to transform them into meaningful information.Visually Processed data. Since the research is based on drug synergy prediction against cancer using a deep learning algorithm, the result was not focused on visually processed data. Instead, they had given high priority to analysed and raw imaging data.
2) **Drug Feature Extraction**. A large number of publications like [7, 11], and [1] have used the auto-encoder for generating high-level features. At the same time, many other publications have used Rdkit and molecular descriptors model for feature extraction. DSeq method, propy generator, molecular graph descriptor have also been used by many authors.
3) **Prediction Technique.** The prediction technique used in most of the publications is a simple deep learning-based framework. Still, some other publications have used a

deep convolutional network that can be described as a more advanced deep learning algorithm.

4) **View**. Many publications have discussed the perception and display subclasses of view taxonomy, but most have not specified the perception location's interaction tools. The deep learning-based algorithm was used for predicting the drug combinations and drug synergy score against cancer treatment. Hence, the majority of the perception location are patients. The prediction was made based on cancer samples found in the database of a cancer patient.
5) **Display**. The majority of the publications have used monitors and microscopes to visualise the generated data to the end-users. Since the monitors or digital screens are already in the model development lab and microscopes are there to show the small drug and chemical compounds, those devices are readily available.
6) **Interaction Tools**. Interaction tools interact the raw data with analysed and visual processing data using hardware and visual interaction tools.

3.2 Classification and Validation of the Components

The papers used in this classification are journal articles from 2017 onwards. Some of the important works that have been considered for this study together with the classification are reported in Table 1. The columns represent each component of the taxonomy and subcomponents of the related components are listed under it.

The model components include data that includes raw data, analyzed data and tools or methods used in the paper. The technique used for prediction of drug target is also

Table 1. Classification of the components

REF	AREA OF STUDY	DATA			DRUG FEATURE EXTRACTION	PREDICTION OF DRUG TARGET	VIEW FOR DRUG COMBINATIONS		
		Raw	Analyzed	Visually processed	Tools/methods	Techniques/Algorithms	Perception Location	Device	Inter action tools
(Celebi et al., 2019)	Anti-cancer	Cancer cell line	Chemical fingerprints Gene expression data	N/G	N/G	Multi-omics data based on machine learning model	Patient	Monitor	N/S
(Preuer et al., 2019)	Anti-cancer	Cancer cell line	Chemical descriptors of drugs, Gene expression data	N/G	Chemopy	Novel deep learning-based method (Deep synergy)	N/S	Microscope	N/S
(Xiaoa et al., 2018)	Lung cancer, Stomach cancer and Breast Cancer	Clinical data	N/G	High-dimensional gene expression data (RNA-seq data)	Auto-encoder	Stacked sparse auto-encoder algorithm based on deep neural network	Patient	N/G	Auto Enco der
(Hakime et al, 2018)	N/A	SMILES Strings data	Drug compound and protein sequence data	N/G	UniProt IDs	Deep learning-based drug-target binding affinity model (DeepDTA)	Patient	Microscope	N/S
(Lingwei et al., 2018)	Cancer		Drug and Gene channel data	N/G	Pubchem ID	Deep learning-based transcriptome data classification model	Real environment	Monitor/ screen	Win dowi ng funct ion
(Xia et al., 2018)	Anti-cancer therapy	Cancer cell line	Gene expression and microRNA data	2D structure data	Molecular feature model, Shared drug descriptor model	Deep neural network Model	Patient	Screen	Data glove

reported for the works that have been considered in this paper. Mainly the works that have been chosen for this paper are the ones that use deep learning-based techniques. Finally, the last component is view, that is used to provide the visualized data to the users. The view can be categorized as perception location, device used, or interaction tools.

We have also identified the components that must be evaluated and validated to display whether there are any added benefits of the system. Validation and evaluation are two different terms in this process, and they are differentiated as: Validation focus on proving the system's accuracy and ensures that the right system is built, on the other side, evaluation focus on showing whether the system is useful and provides greater value. Some of the works such as [1, 3] have used end-system i.e., display to validate their system, yet others utilize prediction technique for this purpose. Few of works, for

Table 2. Evaluation and validation of the components

REFERENCES	AREAS OF STUDY	COMPONENT VALIDATION AND EVALUATION	STUDY CRITERIA	DATASET FOR VALIDATION OR EVALUATION	PROPOSED MATHEMATICAL EQUATION	RESULTS IN TERMS OF INDEPENDENT VARIABLE
(Celebi et al., 2019)	Anti-cancer	Whole system	Accuracy, Training time	Kyoto Encyclopaedia of Genes and Genomes (KEGG) database.	$Common\ Neighbors(x,y) = \lvert\Gamma(x) \cap \Gamma(y)\rvert$ $Jaccard(x,y) = \frac{\lvert\Gamma(x) \cap \Gamma(y)\rvert}{\lvert\Gamma(x) \cup \Gamma(y)\rvert}$ $Adamic/Adar(x,y) = \sum_{z \in \Gamma(x) \cap \Gamma(y)} \frac{1}{log\lvert\Gamma(z)\rvert}$ Where x and y are drug pair features, Γ(y) is neighbors of node x, Γ(y) is neighbors of node y.	It provides accuracy in terms of mean square error and training time in terms of per second.
(Preuer et al., 2019)	Anti-cancer	Prediction process	Accuracy, Balanced accuracy, precision, specificity, Sensitivity	N/G	N/A	This solution provides synergy scores with high accuracy and best prediction in a cross validation set.
(Xiaoa et al., 2018)	Lung cancer, Stomach cancer and Breast Cancer	Whole system	Accuracy, precision and recall	Patient	The mathematical equation is proposed as: Loss function of the classifier $Jsparse(w,b) = J(W,b) + \beta \sum_{j-1}^{s} KL(p \parallel \hat{p}j),$ Where w is weight, b is bias, $\beta \sum_{j-1}^{s} KL(p \parallel \hat{p}j)$, is the sparsity penalty term, $KL(p \parallel \hat{p}j)$ is the Kullback-Leibler (KL), $(p \parallel \hat{p}j)$ is the Bernoulli random variable.	This paper provides accuracy rate of 99.89%, 98.15%, 96.23% in Lung cancer, stomach cancer and breast cancer respectively which is highest than other methods.
(Xiao et al., 2018)	Lung, Stomach and breast cancer	Whole system	Accuracy, Processing time	Patient	Mathematical equation proposed in this work is: $J(W,b) = \frac{1}{m} \sum_{i=1}^{m} J(W,b;x^2,y^2) + \frac{\lambda}{2} \sum_{l=2}^{n_l} \sum_{j=1}^{s_{l-1}} \sum_{i=1}^{s_l} (W_{ij}^{l})^2,$ Where, w is the weight, b is the bias, x and y are the input features, first tem is a mean square error term, second term is a regulation term and λ is the weight decay parameter.	It provides accuracy of 98.80, 98.78 and 98.41 for prediction of lung cancer, stomach cancer and breast cancer respectively.
(Hakime et al, 2018)	N/A	Display	Computational cost, affinity	Davis Kinase binding affinity (Davis dataset) and Kinase inhibitor bioactivities (KIBA dataset)	The proposed mathematical formula are: $MSE = \frac{1}{n} \sum_{i=1}^{n} (P_i - Y_i)^2$ Where MSE is a loss function, p is the prediction vector, and Y corresponds to the vector actual outputs and n is the number of samples.	It provides an affinity of of 0.836 to 0.863 in the KIBA dataset and 0.872 to 0.878 in the Davisis dataset.
(Xia et al., 2018)	Anti-cancer therapy	Whole system	Growth prediction, growth combo score, ranking and variance	Gene expression dataset	Mathematical solution is not provided in this work. $z_i^{AB} = \begin{cases} min(y_i^A, y_i^B), if y_i^A \leq 0 or y_i^B \leq 0 \\ \tilde{y}_i^A \cdot \tilde{y}_i^B, \end{cases}$ Where, y_i^A, y_i^B are the lowest growth fractions, $\tilde{y}_i = min(y_i, 1)$ truncates the growth fraction at 1.	It provides predictive growth of 0.94 in terms of coefficient of determination.

instance, [8, 10] have used whole system for verification purpose. The criteria for validation are mainly accuracy and precision, some other works have also focused on processing/computing cost and time as their criteria. The components used for validations and evaluations for each work are summarized in Table 2.

3.3 Model Verification

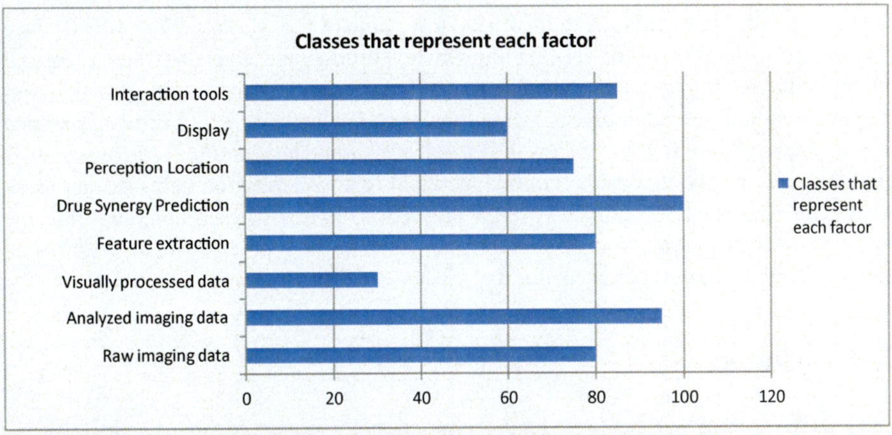

Fig. 2. In the bar graph, the components or classes of the researched paper has been presented in the percentage. The detailed subclasses are shown on Y-axis, and the rate is shown on X-axis. For example, the percentage of drug synergy prediction is 100, as all the publications have proposed the methods to predict accurate drug synergy combinations.

Evaluation of the proposed taxonomy is a critical task to verify the system. For this process, both quantitative and qualitative tools have been used for evaluating the taxonomy. The domain experts estimate the taxonomy based on specific criteria such as accuracy, consistency, sensitivity, completeness, and specificity [10] using a drug bank database or using patient data [8]. Mainly, we analysed overlapping terms between the instances that the components of our proposed taxonomy have. Each factor and the percentage of components/classes described in the chosen publications are shown in Fig. 2.

4 Discussion

In our work, we have proposed the DDPV taxonomy (Data, Drug feature extraction, Prediction of drug target and View) as the system's main components, and we have used deep learning techniques in the cancer domain All the publications researched in this work have focused on deep learning techniques in predicting drug combinations for cancer treatment. Most of the works [1, 2, 9, 10] have considered raw and analyzed image data, on the contrary [7] has only focused on visually processed data. All of the works considered in review, have used drug feature extraction for effective drug interaction prediction. Although all of the publications have used drug, target and cancer cell lines as input and further processed them to predict the accurate drug synergy scores, they have not considered feature extraction and prediction factors; instead, they have focused on classification and detection. For majority of the works considered, perception location is patient or real environment. Some of the works such as [2, 9] did not provide any interaction tools which is essential to see the predicted score by end users. We have also reported evaluation of the reviewed works which shows that most of the works used accuracy as criteria to validate their work. Only some of the works such as [8, 10] have used whole of the system for verification which is promising. Others have only focused on prediction technique, data or display to be used for validation purpose. Based on our proposed taxonomy, evaluation, and validation of system components, it is recommended that different types of raw, analysing and visual data should be identified for drug synergy prediction. Similarly, it is also recommended that feature extraction helps extract high-level drug features for accurate synergy prediction. It is also recommended that the end-users such as pharmacologists and physicians view the predictive synergy scores on the big screen or monitor in the natural environment using interactive tools.

5 Conclusion

The DDPV taxonomy (Data, Drug feature extraction, Prediction of drug target and View) is proposed in this work. Through this taxonomy, the end-users such as physicians and pathologists can see the type of data used, feature extraction tools, prediction techniques and visual display of the synergistic drug combinations. This will further help the pathologists to derive a more accurate drug synergy score which will assist them in smooth anti-cancer treatment.

Overall, the DDPV taxonomy is trying to cover detailed aspects and components that are useful in evaluating and validating the prediction process of anti-cancer. However, there is still more ground for future improvements. Future work can be assessed and validated in a real-world scenario for the guaranteed application of the proposed taxonomy. Moreover, the taxonomy could also be used to test the applicability of the prediction process in cancer types and other medical diseases.

References

1. Chiu, Y.C., et al.: Predicting drug response of tumors from integrated genomic profiles by deep neural networks. GMC Med. Genomics **12**(1), 143–155 (2019)
2. Preuer, K., Lewis, R.P., Hochreiter, S., Bender, A., Bulusu, K.C., Klambauer, G.: DeepSynergy: predicting anti-cancer drug synergy with deep learning. Bioinformatics **34**(9), 1538–1546 (2019)
3. Sharifi-Noghabi, H., Zolotareva, O., Collins, C.C., Ester, M.: MOLI: multi-omics late integration with deep neural networks for drug response prediction. Bioinformatics **35**(14), 501–509 (2019)
4. Chou, T.: Theoretical basis, experimental design, and computerized simulation of syn-ergism and antagonism in drug combination studies. Pharmacol. Rev. **8**(3), 621–681 (2006)

5. Ma, Y., et al.: Predicting cancer drug response by proteomic profiling. Clin. Cancer Res. **12**(15), 4583–4589 (2006)
6. Xia, F., et al.: Predicting tumour cell line response to drug pairs with deep learning. BMC Bioinf. **19**(18), 1471–2105 (2018)
7. Xiao, Y., Wu, J., Zhao, X., Lin, Z.: A deep learning-based multi-model ensemble method for cancer prediction. Comput. Methods Programs Biomed. **153**, 1–9 (2018)
8. Xiao, Y., Zhao, X., Lin, Z., Wu, J.: A semi-supervised deep learning method based on stacked sparse auto-encoder for cancer prediction using RNA-seq data. Comput. Methods Programs Biomed. **166**, 99–105 (2018)
9. Öztürk, H., Özgür, A., Ozkirimli, E.: DeepDTA: deep drug–target binding affinity prediction. Bioinformatics **34**(17), 821–829 (2018)
10. Xie, L., He, S., Song, X., Bo, X., Zhang, Z.: Deep learning-based transcriptome data classification for drug-target interaction prediction. BMC Genomics **19**(I7), 93–102 (2018)
11. Ding, H., Takigawa, I., Mamitsuka, H., Zhu, S.: Similarity-based machine learning methods for predicting drug–target interactions: a brief review. Brief. Bioinform. **15**(5), 734–747 (2014)

Average Power Based EEG Channel Selection Method for Emotion Recognition

Md. Shahriar Rahman[1], Nadia Tasnim Mim[1(✉)], Jonayed Ahmed Riduan[1], Ridwane-Ul-Islam[1], Most. Mahjabin[1], Mohammed Abid Abrar[1], and Mohammad Zavid Parvez[2,3,4]

[1] Department of Computer Science and Engineering, BRAC University, Dhaka, Bangladesh
mimnadiatasnim@gmail.com
[2] Kent Institute Australia, Melbourne, Australia
[3] Engineering Institute of Technology, Melbourne, Australia
[4] Peter Faber Business School, Australian Catholic University, Melbourne, Australia

Abstract. Emotion can be defined as the neurophysiological changes people experience due to significant internal or external occasions. This work applies a channel selection algorithm based on average band power on the preprocessed EEG data frequency bands from the DEAP dataset to select the top 10 EEG channels. DWT is performed to get detail coefficients as features, and a statistical parameter RSS is used to reduce the dimension of the features for both selected and all 32 EEG channels. Finally, valence and arousal are classified using different classification algorithms (like Random Forest, Extra Trees, Naive Bayes, and MLP) to make a performance comparison between selected EEG channels and all EEG channels. The highest test accuracy, 66.8%, was retrieved from the Random Forest (RF) classifier for valence classification. Likewise, Random Forest (RF) and Extra Trees (ET) both achieved the highest test accuracy of 64.84% for arousal classification, which validates the efficiency of the proposed channel reduction technique.

Keywords: Emotion recognition · DEAP · EEG · Channel selection · DWT · RSS

1 Introduction

Emotion is a complex state of human beings. It consists of behavior, feelings, reactions to internal or external stimuli, etc. There is a vital relation between emotion recognition and affective computing. For the identification of human emotion many ways such as speech, facial expressions, behavior or psychological signals, fusion of information using multimodal technique are note-worthy [1–4, 14]. Researchers delineated the reliability of psychological signals as it is a subject independent approach [5]. Moreover, along with the change of emotion, EEG signals quickly capture or respond to the changes and it is better in terms of reliable feature extraction for emotion recognition tasks [6, 7]. Electroencephalogram (EEG) signals are also more insightful especially when any

K. Daimi and A. Al Sadoon (Eds.): ICR 2022, AISC 1431, pp. 270–280, 2022.
https://doi.org/10.1007/978-3-031-14054-9_26

subject can not express his/her desired emotion [13]. Due to the high speed factor, low cost and interaction capability with our central nervous system, most of the HCI/BCI system uses EEG signals along with this many research uses physiological signals to detect human emotions appropriately [8, 12].

A few databases have been constructed with a view to help the study of emotions in recent years. One of the most remarkable datasets here is DEAP dataset that contains physiological signals and electroencephalograms and many research on this database used valence and arousal to measure emotional state [9, 11]. Therefore, it can be claimed that EEG channel selection techniques and feature extraction methods are important factors in increasing the accuracy rate of emotion recognition as well as reducing space and time complexity. A study focusing on only one specific EEG channel F4 showed significant improvement on the accuracy level [21]. On the other hand, another study that uses all 32 channels of EEG signals mainly focuses on feature extraction and performed different experiments to measure the accuracy [20]. Therefore, more focus needs to be put on feature extraction and channel selection in order to predict some good results on different emotional states of human.

In our work, we have proposed a channel selection technique based on average power to select top 10 EEG channels with highest average power values. Furthermore, for the classification task, we have used DWT detail coefficients as feature vector and a statistical parameter Root Sum Square (RSS) to reduce the feature vector dimension.

2 Background of the Study

Emotion plays a very significant role for communicating among humans. In recent years, there has been extensive work on emotion recognition. In the research of Qing et al. [10], they suggested a renewal system, the demonstration curve for the proposed method for emotion prediction using ML and only EEG signal experimenting on the DEAP and SEED data. They extracted features from the EEG signals to construct two coefficients which are entropy and correction. In another study, Wioleta et al. [15] mainly reviewed corporal stimulus, feelings as well as briefly described some of the related research works of the corporal and electrical fields in feelings identification. With the aim of bringing more accuracy in emotion classification, the authors would like to work on gaming and e-related divisions.

In their work, Chen et al. [17] proposed an EEG emotion wave based feature learning and classification technique using deep CNN based on some specific features and fusions of EEG signals in DEAP dataset in order to increase the accuracy. Their experimental outcome indicates that deep CNN's performance was better than any other identifiers. Torres et al. [18] stated that user's emotions can be recognized through EEG based Brain Computer Interfaces (BCI) devices. They also proved that positive emotional states are more easy to detect compared to negative emotional states. Another research showed the statistical analysis of an EEG-based emotion recognition system using a self-organizing map for boundary detection. The proposed method improved the accuracy to 84.5% and it proved that the class difference helps rising the emotion identification accuracy using EEG signals [19]. Ozerdem et al. [22] proposed a positive and negative emotion classification method using five selected EEG channels using the DEAP dataset. The average overall accuracies were 77.14% for MLPNN and 72.92% for KNN. In near future, they plan on using all of the secondary bands individually on their proposed model.

Unlike these studies, we have applied a channel selection technique to select top 10 effective channels on the basis of average power to make any system efficient enough in terms of computational complexity, memory usage and training time. Finally, in the classification task of valence and arousal, a statistical parameter RSS is introduced for the dimension reduction of DWT detail coefficient feature vector.

Table 1. Performance comparison with related works.

Article	Database	Classifiers	No. of EEG channels	Highest test accuracy (%)
Pandey et al. [28]	DEAP	DNN SVM	4	Valence: DNN - 62.50 Arousal: DNN - 61.25
Jirayucharoensak et al. [20]	DEAP	DLN SVM NB	32	Valence: DLN - 53.42 Arousal: DLN - 52.03
Pandey et al. [21]	DEAP	MLP	1	Valence and arousal Average accuracy: 58.5
Zhang et al. [23]	DEAP	SVM	8, 19, 29	Average accuracy of 4 Emotional states: 8 channels: 58.51 19 channels: 59.13 29 channels: 59.98
Yan et al. [29]	DEAP	LSTM RNN	32	Valence and arousal Average accuracy: 59.03
Kumar et al. [30]	DEAP	SVM	2	Arousal: 64.84 Valence: 61.17
Proposed	DEAP	MLP ET NB RF	10	Valence: RF - 66.8 Arousal: RF and ET - 64.84

3 Materials and Methodology

3.1 Database Description

This study is mainly focused on the electroencephalogram (EEG) signals that is used for identifying emotion. Hence, we have used the dataset collected from the DEAP database [16] for extracting the EEG features and perform experiments. It is a multimodal dataset which contains the EEG and circumferential physiologic signals from 32 participants [16]. Data down-sampling rate for all 40 channels are 128 Hz and they are segmented into a 60 s trial where the 3 s pre-trial baseline is removed. Each participant file contains two arrays: data and labels. Data array contains video/trial × channel × data with the shape 40 × 40 × 8064 and the label array contains video/trial × label (valence, arousal, dominance, liking) with the shape 40 × 4 [16]. On this note, we have taken only first 32 EEG channels in consideration for this experiment.

3.2 Methodologies

Our proposed methodology mainly divided into four major steps - dataset preprocessing, EEG channel selection, feature extraction and classification of valence and arousal using all 32 EEG channels and selected 10 EEG channels. The overall methodological illustration of this study is given in Fig. 1.

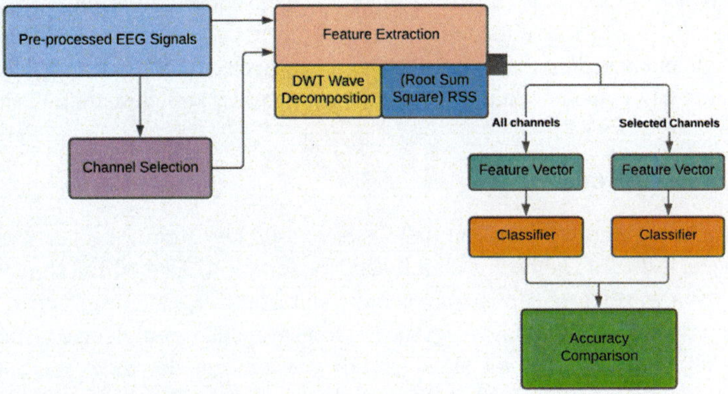

Fig. 1. Proposed methodology.

3.3 Dataset Preprocessing

The valence and arousal target labels are classified as high and low class. The high class is indicated by '1' whereas the low class is indicated by '0'. For both valence and arousal data, where the ratings are in range of 1 to 9, a threshold value of '5' is considered to classify the data, where values less than 5 are classified as low class. On the other hand, values greater than or equal to 5 is classified as high class. Total number of high and low class in valence is 724 and 556, similarly, high and low class in arousal is 754 and 526 respectively. Thus it can be depicted that the dataset is balanced for any classification task.

3.4 Channel Selection

The cortical spectral power activity holds an important statistical significance in analyzing the EEG signals [25]. Different research works relied on three frequency bands-alpha

Table 2. Selected channels from different frequency bands using channel selection algorithm.

Frequency bands	Selected channels
Alpha (8–13 Hz)	Fp2, F7, T7, AF3, Fp1, F8, Cz, AF4, Oz, P7, T8, O1
Beta (13–30 Hz)	Fp2, F7, Fp1, T7, AF3, T8, F8, AF4, O1, Cz, F4, P7
Gamma (>30 Hz)	Fp2, F7, T7, T8, Fp1, AF3, F8, O1, AF4, FC6, F4, P7
10 Common Channels	Fp2, F7, T7, AF3, Fp1, F8, AF4, P7, T8, O1

(8–13 Hz), beta (13–30 Hz) and gamma (>30 Hz) for emotion classification task [26, 27]. In this work, 12 most effective channels from each band are selected using the channel selection Algorithm 1 which is based on average band power and finally, top 10 common channels (Fp2, F7, T7, AF3, Fp1, F8, AF4, P7, T8, O1) from these three frequency bands are taken as shown in Table 2. The proposed algorithm results a time complexity of O($n\ v\ c$) where the number of participants, the number of videos, and the number of channels is denoted as 'n', 'v' and 'c' respectively. The average band power of a particular EEG channel data is calculated using SciPy welch method [24].

3.5 Feature Extraction

For the feature extraction process, at first we have used DWT multilevel decomposition where wavelet is db2 of Daubechies family and the level is 4. As the EEG signals are non stationary data, wavelet transformation is more suitable to extract the effective features. Hence, the proposed methodology uses the Discrete Wavelet Coefficients as it depicts the degree of reciprocity between the signal and the wavelet function at various times [21]. Therefore, four levels of detailed coefficients which are cD1, cD2, cD3 and cD4 has been generated and one approximation coefficient is found [22]. The next feature extraction tasks has been performed on these four detailed coefficients. To reduce the dimension of these detailed coefficient feature vectors and training time of the models, we have implemented a statistical method named Root Sum Square (RSS) which is shown in Eq. 1. Hence, in this method four RSS features are extracted for each EEG channel data. According to our literature knowledge so far, this particular statistical method has not been used on emotion recognition feature extraction tasks using EEG signals.

Algorithm 1 EEG channel selection algorithm based on average power

```
set band range for EEG signal
define the sampling frequency
for participants = 1 to 32 do
  for videos = 1 to 40 do
    for channels = 1 to 32 do
      calculate average band power
      save band powers along with individual channels in a form of mapping
    end for
    append the mapped data in an array or a list
  end for
end for
for each mapped data in the list do
  sort the mapped data in descending order
  select best 10 channels
  append to an array
end for
count the appearance of the channels from the array
select 10 channels with most appearance
```

For generating more information from these detailed coefficients following steps are performed to add four more features for a particular eeg channel data, which are:

a) RSS ratio of cD1 and cD2 is used.
b) RSS ratio of cD3 and cD4 is used.
c) RSS absolute difference between cD1 and cD2 is used.
d) RSS absolute difference between cD3 and cD4 is used.

Finally, the extracted feature dimension for a particular participant is 8 × 32 × 40 (features × channels × videos/trials), after reshaping the dimension which is 40 × 256 (videos/trials × features) for all 32 EEG channels. On the other hand, the feature vector for ten selected channels after reshaping the dimension is found as 40 × 80 (videos/trials × features). As there are 32 participants in the experiment, hence, total rows are counted as 1280 (40 × 32) where the features are constant for all EEG channels and selected channels.

$$X_{RSS} = \sqrt{\sum_{i=1}^{n} x_i^2}; \tag{1}$$

3.6 Classification

In the classification part, we have taken four machine learning classifiers which are Random Forest (RF), Naive Bayes (NB), Multi-layer Perceptron (MLP) and Extra Trees (ET) for observing and comparing the performance of these RSS features on the selected channels. For this task, two feature datasets are shuffled randomly and splitted into training and test set where 80% of the data are taken for training and 20% of the data are utilized for testing the models. Before fitting the data into the models using Scikit-learn [32] package, hyperparameter tuning is done for achieving a standard non-bias accuracy. Finally, the accuracy score and different performance metrics of the classifiers like precision, recall and f1-score are taken in consideration for evaluating the effectiveness of the channel selection algorithm after classifying valence (low/high) and arousal (low/high).

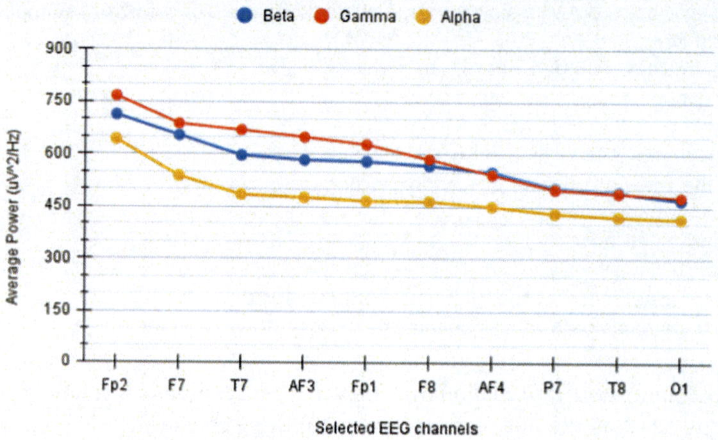

Fig. 2. Average power difference of top 10 EEG channels from alpha, beta and gamma frequency bands.

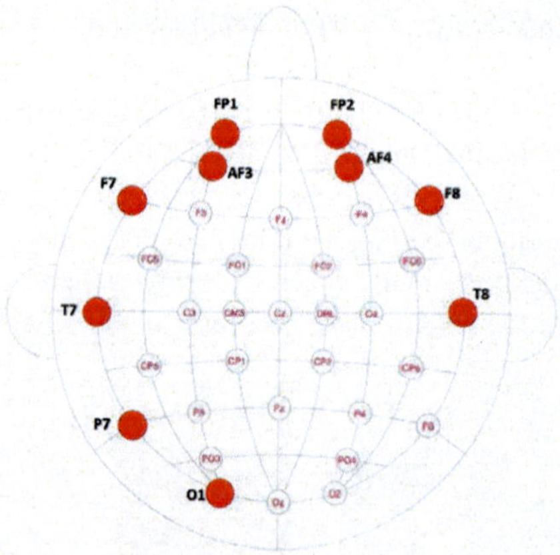

Fig. 3. Selected channel locations based 10–20 standard electrode location system [31].

4 Results Analysis

We have analyzed the performance of the selected channels using some machine learning classifiers. Our work showed a notable difference while experimenting with selected channels. For both valence and arousal classification, selected channels dominates all channels with a better test accuracy. The highest test accuracy is obtained by Random Forest which is 66.8% for valence classification as shown in Fig. 4b. On the other hand, both Extra Trees and Random Forest classifier has performed better than the other algorithms with the highest test accuracy 64.84% for arousal classification as shown in Fig. 4a. Furthermore, precision, recall and f1-score of the selected channels are also have greater values than all channels' metrics as depicted in Table 3. Therefore, this proposed channel selection technique and RSS for feature extraction make this research work efficient in terms of test accuracy and different performance metrics of the classifiers.

Table 3. Comparison of different performance metrics between selected EEG channels and all EEG channels.

Classifiers	Precision score				Recall score				F1-score			
	Selected channels		All channels		Selected channels		All channels		Selected channels		All channels	
	Valence	Arousal	Valence	Arousal	Valence	Arousal	Valence	Arousal	Valence	Arousal	Valence	Arousal
Random Forest	0.68	0.66	0.66	0.65	0.75	0.77	0.75	0.75	0.71	0.71	0.70	0.69
Naïve Bayes	0.55	0.59	0.55	0.59	0.89	0.75	0.86	0.74	0.68	0.66	0.67	0.66
Extra Trees	0.67	0.66	0.67	0.65	0.74	0.77	0.75	0.74	0.71	0.71	0.71	0.69
MLP	0.67	0.65	0.67	0.64	0.73	0.72	0.69	0.69	0.70	0.69	0.68	0.66

In the channel selection task, repeating channels are found from the three frequency bands (alpha, beta, gamma) though the ranking is different. On this note, we have observed the average power of top 10 EEG channels of alpha band is less than beta and gamma band respectively as shown in Fig. 2. Furthermore, most of the selected channels are located in the prefrontal, occipital, temporal and posterior lobe as shown in Fig. 3 which are important locations of the brain in terms of emotion generation [26]. Hence, this channel selection technique can locate the place of emotion generation successfully and these frequency bands are important for emotion recognition task.

While comparing with related works with the same database, our work out-performed some significant researches. Some of the previous works used less channels but they lacked accuracy. With 10 selected channels, we have improved the test accuracy for both valence and arousal binary classification as shown in Table 1. Similarly, the impact of using selective channels is promising as it saves memory space, reduce computational complexity and processing time of this huge data.

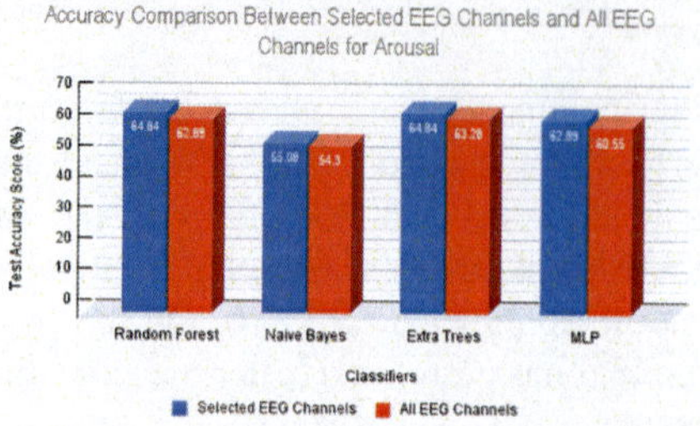

(a) (Left figure)Accuracy comparison for arousal.

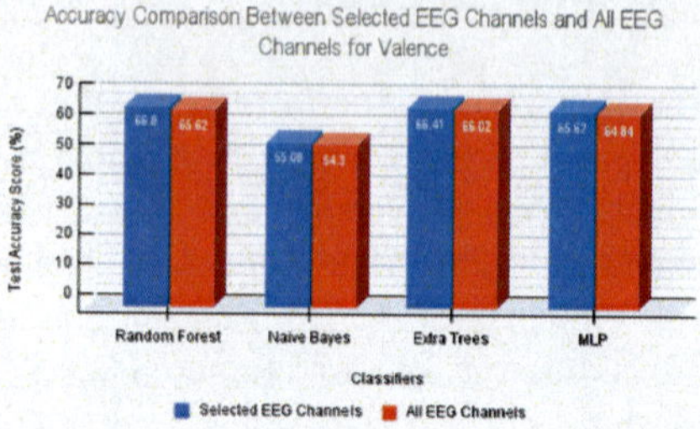

(b) (Right figure)Accuracy comparison for valence.

Fig. 4. Accuracy comparison for arousal and valence.

5 Conclusion

The aim of this study is to classify valence and arousal on the basis of audiovisual stimuli with the help of EEG signals and to compare the efficiency of selected EEG channels with all 32 EEG channels. In this work, we have used DEAP database and have taken preprocessed EEG data of 32 participants to classify valence and arousal. For the feature extraction task, we have used DWT to get detail coefficient feature vectors and then, reduced the dimension of these vectors using Root Sum Square (RSS). Moreover, we have used those features on different machine learning classifiers, ensemble methods and MLP to classify valence and arousal. Top 10 EEG channels (Fp2, T7, AF4, AF3, T8, Fp1, F7, F8, P7, O1) are selected from alpha, beta and gamma frequency band using proposed channel selection algorithm which is based on highest average power. The performance of selected channels in terms of test accuracy is higher compared to all EEG channels as described in the results analysis section. Furthermore, the validation of this study is found while comparing with some recent works on this database. Hence, this proposed channel selection technique is found more efficient in terms of emotion classification on valence and arousal. Finally, it can be depicted that, with selected channels both the training time and memory space is saved as well as performance can be enhanced in this emotion recognition study. Using Root Sum Square (RSS) features from DWT vectors of different frequency bands and average power based channel selection algorithm make this research work unique.

In future studies, channel selection can be done using source localization technique of EEG signals. Blood pressure, respiratory rate, galvanic skin response, body temperature and other signals can be used to analyse their role in this emotion recognition field. Additionally, better machine learning models can be applied for achieving more accuracy in determining different emotions. Lastly, different databases containing EEG signals for emotion recognition can be analyzed with this proposed methodology to compare the performance.

References

1. Petrushin, V.: Emotion in speech: recognition and application to call centers. In: Proceedings of Artificial Neural Networks in Engineering, vol. 710, p. 22, November 1999

2. Anderson, K., McOwan, P.W.: A real-time automated system for the recognition of human facial expressions. IEEE Trans. Syst. Man Cybern. Part B (Cybern.) **36**(1), 96–105 (2006)
3. Pantic, M., Rothkrantz, L.J.M.: Automatic analysis of facial expressions: the state of the art. IEEE Trans. Pattern Anal. Mach. Intell. **22**(12), 1424–1445 (2000)
4. Yin, Z., Zhao, M., Wang, Y., Yang, J., Zhang, J.: Recognition of emotions using multimodal physiological signals and an ensemble deep learning model. Comput. Methods Programs Biomed. **140**, 93–110 (2017)
5. Wang, X.W., Nie, D., Lu, B.L.: Emotional state classification from EEG data using machine learning approach. Neurocomputing **129**, 94–106 (2014)
6. Petrantonakis, P.C., Hadjileontiadis, L.J.: A novel emotion elicitation index using frontal brain asymmetry for enhanced EEG-based emotion recognition. IEEE Trans. Inf. Technol. Biomed. **15**(5), 737–746 (2011)
7. Li, X., Hu, B., Zhu, T., Yan, J., Zheng, F.: Towards affective learning with an EEG feedback approach. In: Proceedings of the First ACM International Workshop on Multimedia Technologies for Distance Learning, pp. 33–38, October 2009
8. Torres-Valencia, C.A., Garcia-Arias, H.F., Lopez, M.A.A., Orozco-Gutiérrez, A.A.: Comparative analysis of physiological signals and electroencephalogram (EEG) for multimodal emotion recognition using generative models. In: 2014 XIX Symposium on Image, Signal Processing and Artificial Vision, pp. 1–5. IEEE, September 2014
9. Koelstra, S., et al.: Deap: a database for emotion analysis; using physiological signals. IEEE Trans. Affect. Comput. **3**(1), 18–31 (2011)
10. Qing, C., Qiao, R., Xu, X., Cheng, Y.: Interpretable emotion recognition using EEG signals. IEEE Access **7**, 94160–94170 (2019)
11. Russell, J.A.: A circumplex model of affect. J. Pers. Soc. Psychol. **39**(6), 1161 (1980)
12. Murugappan, M., Juhari, M.R.B.M., Nagarajan, R., Yaacob, S.: An Investigation on visual and audiovisual stimulus based emotion recognition using EEG. Int. J. Med. Eng. Inform. **1**(3), 342 (2009)
13. Doma, V., Pirouz, M.: A comparative analysis of machine learning methods for emotion recognition using EEG and peripheral physiological signals. J. Big Data **7**(1), 1–21 (2020). https://doi.org/10.1186/s40537-020-00289-7
14. Baratloo, A., Hosseini, M., Negida, A., El Ashal, G.: Part 1: simple definition and calculation of accuracy, sensitivity and specificity. Emergency (Tehran, Iran) **3**(2), 48–49 (2015)
15. Wioleta, S.: Using physiological signals for emotion recognition. In: 2013 6th International Conference on Human System Interactions (HSI), pp. 556- 561. IEEE, June 2013
16. Koelstra, S.: DEAP: A Dataset for Emotion Analysis using Physiological and Audiovisual Signals (2020). http://www.eecs.qmul.ac.uk/mmv/datasets/deap/readme.html. Accessed 6 Oct 2020
17. Chen, J.X., Zhang, P.W., Mao, Z.J., Huang, Y.F., Jiang, D.M., Zhang, Y.N.: Accurate EEG-based emotion recognition on combined features using deep convolutional neural networks. IEEE Access **7**, 44317–44328 (2019). https://doi.org/10.1109/ACCESS.2019.2908285
18. Torres, E.P., Torres, E.A., Hernández-Álvarez, M., Yoo, S.G.: EEG-based BCI emotion recognition: a survey. Sensors **20**(18), 5083 (2020). https://doi.org/10.3390/s20185083
19. Khosrowbadi, R., Quek, H.C., Wahab, A., Ang, K.K.: EEG based emotion recognition using self-organizing map for boundary detection. In: International Conference on Pattern Recognition, pp. 4242–4245 (2010)
20. Jirayucharoensak, S., Panngum, S., Israsena, P.: EEG-based emotion recognition using deep learning network with principal component based covariate shift adaptation. Sci. World J. **2014**, 627892 (2014). https://doi.org/10.1155/2014/627892
21. Pandey, P., Seeja, K.R.: Emotional state recognition with EEG signals using subject independent approach. In: Mishra, D.K., Yang, X.-S., Unal, A. (eds.) Data Science and Big Data

Analytics. LNDECT, vol. 16, pp. 117–124. Springer, Singapore (2019). https://doi.org/10.1007/978-981-10-7641-1_10
22. Özerdem, M.S., Polat, H.: Emotion recognition based on EEG features in movie clips with channel selection. Brain Inform. **4**(4), 241–252 (2017). https://doi.org/10.1007/s40708-017-0069-3
23. Zhang, J., Chen, M., Zhao, S., Hu, S., Shi, Z., Cao, Y.: ReliefF-based EEG sensor selection methods for emotion recognition. Sensors **16**(10), 1558 (2016). https://doi.org/10.3390/s16101558
24. Virtanen, P., et al.: SciPy 1.0: fundamental algorithms for scientific computing in Python. Nat. Methods (2020). https://doi.org/10.1038/s41592-019-0686-2
25. Vecchiato, G., et al.: EEG analysis of the brain activity during the observation of commercial, political, or public service announcements. Comput. Intell. Neurosci. **2010** (2010)
26. Wang, J., Wang, M.: Review of the emotional feature extraction and classification using EEG signals. Cogn. Robot. **1**, 29–40 (2021). https://doi.org/10.1016/j.cogr.2021.04.001
27. Pane, E.S., Wibawa, A.D., Pumomo, M.H.: Channel selection of EEG emotion recognition using stepwise discriminant analysis. In: 2018 International Conference on Computer Engineering, Network and Intelligent Multimedia (CENIM), pp. 14–19. IEEE, November (2018)
28. Pandey, P., Seeja, K.R.: Subject independent emotion recognition from EEG using VMD and deep learning. J. King Saud Univ.-Comput. Inf. Sci. (2019)
29. Yan, J., Chen, S., Deng, S.: A EEG-based emotion recognition model with rhythm and time characteristics. Brain Inform. **6**(1), 1–8 (2019). https://doi.org/10.1186/s40708-019-0100-y
30. Kumar, N., Khaund, K., Hazarika, S.M.: Bispectral analysis of EEG for emotion recognition. Procedia Comput. Sci. **84**, 31–35 (2016)
31. Morley, A., Hill, L., Kaditis, A.G.: 10–20 System EEG Placement. European Respiratory Society, European Respiratory Society (2016)
32. Pedregosa, F., et al.: Scikit-learn: machine learning in Python. J. Mach. Learn. Res. **12**, 2825–2830 (2011)

Deep Learning Algorithm Based Support Vector Machines

Mohamad Naji[1(✉)], Widad Alyassine[1], Qurat Ul Ain Nizamani[2], Lingrui Zhang[1], Xue Wei[1], Ziqiu Xu[1], Ali Braytee[1], and Ali Anaissi[1]

[1] School of Computer Science, The University of Sydney, Sydney, Australia
Mohamad.Naji@sydney.edu.au
[2] School of Computer Science, Kent Institute Australia, Sydney, Australia

Abstract. This paper proposes a new deep learning model which replaces the softmax activation function with support vector machines. To evaluate the performance of the model, we have completed a total of four sets of codes, including the traditional svm classification model, the traditional cnn model, the model of svm behind the fully connected layer, and the model of svm instead of softmax. In order to compare the accuracy of these four groups of models, we trained and tested three data sets, namely the mnist data set, the CIFAR-10 data set and the compass x-ray data set .

Keywords: Deep learning · Support vector machine · Convolution neural network

1 Introduction

The development of artificial intelligence has made considerable progress in the recent years and has been applied in many application domains such as medical treatment, agriculture, finance and aerospace. Furthermore, the image recognition and other destructive innovative technologies have also received a great attention with the advent of AI technologies and deep learning methods such as the deep convolutional neural network (CNN). Since the ImageNet competition in 2012, CNN have excessively used in computer vision applications for image recognition, speech recognition and other aspects.

Traditional CNN uses the Softmax function as its output layer activation function. The limitations of Softmax found in the comparison of research in recent years are that it needs to ensure that the classes of input data are separable. Softmax performs better in data sets like MNIST and ImageNet where all classes are identified in advance. Softmax does not require compactness within classes and separation between classes, therefore, Softmax's results are not very accurate in cases where the training set, such as face recognition, contains far fewer classes than all classes. On the other hand, the support vector machine (SVM) is a very powerful model, it performs well on various data sets, and its

K. Daimi and A. Al Sadoon (Eds.): ICR 2022, AISC 1431, pp. 281–289, 2022.
https://doi.org/10.1007/978-3-031-14054-9_27

kernel function can satisfy the classification of high dimensional data sets. Therefore, SVM itself does not have many restrictions on the types of data sets. For this reason, we use SVM instead of Softmax to reduce the error rate of prediction results and enhance the generalization ability of the model, thus improving the performance of the training model.

In the development of convolutional neural networks, AlexNet is the first network structure that is well known to the public. After winning the competition, many scholars have been deeply studying and learning this model. VGG, RESNET and other networks emerged based on this model. The rationale idea of this work is to replace the Softmax function in CNN with SVM. In this sense, we build three models: Softmax-based CNN model, the simple SVM-based CNN model and our proposed SVM-based CNN model based on AlexNet model.

2 Literature Review

Several researchers use SVM in combination with class probability output networks in neural networks [2]. In this sense, the work in [4] propose an improved technique for CNN, which is to replace the fully connected layer structure in CNN with a global average pool. This can reduce training parameters and reduce the risk of overfitting. In the literatureAnother work in [5] uses three independent models (SVM, CNN, and RNN) to form different ensemble models to compare their performance differences. Similarly, a method based on CNN + SVM is proposed for classifying abnormal audio indoors [6]. The convolutional layer and pooling layer in CNN are used to extract the feature parameters and the SVM for classification. In CNN, the feature parameters of samples are extracted in the convolutional layer for further feature extraction, and the data dimension is reduced in the pooling layer. The data is continuously processed in the convolutional layer and the pooling layer, and finally transmitted to the fully connected, the multi-dimensional vector is converted into a one-dimensional vector, and the SVM is used for classification and output.

In Automatic Diagnosis of Alzheimer's Disease and Mild Cognitive Impairment Based on CNN + SVM Networks with End-to-End Training [7], a three-category classification model is raised. In order to get better classification performance, a novel network model is proposed in the study based on 3D convolution neural networks (CNN) and support vector machines (SVM) by utilizing both the excellent abilities of CNN in feature extraction and SVM in classification. This literature can help us to deal with three-category classification issues. In this article, the structure of the designed 3DCNN network is described in Fig. 1.

In the paper Hybrid SVM-CNN Classification Technique for Human-Vehicle Targets in an Automotive LFMCW Radar [8], they propose a hybrid support vector machine-convolutional neural network (SVM-CNN) approach to address the class-imbalance classification of vehicles and pedestrians with limited experimental radar data available. In another literature, people use AdaBoost method to extract new features and get data pre-trained [9]. Then DeepSVM is used as an ensemble learning way to replace traditional DL methods. Each layer will include several SVM models to create new training data under supervised labels, which will facilitate the final classification. This method focuses on the autoencoder technique and tries to integrate ensemble learning into this procedure, which can be viewed as pre-training in deep learning. The network structure will deal with classifiers in the same layer in each iteration. It has no back propagation and do actually focus on feed forward. The overlapping samples in DeepSVM are much less than that of traditional SVM.

In 'A novel hybrid CNN-SVM classifier for recognizing handwritten digits', people aims to build a new hybrid CNN-SVM system. It replaces the softmax layer with SVM [10]. In our research, this method is also used. After data training in hidden layers, the new feature vector of the last hidden layer outputs will be sent to SVM for classification. The paper gives two SVM classifier, one for two-class classification, the other is used for multi-class data. For multi-class SVM, it uses LIBSVM method to build SVM, which is a one-against-one method. In this network, SVM classifier aims to minimize the generalization errors on the unseen data with a fixed distribution for the training set, by using the Structural Risk Minimization principle. The separating hyperplane is a global optimum solution.

In Improving Image Classification Accuracy using Hybrid Systems of Support Vector Machines and Convolutional Neural Networks literature, which proposes a series of models related to SVM. The author made a comparative study on linear SVM and SVM with kernel function. And based on the convolutional neural network, a new hybrid model is proposed, which is to add SVM classification model after CNN is performed. The SVM takes the fully connected layer in the CNN as input and 128 high-level features extracted from the pre-trained CNN enter. Both weight and bias are weights and inputs that have been trained using traditional CNN. The author also uses the extreme learning machine model to compare with all other models. According to literature, it can be seen that after the data set Mnist is input to each model, the training time of the model that adds SVM after CNN is not the shortest, but the accuracy is the highest. Traditional CNN has a relatively low accuracy rate, but the time is faster. We feel that we can add the traditional CNN plus SVM model proposed in this literature to our research project to compare it with other models we research [11].

3 Method

This work replace the soft-max activation function in CNN with a SVM model to achieve better classification accuracy. In view of the fact that this project is mainly aimed at image classification, in traditional neural networks with hidden layers, a fully connected neural network is generally used to process large-size images directly. The disadvantage of this method is that the image will be expanded into a vector and a lot of space will be lost. Information, and secondly, a large number of parameters will be used in the training process, which will lead to over-fitting and lower training efficiency. In response to these problems, we used a convolutional neural network as a framework for this study. As shown in the figure, the convolutional neural network greatly reduces the number of

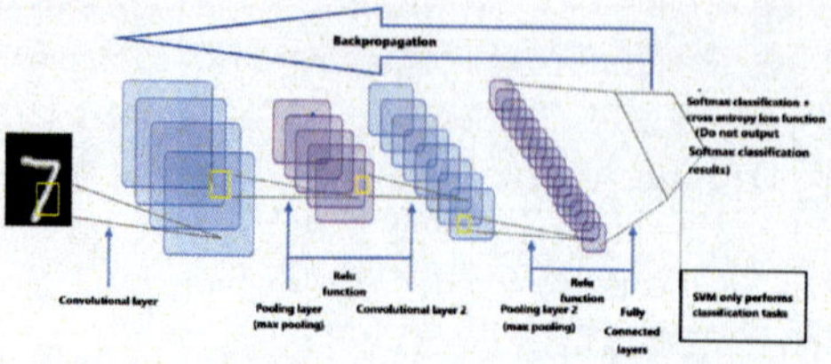

Fig. 1. CNN+SVM principle diagram

picture pixel matrix parameters by changing the conventional neural network to a three-layer structure. The three-layer structure are: Convolutional layer: The convolutional layer is the core layer to construct a convolutional neural network, which generates most of the calculation in the network. It can be regarded as an output of a neuron. Neurons observe only a small part of the input data and share parameters with all neurons on the left and right sides of the space. Thereby reducing the number of parameters. Because convolution has the characteristic of "weight sharing", it can reduce the number of parameters, reduce computational overhead, and prevent over-fitting due to too many parameters.

Pooling layer: Usually a pooling layer is periodically inserted between successive convolutional layers. Its function is to gradually reduce the spatial size of the data volume, so that the number of parameters in the network can be reduced, which reduces the consumption of computing resources and can effectively control over-fitting. In this project, we use maximum pooling, that is, taking the largest feature point in the neighborhood.

Back-propagation: Looking back at the content of back-propagation, the back-propagation of the max(x, y) function can be simply understood as passing the gradient back only along the largest number. Therefore, when propagating forward through the aggregation layer, the index of the largest element in the pool is usually recorded (sometimes this is also called switches), so that the gradient routing is very efficient during back-propagation.

Fully connected layer: After multiple convolutional layers and pooling layers, one or more fully connected layers are connected. Similar to a conventional neural network, each neuron in a fully connected layer is fully connected to all neurons in the previous layer. The fully connected layer can integrate the local information that is distinguished by categories in the convolutional layer or the pooling layer. We chose to use the ReLU function for the activation function of each neuron in the fully connected layer.

3.1 Convolutional Neural Network Combined with Support Vector Machine

The rational idea of our method is to replace the activation function softmax of the output layer in the neural network with the support vector machine algorithm

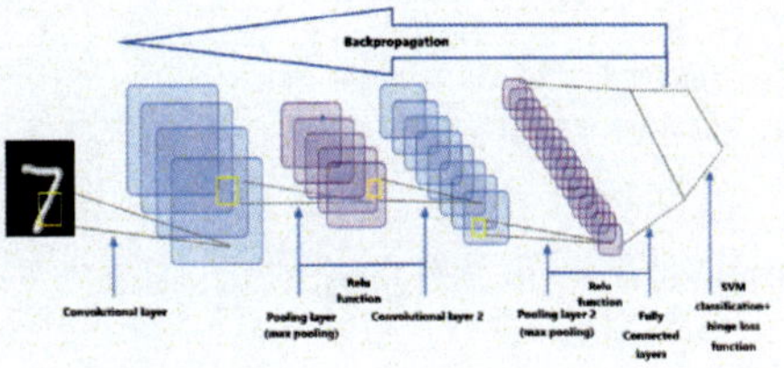

Fig. 2. SVM in CNN principle diagram

for classification. Then our SVM loss is back-propagated to update the parameters through the chain rule. The detailed structure is shown below in Fig. 3. As can be seen, we only keep the first two convolutional layers and the pooling layer along with the fully connected layer of the conventional CNN structure, and then we classify the feature values obtained by the fully connected layer. In this step, we initialize a separating hyperplane matrix according to the number of classes. Then, the weights and parameters of the separation hyperplane matrix are updated at the same time as the neurons are updated in the back propagation. The process of linearly minimizing the loss of the hyperplane matrix is exactly the same as the principle of back propagation. Then we use the hinge loss equation to calculate the loss after SVM classification. In this step, we want to prevent ambiguity caused by multiple weights generated by SVM. We added a preference after the hinge loss equation, as shown in the following formula i.e. adding a regularization penalty to the loss equation will amplify the loss of the classification result with a larger weight, and eventually lead to elimination.

4 Experimental Setup

In this project, we use MNIST, CIFAR-10 and Compass datasets to implement the SVM in CNN model. Also we compare our own model with three other models: traditional SVM model, traditional CNN model and $CNN + SVM$ model. We have two reconstructed models, SVM in CNN and $CNN + SVM$.

For the first model, we replace the softmax layer of CNN with SVM model. After feature vectors are processed by convolutional layers and pooling layers, we set a dropout to avoid over-fitting problem. The outputs of neural network after dropout will be sent to SVM part to derive SVM's weights and biases. At that point, we will get a squared hinge loss calculated by SVM part. The loss will be used for updating convolutional layers' weights and biases, in order to fit the model in a better way. After all the weights and biases updates, we compute the model's final accuracy with all samples.

$CNN + SVM$ is a model with two independent parts. The CNN part will refine its network using the softmax layer. The softmax helps get the neural network's loss to adjust weights and biases of convolutional layers. Then we can get the classification results for SVM's inputs. SVM part takes its own loss to refine the model and gives the final classification for the whole model. For this model, both two parts have their own loss which are calculated independently. It's a combined model rather than reconstructed model as SVM in CNN does.

4.1 Experimental Results on MNIST Dataset

Experiment	CNN	SVM	SVM+CNN	SVM in CNN
1	0.9821	0.8511	0.9862	0.9617
2	0.9814	0.8567	0.9870	0.9643
3	0.9809	0.8645	0.9875	0.9633
4	0.9837	0.8657	0.9870	0.9668
5	0.9807	0.8424	0.9865	0.9648

Fig. 3. Experimental results of different models on the MNIST data set

According to Fig 3, we can find that in five experiments, the process of CNN for feature extraction followed by SVM for classification has the highest accuracy, even higher than the classification results of CNN. Therefore, we can be sure that the classification ability of SVM for the features extracted by the neural network is completely better than the classification ability of Softmax in the traditional CNN. Therefore, we can conclude that support vector machines can get a very impressive performance for classification tasks in neural networks. For some data sets, it even exceeds the performance of the traditional CNN structure.

4.2 Experimental Results on CIFAR-10 Dataset

The performance on loss decreasing also obtained here on CIFAR-10 dataset. We can see that CNN model performs much better than SVM in CNN model, but our model provides a good power in loss decreasing, the model's loss approaching zero is rapid. We get that the accuracy of SVM in CNN is much lower than that of traditional CNN. We expected this may be because SVM requires NxN to use more time to extract feature values for data whose features are not obvious. Hinge The loss calculation for this kind of data has not reached a considerable level.

4.3 Experimental Results on Compass X-ray Dataset

We can find that the accuracy of the two models rises equally fast on Compass X-ray. The accuracy rate is generally higher than that of traditional CNN, but the gap is not very large, which means that SVM in CNN can be used for classification of this type of data set. And in the loss visualization diagram on the right, it can be seen that the loss of CNN is close to 0 at a very fast speed, but the SVM in CNN fluctuates to a certain extent.

[Dataset :Cifar 10; iteration=10000, batch size: 49]			
SVM	SVM IN CNN	CNN	CNN+SVM
0.54	0.35	0.72	0.74

[Dataset :Mnist; iteration:5000, batch size: 64]			
SVM	SVM IN CNN	CNN	CNN+SVM
0.83	0.96	0.98	0.985

[Dataset :Compassxray; iteration=500, batch size: 18]			
SVM	SVM IN CNN	CNN	CNN+SVM
0.90	0.82	0.87	0.875

Fig. 4. **Comprehensive comparison of different data sets**

5 Discussion

We test the performances of four models with three datasets. All datasets are image datasets as our models aim to do image classification tasks. The results show the different performances of traditional machine learning model, general deep learning model and reconstructed models.

Overall, models perform best on MNIST dataset because it's a grey image dataset with a shape size of $28 * 28$. It contains less features than other two datasets, so it will be easier for classification task. We use the grey image dataset of Compass instead of colour dataset. The grey one has less features than colour dataset, and we reshape the sizes of the images, so it will lose some information, which shows to be a lower accuracy than MNIST. We could see that all the models are not good for CIFAR-10 dataset, especially SVM and SVM in CNN model. The CIFAR-10 dataset is a colour image dataset with 3 channels, and it contains noise which causes difficult data processing, so it's much more complex than the other two models, and it's shape size is $32 * 32$, which is larger than MNIST. As CIFAR-10 dataset contains more features, SVM can't deal with its high-dimensional data easily. Besides that, though Compass is a high-dimensional dataset too, it only owns two labels, dangerous or not. Comparing with 10-class CIFAR-10 dataset, Compass will be easier for classification, and we see the results prove it.

Our results show that the SVM model leads to high accuracies with MNIST and Compass dataset. But it does not work well on CIFAR-10 dataset. As we use linear SVM model, it's hard to deal with high-dimensional dataset, and the model is not suitable for large-scaled dataset.

From the form above, we see that $CNN + SVM$ model performs well in all datasets, it seems to get almost the highest accuracies when applying to different situations. $CNN + SVM$ model is a twice classification model. The raw data will be processed to fit in CNN part. CNN model will eliminate the useless information and get the first classification results. And then the results as inputs will be sent to the SVM part, which is aimed for the second classification. As some invalid and unimportant features are pruned by CNN model, the features vectors of SVM will focus on the main effective features, which helps SVM model get a more precise result. Besides that, as our datasets are images, they're high dimensional. SVM will do the second features processing after CNN classification, which will also contribute to finding important information.

For the SVM in CNN model, SVM model is used to replace the softmax layer of CNN model. Using softmax layer as convolutional neural network classifier will lead to a lack of generalization ability of image classification and recognition, which is not suitable for image classification tasks. The model aims to retain the advantage that the convolutional network can automatically extract features, it also adds the SVM part to enhance model robustness and generalization. From the visualizations we could see that SVM in CNN model has fluctuations as accuracy increasing. It does not work well on CIFAR-10 dataset as CNN model's accuracy is double of it. With 10000 iterations, we can still see a rising trend of accuracy line of SVM in CNN model, so it needs much longer training process to view the final result. As we use SVM's hinge loss to do back propagation for CNN framework, the loss line is rapidly approaching zero, it will cause weights and biases update to be too slow. When the network does not perform well during initialization, it will take a long time for the model to be an ideal one. Beside that, the SVM in CNN model performs well when testing on MINST and COMPASS datasets. As the accuracy of CNN model has reached a relatively high level, all three CNN-related models' accuracies are very close. Though it's a little lower with the Compass dataset, there're drastic fluctuations of accuracy lines viewing from the figures. As the models stabilize, the accuracies will be almost the same. SVM in CNN model has a good promotion as figures of loss shown. It brings a big boost on loss decreasing. The model's loss falls down approaching to zero rapidly and it's proven to be effective with three different datasets.

Our model carries out a boost of loss decreasing, and it shows to work well for enhancing generalization ability. When general classification models has already to be precise, we could do little to get accuracy improvement in a high level. The promotion of loss decreasing can help the model train in a few times, and it still ensures a high accuracy. For applications, the model can be applied with fast emergency classification when there's no time for enough training times. For example, when epidemic bursts out, the model can be used for temporary test of suspected cases. However, as we replace softmax layer with SVM model, we should be aware of the negative sample problem of SVM. SVM is trained with all samples, so there will be more and more negative samples as iterations go on. Erroneous judgements take the negative samples with highest scores to the negative training set during iterations, which leads to a over-fitting. So SVM is suitable for small-scale dataset. Due to that, our SVM in CNN model also faces the challenge, the model fits in small-scale datasets and does not work well if a dataset is too large.

As the SVM part of our reconstructed model is linear SVM, it might have a hard time dealing with high-dimentional data. We can improve model accuracy if we do more detailed feature reprocessing or extend convolutional neural network architecture. Also we could use kernel funtions in SVM part. Kernel functions could handle the situations as they do dimentionality reduction for high-dimentional data. They will transform the data into simplified feature vectors for SVM to do classification. In that way, the SVM in CNN model can deal with high-dimensional data easily, which leads to a promotion in accuracy.

6 Conclusion

We popose a one-vs-rest SVM model for replacing the softmax layer in CNN. We evaluate our model on three data sets MNIST, Cifar-10 and Compass X-ray datasets. Based on the analysis of the experimental results, we found that the performance of the new model that replaces Softmax and uses SVM in CNN outperformed the other start-of-the-art methods in image classification tasks.

References

1. Tang, Y.: Deep learning using support vector machines. CoRR, abs/1306.0239, 2 (2013)
2. Kim, S., Yu, Z., Kil, R.M., Lee, M.: Deep learning of support vector machines with class probability output networks. Neural Networks **64**, 19–28 (2015)
3. Elleuch, M., Maalej, R., Kherallah, M.: A new design based-SVM of the CNN classifier architecture with dropout for offline Arabic handwritten recognition. Procedia Comput. Sci. **80**, 1712–1723 (2016). https://doi.org/10.1016/j.procs.2016.05.512
4. Gong, C., Zhang, Z., Wang, G., Wang.: A novel deep learning method for intelligent fault diagnosis of rotating machinery based on improved CNN-SVM and multichannel data fusion. Sensors, **19**(7), 1693 (2019). https://doi.org/10.3390/s19071693
5. Peng, Y., Rios, A., Kavuluru, R., Lu, Z.: Extracting chemical-protein relations with ensembles of SVM and deep learning models. Database, **2018** (2018)
6. Liu, J., Ning, S., Wang, S., Yi, J., Zhao, M.: A method based on CNN + SVM for classifying abnormal audio indoors. In: Li, Y., Zhu, Q., Qiao, F., Fan, Z., Chen, Y. (eds.) ISSPM 2020. AISC, vol. 1305, pp. 385–394. Springer, Singapore (2021). https://doi.org/10.1007/978-981-33-4575-1_37
7. Wu, Q., Gao, T., Lai, Z., Li, D.: Hybrid SVM-CNN classification technique for human-vehicle targets in an automotive LFMCW radar. Sens. (Basel, Switz.) **20**(12), 3504 (2020). https://doi.org/10.3390/s20123504
8. Sun, M., Huang, Z., Guo, C.: Automatic diagnosis of Alzheimer's disease and Mild cognitive impairment based on CNN+SVM networks with end-to-end training. In: 2021 13th International Conference on Advanced Computational Intelligence (ICACI), pp. 279–285 (2021). https://doi.org/10.1109/ICACI52617.2021.9435894
9. Qi, Z., Wang, B., Tian, Y., Zhang, P.: When ensemble learning meets deep learning: a new deep support vector machine for classification. Knowl.-Based Syst. **107**, 54–60 (2016). https://doi.org/10.1016/j.knosys.2016.05.055
10. Niu, X., Suen, C.: A novel hybrid CNN-SVM classifier for recognizing handwritten digits. Pattern Recogn. **45**(4), 1318–1325 (2012). https://doi.org/10.1016/j.patcog.2011.09.021
11. Macedo, D.: Improving Image Classification Accuracy using Hybrid Systems of Support Vector Machines and Convolutional Neural Networks [Blog] (2016). https://github.com/dlmacedo/SVM-CNN/blob/master/svm-cnn-article.pdf
12. Barnes, G., Lauro, K.: Image processing in digital radiography: basic concepts and applications. J. Digit. Imaging **2**(3), 132–146 (1989). https://doi.org/10.1007/bf03168032

Computer and Network Security

Blockchain Potentials in the Maritime Sector: A Survey

Rim Abdallah[1,2](✉), Cyrille Bertelle[1], Claude Duvallet[1], Jérôme Besancenot[2], and Frédéric Gilletta[2]

[1] Normandie Univ., UNILEHAVRE, LITIS, SFlog, 76600 Le Havre, France
rim.abdallah@etu.univ-lehavre.fr,
{cyrille.bertelle,claude.duvallet}@univ-lehavre.fr
[2] HAROPA PORT, 71 Quai Colbert, 76600 Le Havre, France
{rim.abdallah,jerome.besancenot,frederic.gilletta}@haropaport.com
https://www.haropaport.com

Abstract. Digitalization is becoming more omnipresent in the maritime sector, and actors are increasingly using technological solutions to gain competitiveness and efficacy. Generally, entities use distinct heterogeneous systems, making it challenging to integrate them into a commonly advantageous single and secure interconnected system. While maritime actors show interest in Blockchain, given that its features align with the industry's needs, they remain reluctant to allocate the needed resources to explore the technology's revolutionizing potentials. In this paper, we present insights related to Blockchain applications in the maritime sector and the technology's capabilities in revolutionizing and accelerating the global digitization of the shipping industry. We explore Blockchain literature and bring forward the advantages of its innovative applications in the sector.

Keywords: Blockchain · Digitalization · Maritime sector · Shipping industry · Connected ports

1 Introduction

We live in a world where the fast development of communication, information and transport technologies has sped up internationalization and liberalization. Organizations are no longer restricted by regions' borders but instead are operating in a worldwide market where shipping handles 90% of traded goods [42]. This evidently has had a significant impact on companies' strategies in order to enhance their competitiveness and logistics infrastructure, increase their efficiency, and bounce back from the 2008 economic crisis that took its toll on the maritime global trade market [23,24,54]. However, the involvement of multiple entities in a single shipment increased the conundrum's complexity. Each party must deal with a considerable number of physical documents which will eventually decrease the efficiency, slow the process, and increase costs [2,30]. Supply

K. Daimi and A. Al Sadoon (Eds.): ICR 2022, AISC 1431, pp. 293–309, 2022.
https://doi.org/10.1007/978-3-031-14054-9_28

chains processes and logistics management rely on the secure and authentic continuous flow of data which is why entities in the shipping industry are headed towards digitization to facilitate the data exchange between the considerable number of parties involved.

1.1 Toward Maritime Digitization

The growing inter-correlation of economies and populations and consequently increased international trade has accelerated digitization. It also has accentuated the necessity for implementing integrated information and communication systems in ports to sustain high competitiveness and efficiency [51]. Moreover, port success is increasingly measured by efficiently managing interactions between relevant stakeholders, in addition, to previous success variables such as its infrastructure and superstructure [21]. This widespread evolution over the last decades of integrating technological advancement in each port interconnecting several relevant stakeholders transformed data port processing systems into port community systems (PCS) that aimed to reduce communication costs and enhance its users' competitiveness (see Fig. 1 below).

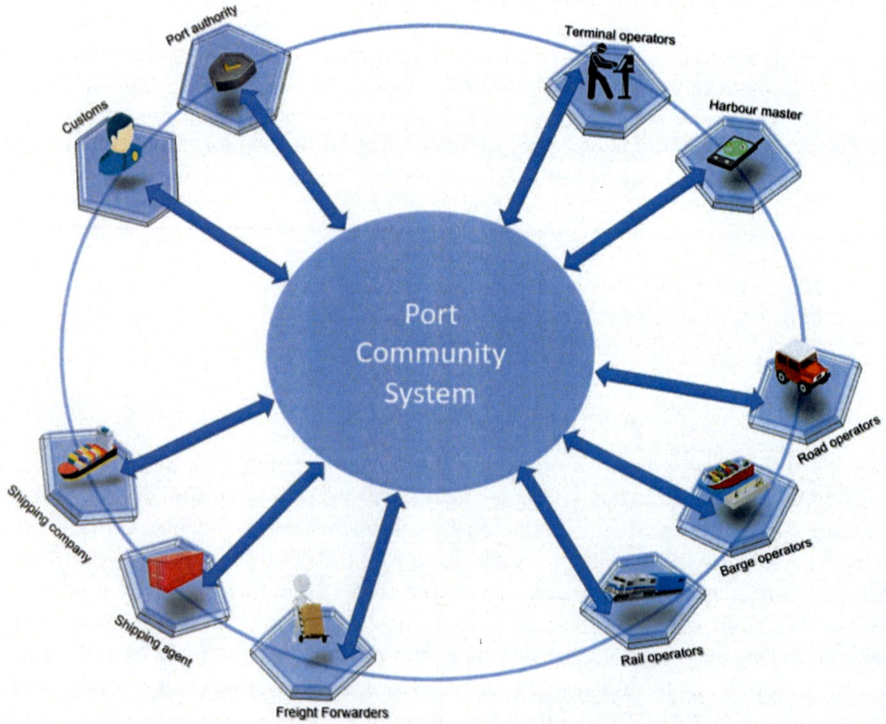

Fig. 1. A port community system network

PCS is defined by the International Port Community System Association as a neutral and open electronic platform that allows secure information exchange amongst port-related stakeholders to generate more competitive advantages for the port [6]. The PCS's functionalities are difficult to list since they vary depending on relevant metrics to the stakeholders in each port community [10]. Generally, PCSs have been known to increase efficiency and streamline the enforcement of regulations and are usually at the center of port governance models [15]. There are different port governance models (public service, tool, landlord, and private port) where the infrastructure, superstructure, labor, and other functionalities are managed by different types of actors (public sector, private sector, delegation ....) [52]. Therefore, actors and their roles might differ from one port community to another, and this accentuates the importance of using a distributive collectively maintained platform that facilitates the shift toward a homogeneous globally connected communication system.

In general, the actors' roles revolve around maintaining the business, informational, capital and logistics flow with the help of technological advancements and solutions such as PCS designed to digitize information exchanges and eliminate avoidable processes that might halt shipments processing. For example, when a ship enters a port, the cargo documentation is managed by its agent who sends it to the PCS. And the PCS will distribute the data across its network to expedite containers processing. Thus, the PCS plays the role of a data Hub between its network's actors. Typical network participants are port authorities, shipping agents, customs agents, shippers, stevedores, and freight forwarders. And the digitized information exchange platforms commonly assure operations including Cargo inspections (request, instructions, and response), Cargo control (release, approval, and movement), Cargo logistics (Transport orders, deliveries, pick-ups, loading, and unloading), Vessel operations (manifest, cargo list, hazardous cargo, and berth requests) and E-commerce operations (Bookings, Invoicing, Payments) amongst other services [52].

However, the steps of processing a shipment through its entire journey are not all connected consistently to all parties, and not all parties relevant to the shipment are included in the PCS network [53]. When a shipment arrives at a port, prior PCS data are not collected since there is generally no communication between different port communities. This lack of coordination and communication can severely affect efficiency and leave room for improvement in addition to fragmenting accountability and governance on the shipment's journey. Moreover, inter-organizational information exchange remains mostly manual and behind-hand. Despite the thorough standardization of the physical documents used across the supply chain (such as Bill of Lading, certificate of origins, and customs declaration), document handling remains in its physical manual form. And shipping companies participate only partially in digitization for confidentiality is a key factor for their success and with no clear information security guarantees, they remain reluctant to fully digitize and divulge data despite important digitization advantages. This redundancy of document processing across the supply chain leads to numerous problems and increases costs. As a result, the absence of readily available information also leads to halting the container for nearly half of its shipping journey [22]. Additionally, transparency in the supply chain is at its minimum. An enormous volume of data circulating in PCSs can expose data to economic intelligence risks for both public and private stakeholders. Thus, a prevalent lack of trust remains across the shipping supply chain where parties remain hesitant to share data and coordinate amongst each other and this could be troublesome. For example, for governmental entities, information ambiguity or inaccuracy can lead to security risks and enforce additional scrutiny that results in additional delays.

Therefore, organizations involved in global trade started to look for more efficient solutions [28]. However, achieving efficient inter-organizational digitization of information exchanges needs to overcome the multitudinous of actors in the supply chain, the complexity of different regulations and relations, and other barriers in order to result in an optimum efficiency that can cut costs significantly for all participants. And this is what drove, in 2013, Maersk, one of the biggest shipping companies to shift its interest from intra-organizational solutions that increase efficiency and cost handling per container to researching promising inter-organizational solutions that enable overall trade shipping and improve container shipping as a part of the enterprise's sustainability agenda [23]. An optimal digitized solution should allow real-time cargo information access to all relevant parties from departure to destination creating an international digitized port with full digitization of document exchanges. Even though it poses diverse challenges, this can now be achieved using a 21st-century surging technology called "Blockchain".

Blockchain emergence can be traced back to 2008, to an academic paper by an unknown entity under the name of Satoshi Nakamoto [34]. It was introduced as the technological infrastructure of the bitcoin cryptocurrency. A Blockchain is a distributed encrypted ledger used to record transactions of various nature. The distributed network uses a consensus mechanism across nodes to validate data recorded on the append-only ledger. Transactions are grouped by blocks and blocks are cryptographically and chronologically linked together to form an extremely hard to alter chain of data. Encrypted data recorded on the ledger can be accessed by all networks participants. The network can be public, accessible to all, or private, with rules and permissions managed by a network authority [43]. The technology has been acknowledged for its versatility and revolutionary innovation that can profoundly impact many fields in our society, particularly the shipping industry. And Blockchain technology has been progressively recognized by the maritime sector for its potential to increase efficiency, digitize data exchanges with real-time traceability, and decrease costs while maintaining prominent levels of visibility, security, and transparency. Nevertheless, the technological adoption of Blockchain in the industry remains at its early stage impeding the harness of its full potential due to many reasons. In an interview that dates back to 2017, the reputable British economist, Dr. Martin Stopford expresses the importance of digitization in the shipping industry emphasizing the role of smart logistics. He also argues that performance improvement is crucial for Blockchain adoption and application [8]. This document dissects the potentials of Blockchain technology and its performance improvement axes in the maritime sector.

2 How Can Blockchain Improve Performance in the Maritime Sector

2.1 Build a Scalable Global Maritime Decentralised Communication System

Viewing the Global Shipping Network (GSN) from a global perspective emphasizes unconventional results in the shipping map structure, which encourages to shift from traditional studies that define ports as nodes of the shipping network towards a more innovative approach where we consider shipping areas as nodes and connections between them as its edges. Studies show that the influence of shipping areas on the GSN has a much higher impact than any single port [29] which explains the technological research shift towards decentralized border-crossing digitized solutions.

What halted the development of a global shipping communication system and prevented unlocking the full potential of shipping areas is that they are fragmented across multiple governmental authorities that are often hesitant to trust one another. Also, traditional centralized fragmented systems are highly susceptible to a single point of failure. Using Blockchain technology can allow the development of a scalable, trusted, and interconnected system. Its infrastructure can be distributed across these nodes, without the need for a trusted centralized authority. Infrastructural maintenance, processing, and auditings such as decision making, transactions approvals, and data validation can be collective. In Blockchain, trust is established through the secure technological infrastructure that relies on chronological chaining, encryption, and consensus protocols. The need for centralized trusted entities and databases is thus eliminated. However, we can control the level of decentralization that aligns with the environment's needs. Using Blockchain does not necessarily mean sharing all of the maritime sensitive data to public networks, even if it can be encrypted. We can alternate between public, private, and consortium Blockchains [12] depending on the system's wanted characteristics and limiting access to shared data. Different Blockchain types have different characteristics (see Table 1). Using a public Blockchain, we can establish a fully decentralized environment. Whereas using a permissioned Blockchain, limits the level of decentralization, since only authorized members are part of the network. It is important to choose wisely the level of decentralization because it has a direct impact on the ledger's immutability. A Blockchain-based system maintains data authenticity through ledger replication across multiple network nodes. Moreover, each block of appended data contains the hash of its previous, creating a hard to alter chain of information [13]. Therefore, the more nodes in the network, the more time and computational power are required to alter the ledger. This is why private and permissioned Blockchains are considered much less immutable than public ones. Hence, we need to find the optimal decentralization to immutability ratio to establish a successful, secure, and efficient global maritime communication environment.

Table 1. Characteristics of different types of blockchain

Characteristic	Public	Private or Consortium
Network access	Permission less	Permissioned
Identity	Anonymous	Identified
Trust Level	Low (nodes could be malicious)	High (nodes are generally trusted)
Decentralisation	Total	Partial
Decision making	Collective	Restricted to a number of nodes
Energy consumption	Higher	Lower
Finality	Non achievable	Is achievable
Transaction validation time	Longer	Shorter

2.2 Increase the Overall Operational Efficiency

Despite the technological advancement and widespread use of PCSs and centralized data-driven tools to increase operational efficiency and manage logistics in the shipping industry, goods flow across the supply chain, remains relatively expensive and slow due to poor global transparency and poor global data management [8]. Paper documentation remains required across the supply chain, and processes often need physical validation of documents which causes time delays, increase costs, and might add additional validating third parties to the already long list of actors involved in the shipment (i.e. importers, exporters, port terminals, shipping agents, freight forwarder, customs, and governmental authorities....). Moreover, none of these parties have continuous real-time access to required information throughout the whole supply chain and the accountability level for inefficiencies and fraudulent activity is at its minimal [3].

Introducing Blockchain to the equation can make all these processes impressively more efficient and smoother. The global replication of the ledger across network nodes beyond border restrictions and PCS networks can significantly increase transparency, and allow better cargo traceability. Data collection can be done through all relevant data points, and all relevant participants can, therefore, access the data shared on the ledger to be viewed or verified. A conceptual blockchain architecture including some maritime actors and exemplary transactions is represented in the Fig. 2 below. All relevant information or documents such as bills of lading, clearance forms are accessible to all relevant parties. Data is recorded into blocks to form a transparent secure source of information. Inherently increasing transparency and traceability reduces transactions fees and other costs such as accounting and auditing fares [17].

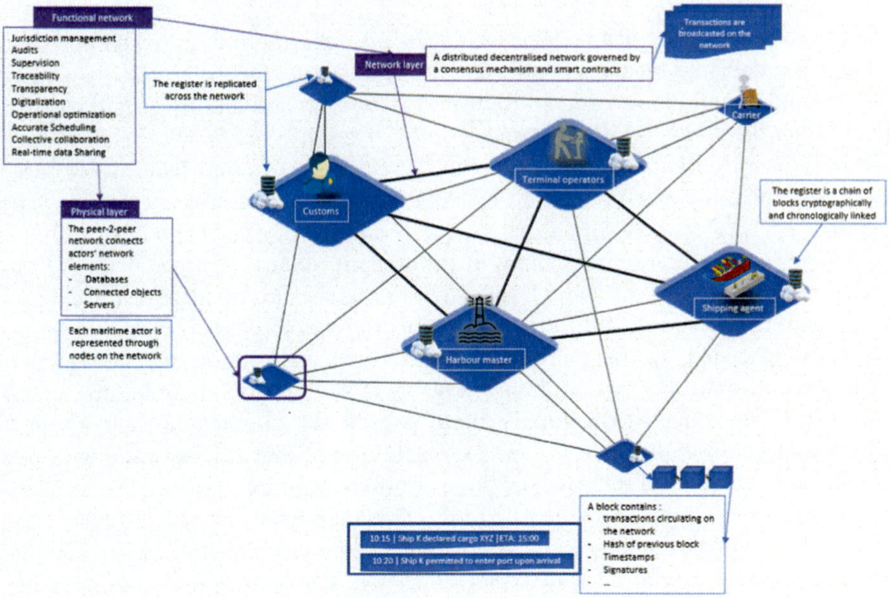

Fig. 2. A conceptual blockchain architecture for the maritime sector

Moreover, regulatory quality and safety requirements in the shipping industry are anticipated to become increasingly severe after the trade union's economic disintegration of primal powers. This will further complicate documentation processes and transactions [11]. Similarly, Blockchain can simplify the administrative documentation of Implementation of International Safety Management (ISM) and International Organisation for Standards (ISO) related to quality and safety management respectively.

Additionally, several trade goods in the shipping industry require particular conditions to ensure safety or efficacity. According to the World health organization, temperature variation causes the degradation of approximately 40% of transported vaccines. The use of Blockchain-enabled containers that manage temperature could be particularly useful and considerably increase efficacity, temperature and location are monitored through sensors along with passive cooling systems to ensure temperature regulation. The real-time temperature monitoring allows immediate intervention in case it drops beyond a threshold limiting goods degradation [11]. These containers are currently used in air transport therefore their use in the shipping industry can be deemed feasible [20]. And the recorded data can ensure the validity of the transported goods along with other required documents. This allows us to reflect on the use of the internet of things (IoT) to ensure full traceability of goods across the shipping supply chain. Currently, IoT's use in the shipping industry is limited to GPS tracking that provides real-time cargo and vessel tracking. However, there are significant security concerns surrounding its use. The IoT devices have relatively delimited computational power with connection to the internet and are not often updated. This poses multiple security risks [25]. Blockchain can thus be coupled with IoT devices and document recorded data from IoT sensors and monitors on its ledger. It also can be coupled with the smart contract feature of the Blockchain which could allow autonomous actions eliminating third parties and facilitating cargo movement across the supply chain which will eventually decrease cost and time delays [11].

Furthermore, the use of hashing in Blockchain reduces storage fares. All relevant parties can connect using Blockchain infrastructure to a decentralized system where they can verify information authenticity whereas the current systems are being impeded by the ever-increasing hard to verify data storage size that halts the information flow and are susceptible to singular points of failure. In the majority of steps across the supply chain data is not shared real-time amongst all relevant entities and data inflow can reach up to 35 zeta bytes per day [8,33]. Blockchain can offer all relevant parties a secure connection to a single decentralized system to overcome this. It provides real-time access to verified information recorded in the Blockchain which aligns with the collective acknowledgment of the need for a secure borderless connected system where data is shared instantly across all relevant parties.

This technological advantage is of high interest in the maritime sector where all kinds of goods are exchanged and there is a need for prominent levels of traceability and transparency, especially for food, medicine, and hazardous goods.

2.3 Adjoin Supplementary Security Privileges

The increased shift towards digitization, automation, data-driven tools, PCS, and technologically connected vessels and cargos introduces new security challenges to the industry and new vulnerabilities. Therefore, not only ports are susceptible to security challenges, but nowadays ships implement onboard connected systems allowing more efficient operations and communication such as Electronic Chart Display and Information System (ECDIS), digitized connected compasses and steering, radars and automating radar plotting aid, and automatic identification system (AIS). Researchers have shown that ships onboard connected systems can be hacked, data records can be erased, and continuous communication can be halted with signal jammers [14]. Therefore, despite the advantages of incremented digitization in the maritime sector, security attacks, and accidental errors can have immense impacts on several levels varying from environmental to financial damages. For example, a ransomware attack on one of the largest shipping companies "Maersk" resulted in an estimated loss of 250 million dollars [33]. Hence, with increased digitization rise the need for more cyber scrutiny to minimize risks. Blockchain can alleviate this cyber burden that lies in centralized systems with a single point of failure and prevents data alteration through its replicated encrypted cryptographically chronologically chained ledger. Decentralized distributed systems are generally considered more secured than centralized ones [11]. Blockchain combined with connected devices can provide a more scalable infrastructure where data provided can be traced to an identified device on the system and fraudulent devices can be more efficiently detected due to the ledger's immutability with great automatization potential without the need for centralized servers. Devices can directly interact with one another [39].

2.4 Prevent and Potentially Decrease Pollution

Despite being one of the least energy-wasteful means to transport large cargos, shipping emits considerable amounts of various gazes such as NOx, SOx, carbon dioxide, and particulate matter into the atmosphere. And even though shipping emissions were not included in the 2015 Paris global climate change agreement [44], the international maritime organization (IMO) is increasingly introducing more stern rules to limit the polluting effect of the shipping industry on our environment and restrict harmful emissions into our environment. Since 1980, and particularly after many disastrous incidents, the pernicious effect of noxious liquids released into the ocean were acknowledged and restricted [18]. Similarly, air emissions restrictions were announced in 1997 and enforced in 2005. From 2013, the IMO focused more and more on pollution in the maritime sector. As of 2020, the IMO restricted each ship's fuel to 0.5% of sulfuric content compared to a previous 3.5%. This will oblige ships to change to low-sulfur fuel or use scrubbers. Moreover, in 2018, ships without scrubbers have been banned from high-sulfuric fuel carriage, and starting in 2016 shippers were required to present as a condition for ships loading, for every container, a Verified Gross Mass (VGM) alongside the standards certifications. These regulations are estimated to prevent around half a million preterm death in the next five years [38,45]. Howbeit, the enforcement of these regulations is significantly challenging to authorities along with tracing substances, monitoring, and prevention of violation on a global scale. And the approximate voluntary violation recorded in 2018 was between 10% and 30% of fuel consumption in the shipping industry [19].

There is no significant technological literature coverage for this issue in the maritime sector. One study has been conducted to explore the possibility of using Blockchain technology to reduce and prevent pollution in the maritime sector including the willingness of actors in the shipping industry to use innovative technologies for environmental benefits. The study shows a direct correlation between increased costs and innovation barriers. For a modern technology adoption and increased innovative costs there should be a reverse effect on overall costs [8]. Despite the lack of coverage on pollution prevention using Blockchain in the maritime sector, considerable studies have been conducted in other sectors that highlighted Blockchain's potential in reducing and preventing pollution. Particularly the combination of IoT and smart sensors with Blockchain and smart contracts to audit air pollution in China. This new generation technology allowed real time monitoring and data collection of air quality facilitating the continuous auditing process for government officials [9]. Blockchain can be used not only in air pollution prevention and air quality monitoring but also with other harmful substances. This was demonstrated through the open litter map launched in 2017, that helps keep tracks of pre-defined polluting substances such as glass, plastic, cans, and others. This is done via a Blockchain infrastructure that relies on the use of its application on a global scale. Users that collect data, maps, process and produce open geospatial data are rewarded with the Littercoin cryptocurrency. Despite its promising idea that empowers any global user with a smart phone to help save our environment and be rewarded with a cryptocurrency, in order for this innovation to survive it will need significant support from the global community [32]. Similarly, another study proves the feasibility and the brilliant potential of the IoT-Blockchain combination to trace in real-time water pollution sources [50]. One more study also researched the possibility to monitor air quality using Blockchain, where they proposed a prototype for a public global immutable system based on the public Blockchain Ethereum coupled with the distributed file system called interplanetary File system (IPFS) and uPort (for identity management and permissions). The idea behind IPFS was to cut costs to a minimum. At the time of the study, time storing 1 Gb of data on the Ethereum Blockchain would cost a million dollars. Their solution reduced the cost by storing the same amount of data suing only 21.33 kb on the Blockchain that results in a highly affordable price of 21.88 us dollars. The prototype proved highly effective with room for improvement specially with pre-validation of data and user verification [50].

Based on these studies we can deduct that Blockchain has immense potential in preventing and reducing pollution in the shipping industry from gas emission control to water and air pollution prevention and monitoring, especially when combined with IoT technology. Moreover, storage size issues, cost issues, and scalability problems can be reduced by alternating between public and private Blockchain and using distributed storage protocols [55].

2.5 Fight Fraud and Prevent Corruption

The previous discussion of secured distributed systems with real-time transparency and traceability allowed us to also reflect on the possibility of using Blockchain and smart contracts to prevent corruption and detect fraud. There have been many studies in the literature that demonstrated the efficiency of such systems in various sectors, allowing real-time traceability with a reduced cost while preserving privacy and security [4,27,41,46].

The ongoing fight against corruption made use over time of technological advancement to tip the scale and defeat fraudulent activities. There are numerous studies that prove that technical and IT advancement restraint corruption [1,31,47]. Using Blockchain not only prevents fraud but simplifies transactions authentication and validation. The transparency of the encrypted replicated ledger makes it tamper-proof and facilitates the identification of malicious activities. Moreover, the use of smart contracts allows processes automation limiting the margin for any accidental or deliberate errors. And this was clearly expressed in a study that emerged in 2019 [40]. There are several types of literature coverage related to the use of Blockchain in the fight against corruption from abstract oriented and technical studies [35,37,49] to more case-specific studies covering IoT [7], the maritime sector [23,36] and others [26,48,56].

Fraud and corruption have always been major concerns in the maritime sector. Its global coverage, complex structure, and multitudinous actors increase fraud and corruption scopes. It can include various malicious acts such as document falsification, illicit payments, bribes, invoice falsification (under or over). These acts are estimated to raise shipping costs by at least 10% [11]. Actors in the sector have recognized technological advancements as a powerful weapon against corruption. It started in the 1980s with the widespread adoption of digitized management and financial intra-organization systems. Later on, it evolved to partial inter-organizational digitization with the "e-government" notion. Where certain exchanges are digitized to allow a more fluid shipping process and narrow malicious horizons. However, digitization projects remain fragmented and still have not managed to be adopted on a global scale till now. This fragmentation can be blamed on various reasons, notably the use of centralized systems. Actors remain hesitant to share data as a part of risk management prevention in case of data leaks or cyber-attacks. This data fragmentation can be beneficial for malicious acts where transparency is at its minimum.

Blockchain, in theory, can help consolidate the digitization process. Its encrypted decentralized infrastructure coupled with the current existing technologies could revolutionize the shipping industry. It overcomes the uncertainty and lack of visibility across supply chains. The decentralized and distributed nature of Blockchain allows to information sharing across relevant actors. Its cryptographic linkage and encryption allow diminishing ambiguity and easier validation and authentication. The added transparency and immutable ledger make it easier to corroborate transactions and identity, spot double claims, and identify fraudulent patterns. Moreover, using permissioned or private Blockchain, we add permissions and restrictions, enforcing system regulations while maintaining a certain level of decentralization for supplementary transparency and fluidity. Blockchain can unleash a collaborative action amongst actors of the maritime sector to reduce fraud.

Nevertheless, Blockchain cannot be seen as the magical solution for all existing problems. And due to the diverse types of fraud in the maritime sector, we cannot expect a technological advancement, despite its great fraud-prevention and fraud-detection potential, to solve all corruption practices across the industry but it can minimize it.

2.6 Eliminate Unnecessary Intermediaries

In general, in order to complete any transaction in centralised systems third parties are often required for verification. Intermediaries charge extra fees which significantly increase the cost of transactions. This particularly applies to the maritime sector. The need for physical documentation, brokers and couriers increase substantially costs. Blockchain not only allow document digitization but also remove the need for any third party without significantly increasing cost. Moreover, the global nature of maritime shipping can benefit from the borderless technology. It can provide borderless electronic payments as opposed to traditional fiat currencies, banks, or other intermediaries. The shipping industry has already recognised this potential and started acting upon it. After the SOLAS treaty on 1st July 2016 that introduced new VGM (Verified Gross Mass) requirements to packed containers. MTI (Marine Transport International) announced using a public Blockchain called TrustMe to record VGM data. Hence, making records easily available and verifiable to all relevant parties from port authorities to cargo owner and shippers. This innovative approach was quickly deemed highly efficient as compared to old systems where data were ingrained causing delays and halting development of new capabilities and services. Unnecessary data third parties were eliminated. The Blockchain structure being a public secure hard to alter ledger made data available to relevant parties through any device without the need of an expensive infrastructure [16].

2.7 Minimize Costs and Delays

The aforementioned Blockchain potentials consequently result in increasing the global shipping process efficiency, eliminating unnecessary delays, reducing the overall shipping journey duration, and inherently costs. Introducing Blockchain to the maritime sector will potentially fast forward digitization efforts overcoming physical documents redundancy, relatively slow processing, and allowing additional automation using smart contracts. IBM reckons that full digitization of documents through the supply chain in the shipping industry can economize thirty-eight billion dollars per year to ship carriers [17]. Moreover, the elimination of third parties through direct interaction between essential shipping actors, the use of smart contracts to automate business logic, and the added transparency and traceability feature through an immutable secure ledger will obviously reduce time delays. For example, automatic payments will be automatically made from the importer to banks upon cargo arrival, without the need for an insurer. The access from the port parties to a ledger where transactions are recorded and validated in addition to real-time monitoring of the cargo status accessible for the importer, with no need to re-contact banks or double verify will ensure a faster cargo release. This saves time for all relevant parties and also saves costs allowing optimal efficiency.

3 Conclusion

We have detailed the potential use of the Blockchain in the maritime sector with the related literature and gaps. The lack of full academic literature about the innovative technology potentials in the maritime sector was the key motive behind this research. The main research question driving this study is to shift the concept of Blockchain application in the maritime industry from theory to demonstration. This study came from the perception that the maritime industry recognizes partial potentials of Blockchain but remains hesitant to allocate enough resources to allow mass adoption of the revolutionizing technology. And identifying and listing all potentials allow establishing axes of possible amelioration for existing technologies to start working towards conceptualizing a Blockchain solution and demonstrate these potentials, and their benefits allowing more efficiency, competitiveness, cost, and delay reduction. This paper answers why should companies re-consider the effort to adopt Blockchain technology. Innovative technology should be able to cut costs respecting lucrative motifs of the industry while maximizing efficiency through digitization and process fluidity. Moreover, requirements and legislation should be met and respected with the ability to establish accountability.

The application of Blockchain technology to existing technologies and architectures allows maritime actors to keep a cryptographically protected immutable ledger that can be shared trustfully within a network of selected actors. The scalability that a peer-to-peer network offers can immensely affect port efficiency. Prior study such as [5] has successfully identified a proportional relation between the number of network partners and port efficiency. With Blockchain features the idea of creating larger networks incorporating not only port agents but all supply chain actors in a trusted environment where they can trustfully share data is now feasible. More scalable solutions within a larger spectrum of potential actors without third parties can now be achieved through a Blockchain-based solution overcoming the complexity of the shipping industry. With more scalability comes additional advantages that also reduce costs. A larger secure network will increasingly alleviate barriers between actors and decrease processing redundancy, thus cutting more costs and delays. Moreover, the motivation behind Blockchain adoption surpasses financial gains and operational efficiency to environmental preservation. In addition to enhancing cyber security in the maritime sector, preventing fraud and corruption.

The shipping industry is mostly driven by costs and gains to adopt technological advancements. And Blockchain's adoption rate in the maritime sector is still relatively slow. This can be related to the lack of knowledge of the opportunities spectrum that this technology can present in the maritime sector. Blockchain-based solutions have a broad range of applications within this industry. This study contributes to enriching the maritime culture about this innovative technology and identifies all its potentials in the industry detailing possible axes of application. Enriching the culture can accelerate Blockchain adoption in the sector that will unleash the full potential of the distributed replication power of this revolutionary technology for optimal efficiency. But, as it is important to innovate, pre-existing technologies should not be undermined. A successful and effective operational evolution should leverage the strength of existing solutions and improve them by integrating innovative technologies such as Blockchain.

We hope that this study contributes as a foundation stone for future research and projects on Blockchain in the maritime sector. And despite deeply exploring the utilization of the innovative technology, it is important to also understand the technology's limitations in general and sector-specific technological obstacles to evade them, explore solutions and eschew inadequacies for a smoother technological adoption when interpreting our findings. Moreover, it is crucial not to undermine existing functional technologies, which promote the integration of those solutions.This directs future research toward testing the successful integration of prior systems and the formulation of widespread technological and operational standards.

References

1. Arayankalam, J., Khan, A., Krishnan, S.: How to deal with corruption? examining the roles of e-government maturity, government administrative effectiveness, and virtual social networks diffusion. Int. J. Inf. Manag. **58**, 102203 (2021). https://doi.org/10.1016/j.ijinfomgt.2020.102203
2. Bonuedi, I., Kamasa, K., Opoku, E.E.O.: Enabling trade across borders and food security in Africa. Food Secur. **12**(5), 1121–1140 (2020). https://doi.org/10.1007/s12571-020-01095-y
3. Botton, N.: Blockchain and trade: not a fix for brexit, but could revolutionise global value chains (if governments let it). ECIPE Policy Brief 1/2018, European Centre for International Political Economy, Brussels (2018). http://hdl.handle.net/10419/174812
4. Cai, Y., Zhu, D.: Fraud detections for online businesses: a perspective from blockchain technology. Financ. Innovation **2**(1), 1–10 (2016). https://doi.org/10.1186/s40854-016-0039-4
5. Caldeirinha, V., Felício, J.A., Salvador, A.S., Nabais, J., Pinho, T.: The impact of port community systems (pcs) characteristics on performance. Res. Transp. Econ. **80**, 100818 (2020)
6. Carlan, V., Sys, C., Vanelslander, T.: How port community systems can contribute to port competitiveness: developing a cost–benefit framework. Res. Transp. Bus. Manag. **19**, 51–64 (2016). https://doi.org/10.1016/j.rtbm.2016.03.009
7. Chanson, M., Bogner, A., Bilgeri, D., Fleisch, E., Wortmann, F.: Blockchain for the iot: privacy-preserving protection of sensor data. J. Assoc. Inf. Syst. **20**(9), 1274–1309 (2019)
8. Czachorowski, K., Solesvik, M., Kondratenko, Y.: The application of blockchain technology in the maritime industry. In: Kharchenko, V., Kondratenko, Y., Kacprzyk, J. (eds.) Green IT Engineering: Social, Business and Industrial Applications. SSDC, vol. 171, pp. 561–577. Springer, Cham (2019). https://doi.org/10.1007/978-3-030-00253-4_24
9. Dai, J., He, N., Yu, H.: Utilizing blockchain and smart contracts to enable audit 4.0: from the perspective of accountability audit of air pollution control in china. J. Emerg. Technol. Account. **16**(2), 23–41 (2019). https://doi.org/10.2308/jeta-52482
10. Desiderio, D.: Port community systems, customs one-stop-shops and their possible combination with a single window. J. Customs Trade **3**, 3–14 (2011)
11. Di Gregorio, R., Nustad, S.S., Constantiou, I.: Blockchain adoption in the shipping industry. A study of adoption likelihood and scenario-based opportunities and risks for IT service providers, Copenhagen business school, Number of STUs 272 (2017)
12. Dib, O., Brousmiche, K.L., Durand, A., Thea, E., Hamida, E.B.: Consortium blockchains: overview, applications and challenges. Int. J. Adv. Telecommun. **11**(1&2), 51–64 (2018)
13. Dib, O., Toumi, K.: Decentralized identity systems: architecture, challenges, solutions and future directions. Annals of Emerging Technologies in Computing (2020)
14. DiRenzo, J., Goward, D.A., Roberts, F.S.: The little-known challenge of maritime cyber security. In: 2015 6th International Conference on Information, Intelligence, Systems and Applications (IISA), pp. 1–5. IEEE (2015)
15. Fedi, L., Lavissiere, A., Russell, D., Swanson, D.: The facilitating role of IT systems for legal compliance: the case of port community systems and container verified gross mass (VGM). Supply Chain Forum Int. J. **20**(1), 29–42 (2019). https://doi.org/10.1080/16258312.2019.1574431

16. Finextra: marine transport international applies blockchain to shipping supply chain (2016)
17. Ganne, E.: Can blockchain revolutionize international trade? World Trade Organization Geneva (2018)
18. Gold, E.: Learning from disaster: lessons in regulatory enforcement in the maritime sector. Rev. Eur. Comp. Int'l Envtl. L. **8**, 16 (1999)
19. Grimmer, R.: Imo 2020 part 5: enforcement (2018). https://stillwaterassociates.com/imo-2020-part-5-enforcement/
20. Hampstead, J.: Swiss firm brings blockchain to the biopharmaceutical cold chain. Freightwaves (2018)
21. Henesey, L., Notteboom, T., Davidsson, P.: Agent-based simulation of stakeholders relations: an approach to sustainable port and terminal management. In: Multi-Agent Systems for Container Terminal Management, vol. 99 (2003)
22. Jensen, T., Bjørn-Andersen, N., Vatrapu, R.: Avocados crossing borders. In: Proceedings of the 5th ACM International Conference on Collaboration across Boundaries: Culture, Distance Technology, pp. 15–24. ACM Press (2014). https://doi.org/10.1145/2631488.2631500
23. Jensen, T., Hedman, J., Henningsson, S.: How tradelens delivers business value with blockchain technology. MIS Q. Executive **18**(4), 221–243 (2019)
24. Kalgora, B., Christian, T.M.: The financial and economic crisis, its impacts on the shipping industry, lessons to learn: the container-ships market analysis. Open J. Soc. Sci. **4**(1), 38–44 (2016). https://doi.org/10.4236/jss.2016.41005
25. Khan, M.A., Salah, K.: IoT security: review, blockchain solutions, and open challenges. Futur. Gener. Comput. Syst. **82**, 395–411 (2018). https://doi.org/10.1016/j.future.2017.11.022
26. Köhler, S., Pizzol, M.: Technology assessment of blockchain-based technologies in the food supply chain. J. Cleaner Prod. **269**, 122193 (2020). https://doi.org/10.1016/j.jclepro.2020.122193
27. Kshetri, N., Voas, J.: Blockchain in developing countries. IT Prof. **20**, 11–14 (2018). https://doi.org/10.1109/MITP.2018.021921645
28. Lehmacher, W.: Why blockchain should be global trade's next port of call. In: World Economic Forum, vol. 23 (2017)
29. Li, Z., Xu, M., Shi, Y.: Centrality in global shipping network basing on worldwide shipping areas. GeoJournal **80**(1), 47–60 (2014). https://doi.org/10.1007/s10708-014-9524-3
30. Lieber, A.: Trust in trade: announcing a new blockchain partner (2017). www.ibm.com/blogs/blockchain/2017/03/trust-trade-announcing-new-blockchain-partner/
31. Lio, M.C., Liu, M.C., Ou, Y.P.: Can the internet reduce corruption? a cross-country study based on dynamic panel data models. Gov. Inf. Q. **28**(1), 47–53 (2011). https://doi.org/10.1016/j.giq.2010.01.005
32. Lynch, S.: OpenLitterMap.com – open data on plastic pollution with blockchain rewards (Littercoin). Open Geospatial Data Softw. Stand. **3**(1), 1–10 (2018). https://doi.org/10.1186/s40965-018-0050-y
33. Mathews, L.: Notpetya ransomware attack cost shipping giant maersk over 200 million (2017). www.forbes.com/sites/leemathews/2017/08/16/notpetya-ransomware-attack-cost-shipping-giant-maersk-over-200-million/
34. Nakamoto, S.: Bitcoin: a peer-to-peer electronic cash system. In: Decentralized Business Review, p. 21260 (2008)
35. Narayanan, A., Bonneau, J., Felten, E., Miller, A., Goldfeder, S.: Bitcoin and Cryptocurrency Technologies: A Comprehensive Introduction. Princeton University Press (2016)

36. Pu, S., Lam, J.S.L.: Blockchain adoptions in the maritime industry: a conceptual framework. Marit. Policy Manag. **48**(6), 777–794 (2020). https://doi.org/10.1080/03088839.2020.1825855
37. Rauchs, M., Hileman, G.: Global Cryptocurrency Benchmarking Study. Cambridge Centre for Alternative Finance Reports, Cambridge Centre for Alternative Finance, Cambridge Judge Business School, University of Cambridge (2017). https://econpapers.repec.org/bookchap/jbsaltfin/201704-gcbs.htm
38. Reuters: factbox: imo 2020 - a major shake-up for oil and shipping (2019). www.reuters.com/article/us-shipping-imo-enforcement-rules-factbo-idCAKBN1YN1UZ
39. Reyna, A., Martín, C., Chen, J., Soler, E., Díaz, M.: On blockchain and its integration with IoT. Challenges and opportunities. Future Gener. Comput. Syst. **88**, 173–190 (2018). https://doi.org/10.1016/j.future.2018.05.046
40. Santiso, C.: Will blockchain disrupt government corruption? Stanford Social Innovation Review (2018). https://doi.org/10.48558/B59A-8P46
41. Sarda, P., Chowdhury, M.J.M., Colman, A., Kabir, M.A., Han, J.: Blockchain for fraud prevention: a work-history fraud prevention system. In: 2018 17th IEEE International Conference On Trust, Security And Privacy In Computing And Communications/ 12th IEEE International Conference On Big Data Science And Engineering (TrustCom/BigDataSE), pp. 1858–1863 (2018). https://doi.org/10.1109/TrustCom/BigDataSE.2018.00281
42. Schiffling, S., Valantasis Kanellos, N.: Ship happens: ever given and forgotten. World Infrastructure Journal (2021). https://doi.org/10.21427/31Z0-JN78
43. Singhal, B., Dhameja, G., Panda, P.S.: How blockchain works. In: Beginning Blockchain, pp. 31–148. Apress (2018). https://doi.org/10.1007/978-1-4842-3444-0_2
44. Sites, U.: Platforms: the paris agreement (2016). https://unfccc.int/process-and-meetings/the-paris-agreement/the-paris-agreement
45. Sofiev, M., et al.: Cleaner fuels for ships provide public health benefits with climate tradeoffs. Nat. Commun. **9**(1), 1–12 (2018). https://doi.org/10.1038/s41467-017-02774-9
46. de Souza, R.C., Luciano, E.M., Wiedenhöft, G.C.: The uses of the blockchain smart contracts to reduce the levels of corruption. In: Proceedings of the 19th Annual International Conference on Digital Government Research: Governance in the Data Age. ACM (2018). https://doi.org/10.1145/3209281.3209408
47. Srivastava, S., Teo, T., Devaraj, S.: You can't bribe a computer: dealing with the societal challenge of corruption through ict. MIS Q. **40**, 511–526 (2016). https://doi.org/10.25300/MISQ/2016/40.2.14
48. Sullivan, C., Burger, E.: E-residency and blockchain. Comput. Law Secur. Rev. **33**(4), 470–481 (2017)
49. Sun Yin, H.H., Langenheldt, K., Harlev, M., Mukkamala, R.R., Vatrapu, R.: Regulating cryptocurrencies: a supervised machine learning approach to de-anonymizing the bitcoin blockchain. J. Manag. Inf. Syst. **36**(1), 37–73 (2019). https://doi.org/10.1080/07421222.2018.1550550
50. de Tazoult, C.T., Chiky, R., Foltescu, V.: A distributed pollution monitoring system: the application of blockchain to air quality monitoring. In: Nguyen, N.T., Chbeir, R., Exposito, E., Aniorté, P., Trawiński, B. (eds.) ICCCI 2019. LNCS (LNAI), vol. 11684, pp. 688–697. Springer, Cham (2019). https://doi.org/10.1007/978-3-030-28374-2_59
51. Tijan, E., Agatić, A., Hlača, B.: The necessity of port community system implementation in the croatian seaports. PROMET-Traffic Transp. **24**(4), 305–315 (2012)

52. Tijan, E., Jović, M., Panjako, A., Žgaljić, D.: The role of port authority in port governance and port community system implementation. Sustainability **13**(5), 2795 (2021). https://doi.org/10.3390/su13052795
53. Weernink, M.O., van den Engh, W., Thorborg, M.F.F.: The blockchain potential for port logistics. Whitepaper, Smart Port, the Port of Rotterdam Authority, TU Delft (2017)
54. Yang, C.S.: Maritime shipping digitalization: blockchain-based technology applications, future improvements, and intention to use. Transp. Res. Part E Logistics Transp. Rev. **131**, 108–117 (2019)
55. Zheng, Q., Li, Y., Chen, P., Dong, X.: An innovative ipfs-based storage model for blockchain. In: 2018 IEEE/WIC/ACM International Conference on Web Intelligence (WI), pp. 704–708 (2018). https://doi.org/10.1109/WI.2018.000-8
56. Ziolkowski, R., Miscione, G., Schwabe, G.: Decision problems in blockchain governance: old wine in new bottles or walking in someone else's shoes? J. Manag. Inf. Syst. **37**(2), 316–348 (2020). https://doi.org/10.1080/07421222.2020.1759974

Decentralized Blockchain Based IoT System to Enhance Security in Smart Homes

Shijon Das[1](✉), Mushaidul Islam[1], Mohammad Sayeem Sadat Hossain[1], Abdussalam Mohamad Ali[2], and Mohammad Zavid Parvez[2,3,4]

[1] Department of Computer Science and Engineering, Brac University, Dhaka, Bangladesh
{shijon.das,mushaidul.islam, mohammad.sayeem.sadat.hossain}@g.bracu.ac.bd
[2] Kent Institute Australia, Sydney, Australia
abdussalam.ali@kent.edu.au
[3] Engineering Institute of Technology, West Perth, Australia
[4] School of Behavioural and Health Sciences, Australian Catholic University, Banyo, Australia

Abstract. Smart houses are more about being environmentally conscious and offering security. Smart home technologies can make homes more energy-efficient and allow users to save money. This concept of making the life of the common people easier has increased the demand for smart homes. However, the rising demand also calls for security concerns. Many approaches have been taken to enhance IoT installation security, but most of the issues concerned with its protection are still left to deal with.

On the other hand, the rise of the popularity of Blockchain, because of the security of data it ensures, has made it a potential component to pair up with IoT. Along with the many benefits of Blockchain integration, it also ensures the decentralization of data. This paper aims to discuss the need for Blockchain-based IoT and its limitations. Further, along with the paper, we consider the past implementations. To support our work, we proposed a model that enhances security in smart homes using blockchain by verifying the incoming requests and giving access to only authorized users.

Keywords: Smart home · IoT · Blockchain · Consensus protocol · Security

1 Introduction

The Internet of Things (IoT) is a generic term for an increasing number of electronic devices that connect to the Internet to send data, receive instructions, or both, rather than traditional computing devices [1]. Internet of Things (IoT) successfully achieves trust and popularity amongst the masses due to a significant rise in network speed and smart devices [15]. The IoT plays an essential role in the implementation of smart home systems. A smart home, also known as a connected home or eHome, is a highly developed automated system [2]. The overall idea of a smart home is to make everyday life more accessible, and the IoT will help you realize that vision by connecting every device in

K. Daimi and A. Al Sadoon (Eds.): ICR 2022, AISC 1431, pp. 310–320, 2022.
https://doi.org/10.1007/978-3-031-14054-9_29

your home to the Internet. However, as the existence of IoT objects and visibility from the Internet increases, security, i.e., access to authorized user resources, is a significant issue [3]. Here, the use of blockchain comes to play. A blockchain is essentially a digital ledger that is duplicated and distributed over the blockchain's network of computer systems. Each square in the chain contains countless exchanges. Each time another exchange happens in the blockchain, a record of that exchange is added to every member's catalog [5]. When implemented decentralized, storing information in the blockchain makes the data an invariant timeline.

1.1 Problem Statement

The IoT-Internet of Things has taken a toll on our lives quite steadily and invisibly as smart devices and high-speed networks saw rapid growth. In 2017 worldwide, almost 10 billion connected things joined this network and are expected to reach nearly 20 billion by 2020 [7]. Henceforth, it is necessary to consider the massive number of IoT devices connected and ensure their orderly sharing of information and expected functionalities. Moreover, centralization is an alarming issue, leading to isolated vulnerability and security violations [13]. Unfortunately, during primitive times, this security was not considered a mandatory objective while designing those devices. As a result, data breach was a common problem in these appliances.

Furthermore, IoT-enabled devices provide only the required basic functionalities that the users ask for. They are designed so that selling is prioritized more than their security. These devices are there only to meet basic needs such as temperature regulation, light regulation, etc. As a result, safe and secure entrance control is regarded as one of the most critical technologies for ensuring IoT privacy and security [7]. Due to the IoT, the network environment of smart homes is considered an essential factor. Communications now are shifting from wired to wireless as the network structure of smart homes, consisting mainly of embedded computers, is connected to various IoT devices on the internet [8].

The gateway is responsible for controlling and monitoring the communication of multiple devices, which the smart home collectively consists of. This network configuration is harmful as it can leak data of the house, breach privacy, malfunction devices, and harm users. When a user logs in to a smart home network that explores our model's demonstration and testing in a household, there is always a probability of data collected by devices being leaked [8]. Difficulties arise when we bring in different heterogeneous devices, but smart home and appliance security standards are missing, preventing the smooth handing over of various smart devices to users.

1.2 Research Objective

A blockchain allows the data in a database to be distributed across several network nodes in different places. This adds redundancy to the database and ensures that the data is accurate. If one node of the database is updated, the other nodes are not affected, preventing a bad actor from doing so. If one user tampers with Bitcoin's transaction record, all other nodes will cross-reference, making it easy to find the node with erroneous data. This system aids in the establishment of a precise and visible sequence of occurrences. In this manner, no one node in the network may change the data it contains.

Most of the current implementation involves a centralized IoT system, where a network of IoT is built around a central server to manage all the nodes in the system. This server handles requests from nodes and assigns roles to the nodes. However, this approach brings with it the risk of single-point failure. On the other hand, implementing a Blockchain system for the network of IoT will create a decentralized system that prevents such risks from arising. Thus, in this paper, we proposed a model that enhances security in smart homes using blockchain by verifying the incoming requests and giving access to only authorized users.

1.3 Research Outline

Exploring a Blockchain-based IoT model which provides a decentralized network and handles authentication is the primary focus of our research. Section 2, "Literature Review" explains the IoT system, defines Blockchain, and provides applicable related definitions of terms that have been used throughout the paper. Furthermore, research papers on issues similar to the topic of this paper are discussed. Section 3, "Architecture of the Proposed Model," introduces the proposed model and provides relevant diagrams to understand the model. Section 4, "Experimental Progress," the details of the technical arrangements used in this research are explored in addition to the model's demonstration and testing. Section 5, "Analysis and Results", analyzes model's performance, storage handling, and cost-benefit. Finally, the paper is concluded in Sect. 6.

2 Literature Review

In [9], the three primary layers of IoT have been described: The application layer, the Network layer, and the Physical layer. This paper sheds light on the security risks and internet attacks that could take place in an IoT ecosystem. Due to the presence of the low power devices, the protocols of the TCP/IP Stack cannot be applied to an IoT system despite having homogenous architecture. Physical layer attacks include but are not limited to Physical damage, Node jamming, Malicious node injection, Node Tampering, RF interface, Sleep deprivation, Social Engineering, etc. Likewise, in the network layer, we have DOS, Sinkhole attack, RFID spoofing, Sybil, Man in the middle attack, RFID cloning, DDOS, Sybil attacks, etc. The application layer consists of spyware, Malware, Adware, DOS, viruses and worms, Trojan horse, etc. They provided a few layer-specific protections to secure the layers from the threats mentioned here. The physical layer is kept secure with the help of fast booting of IoT devices using cryptographic hash algorithms, authenticating devices with the support of less power consumption, securing data before transmission where data of each device is encrypted, and anonymity where sensitive data like identity and location of nodes is kept anonymous. The network layer uses authentication mechanisms and point-to-point encryption to prevent access to the sensor nodes for counter-attacking incoming threats. In this way, the privacy of data is maintained.

Furthermore, multiple paths ensure the information is routed securely, enhancing the system's error detection ability and performing even when a failure is detected. Finally, the application layer uses Firewalls and protective software like antivirus or anti-adware to counter threats and ACLs. However, to ensure that an IoT system functions smoothly, it is mandatory to continue applying patches and updates, upgrading systems, providing improvements, monitoring devices, finding threats, using IDS (Intrusion Detection System), Trust management, Securing IoT physical premises, etc.

This paper [10] guided us on how blockchain technology can make a secure and trustworthy IoT model as blockchain is revolutionizing IoT security. The four pillars of blockchain in enhancing IoT security. First is the consensus responsible for providing the proof of work (PoW) and confirming the activities in the networks. Second, comes the ledger, which contains the details of transactions within networks. At the same time, the third pillar, Cryptography, ensures all information in the ledger and networks are encrypted and provides access to decrypt the information only to the authorized user. Lastly, the smart contract verifies and confirms the participants of the network. Several patterns are being used for implementing blockchain-based IoT. This paper defined three such ways. First is the communication model, where three primary functions of the blockchain network are applied: peer-to-peer messaging, distributed data sharing, and autonomous coordination with the device. However, this model is challenging to implement due to its drawbacks, such as slow processing, since blockchain networks need high configuration CPU and memory to function correctly as the size of the ledger increases with time. The second model discussed here connects multiple blockchain networks, and the third is Discovering legitimate IoT at a large scale.

In another paper [6], we came across techniques for securing our online transactions, vitality exchanging, digital money/cryptocurrency, industrial IoT, etc. While working over the internet, it is crucial to ensure network layer security as data security is necessary to safeguard a system from hackers. To achieve this, at first, the data is secured from unauthorized access and protected from hackers. This is done by storing all data in blocks linked together and maintaining a sequence to make a continuous chain. Here, blockchain is applied to safeguard transactional data. The existing blockchain nodes validate the blocks containing transactions.

However, these procedures contain specific challenges and limitations too. The energy and costs associated with it are very high, and there is a high chance of people not being familiar with blockchain as it is an emerging technology. Blockchain-based applications in IoT focus on the security and privacy issues the most since we know that the biggest concern for IoT is the centralization of the Server continuously interacting with the devices connected to it, for which multiple attacks by intermediary entities are possible [11]. Hence, the numerous proposed solutions to those problems, upsides, and challenges are discussed below. Most models use Ethereum-based blockchain and smart contracts to develop a viable solution.

3 Architecture of the Proposed Model

As mentioned in [14], the Internet of Things will soon take over the whole array of digital devices as they will tend to depend more on the Internet for their specific operations. For this reason, a central or general architecture representing IoT as a whole is quite near impossible. As a result, this section contains the description of the architecture to be implemented by focusing on the shortcomings we experienced in the existing architectures based on blockchain.

3.1 Existing Works

Implementation of the current architectures based on blockchain is complex since the network on which public blockchain works is open to all and lacks scalability. Taking this into account, new private and consortium blockchain implementations have emerged. However, these architectures are prone to attack as they are known to make maximum use of cloud storage; this results in compromising the user's privacy, potentially increasing the cost of implementing the solution. Moreover, smart contracts that use Ethereum-based models are not cost-effective for smart home systems.

Recent literature rarely contains the real-life implementation of the models they propose. Additionally, the TX verification requires an extra node (user node). Therefore, whenever a node wishes to get connected to the home network, the TX created by the associated node needs to be validated by the other nodes; this is troublesome for a single homeowner.

We developed a solution for smart homes that work on a private local blockchain considering all these issues. Here, in place of the user nodes, the IoT devices play the role of a node in the blockchain process and actively participate during the transaction verification. A separate process known as RESTful API is used to authorize the users. The security and privacy of the architecture are enhanced by implementing the core blockchain process through Proof of Work together with additional checking for verification and security that increases the system's integrity and safety. The solution provides a design that can be implemented simply. It is also cost-effective, safe, and consumes less amount of time. The following subsection contains a detailed description of the architecture.

3.2 Building Blocks

- Super Node (*SN*): Super Node (*SN*) is described as a storage for all the ledgers in the blockchain, done by a Peer-to-Peer server. By communication with the sensor nodes (*SeNs*), this node is utterly responsible for the transaction verification process of the users connected to the smart home environment. Moreover, the super nodes help a user verify themselves in the smart home network, and in the process, the registered user's data is stored for future use. It connects to the users through RESTful (Representational State Transfer).

  A safe and secure API that applies the principles of REST architecture for services provided by the web, and hence it ensures us with a secured communication process over the internet.
- Sensor Nodes (*SeN*): Sensor Nodes are equally crucial for user authorization and transaction verification by communicating with the *SN*s. The Sensor Nodes receive the broadcasted transactions made by the *SN*s; these are being called miners. When a transaction is created when a new user enters the intelligent home network, a block is made by the miners. This block needs to verify a PoW by other miners before finally adding the block into the blockchain storage.

Blockchain, Sensor Nodes (*SeN*), Users, and Super Node (*SN*) are used to create the building blocks in the proposed model. All *SeNs* and *SN* use the mesh network topology to communicate inside the smart home network. A renewed version of blockchain called consortium blockchain has been used to design the solution. Here, the pre-chosen nodes generate the blocks and participate in consensus; hence, all nodes do not need to participate in consensus. The reason for choosing consortium blockchain was its ability to reduce the load on the network and communication overhead, which are considered ideal for smart home environments. This proposed model has eliminated the concept of using a user's performance as a node. Instead, mining occurs through the participation of all the smart devices present inside the smart home, where they play the role of a node. Nonetheless, if the number of devices increases, the user will have the liberty to choose two devices for mining where $N = 2$ (N represents the number of nodes).

We are defining the total number of miners by Q which contains a combination of selected $SeN \in \mathbf{N}$ and $SN \in \mathbf{N}$. Mathematically we represent it using the equation below.

$$Q = \sum\nolimits_{i=1}^{N} (SeN_i) + SN \tag{3.1}$$

Furthermore, the communication between sensor nodes is shown using p_{ij}. Here p is used to indicate the packet containing the data being sent from node i to node j where i, $j \in N$. The network model with *SeNs* and *SN* is analogous to a strategic game which has a set of N players (network sensor nodes). Participation rules for transaction verification are dictated by *SN* for $SeNs \in \mathbf{N}$. The role of each *SeN* is to ensure that its participation is maximum in the verification process. The greater the number of nodes, the greater the time to complete a transaction. Let T denote the total time it takes for a transaction to complete, which includes the time Q miners take given by Eq. 3.1, and mathematically can be expressed as,

$$T_Q = \sum\nolimits_{i=1}^{Q} (t_i) \tag{3.2}$$

Next, we observe the crucial building blocks for the proposed model.

3.3 Process for Verifying Transactions

If a block, b_i, wants to get recognized by participants in the network and be a part of the blockchain, the miner (sensor nodes), Q, needs to complete PoW. The creation of blocks is slowed down using PoW since it gets challenging to tinker, as tinkering with one block means the offender needs all blocks' PoW calculation, which is nearly impossible. The process requires significant time since PoW covers the entire data needed for mining in block b_i. A complex mathematical problem is resolved for initiating PoW, a unique transaction for each block. As the mathematical problems to each block are unique, a mathematical problem that is unique for the block they made is attempted by each miner, with each of these problems having equal amounts of difficulty when it comes to fixing. Sufficient computer power is required for solving this mathematical problem [24]. However, for cases including turning on/off lights, locking, and unlocking doors, it is not regarded as optimal as they need to be performed quickly. Despite this, it is a significantly proven effective technique known to provide the highest level of safety in systems involving blockchain. Hence, considering the security measures of a smart home, PoW is given a difficulty target of 1 for creating a reasonable delay. *SN* looks at the blockchain ledger in its database when the authorized user sends a command to perform an activity. After *SN* generates a block transaction, the old ledger is updated if the old ledger is found. Through the P2P server, a new block is broadcasted to all *SeNs*. The *SeNs* (miners) are detected automatically by the *SN* based on which *SeN* is readily available and has robust network connectivity.

The new block is being validated against the last five blocks they previously had in the blockchain by the *SeNs*. After this validation process, mining will be performed by the *SeNs* by generating a hash output to verify the data in its block with the difficulty target 1. All *SeNs* check the intended referenced device upon completion of the incoming request. The activity then gets accepted by the targeted *SeN* and performs the requested action while waiting for other *SeNs* to acknowledge it. Multiple security checks are carried out on the user's device's request before block mining and creating the transaction.

3.4 Ensuring Security on Incoming Requests

In almost all of the IoT networks, the users are aware of the interconnecting devices, i.e., a thermostat comes with an IoT enables air conditioner where the thermostat is responsible for controlling the temperature of the surrounding after measuring the temperature; similarly, an IoT enabled motor is connected with a depth sensor which delivers signals to turn the motor on or off.

The architecture will consist of a decentralized server where every device will possess an instance of a consortium and local blockchain, which is granted only to a group of approved individuals and is regarded as the firmest system when it comes to immutability. The unique Ethereum address of each node (here, devices are called nodes) will be contained in a smart contract. This unique address will be required by nodes or devices to connect with the blockchain instance to carry out their functions. The devices on our network cannot establish communication with nodes whose addresses are missing from our smart contract. This, in turn, ensures that our IoT devices are secured from malicious attacks.

Here, the owner of the Ethereum account can only make changes to the blockchain network, that is - add or delete a device. The owner here is called the 'Home Miner' who only has the authority to decide which node can establish communication. The secured model will be run using a local private blockchain, and hence every IoT device connected to the safe architecture will need to install an instance of this blockchain. The system can process only three types of requests for a device from the home miner: add, delete, and the last is where it checks connectivity. The first two is valid only upon requests of the home miner. A device needs to send an address of an Ethereum account that is valid coupled with a random message regardless of the nature of the request. Both, in turn, form an encrypted signature allowing the system to get the signature associated with the message that is hashed upon the message being sent over by the requester. The signature can be decrypted through this process by our smart contract and obtain the sender's Ethereum address.

If the request for add or delete has been sent by any other node other than the home miner, then our system will not go through with the request and report possible intrusion. This identification of intrusion was possible because our system is already aware of the Ethereum address of the home miner. On the contrary, the address shall be verified if the home miner made the request. The verification is carried out to add or delete from the network. The blockchain will be updated with a transaction where it will have the address and information regarding the device.

3.5 Checking Connectivity

A request for check connectivity is carried out to verify if any device from outside is part of our network or not. To put it simply, this request is made when an IoT device wants to establish communication with another IoT device carrying the provided Ethereum address. The smart contract first checks the requester's account address to execute this request. When it matches with the home miner, it indicates a valid request. The home miner then determines whether a communication needs to be established with the sent address. Following this, a security check is carried out by the smart contract to verify whether the address that was requested exists on our list. A true or false is sent as a result after confirming. If the sender is not our home miner, the system will realize that someone from outside of our system is looking for access and hence will count this as intrusion before taking the appropriate steps.

Elliptic-curve cryptography is used to verify the home miner, a well-known algorithm for verifying digital signatures. It is Public-key cryptography where the structure of elliptic curves is used over finite fields. Here, a public key is used to verify the signature of a sender, where the only possible way of generating the signature is by using the sender's private key.

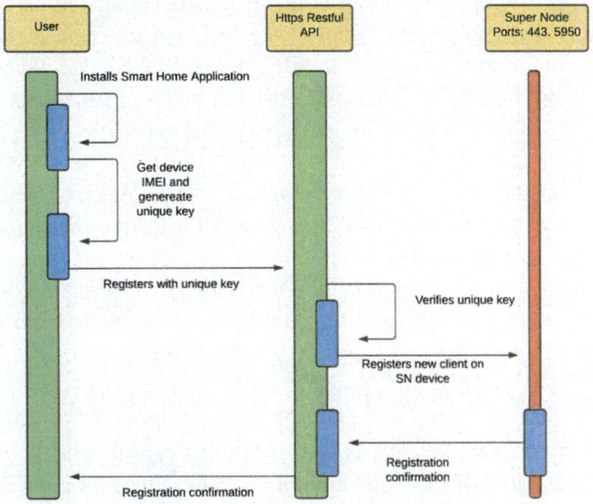

Fig. 1. User authentication process

3.6 User Authentication

This subsection describes how a user is verified after entry has been authorized. *SN* takes the help of RESTful API (Representational State Transfer) to ensure users are allowed [26]. A RESTful API is responsible for transferring data securely from one system to another over the internet. It designs web services through which the system can access its resources by applying predefined rules. The architectural constraints make the RESTful API suitable for transferring data safely in the proposed model. The smart home system will have two users - Admin and General Users. At first, the *SN* registers the admin user because the admin user is pre-authorized. General users can be a part of the smart home network if the admin user adds them by providing the admin user with the IMEI of their device. The admin user initially installs the smart home application as an authorized user, and a request is sent through the application to add general users. The application will generate the particular user's unique key. RESTful API then sends the unique key to *SN*. *SN* then verifies the key; *SN* registers the user as a new client through its unique identifier. For further communication, the general user is provided with a username and password by the admin user. The unique key, stored in *SN's* database, gets identified through its unique key whenever the user requests the *SN*. Figure 1 represents the proposed architecture's user authorization process.

4 Experimental Progress

4.1 Experimental Implementation of the Model

A genesis block can be created to deploy a private blockchain on our computer, through which we will be able to run an instance of the private blockchain and carry out the rest of the procedure after deploying our smart contract. But instead, Ganache is used, a truffle framework to make the process easier. Truffle developed Ganache which is a personal blockchain for deploying or developing dApps. Ten ethereum accounts are given after starting, where each of them containing 100 ethers. The entire process is run on a private blockchain.

Our blockchain needs an intelligent contract to be deployed while running on Ganache. This is done using the Remix IDE. ABI is collected after writing and compiling the solidity code on the Remix IDE. After this, the smart contract was deployed on our ganache blockchain, which gave us a deployment address. The smart contract uses this deployment address for transferring virtual ethers to complete the required transaction.

4.2 Experimental Testing of the Model

An outsider can't enter our network as we run a local private Ethereum network. We deliberately altered a digit of the smart contract's address to test our application.

5 Analysis and Results

In this chapter, we will analyze the performance, capacity, and implementation cost of the proposed model.

5.1 Performance

It takes 10 min for the bitcoin blockchain to generate transactions, while Ethereum can affect up to 20 transactions per second. Twenty inputs per second should be ideal for the model we proposed. We need only take speed when admitting devices are greater than 20 per second. Getting 20 Ethereum address inputs per second is quite impractical for humans. Hence, this won't be a drawback for our proposed model.

When a request for a valid transaction appears during mining of a block by a node, then mempool stores the incoming request. Mempool is the place where the transaction for a node waits. The transaction is processed upon completion of mining. To put it simply, the probability that a mempool will hold the transactions is directly proportional to the time a block takes for mining. The time to mine a block is based upon a blockchain's difficulty level. Since we are running an instance of a private blockchain, we can adjust the difficulty level to low, ensuring that the time taken to process a transaction is minimal. This ensures that it can run smoothly on high-configuration devices and low-configuration devices.

The performance of this model is further enhanced through the use of Ganache for the web version. Normally, when we implement transactions using Ethereum, there is a high probability of transactions getting stuck. This arises because the transactions are not getting picked up by a miner. This problem is solved when we implement Ethereum using Ganache.

Most of the models that we saw used public blockchain. As a result, performance was compromised in those models since public blockchain require more energy than private blockchain. This happens due to public blockchain requiring large amounts of electrical resources for functioning.

Public blockchain are inherently slower as they need to process multiple transactions at a time since everyone on the internet can access them. On the contrary, a selected few can only access the private blockchain. Hence, the speed remains the same.

5.2 Storage Handling

A primary concern regarding blockchain is storage. Approximately 1.498 GB is the capacity of the Ethereum blockchain currently. The power is increasing every day, with additional blocks getting added. Here, a string containing a list of Ethereum addresses is saved only. It can be deduced that there won't be a large number of blocks due to the architecture of the model we proposed, and hence it is safe to say that storage won't act as a hindrance to the proposed architecture.

5.3 Cost-Benefit Analysis

It is practically possible to run this model at zero cost as a private blockchain is free. Thus, IoT devices can have private blockchain instances running for free on a 24/7 basis after deploying smart contracts. Virtual ethers are used on the local blockchain and will not cost a penny to the device owner.

The prices for models that run on public blockchain rise drastically as it contains more nodes and receives numerous requests every second, which significantly increases the transaction cost. Our model is cheaper than the models we have come across so far as most of the models used public blockchain, which is quite expensive and is mainly used for large-scale applications, i.e., intelligent power grids, smart cities, etc.

6 Conclusion and Future Works

The cost of this model makes it an ideal choice for a smart clinic where data that is not so important can be kept on a cloud server. The blockchain is attached to the cloud server so that the blockchain does not have to hold onto unnecessary data. In our report, we researched previous work that has been done on smart home security using blockchain. Taking the drawbacks into account, we took a simpler step where we focused on user verification and emphasized security in incoming requests. Most of the architectures we came across used public blockchain, which is costly and possesses a lot of security threats since it is open to everyone. Hence, we pivoted our model to a private blockchain that only allows authorized users. It ensures a smooth run on both low and high-end devices and comes at a total free of cost. In the future, we hope to carry out further research on it and test the performance using Raspberry Pi.

References

1. Fruhlinger, J. What is IoT? The internet of things explained. Network World (2020). https://www.networkworld.com/article/3207535/what-is-iot-the-internet-of-things-explained.html
2. Malche, T., Maheshwary, P.: Internet of things (IoT) for building smart home system. In: 2017 International Conference on I-SMAC (2017)
3. Panarello, A., et al.: Blockchain and IoT integration: a systematic survey. Sensors **18**(8), 2575 (2018). MDPI
4. Islam, M.A., Madria, S.: A permissioned blockchain-based access control system for IOT. In: IEEE International Conference on Blockchain (Blockchain) (2019)
5. What is blockchain? Blockchain Explained: What is blockchain?—Euromoney Learning (n.d.). https://www.euromoney.com/learning/blockchain-explained/what-is-blockchain
6. Arif, S., et al.: Investigating smart home security: is blockchain the answer? IEEE Access **8**, 117802–117816 (2020)
7. Sun, S., et al.: Blockchain-based IoT access control system: towards security lightweight and cross-domain. IEEE Access **9**, 36868–36878 (2021)
8. Lee, Y., et al.: A blockchain-based smart home gateway architecture for preventing data forgery. Hum. Cent. Comput. Inf. Sci. **10**(9), 1–14 (2020)
9. Andrea, I., Chrysostomou, C., Hadjichristo, G.: Internet of things: security vulnerabilities and challenges. In: 2015 IEEE Symposium on Computers and Communication (2015)
10. Singh, M., et al.: Blockchain: a game-changer for securing IoT data. In: 2018 IEEE World Forum on Internet of Things (2018)
11. Kshetri, N.: Can blockchain strengthen the internet of things? IT Prof. **19**(4), 68–72 (2017)
12. Papadodimas, G., et al.: Implementation of smart contracts for blockchain-based IoT applications. In: IEEE International Conference on the Network of the Future (NOF) (2018)
13. Ray, P.P., et al.: Blockchain for IoT-based healthcare: background, consensus, platforms, and use cases. IEEE Syst. J. **15**(1), 85–94 (2021)
14. Zanella, A., et al.: Internet of things for smart cities. IEEE Internet Things J. **1**(1), 22–32 (2014)
15. Khan, M.A., Salah, K.: IoT security: review, blockchain solutions, and open challenges. Futur. Gener. Comput. Syst. **82**, 395–411 (2018)

Towards an Error-Detecting Code

Natasha Ilievska(✉)

Faculty of Computer Science and Engineering, Ss. Cyril and Methodius University, Skopje, Republic of North Macedonia
natasa.ilievska@finki.ukim.mk
https://www.finki.ukim.mk/en/staff/natasa-ilievska

Abstract. In this paper we consider an error-detecting code that we have previously defined using quasigroups. The code is defined in the following way: Each input block $a_0a_1 \dots a_{n-1}$ of symbols from the quasigroup used for coding is extended into block $a_0a_1 \dots a_{n-1}d_0d_1 \dots d_{n-1}$, where the redundant symbols $d_i, i \in \{0, 1, \dots, n-1\}$, are calculated using the quasigroup operation $*$, i.e., $d_i = a_i * a_{i+1\ (mod\ n)}$. In our previous work we classified the quasigroups of order 4 according to their probability of undetected errors. Since in our previous work we showed that the quasigroups in the first two classes give almost equal probabilities of undetected errors, now we will compare the quasigroups from these two classes according to the number of errors that the code surely detects when they are used for coding. In order to do this, first using simultions we will obtain the number of errors that the code surely detects when for coding is used a quasigroup from the second best class of quasigroups of order 4 for coding. We will show that from the aspect of the number of errors that the code surely detects, these quasigroups are equally good for coding as the quasigroups from the best class of quasigroups when the length of the input blocks is at least three characters from the quasigroup of order 4.

Keywords: Error-detecting code · Number of surely detected errors · Error-detecting capability · Quasigroup

1 Introduction

In [1] we have defined an error-detecting code in the following way. Let for coding be used the quasigroup $(Q, *)$. The input message over the alphabet Q is divided in blocks (further input blocks) of length n and each block is coded separately. Let one such input block be $a_0a_1 \dots a_{n-1}$ ($a_i \in Q$ for all $i \in \{0, 1, ..., n-1\}$). Then, the redundant characters are defined with the equation

$$d_i = a_i * a_{i+1}, i \in \{0, 1, \dots, n-1\} \tag{1}$$

where the operations in indexes are modulo n. The binary form of the extended block $a_0a_1 \dots a_{n-1}d_0d_1 \dots d_{n-1}$ is transmitted through the binary symmetric channel. Since there are noises in the channel some of the characters may not be correctly transmitted. Let denote the output block with $a'_0a'_1 \dots a'_{n-1}d'_0d'_1 \dots d'_{n-1}$.

K. Daimi and A. Al Sadoon (Eds.): ICR 2022, AISC 1431, pp. 321–330, 2022.
https://doi.org/10.1007/978-3-031-14054-9_30

In order to check if there are some errors in transmission of the block, the receiver checks whether

$$d'_i = a'_i * a'_{i+1}, i \in \{0, 1, \ldots, n-1\} \tag{2}$$

If (2) is satisfied for all $i \in \{0, 1, \ldots, n-1\}$, the receiver accepts the block as correctly transmitted. If there is some $i \in \{0, 1, \ldots, n-1\}$ for which (2) is not satisfied, the receiver concludes that there is some error in transmission of the block and asks for repeated transmission of that block. But, since the redundant characters are also transmitted through the channel, they can be incorrectly transmitted, too. Therefore, it is possible to have undetected errors in transmission. For that reason it is important to know the error-detecting capability of the code. It is determined by its probability of undetected errors and the number of errors that the code surely detects.

We analyzed the code in a few papers [1–6]. In [1] and [2] we concluded that the probability of undetected errors depends on the quasigroup used for coding. Therefore, we classified the quasigroups of order 4 such that the quasigroups in a same class give equal probabilities of undetected errors. For the quasigroups in each class we obtained this probability. There are 576 quasigroups of order 4. They are divided in seven such classes. The quasigroups in the best class give smallest probability of undetected errors. We compared this probability with that of the most commonly used error-detecting code - CRC. This code is defined by Peterson and Brown in 1961 [7]. Many variants of this code have been proposed since then ([8–13] and many others). In the last decade, there are ideas for using CRC as error-correcting codes or in combination with some error-correcting codes as polar, turbo, convolutional and other codes in order to enhance their performance [14–22]. We compared the probabilities of undetected errors of this quasigroup code with few CRC codes when they are used as error-detecting codes. The error-detecting code based on quasigroups, as the name itself says, use the algebraic structure quasigroup in the coding process. From (1) and (2) we can see that the coding and checking for errors consists of quasigroup multiplication. On the other hand, CRC codes use polynomial, i.e., the coding and checking for errors is based on polynomial division. But, both codes are very fast and have simple implementation. While in the quasigroup code the length of the redundancy is equal to the length of the information block, CRC are codes with fix length redundancy, i.e., they add fixed number of redundant bits regardless of the length of the input block. Therefore, in our previous work we compared their probabilities of undetected errors when the code rates of the both codes are equal, and also the lengths of the input blocks for both codes are equal. Since our code gave smaller probability of undetected errors than some CRC codes when for coding is used a quasigroup from the best class of quasigroups of order 4, we continued our investigation of the code. We obtained the number of errors that the code surely detects when for coding is used a quasigroup from the best class of quasigroups of order 4 for which the constant term in the linear representation is zero matrix [4–6]. We also showed that the difference in the probability of undetected errors between the quasigroups from the best and those from second best class is negligibly small. This means that the quasigroups from the second best class have practically equal probability of undetected errors as the quasigroups from the best class. For this reason, it deserves to check whether these quasigroups are equally good for coding as those from the best class from the aspect of the number of surely detected incorrectly transmitted bits, too. This is the goal of this paper. Since of particular interest are the linear quasigroups for which the constant term in the linear representation is zero matrix, we will be focused on those quasigroups from the second best class that satisfy this condition. Namely, in this paper we will obtain the number of errors that the code surely detects in the case when for coding is used arbitrary quasigroup from the second best class of quasigroups of order 4 for which the constant term in the linear representation is zero matrix and we will compare the results in these two cases (when for coding is used a quasigroup from the best and when it is used a quasigroup from the second best class of quasigroups of order 4 for coding).

The paper is organized in the following way: In Sect. 2 we give the basic mathematical definitions. In Sect. 3, first we give a brief view on the simulation procedure (Subsect. 3.1). Then, in a same section we present the obtained simulation results for the number of errors that the code surely detects when for coding is used arbitrary quasigroup of order 4 from the second best class of quasigroups of order 4 for which the constant term in the linear representation is zero matrix (Subsect. 3.2). In Sect. 4 we compare the obtained results with those for the quasigroups from the best class of quasigroups. At the end, we conclude the paper.

2 Mathematical Preliminaries

Since the code is defined using quasigroups, in this section we will give the definition of this algebraic structure.

Definition 1. *Quasigroup is algebraic structure* $(Q, *)$ *such that*

$$(\forall u, v \in Q)(\exists! x, y \in Q) \ \ (x * u = v \ \& \ u * y = v) \tag{3}$$

From the definition follows that the body of the quasigroup is a latin square. A special class of quasigroups, so-called linear quasigroups, is of interest for the code considered in this paper. The definition of this kind of quasigroups is as follows.

Definition 2. *The quasigroup* $(Q, *)$ *of order* 2^q *is linear if there are non-singular binary matrices* A *and* B *of order* $q \times q$ *and a binary matrix* C *of order* $1 \times q$*, such that*

$$(\forall x, y \in Q) \ \ x * y = z \Leftrightarrow \boldsymbol{z} = \boldsymbol{x}A + \boldsymbol{y}B + C \tag{4}$$

where $\boldsymbol{x}$, $\boldsymbol{y}$ *and* $\boldsymbol{z}$ *are the binary representations of* x, y *and* z *as vectors of order* $1 \times q$ *and* $+$ *is a binary addition.*

Therefore, when we work with a linear quasigroup, instead to work with a latin square, we can simply work with binary matrices.

3 The Number of Errors that the Quasigroups from the Second Best Class Surely Detect

The second-best class of quasigroups of order 4 is obtained in [1] and [2]. It contains 16 quasigroups and all of them are linear. In [2], the quasigroups from this class are given with their number according the lexicographical ordering of the quasigroups of order 4. Using Definition 2, we obtained the matrices A, B and C that define these quasigroups. There are four pairs of matrices A_i and B_i, $i = 1, 2, 3, 4$. They are given in Fig. 1. Each combination of the four pairs A_i and B_i, $i = 1, 2, 3, 4$ with one of the four binary matrices C of order 1×2, give one of the sixteen quasigroups from the second best class.

$$A_1 = \begin{bmatrix} 0 & 1 \\ 1 & 1 \end{bmatrix}, B_1 = \begin{bmatrix} 1 & 1 \\ 0 & 1 \end{bmatrix}$$

$$A_2 = \begin{bmatrix} 1 & 0 \\ 1 & 1 \end{bmatrix}, B_2 = \begin{bmatrix} 1 & 1 \\ 1 & 0 \end{bmatrix}$$

$$A_3 = \begin{bmatrix} 1 & 1 \\ 0 & 1 \end{bmatrix}, B_3 = \begin{bmatrix} 0 & 1 \\ 1 & 1 \end{bmatrix}$$

$$A_4 = \begin{bmatrix} 1 & 1 \\ 1 & 0 \end{bmatrix}, B_4 = \begin{bmatrix} 1 & 0 \\ 1 & 1 \end{bmatrix}$$

Fig. 1. The second best class of quasigroups of order 4

Using simulation, for each of the four pairs of matrices A_i and B_i, $i = 1, 2, 3, 4$ we obtain the number of errors that the code surely detects. For each of these four pairs of matrices, we take the constant term C in (4) to be a zero matrix.

In the simulation process, we use quasigroup Q of order 4 for coding, the length of the input blocks is n characters from Q and the probability of bit-error in the binary symmetric channel is p. Using simulation for different values of the input blocks, we obtain the number of blocks with k incorrectly transmitted bits $e[k]$ and the number of such blocks in which the error in transmission is not detected $ue[k]$ for every k from 1 to the length of the coded blocks in a binary form.

3.1 The Simulation Procedure

In this subsection we will give short description of the simulation process. In order to obtain the number of blocks with k incorrectly transmitted bits $e[k]$ and the number of such code words in which the error is not detected $ue[k]$ for a given length of the input blocks n characters from the quasigroup Q, we use the following simulation process. First, we generate a long input message, for example around 2000000 characters from the alphabet Q. Then, this message is separated into blocks with length n characters and each block is coded separately.

Each coded block has length $2n$ characters from the quasigroup of order 4. This coded message is turned into binary form. Since each character from the quasigroup of order 4 is represenred with 2 bits in a binary form, each coded block from this coded message has length $4n$ bits. We generate the noise in the binary symmetric channel, which is a binary string with length equal to the length of the coded input message turned into binary form. The noise string is generated such that the probability of occurrence of 1 in this string is p. The positions in the noise string to which there is 1 are the positions on the coded input message in a binary form that are incorrectly transmitted. The output message is calculated with simple adding per modulo 2 the coded input message in a binary form and the noise string. Now, from the noise string, for every $k \in \{1, 2, \ldots, 4n\}$, we count the number of incorrectly transmitted coded blocks with k incorrectly transmitted bits ($e[k]$). For each incorrectly transmitted block, using the output message we check whether the code detects the error. With this we obtain the number of incorrectly transmitted coded blocks with k incorrectly transmitted bits in which the error is not detected ($ue[k]$).

The number of errors that the code surely detects for a given length of the input block is the largest integer s, such that the code detects all incorrectly transmitted blocks with $k \leq s$ incorrectly transmitted bits, but there are blocks with $s+1$ incorrectly transmitted bits in which the error is not detected. This means that the number of incorrectly transmitted bits that the code surely detects is $s = max\{k|ue[i] = 0 \text{ for all } i \leq k\}$.

The number of errors that the code surely detects does not depend on the probability of bit-error p in the binary symmetric channel. Therefore, in order to obtain accurate results, for each length of the input blocks, we adjusted the values of p in order to obtain a large numbers of incorrectly transmitted blocks $e[k]$ for each k.

3.2 The Results for the Number of Surely Detected Errors

We performed the simulation process for each of the four pairs of matrices (A_i, B_i), $i = 1, 2, 3, 4$ from Fig. 1. For matrix C we take the zero matrix of order 1×2. The results are given in Table 1, 2, 3 and Table 4. Thereby, in Table i are given the obtained results when for coding is used a quasigroup represented with the pair of matrices (A_i, B_i), $i = 1, 2, 3, 4$. In the first column of each table is given the length of the input blocks expressed in characters from the quasigroup of order 4. As explained earlier, when the length of the input block is n characters from the quasigroup, the length of the coded block (i.e., the codeword) is $4n$ bits. In the tables are given results for the lengths of the input blocks up to 18 characters from the quasigroup, i.e., the lengths of the codewords up to 72 bits. In the $2k$-th column, is given the number of blocks with k incorrectly transmitted bits $e[k]$, while in the $2k+1$-th column is given the number of blocks with k incorrectly transmitted bits in which the error is not detected $ue[k]$, $k = 1, 2, ..., 6$. Due to space limitation, the results for larger values of k are not given. But, since we are looking for the smallest k such that $ue[k]$ is not equal to zero, the results for larger values of k are not important.

Table 1. Number of incorrectly transmitted coded blocks with i incorrectly transmitted bits $e[i]$ and the number of such coded blocks in which the error is not detected $ue[i]$ when the length of the input block is n characters from the quasigroup of order 4. For coding is used the quasigroup defined with the matrices A_1 and B_1 from Fig. 1.

n	e[1]	ue[1]	e[2]	ue[2]	e[3]	ue[3]	e[4]	ue[4]	e[5]	ue[5]	e[6]	ue[6]
2	312063	0	69426	**5125**	219028	0	273219	34868	218727	0	109187	15623
3	242395	0	85538	0	35863	0	80440	**2888**	128807	0	150429	3942
4	189447	0	90223	0	27566	0	13879	**139**	33668	0	60933	389
5	147916	0	89987	0	34238	0	9294	**46**	5751	0	14869	30
6	94025	0	94132	0	59824	0	27732	**67**	9534	0	2655	0
7	67648	0	79840	0	59274	0	31967	**42**	13370	0	4510	0
8	48734	0	65550	0	57081	0	35114	**35**	16826	0	6634	1
9	34413	0	53503	0	52286	0	37091	**21**	20098	0	9056	0
10	43602	0	53985	0	43299	0	37025	**17**	22877	0	11550	0
11	33693	0	46519	0	41224	0	26789	**22**	13467	0	5750	1
12	26268	0	39812	0	38774	0	27430	**5**	15177	0	6959	0
13	24397	0	36928	0	35820	0	25223	**2**	13619	0	6273	0
14	24111	0	34888	0	32676	0	22574	**5**	25555	0	18549	0
15	28841	0	36091	0	28349	0	16639	**2**	24347	0	19115	0
16	19845	0	29630	0	28911	0	22131	**4**	23048	0	19625	0
17	31002	0	44024	0	40455	0	26480	**4**	31967	0	28880	0
18	26732	0	39445	0	38421	0	24678	**4**	29096	0	28005	0

Table 2. Number of incorrectly transmitted coded blocks with i incorrectly transmitted bits $e[i]$ and the number of such coded blocks in which the error is not detected $ue[i]$ when the length of the input block is n characters from the quasigroup of order 4. For coding is used the quasigroup defined with the matrices A_2 and B_2 from Fig. 1.

n	e[1]	ue[1]	e[2]	ue[2]	e[3]	ue[3]	e[4]	ue[4]	e[5]	ue[5]	e[6]	ue[6]
2	311732	0	69442	**4989**	219018	0	273166	34864	218985	0	109685	15607
3	242854	0	85408	0	36105	0	80962	**2904**	128642	0	149627	3841
4	189220	0	90862	0	27133	0	13931	**154**	33429	0	60871	392
5	148046	0	89901	0	34319	0	9343	**41**	5948	0	14764	21
6	93947	0	93863	0	60324	0	27222	**72**	9582	0	2675	3
7	67848	0	79420	0	59644	0	32027	**39**	13323	0	4599	2
8	48342	0	66090	0	56707	0	35269	**39**	16870	0	6846	2
9	34686	0	52972	0	52253	0	37103	**28**	20444	0	9204	0
10	43094	0	54219	0	43398	0	37028	**10**	22751	0	11592	0
11	33777	0	46667	0	41581	0	26500	**10**	13274	0	5666	0
12	26323	0	40151	0	38531	0	27274	**16**	15124	0	6941	0
13	24561	0	36903	0	35688	0	24883	**5**	13914	0	6439	0
14	23701	0	34878	0	32867	0	22537	**3**	25561	0	18148	0
15	29039	0	35903	0	28447	0	16620	**4**	24484	0	19263	0
16	19804	0	29949	0	29029	0	20380	**1**	23097	0	19251	0
17	31142	0	44149	0	40302	0	26664	**1**	32262	0	28909	0
18	26499	0	39657	0	38432	0	26944	**2**	28820	0	28158	0

Table 3. Number of incorrectly transmitted coded blocks with i incorrectly transmitted bits $e[i]$ and the number of such coded blocks in which the error is not detected $ue[i]$ when the length of the input block is n characters from the quasigroup of order 4. For coding is used the quasigroup defined with the matrices A_3 and B_3 from Fig. 1.

n	e[1]	ue[1]	e[2]	ue[2]	e[3]	ue[3]	e[4]	ue[4]	e[5]	ue[5]	e[6]	ue[6]
2	310929	0	69642	**4919**	218874	0	272979	35091	218652	0	109438	15464
3	242993	0	85648	0	35909	0	80603	**2945**	129048	0	150158	3879
4	189921	0	91031	0	27060	0	14004	**114**	33341	0	60871	358
5	148175	0	89769	0	34404	0	9367	**44**	5831	0	14831	23
6	94177	0	94024	0	59782	0	27210	**61**	9504	0	2683	1
7	67844	0	79324	0	59726	0	31896	**51**	13638	0	4448	1
8	48324	0	65607	0	57056	0	35114	**28**	17192	0	6845	0
9	34684	0	53401	0	52199	0	36700	**35**	20186	0	9273	0
10	43512	0	53918	0	43072	0	36870	**13**	22820	0	11453	0
11	33631	0	46728	0	41309	0	26599	**9**	13307	0	5754	0
12	26273	0	40017	0	38816	0	27298	**16**	15197	0	6864	0
13	24416	0	36960	0	35700	0	25151	**6**	13908	0	6229	0
14	23748	0	34796	0	32932	0	22876	**3**	25338	0	18630	0
15	29147	0	35794	0	28618	0	16536	**2**	24582	0	19265	0
16	19782	0	29613	0	28787	0	20668	**2**	23271	0	192506	0
17	31200	0	44443	0	40166	0	26507	**2**	31811	0	28899	0
18	26423	0	39855	0	38305	0	27075	**2**	15119	0	7033	1

Table 4. Number of incorrectly transmitted coded blocks with i incorrectly transmitted bits $e[i]$ and the number of such coded blocks in which the error is not detected $ue[i]$ when the length of the input block is n characters from the quasigroup of order 4. For coding is used the quasigroup defined with the matrices A_4 and B_4 from Fig. 1.

n	e[1]	ue[1]	e[2]	ue[2]	e[3]	ue[3]	e[4]	ue[4]	e[5]	ue[5]	e[6]	ue[6]
2	311596	0	70220	**5015**	218899	0	272752	35143	219866	0	108919	15722
3	243521	0	85380	0	35849	0	80758	**2898**	128944	0	150266	3910
4	190428	0	90716	0	26910	0	13724	**141**	33252	0	61214	377
5	148314	0	89628	0	34288	0	9411	**36**	5885	0	14776	31
6	94443	0	93660	0	60118	0	27486	**67**	9568	0	2652	1
7	67796	0	79785	0	59222	0	32040	**35**	13390	0	4574	1
8	48388	0	65593	0	57009	0	35366	**22**	16915	0	6751	1
9	34530	0	53034	0	52303	0	37099	**28**	20485	0	9062	0
10	43158	0	54105	0	43366	0	36873	**15**	22739	0	11367	1
11	33687	0	46870	0	41331	0	26400	**22**	13426	0	5657	1
12	26120	0	39902	0	38546	0	27566	**1**	15237	0	6939	0
13	24577	0	37170	0	35676	0	24945	**2**	16713	0	8237	0
14	23829	0	34887	0	32815	0	22427	**3**	25338	0	18360	0
15	29015	0	35850	0	28346	0	16549	**6**	24551	0	19135	0
16	19561	0	29821	0	29052	0	20581	**1**	22837	0	19506	0
17	31043	0	44184	0	40150	0	26795	**3**	31791	0	28570	0
18	26653	0	39983	0	37964	0	24986	**3**	29141	0	27970	0

As we can see from the tables, the number of errors that the code surely detects is equal for all four quasigroups. When the length of the input block is 2 characters (i.e., codewords with length 8 bits), the code detected all incorrectly transmitted coded blocks (codewords) with one incorrectly transmitted bit, but there are coded blocks with two incorrectly transmitted bits in which the error is not detected. Therefore, when the length of the input block is two characters, the code surely detects one incorrectly transmitted bit, regardless which of the four quasigroups from the second best class of quasigroups of order 4 for which the constant term C in the linear representation is zero matrix is used for coding. When the length of the input block is greater than or equal to three characters (i.e., codewords with length greater than or equal to 12 bits), the code surely detected all incorrectly transmitted blocks with one, two and three incorrectly transmitted bits. But, there are blocks with four incorrectly transmitted bits in which the error is not detected. Hence, when the length of the input block is greater than or equal to three characters, the code surely detects up to three incorrectly transmitted bits, regardless which of the four quasigroups from the second best class of quasigroups of order 4 for which the constant term C is zero matrix is used for coding.

Another thing that obtained results suggest is that the code detects all odd number of incorrectly transmitted bits, regardless of the length of the input block.

4 Comparison of the Results for the Quasigroups from the Best and the Second Best Class

In [4–6] we showed that when for coding is used a quasigroup from the best class of quasigroups of order 4 for which the constant term C in the linear representation is zero matrix, the code surely detects up to three incorrectly transmitted bits, regardless of the length of the input blocks. On the other hand, in [1] and [2] we showed that the quasigroups from the best and second best class of quasigroups of order 4 give practically equal probabilities of undetected errors (the difference is inconsiderable, imperceptibly small).

With the results described in previous section, we can conclude that the quasigroups from the second best class are practically equally (or almost equally) good for coding as the quasigroups from the best class when the length of the input blocks is greater than or equal to three characters from the quasigroup of order 4. If the length of the input blocks is two characters from the quasigroup of order 4, the quasigroups from the best class for coding are superior, since in this case they surely detect more incorrectly transmitted bits.

5 Conclusion

In this paper we analyzed the number of errors that the code surely detects when for coding is used a quasigroup from the second best class of quasigroups of order 4 for coding for which the constant term in the linear representation is zero matrix. The results obtained with simulation show that when such quasigroup is used for coding, the code surely detects one incorrectly transmitted bit when the length of the input block is two characters from the quasigroup of order 4. When such quasigroup is used for coding and the length of the input block is greater than or equal to three characters from the quasigroup of order 4, the code surely detects up to three incorrectly transmitted bits. In our previous work, we have proven that when a quasigroup from the best class of quasigroups of order 4 is used for coding, the code surely detects up to three incorrectly transmitted bits, regardless of the length of the input blocks. Therefore, when the length of the input blocks is greater than or equal to three characters from the quasigroup of order 4, the best and the second best class of quasigroups of order 4 are equally good for coding from the aspect of the number of errors that the code surely detects.

In our previous work we also showed that the difference in the probabilities of undetected errors between the quasigroups in the best and the second best class is insignificantly small, i.e., they are practically equal. With the results in this paper, we show that the quasigroups from the second best class are practically equally good for coding as the ones from the best one when the length of the input block is grater than or equal to three characters.

Our next step is to give a theoretical proof of the results in this paper.

Acknowledgments. This work was partially financed by the Faculty of Computer Science and Engineering at the "Ss.Cyril and Methodius" University.

References

1. Ilievska, N., Bakeva, V.: A Model of error-detecting codes based on quasigroups of order 4. In: 6th International Conference for Informatics and Information Technology, pp. 7–11. Bitola (2008)
2. Bakeva, V., Ilievska, N.: A probabilistic model of error-detecting codes based on quasigroups. Quasigroups Relat. Syst. **17**, 135–148 (2009)
3. Ilievska, N., Gligoroski, D.: Quasigroup redundancy check codes for safety-critical systems. In: 11th Advanced Internetional Conference on Telecommunications IARIA-AICT, pp. 72–77. Brussels (2015)
4. Ilievska, N.: Number of errors that the error-detecting code surely detects. In: Trajanov, D., Bakeva, V. (eds.) ICT Innovations 2017. CCIS, vol. 311, pp. 219–228. Springer Nature (2017). https://doi.org/10.1007/978-3-319-67597-8_21
5. Ilievska, N.: Simulating the error-detecting capability of the error-detecting code. In: 41st International Convention on Information and Communication Technology, Electronics and Microelectronics (MIPRO), pp. 528–533. IEEE (2018). https://doi.org/10.23919/MIPRO.2018.8400091
6. Ilievska, N.: A note on an error-detecting code. In: 15th International Conference for Informatics and Information Technology, pp. 53–57. Mavrovo (2018)
7. Peterson, W.W., Brown, D.T.: Cyclic codes for error detection. In: IRE 1961, vol. 49, no. 1, pp. 228–235. IEEE (1961). https://doi.org/10.1109/JRPROC.1961.287814

8. Perez, A.: Byte-wise CRC calculations. IEEE Micro **3**, 40–50 (1983). https://doi.org/10.1109/MM.1983.291120
9. Ramabadran, T.V., Gaitonde, S.S.: A tutorial on CRC computations. IEEE Micro **8**, 62–75 (1988). https://doi.org/10.1109/40.7773
10. Koopman, P.: 32-Bit cyclic redundancy codes for internet applications. In: The International Conference on Dependable Systems and Networks, pp. 459–468. IEEE (2002). https://doi.org/10.1109/DSN.2002.1028931
11. Koopman, P., Chakravarty, T.: Cyclic redundancy code (CRC) polynomial selection for embedded networks. In: International Conference on Dependable Systems and Networks, pp. 145–154. IEEE (2004). https://doi.org/10.1109/DSN.2004.1311885
12. Richardson, A.: WCDMA Design Handbook. Cambridge University Press, Cambridge (2005)
13. Jones, D. T.: An improved 64-bit cyclic redundancy check for protein sequences. University College London (2009)
14. Niu, K., Chen, K.: CRC-aided decoding of polar codes. IEEE Commun. Lett. **16**, 1668–1671 (2012). https://doi.org/10.1109/LCOMM.2012.090312.121501
15. Li, B., Shen, H., Tse, D.: An adaptive successive cancellation list decoder for polar codes with cyclic redundancy check. IEEE Commun. Lett. **16**, 2044–2047 (2012). https://doi.org/10.1109/LCOMM.2012.111612.121898
16. Wei, Y., Jiang, M., Xia, B., Chen, W., Yang, Y.: A CRC-aided hybrid decoding algorithm for turbo codes. IEEE Wirel. Commun. Lett. **2**, 471–474 (2013). https://doi.org/10.1109/WCL.2013.052813.130259
17. Lou, C., Daneshrad, B., Wesel, R.D.: Convolutional-code-specific CRC code design. IEEE Trans. Commun. **63**, 3459–3470 (2015). https://doi.org/10.1109/TCOMM.2015.2459058
18. Tonnellier, T., Leroux, C., Le Gal, B., Gadat, B., Jego, C., Van Wambeke, N.: Lowering the error floor of turbo codes with CRC verification. IEEE Wirel. Commun. Lett. **5**, 404–407 (2016). https://doi.org/10.1109/LWC.2016.2571283
19. Zhang, Q., Liu, A., Pan, X., Pan, K.: CRC code design for list decoding of polar codes. IEEE Commun. Lett. **21**, 1229–1232 (2017). https://doi.org/10.1109/LCOMM.2017.2672539
20. Chaki, P., Kamiya, N.: A novel design of CRC-concatenated polar codes. In: International Conference on Communications (ICC) 2019, pp. 1–6. IEEE (2019). https://doi.org/10.1109/ICC.2019.8761833
21. Geiselhart, M., Elkelesh, A., Ebada, S., Cammerer, S., Brink, S.: CRC-aided belief propagation list decoding of polar codes. In: International Symposium on Information Theory (ISIT) 2020, pp. 395–400. IEEE (2020). https://doi.org/10.1109/ISIT44484.2020.9174249
22. An, W., Medard, M., Duffy, K. R.: CRC codes as error correction codes. In: International Conference on Communications (ICC) 2021, pp. 1–6. IEEE (2021). https://doi.org/10.1109/ICC42927.2021.9500279

Classification of Encrypted Data Using Deep Learning and Legendre Polynomials

Emad M. Alsaedi[1](✉), Alaa Kadhim Farhan[1], Mayadah W. Falah[2], and Bashra Kadhim Oleiwi[1]

[1] Computer Sciences Department, University of Technology, Baghdad, Iraq
cs.19.71@grad.uotechnology.edu.iq, {110030, bushra.k.oleiwi}@uotechnology.edu.iq

[2] Building and Construction Engineering Technology Department, AL-Mustaqbal University College, Hillah 51001, Iraq
mayadahwaheed@mustaqbal-college.edu.iq

Abstract. Problems involving the classification of sensitive cloud data, such as medical or financial records, can be solved using a convolutional neural network (CNN) approach. Data privacy and security, however, require extra care. Homomorphic encryption is a potential security solution to allow CNNs to classify cypher data. The convolution layer, for example, is a computation that can be fully homomorphically evaluated; however, non-linear functions, such as the activation layer, cannot be fully homomorphically assessed since they do not follow a linear pattern. This paper uses low-degree polynomials to approximate these non-linear functions. We compare various polynomial approximation approaches to achieve the optimal approximation function for activation functions such as Relu. Finally, we use a proposed CNN and the MNIST dataset to demonstrate the effectiveness of our approximation functions. The resulting proposed CNN achieved a 99.80% accuracy rate.

Keywords: Cloud-based machine learning as a service · Convolution neural network · Homomorphic encryption · Polynomial activation function

1 Introduction

Deep learning (Dl) services that use cloud computing are becoming more common. Dl algorithms need to see original data, putting people's security and privacy at risk [1]. Cryptography is a branch of mathematics that uses complex algorithms to ensure the confidentiality of information while it is transmitted and stored. Several new public-key cryptosystems have been created, these cryptosystems are very safe and contain considerable essential space, but it been regarded as expensive and slow [2, 3]. Data security is an essential requirement in our time. As a result of the rapid development of unsecured computer networks, personal data should be protected from unauthorized persons [4]. The security and protection of sensitive data have been an issue of concern for decades as the open nature of the internet makes it vulnerable to attacks [5]. Data

K. Daimi and A. Al Sadoon (Eds.): ICR 2022, AISC 1431, pp. 331–345, 2022.
https://doi.org/10.1007/978-3-031-14054-9_31

and information are the most important assets of any organization. Their protection from intruders has become a necessity of today's life as the attackers may use captured data for malicious activities [6]. However, the client owns the data. Therefore, a client's data is shared between the client and the cloud, or the cloud must show the client how it works. Privacy-preserving machine learning (PPML) is a field of study that tries to find methods to solve this problem [7]. PPML research typically takes one of three approaches—first, Multiple-Party Computation (MPC) [8] and Secret Sharing (SS) [9]. Second, Homomorphic Encryption (HE) is another option [10, 11]. Third, a dependable execution environment [12] is required. This research will focus on the second method HE. CryptoNet [14] is the first network in privacy-preserving achieved accuracy rate on the MNIST dataset was 98.95. Later two works [15] and [16] relied on CryptoNets, but they achieved higher accuracy than CryptoNets. Chabanne et al. [15] achieved an accuracy rate of 99.30%, while CryptoDL [16] achieved 99.52%. Chou et al. [1] present and evaluate new methods for speeding up CryptoNets. This work relies on efficient polynomial approximations for the activation functions and pruning and quantization. As a result, this proposed network was Faster than CryptoNets. An alternative FHE-DiNN approach for homomorphic prediction in neural networks was recently presented by Bourse et al. [17] Compared with Cryptonet, the accuracy was low (96.35%). In recent decades, the polynomial function support for CNN evaluation on homomorphically encrypted data has been necessary research. These researches [1, 14, 15], and [16] have been used low-degree polynomial approximations of activation have so far been used to build HE-friendly alternatives, as illustrated in Table 1.

Table 1. Polynomial approximations of activation function to related works

Related works	Methods of the polynomial approximation
[14, 15]	Square polynomial
[1]	Taylor-series polynomials
[16]	Chebyshev polynomials and Taylor series approach

This paper aims to build an effective HE-friendly polynomial activation function for CNNs. The following contributions were fought toward this aim:

1- suggest new activation functions based on polynomial dominos, equivalent to the standard activation functions such as Rectified linear unit (Relu) and Softmax.
2- propose a CNN, namely MnistCNN; this network was trained on the Mnist dataset once with the Relu activation function and again with a HE-friendly polynomial.
3- increase cloud computing privacy by storing customer data in an encrypted form within the cloud.

2 Proposed System

There are multiple steps illustrated in Fig. 1 used to achieve the above aim. First, the CNN is trained cloud-side on unencrypted data based on a global dataset from the same field of research used for model generation, such as the MNIST dataset. The client then generates the public and private keys based on its chosen set of variables. After that, the weights that result from the training process based on the public key sent by the client are encrypted in the cloud. Next, the client chooses which encrypted data must be classified and uploads it to the cloud. Finally, the cloud classifies the encrypted data based on the encrypted weights by applying the principles of HE, which allow the use of addition and multiplication operations on the encrypted data. The result of this step is the encrypted class corresponding to the client's data. This encrypted class is then sent to the client and decrypted using the private key to produce an inference result.

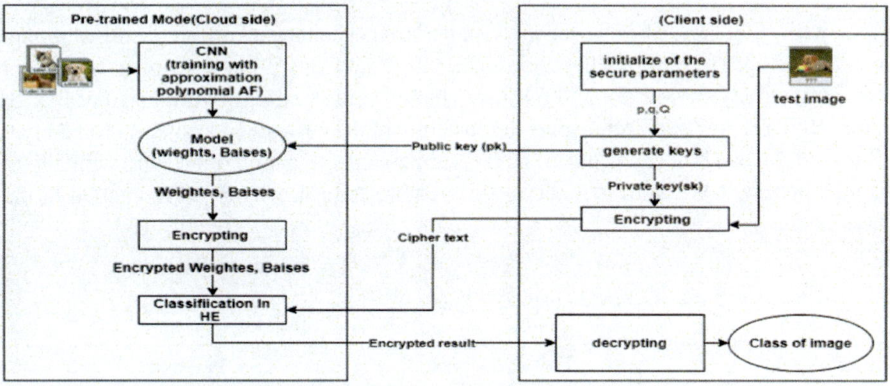

Fig. 1. Inference of the encrypted data in cloud computing.

Table 2. Polynomial approximations of activation functions and related works

Related works	Methods of approximation
[14, 15]	Square
[1]	Taylor-series
[16]	Chebyshev and Taylor

2.1 Datasets

The MNIST dataset is used in this project, which was constructed from the original NIST database. It contains 70,000 images, of which 60,000 training images and 10,000 are test images. These black and white digits are size-normalized and centred in a fixed-size image where the centre of gravity of the intensity lies at the centre of images of size 28 * 28 pixels [18]. The key specifications of this dataset are summarized in Table 2.

Table 3. Specification of MNIST Datasets

Properties	Values
Complexity	Easy
Image type	Grayscale
Image dimension	28 × 28
Number of classes	10
Training set size	60,000
Test set size	10,000

2.2 Network Architecture

As shown in Table 3, the CNN used in the paper's experiment uses different convolutional layers. The input size of this network is 28 * 28 * 1. 'Conv32' and 'Conv64' represent convolutional layers with 32 and 64 filter channels, respectively, with a size of 3 × 3. 'Conv-BN-Act-AvgPool' represents the structure of the network as a convolutional layer followed by a batch normalization (BN) layer and an activation (Act) layer, with a final average pooling (AvePool) layer. Two fully connected (FC) layers were applied in the networks.

Table 4. MNISTNet: CNN network of the MNIST dataset

Layer (type)	Output shape	Param #
Convolution	(None, 26, 26, 32)	320
Batch normalization	(None, 26, 26, 32)	128
Activation function	(None, 26, 26, 32)	0
Average pooling	(None, 13, 13, 32)	
Convolution	(None, 11, 11, 64)	18,496
Batch normalization	(None, 11, 11, 64)	256
Activation function	(None, 11, 11, 64)	0
Convolution	(None, 9, 9, 64)	36,928
Batch normalization	(None, 9, 9, 64)	256
Activation function	(None, 9, 9, 64)	0
Average pooling	(None, 4, 4, 64)	0
Flatten	(None, 1024)	0
Dense	(None, 100)	102,500
Dense	(None, 10)	1,010

2.3 Finding Practical Polynomial Activation Functions

Activation functions should be monotonic, differentiable, and quickly converge to weights for optimization purposes [19]. This paper will propose an approximation activation function of an essential activation function, namely the rectified linear unit (ReLU), which is the most popular activation function for updating the hidden layers. ReLU returns 0 when it is passed a negative value and returns the value itself for any positive input. This function is defined as [20]:

$$f(x) = \max(0, x) \tag{1}$$

The function and its derivative are shown in Fig. 2.

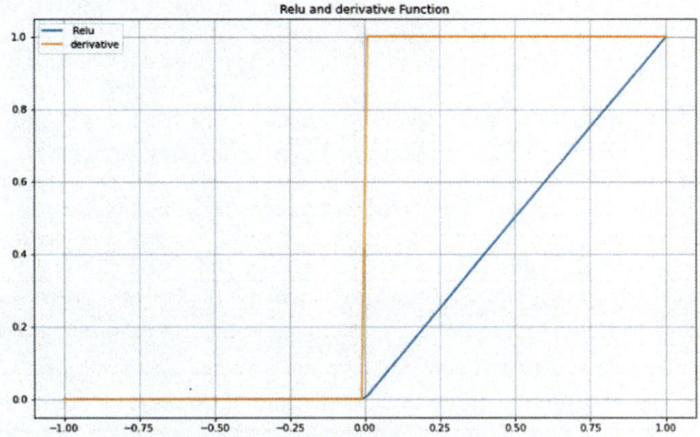

Fig. 2. ReLU function and its derivative.

As shown above, the function outputs 0 for any value less than zero, while the function is monotonic and continuous for positive values. In addition, the function's derivative is 0 for $z < 0$ and 1 for z>; however, the function is not differentiable at $z = 0$. Therefore, it is not differentiable for negative inputs and the derivative is 0. This research converted several ReLU functions to approximate polynomial functions with different ranges and degrees, as shown in Table 4.

Table 5. Approximation polynomial activation functions

Standard activation function	Approximation method	X-axis range to be fitted	Degree	Error LSE	Error RMSE	Proposed approximated polynomial function
Legendre	Relu	[−1, 1]	2	0.08969	0.00132	$0.24939994 + 0.5 * x + 0.30940594 * x^2$
			4	0.05421	0.00033	$0.250295492 + 0.5 * x + 0.313927337 * x^2 - 0.0910565796 * x^4$
			6	0.03822	0.00012	$0.249843075 + 0.5 * x + 0.311644182 * x^2 - 0.095254539 * x^4 + 0.0484619548 * x^6$
		[−2, 2]	2	0.17938	0.00530	$0.26674542 + 0.5 * x + 0.15470297 * x^2$
			4	0.10843	0.00132	$0.243804095 + 0.5 * x + 0.242329212 * x^2 - 0.0113820725 * x^4$
			6	0.07644	0.00051	$0.245615429 + 0.5 * x + 0.293395872 * x^2 - 0.0323517046 * x^4 + 0.00151443609 * x^6$
		[−4, 4]	2	0.35877	0.02121	$0.41746362 + 0.5 * x + 0.07735149 * x^2$
			4	0.21687	0.00528	$0.303193608 + 0.5 * x + 0.131835299 * x^2 - 0.00142275906 * x^4$
			6	0.15288	0.00205	$0.263663638 + 0.5 * x + 0.178536179 * x^2 - 0.00468286579 * x^4 + 0.0000473261277 * x^6$
Taylor	Softmax		2	0.00169	0.0000002	$(1 + x + 0.5 * x^2)/\sum(1 + x + 0.5 * x^2)$

The results of the proposed approximate polynomial functions in Table 4 are shown in Fig. 4. Note that the outputs of the proposed functions are identical to those of the original functions. This comparison suggested that each function is implemented within different degrees and ranges because the network's data may occur within different ranges. However, from Fig. 3, we note that despite the different ranges, the shape of all the functions is very similar, indicating that the proposed functions perform the same work as the original functions when applied within a network.

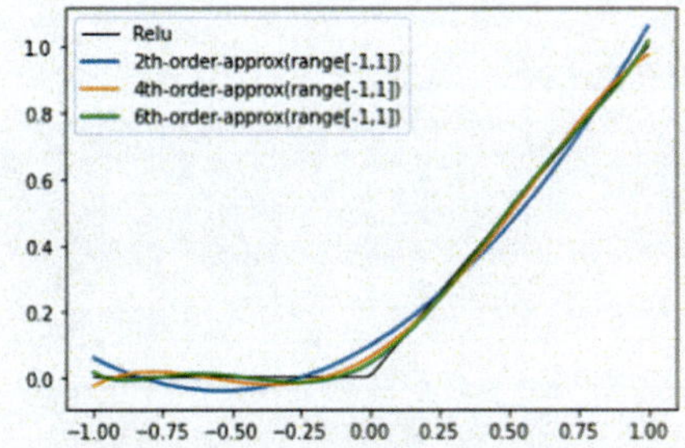

A: ReLU and its approximation for range[-1,1]

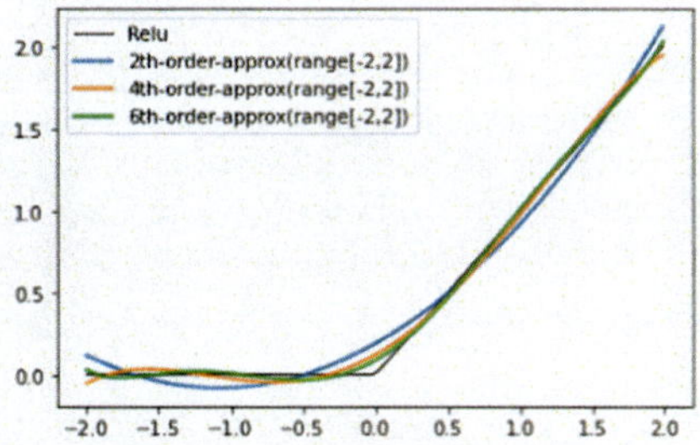

B: ReLU and its approximation for range[-2,2]

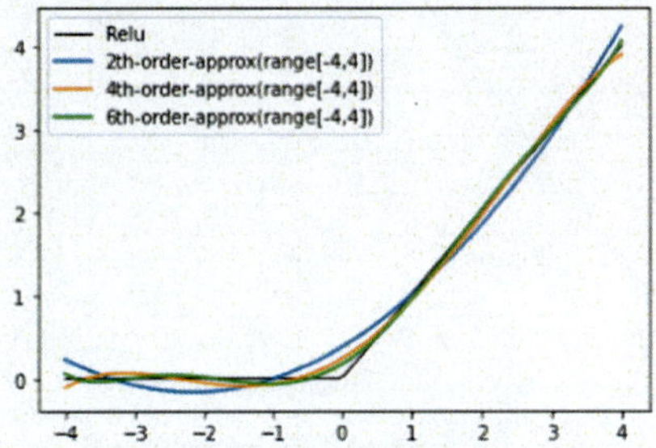

C: Relu and its approximation for range [-4,4]

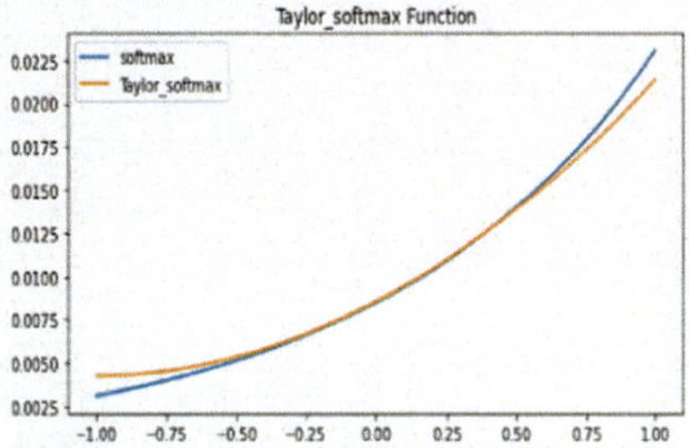

D: Softmax and its approximation for range [-1,1]

Fig. 3. Standard activation functions and their approximations

Differentiable

For neural networks, backpropagation is a common and effective training method. The gradients functions employed in a network are used in this training method to determine how much weight to modify during optimization. As a result, differentiability in the activation function is essential [13].

Figure 5a shows the ReLU function and its derivative over the range [−1, 1]. The function and its derivative converge only in the region less than zero, with divergence at zero and subsequent convergence towards unity. We note that in Fig. 5b, convergence exists along with the same range. The LSE and RMSE values for standard ReLU and its derivative were 0.98989 and 0.16498, respectively, while the equivalent values of the approximated function and its derivative were 0.262005 and 0.03479, respectively (Table 5). The authors note that the approximation function gave a nominal error rate. Thus, Fig. 5 and Table 5 demonstrate that the approximation function is better differentiable than the standard function.

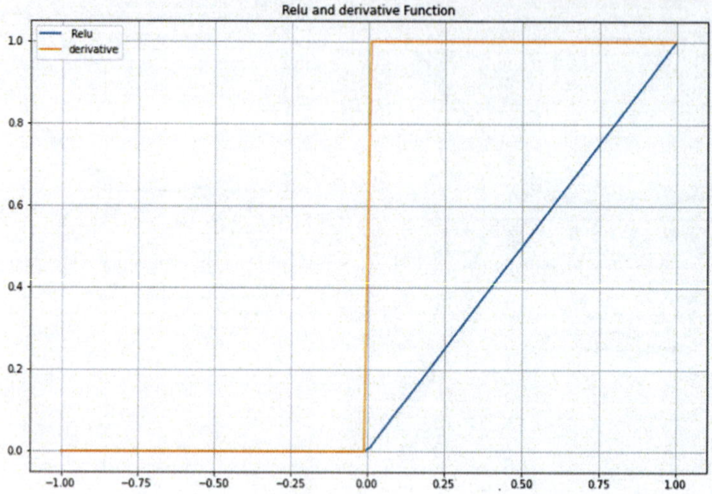

a. ReLU function and its derivative in the range [-1,1] with degree 2

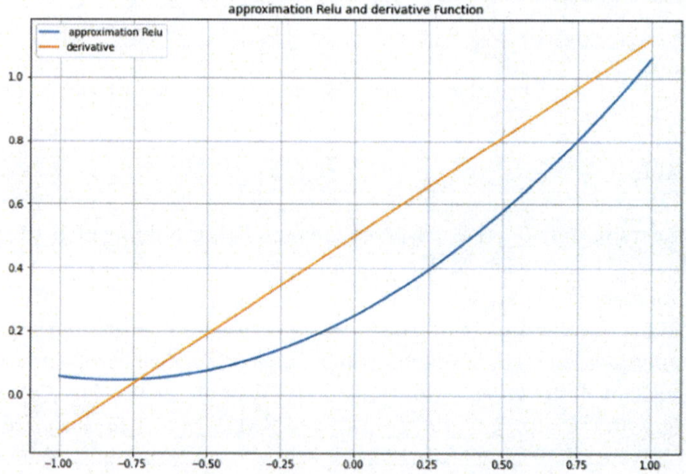

b. Approximations of the ReLu function with its derivative in the range [-1,1] with degree 2

Fig. 4. Activation functions and their derivatives

Table 6. The error between the activation function and its derivative

Activation function	LSE	RMSE
Standard ReLU	0.98989	0.16498
Approximate ReLU	0.262005	0.03479

Continuous

There are two approaches to assess whether a function is continuous or not; the first is based on graphs, while the second is based on the limit function. In the first method, for some function f(x), the continuity between points a and b can be simply assessed if the graph of f(x) over this region could be plotted without lifting one's hand from the graph paper. In the second method, some function f(x) can be said to be continuous at a given point x0 if $\lim_{x \to x0} f(x) = f(x0)$, while function f(x) is said to be continuous in the open interval (a, b) if at any point in the given interval the function is continuous. For the case of closed interval [a, b], the function is said to be continuous if f(x) is continuous in the open interval (a, b) [21]:

$$\operatorname{Lim}_{x \to xa} f(x) = f(a) \tag{2}$$

$$\operatorname{Lim}_{x \to xb} f(x) = f(b) \tag{3}$$

Based on these two methods, all the functions shown in Table 4 are continuous. Through the graphs shown in Fig. 4, we note that all the functions when drawn over their corresponding ranges (i.e. [−1, 1], [−2, 2], [−4, 4]) showed no interruption in the line drawn between a and b where a is the lower value and b is the higher value. By applying Eqs. (1) and (2) to all the equations shown in Table 4, the output values extracted from f(x) are close to $\lim_{x \to [a,b]} f(x)$. For example, consider 0.24939994 + 0.5 * x + 0.30940594 * x^2 for values of x in the range [−1, 1]. The values of this equation when applied to the range [1, −1] and those corresponding to the limit function are shown in Table 6. The consistency in results is demonstrated by the zero differences recorded between the values of the original equation and the limit function.

Table 7. Continuous of approximation function

f(x) = 0.24939994 + 0.5 * x + 0.30940594 * x^2	$Lim_{x \to xa,b} f(x)$
0.0588058	0.05880588
0.05653192	0.05653192
0.99213558	0.99213558

Monotonic

A function *f* is described as monotonic when it changes consistently in a single direction, either by increasing or decreasing [22]. There are two methods to assess whether a function is monotonic or not, as follows. Graphically, it is trivial to assess whether a function is increasing, decreasing or neither. Notice that all the functions graphed in this study change in one direction, i.e. up or down. If the function graph is not available, a function can be determined as monotonic or not by applying the following conditions to the function's derivative. Let i be an open interval and let f: i → real number(r) be differentiable. Case (i): if $f'(x) \leq 0$ for all x in i, then the function f is decreasing. Alternatively, in case (ii), if and only if $f'(x) \geq 0$ for all x in i, then function f is increasing. **Theorem 1:** An interval in which a function has a changing sign indicates that said function is not monotonic. It is sufficient to demonstrate that f′ takes on distinct signs at various places to prove that a function is not monotonic.

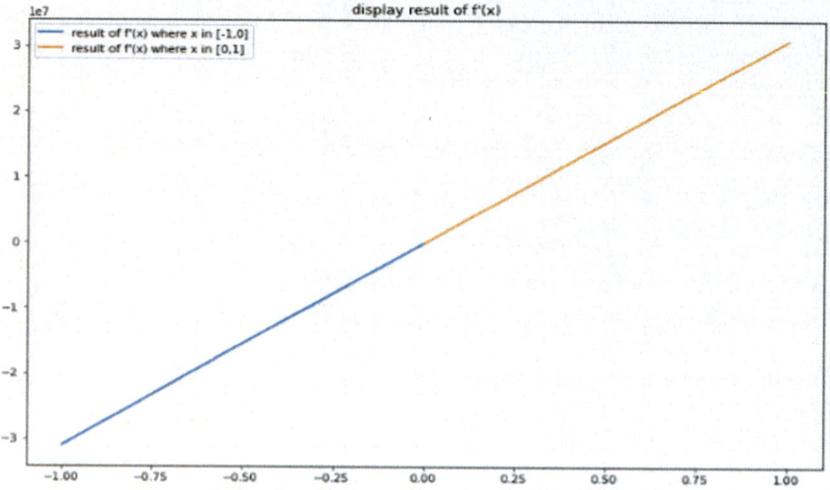

Fig. 5. Results of f(x) for x between [−1, 1]

For more data to prove the validity of theorem 1, a set of data was considered between [−1, 1]. The derivative equation *f'(x)* was applied to the data between [−1, 0] for 100 real number values. The results showed that all values are negative values less than zero, corresponding to case (i) above, where the result appears from the lowest value (around -3.09×10^{-7}) to the highest value (approx. -3.12×10^{-5}), which indicates that the derivative of the function with negative values is increasing. Also, notice that all the results are positive and increase when taking 100 values between [0, 1]. The results in Fig. 6 and comparison with Theorem 1 indicates that the approximation polynomial function is monotonic.

Bounded Derivative

Activation functions with bounded derivatives lead neural networks to perform effectively due to the bounded derivatives restricting the training algorithm from updating the network's weights [20]. If this phenomenon is not prevented, there will be large resultant variations in the network's weights and instability in the training process. As an example, Fig. 5 shows that ReLU and its approximation functions are bounded derivative functions because all values of the derivative fall between 0 and 1.

2.4 Accuracy in Plaintext Using Different Activation Functions

The Keras framework was used to train the CNN network using various activation functions. With a Nesterov momentum of 0.9, the Adam optimizer was employed for learning.

The learning rate was 0.1, with a 10^{-6} decrease in the decay rate with each update. Table 8 shows the accuracy, loss, and confusion matrix of the MNISTNet models. In this table, the training and validation results shown are based on the standard Relu activation function for all convolution layers and the Softmax function in the Fully connected layer. In addition, a configuration is shown with the proposed approximate ReLU functions for the convolution layers and proposed Taylor Softmax for the fully connected layers. As shown in Table 3, the MNISTNet model has three convolutional layers with 32, 64 and 64 filter channels. Our approximate ReLU activations and the Taylor Softmax function achieved better results than the ReLu activation and Softmax configuration, illustrating the excellent expressiveness of polynomial activations in MNISTNet. Both versions of our polynomial activations during the training process gave higher testing accuracy and lower testing loss than the standard activation functions. These results show that the accuracy of approximation functions is close to that of ReLU. Compared to the ReLU function, the proposed model achieved the best validation accuracy with a second-degree function.

Table 8. Performance of standard and approximate activation functions

Activation function	X-axis range to be fitted		Degree	validation		Training	
				Loss	Accuracy	Loss	Accuracy
ReLU	-	-	9	0.037	0.989	0.0379	0.989
		2	4	0.039	0.992	0.0204	0.998
	[-1,1]	4	0	0.060	0.983	0.0309	0.994
		6	9	0.743	0.777	0.760	0.776
		2	8	0.034	0.993	0.0246	0.997
Approximation method	[-2,2]	4	0	0.058	0.992	0.0368	0.996
		6	9	1.886	0.559	0.0379	0.992
		2	7	0.075	0.989	0.0467	0.993
	[-4,4]	4	0	0.049	0.993	0.0349	0.996
		6	1	0.066	0.991	0.0366	0.995

2.5 Accuracy in Ciphertext Using Approximation Activation Functions

We used approximate activation functions with degree two, range $[-1, 1]$ and Taylor Softmax in our model because these functions provided greater plaintext prediction accuracy; using this configuration, a detailed investigation was performed on encrypted data. In addition, the prediction performance of the MNISTNet model was examined. The inference phase of the CNN was performed over HE using Microsoft's Simple Encrypted Arithmetic Library (SEAL), which implements the CKKS scheme based on pre-training models resulting from MNISTNet. This inference phase begins when the client generates the public and private keys to encrypt the image(s) and later sends the encrypted image(s) to the server. In this phase, using CKKS as the FHE algorithm, the client initially takes the image as a message and converts it to cypher vectors ([⟨ct1, pk⟩]%q, [⟨ct2, pk⟩]%q), where ct1 and ct2 are ciphertexts represented in polynomial form, pk represents the public key, and q refers to the ciphertext modulus. On the server-side, the image inference process uses the pre-training model (M), which has already been trained on plain images using MNISTNet with the MNIST dataset. After receiving the encrypted data with the public key by the server, a model is encrypted using the public key. All operations are then performed through ciphertext–ciphertext multiplication or ciphertext–ciphertext addition to extract the class of the encrypted image(s).

Table 9. Experiment results on encrypted data Models

Models	Conv structure	Circuit depth	Poly modules	Prediction time (s)	accuracy
[14]	5-10	2	8192	0.39	98.95%
[15]	32-32-64-64-128-128	6	16384	100	99.30%
[16]	32-32-64-64-128-128	6	16384	50	99.52%
Our MINSTNet	32-64-64	3	16384	43	99.80%

Table 9 compares three different models, i.e. the CrytoNets[14] model, which uses square activation, in addition to the model in study[15] and CryptoDL[16], which make use of non-trainable polynomial activations. Comparing the three models shows that the proposed activations in MNISTNet achieve higher prediction accuracy with considerably less computing resources required than the models in [15] and [16] but with more resource requirements than the model from [14].

2.6 Evaluation of CNN

Table 9 shows the results of the classification of the MNIST dataset. As a result of the evaluation, we achieved the best classification accuracy of 99.8%, a value of 0.28% greater than that achieved by the next-best model, i.e. the model from study [16]. We classified 8,192 images with one inference; thus, the amortized time (i.e. inference execution time per image) in the proposed method achieved the best value of 3.20 ms (approximating Swish with a second degree polynomial in the range [−1, 1]). The CNN was evaluated using a confusion matrix, shown in Fig. 6a. The accuracy and loss functions of the training and validation are also shown in Fig. 6b and c.

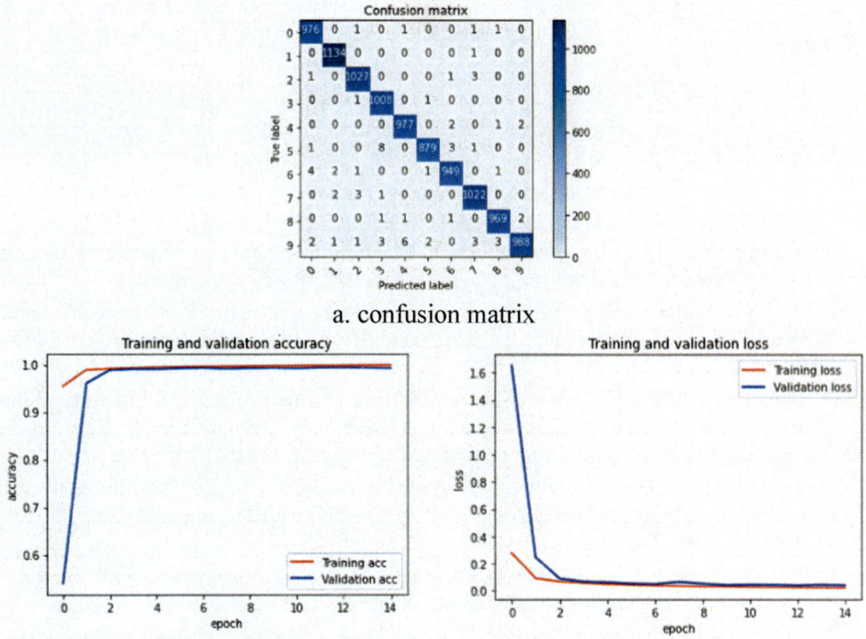

a. confusion matrix

b. Accuracy

c.Loss

Fig. 6. Evaluation of CNN (MINSTNet) with degree 2 and range [1, −1]

3 Conclusions

This paper proposes a method for improving the classification accuracy for CNN inference using HE by adopting BN with a polynomial approximated activation function as an activation function instead of the square function. We apply the polynomial approximated activation function's layer combination and coefficient manipulation to reduce the multiplicative depth. For CNN inference, an approach that replaces the ReLU and Softmax activation function with polynomial approximated versions was presented; using batch normalization before each function led to improved classification accuracy. Several approximation methods were compared to identify the best-performing approach. The proposed approach achieved a classification accuracy of 99.80% for the MNIST dataset, outperforming other related studies by 0.28%. In the future, we plan to reduce memory use during inference and extend these techniques to more complex network models.

References

1. Chou, E., Beal, J., Levy, D., Yeung, S., Haque, A., Fei-Fei, L.: Faster CryptoNets: leveraging sparsity for real-world encrypted inference. arXiv, November 2018. https://arxiv.org/abs/1811.09953. Accessed 14 Nov 2021
2. Denning, D.E.R.: Cryptography and data security (1982)
3. Yassein, H.R., Al-Saidi, N.M.G., Farhan, A.K.: A new NTRU cryptosystem outperforms three highly secured NTRU-analog systems through an innovational algebraic structure. J. Discret. Math. Sci. Cryptogr. (2020). https://doi.org/10.1080/09720529.2020.1741218
4. Kadhim, A.F., Kamal, Z.A.: Generating dynamic S-box based on particle swarm optimization and chaos theory for AES. Iraqi J. Sci. **59**(3), 1733–1745 (2018). https://doi.org/10.24996/IJS.2018.59.3C.18
5. Alhudhaif, A., Ahmad, M., Alkhayyat, A., Tsafack, N., Farhan, A.K., Ahmed, R.: Block cipher nonlinear confusion components based on new 5-D hyperchaotic system. IEEE Access **9**, 87686–87696 (2021). https://doi.org/10.1109/ACCESS.2021.3090163
6. Zahid, A.H., et al.: Efficient dynamic S-box generation using linear trigonometric transformation for security applications. IEEE Access **9**, 98460–98475 (2021). https://doi.org/10.1109/ACCESS.2021.3095618
7. Podschwadt, R., Takagi, D., Hu, P.: SoK: privacy-preserving deep learning with homomorphic encryption (2021). http://arxiv.org/abs/2112.12855
8. Yao, A.C.C.: How to generate and exchange secrets. In: Annual Symposium Foundations of Computer Science, no. 1, pp. 162–167 (1986). https://doi.org/10.1109/sfcs.1986.25
9. Shamir, A.: How to share a secret. Commun. ACM **22**(11), 612–613 (1979). https://doi.org/10.1145/359168.359176
10. Gentry, C.S.: Fully homomorphic encryption from approximate ideal lattices. Ruan Jian Xue Bao J. Softw. **26**(10), 2696–2719 (2015). https://doi.org/10.13328/j.cnki.Jos.004808
11. Cheon, J.H., Han, K., Kim, A., Kim, M., Song, Y.: Bootstrapping for approximate homomorphic encryption. In: Nielsen, J.B., Rijmen, V. (eds.) EUROCRYPT 2018. LNCS, vol. 10820, pp. 360–384. Springer, Cham (2018). https://doi.org/10.1007/978-3-319-78381-9_14
12. McKeen, F., et al.: Innovative instructions and software model for isolated execution. In: Proceeding of the 2nd International Workshop HASP (2013). https://doi.org/10.1145/2487726.2488368
13. Obla, S., Gong, X., Aloufi, A., Hu, P., Takabi, D.: Effective activation functions for homomorphic evaluation of deep neural networks. IEEE Access **8**, 153098–153112 (2020). https://doi.org/10.1109/ACCESS.2020.3017436
14. Dowlin, N., et al.: CryptoNets: applying neural networks to encrypted data with high throughput and accuracy - Microsoft research. Microsoft Res. TechReport **48**, 1–12 (2016). http://proceedings.mlr.press/v48/gilad-bachrach16.pdf. http://research.microsoft.com/apps/pubs/?id=260989
15. Chabanne, H.: Privacy-preserving classification on deep neural network. Med. Today **4**(7), 59–64 (2017)
16. Hesamifard, E., Takagi, H., Ghasemi, M.: CryptoDL: deep neural networks over encrypted data, pp. 1–21 (2017). http://arxiv.org/abs/1711.05189
17. Bourse, F., Minelli, M., Minihold, M., Paillier, P.: Fast homomorphic evaluation of deep discretized neural networks. In: Shacham, H., Boldyreva, A. (eds.) CRYPTO 2018. LNCS, vol. 10993, pp. 483–512. Springer, Cham (2018). https://doi.org/10.1007/978-3-319-96878-0_17
18. Deng, L.: The MNIST database of handwritten digit images for machine learning research. IEEE Signal Process. Mag. **29**(6), 141–142 (2012). https://doi.org/10.1109/MSP.2012.2211477

19. Ohn, I., Kim, Y.: Smooth function approximation by deep neural networks with general activation functions. Entropy **21**(7), 1–24 (2019). https://doi.org/10.3390/e21070627
20. Maennel, H., Bousquet, O., Gelly, S.: Gradient descent quantizes ReLU network features, arXiv, vol. abs/1803.0 (2018)
21. Harrou, F., Zeroual, A., Sun, Y.: Calcuas. In: Proceedings of the American Control Conference, vol. 2018-June, pp. 604–609 (2018). https://doi.org/10.23919/ACC.2018.8431387
22. Obla, S., Gong, X., Aloufi, A., Hu, P., Takabi, D.: Effective activation functions for homomorphic evaluation of deep neural networks (2020)

Real-Time Detection of TOR Attacks from the Dark Web

Selahattin Hürol Türen[1,2](✉), Kenneth Eustace[1,2], Rafiqul Islam[1,2], and Geoffrey Fellows[1,2]

[1] Charles Sturt University, Wagga Wagga, Australia
hturen@csu.edu.au
[2] Charles Sturt University, Albury, Australia

Abstract. This paper discusses a case study project in cybersecurity on the Dark Web that uses quantitative data science research methods and techniques. Beginning with a comparative analysis of dark web forum data sets using data science techniques and then adding an experimental research design that includes machine learning techniques and strategies for training and development of a model.

After the gap analysis was identified from an extensive literature review, the authors suggest that it is possible to try to extend or modify these algorithms or the applied techniques. This hybrid experimental research methodology will lead to a proposal on mitigating risks via a model for real-time detection, evaluation, and response by cybersecurity professionals.

Keywords: Dark web · Threat analytics · Machine learning algorithms · Real-time detection · Hybrid experimental research

1 Introduction

The dark web is an encrypted subset of the deep web, whose content cannot be indexed by search engines [1]. Dark web pages can be accessed from private networks such as TOR (The Onion Routing), I2P (Invisible Internet Project), Freenet. TOR is widely used by the dark web users in a domain defined by.onion extension. Dark web users can communicate with each other without using their identifications. However, the anonymity of the users encourages them to perform illegal activities.

There are two issues to be considered in the dark web. First, it is important to monitor the illegal activities, which can give global damage. Second, it is important to protect the identity of users, who use TOR just to hide their identity without performing illegal activities. This is also as much as important to monitor illegal activities.

Dark web users can communicate with each other without using their identities. However, the anonymity of the users encourages them to perform illegal activities.

The worst illegal activities are about terror activities such as how to build a bomb or how and where to perform suicide bombing. Human trafficking [2] and child pornography [3] can also be seen as the worst illegal activities. Drug dealing [4] and DDOS (Distributed Denial of Service) activities [5] can follow these worst illegal activities.

K. Daimi and A. Al Sadoon (Eds.): ICR 2022, AISC 1431, pp. 346–355, 2022.
https://doi.org/10.1007/978-3-031-14054-9_32

Crypto currency stealing, distributing fake ids are also bad enough for the people and communities.

Another big issue is the usage of the Dark Web in a war. During a war between two or more countries, hackers use the Dark Web to destroy the information systems of the enemy. This can be called as a Cyber Warfare.

For instance, hackers have hacked the SyTech is one of the contractors of FSB which is the Russian National Intelligence Service. These hackers wanted to gather the internal company project information of SyTech which are related to FSB [6]. They were successful to steal 7.5 TB data from SyTech.

An interesting example comes from Twitter. During the war between Russia and Ukraine, the Russian government has restricted the social media companies like Facebook and Twitter. Twitter has overcome this restriction by using TOR to launch a privacy protected site [7].

The following are the objectives of this paper. These objectives are the main issues of the further research.

1) Introduce some machine learning and AI algorithms which have already applied to monitor the illegal activities in the Dark Web. This also includes the attacks in the Dark Web to deanonymise the users. This is very important, because many users are leaving TOR network, because they are afraid to be exposed during such attacks.
2) Introduce a cyber forensic maturity model, which can make possible to monitor and detect the illegal activities in the Dark Web in real-time by optimising machine learning algorithms.

2 Background

There are two types of threat which should be concerned in the TOR network. One of them is the attacks on TOR Network from adversaries, whose aim is to deanonymise the users. Another threat is revision of dark web activities detection methods which explains different machine learning algorithms to monitor the illegal forum activities on TOR Network. These forum activities can trigger cybercrime events in the future, that's why it is important to monitor and detect them on time.

2.1 Attacks on TOR

Anonymity is the most important feature of TOR. That is why the user should not get worried about the exposure of his location and his identity. A weakness of TOR network is that TOR has a decentralised architecture which makes it possible for adversaries to launch Distributed Hash Table attacks (DHT). [8] A distributed hash table is a hash table, which includes key value pairs of the connected nodes in a network. That is why it is quite easy to find the value of each connected node with its given key. It is quite easy to find the value of a connected node from its key. That is the big advantage of a DHT. It is possible to group these attacks as Eclipse Attacks, Website Fingerprint Attacks and RAPTOR (Routing Attacks on Privacy in TOR).

Eclipse Attacks Against TOR Hidden Services. In an Eclipse attack an adversary captures the DHT, receives the information of the onion router key value pairs and monitors and blocks the incoming and outcoming communication of the users, so that they cannot communicate with the rest of the onion routes in the network. The hidden services in TOR are kept as their descriptors in the Hidden Service Directories (HSDirs) [8].

If a user wants to be connected to a hidden service, this user should grab a hidden service descriptor. This descriptor includes short messages about the hidden service, which is updated periodically. A short message includes important information about nodes like their descriptor ids. A descriptor id is a hash code, which is updated every day [9]. A HSDir can save the descriptor of a hidden service according to the smallest XOR – distance between the HSDir fingerprint list and descriptor ids. If the adversary has a good algorithm, it is possible for him to calculate and collect such HSDirs to block user, which makes it impossible for them to reach the right hidden service. An Eclipse attack on a TOR hidden service has the following phases:

Phase 1: Calculation of the hidden service's descriptor ids. Every TOR Hidden Service has descriptors, and these descriptors make it possible for the user to connect with their hidden services anonymously. A descriptor contains information from the hidden service. Those are the introduction points of hidden services. An adversary can predict these introduction points easily. That's because some TOR networks can upload these descriptors with their HSDir flags. These relays with HSDir flag have the form of a DHT and they are called as Hidden Service Directory Servers (HSDirs). These servers can be considered as a DNS of TOR Network. The HSDirs includes onion router (OR) information which the user wants to connect. That's why these HSDirs are very important for the adversaries.

Phase 2: Take over the Hidden Service Directories and start an Eclipse attack. The HSDirs have the descriptor Ids and onion router fingerprints, which makes it possible for a user to connect with its hidden service. If an adversary can calculate the descriptor ids, he or she can obtain the hash table of the given descriptor ids with their fingerprints, and it is good enough to start an Eclipse attack on TOR. The attacker can collect the private key in a secret Id key file. A TOR instance can be restarted with a Data Directory (DataDir) which contains the secret Id key file in a key directory. The TOR instance runs with the ORs fingerprints, which are provided via the descriptor Ids. The attacker runs this process 96 h long to grab the HSDir flags. Then it is possible for the adversary to take control over the hidden service directories. The attacker can modify the TORs source code before the ORs are running and this blocks the user to get the appropriate data from the target hidden data descriptor. This is a DOS attack. An Eclipse attack can be persistent. That's possible by mocking the HDirs and having a high secrecy for the mocked data for a long period of time. The attacker should know how many instances he or she needs to run to manage a persistent Eclipse attack.

It is viable to perform a shadowing technique to make an Eclipse attack persistent. [10] If the attacker sets up the nodes to receive descriptor Ids from the HSDirs, it will take longer than 96 h to gather all relays with their HSDir flags.

Website Fingerprinting Attack. A website fingerprinting attack determines the URLs of the visited websites of a user by using the TOR browser. That is a kind of monitoring of the communication of the web sites in the TOR network to describe the network traffic of the users in the TOR network. It is possible to determine what kind of user visit which web sites or forums in the dark web. [11] Static and dynamic web sites exist in the TOR network. The research studies investigated mostly the website fingerprinting attacks on the static web sites.

The advantage of stream mining algorithms is that they could renew their models frequently. Another advantage of these stream mining algorithms is that they can recognise concept drifts. This feature gives them the opportunity to be applied for the website fingerprinting attacks against the websites with dynamic contents. The research of [11] has used the stream mining algorithm for the following methods to see, which method is the best for a website fingerprinting attack.

These following four Hoeffding Tree-based algorithms are examined by [11] and Adaptive Hoeffding Tree gives the best detection rate, because it updates its model, and this makes the model adaptable for the new data, as shown in Table 1. Adapting Hoeffding Trees can learn from constant content updates, and this makes them to have a better recognition rate by the detection of the visited websites.

Table 1. The results of stream mining algorithms [11].

Methods	Window	Precision%	Recall%	Accuracy%	Kappa%
Adaptive Hoeffding tree	1000	97.97	99.00	98.97	97.80
	5000	98.74	98.99	98.87	98.77
	8000	98.99	99.12	99.20	98.81
EFDT	1000	98.00	98.10	98.20	98.14
	5000	98.10	98.13	98.20	98.13
	8000	98.15	98.14	98.20	98.14
OzaBag	1000	98.07	98.04	98.02	98.04
	5000	98.25	98.40	98.85	97.93
	8000	98.24	98.69	98.88	98.79
CVFDT	1000	98.00	98.14	98.26	98.15
	5000	98.13	98.17	98.24	98.17
	8000	98.11	98.17	98.27	98.16

Adaptive Hoeffding Tree: This kind of Hoeffding tree has additional feature to expose changes in the data streams. These changes make the stream module to adapt itself during the changes in the data streams [12].

Extreme Fast Decision Tree (EFDT): EFDT is another kind of Hoeffding tree which is the implementation of Hoeffding Anytime Tree (HATT). EFDT has a higher predictive sequential accuracy than VFDT (Very Fast Decision Tree) [13] HATT has only one difference from a Hoeffding tree. It applies a Hoeffding Bound to separate the attribute to examine if the separated attribute is better than the non-separated attribute.

OzaBag: This is a part of MOA (Massive Online Analysis) API, which is developed at the University of Waikato in New Zealand. It is a typical bagging and boosting learning method which is applied to data streams. Hoeffding trees are used as data streams in this situation.

Concept Adapting Very Fast Decision Tree (CVFDT): As it is clear from its name, this method is based on VFDT (Very Fast Decision Tree) and Hoeffding Tree algorithms. CVFDT takes the old data and builds another tree for it. It also builds another three for the new data. If the new data is more accurate than the old data, then the model replaces the old data with the new data in the alternative tree [14].

RAPTOR (Routing Attacks on Privacy in TOR). RAPTOR attacks are also threatening the anonymity of the user in the TOR network. That's why [15] wanted to protect the TOR network from RAPTOR attacks. [15] This research group has found out that Autonomous Systems (AS) adversaries exist almost 30% of entry exit pairs of Onion Routes. That's why, according to their research AS network adversaries are a big threat in the TOR network. It is possible for them to expose the identity of the anonymised users in TOR network by applying BGP (Border Gateway Protocol) hijacking attacks. These BGP hijacking attacks exist between entry and exit points in the TOR network. Therefore, they are called as RAPTOR attacks.

[15] tried to build a proactive defence against BGP attacks. That's why they have built a live monitoring system to monitor TOR relays in a real time to detect BGP hijacking attacks. It was important to find the resilience of TOR relays to prefix interception attacks and BGP hijack attacks.

How is it possible to describe the resilience of an AS?

Assume that there is source AS as s, a false origin as f which BGP hijack attack launches, and a true origin AS as t. If s is not deceived by f and it sends the traffic to t, then the AS is resilient against a BGP hijack attack. [15] has created an algorithm to calculate the resilience of an AS.

The following figure (see Fig. 1) shows Cumulative Distribution Function of different sort of AS resilience distributions:

According to the recent research passive AS level adversaries can adopt new algorithms which take care of asymmetric routing, relay capacity of TOR network and it is also important to collude ASes. Astoria is such a TOR client whose clients consider passive AS -level adversaries [16].

2.2 The Dark Web Activities Detection Methods

MLP (Machine Learning Perceptron). It is possible to apply MLP (Machine Learning Perceptron) to learn and train data from the Dark Web. The doc2vector method is useful for feature extraction. The author of [17] have optimised MLP hyperparameters via grid search which could divide hyperparameter search space into grids and it tests the all the hypermeter combinations of these grid intersections. Stratified k-fold cross validation is used to evaluate datasets. Cross validation methods split data so that ratio between evaluated and trained data stays same. Sixgill (https://www.cybersixgill.com)

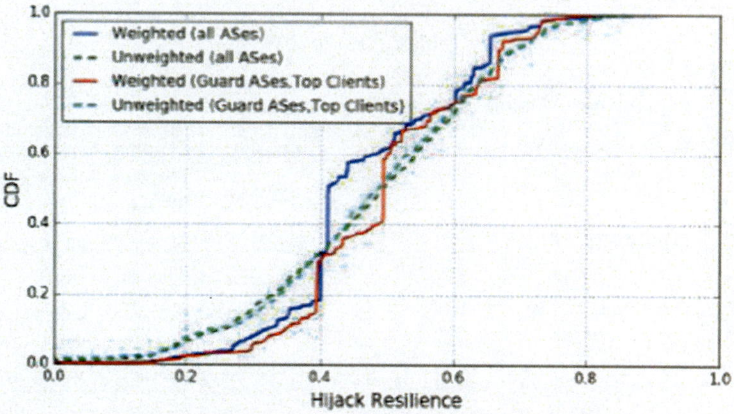

Fig. 1. Hijack resilience of TOR-Related ASes [15]

is used to collect data from the Dark Web. Sixgill provides very good search functionalities. MLP with optimised hyperparameters is applied to the dataset obtained by Sixgill and the classification result had 79.4% accuracy [17].

Black Widow. Black widow is a tool, which can parse raw data into HTML form, and it can also translate the data by using Google translator. [18] This tool is very helpful to extract and train the data with an ML model to learn from it to detect the illegal forum activities in TOR network. Black Widow has the following lifecycle: Planning and requirements, Collection, Processing and Dissemination.

The following Table 2 categorise these forums with the help of data processing by Black Widow [18]. Because of privacy issues, they didn't give the name of the forums.

Table 2. Categories of dark web forum [18].

Forum	Forum type	Online as of 12/2018	Language	Categories
Forum 1	Deep Web	Yes	English	News, Porn, Software, Drugs
Forum 2	Deep Web	No	Russian	Marketplace, Electronic Money, Hacking
Forum 3	Dark Web	No	French	Drugs, News, Porn, Technology
Forum 4	Dark Web	Yes	Russian	Marketplace, General Discussions, Hacking, Security

(*continued*)

Table 2. (*continued*)

Forum	Forum type	Online as of 12/2018	Language	Categories
Forum 5	Deep Web	Yes	English	Gaming, Leaks, Cracking, Hacking, Monetizing Techniques, Tutorials
Forum 6	Dark Web	No	French	News, Frauds, Conspiracy Theories, Drugs, Crime
Forum 7	Deep Web	Yes	Russian	Software, Security & Hacking, DDoS Services, Marketplace

3 Predictive Analysis and Real-Time Detection Model (PARTD)

Our experimental Machine Learning research will develop and combine the predictive analysis of Dark Web forum data sets with the capture and detection of real-time threat activity, even though results can appear as being asymptotic to a 'best practice' response and recovery. The model is an adaptable and expandable framework that learns from historical cases and goes beyond building a database of storing incoming real-time messages. The model has a machine learning framework that includes acceptance of predictive cases and the limiting and asymptotic behaviour in the run-time analysis. The performance of machine learning algorithms depends upon the relative latencies when using real-time vs near real-time network traffic as input data which in turn, requires rapid detection and response to each threat case.

In an analogous situation, consider the real-time or near real-time credit or debit card fraud detection at banks, as handled by the bank's fraud response team, monitoring online purchases. Once an anomalous behaviour is detected, the purchase transaction is suspended by a team member until they ring the consumer personally to verify. This can take 15–30 s after clicking the submit button. An analysis of the threat behaviour from the Dark Web can be incremental and build on current processes. However, as the model evolves with the latest infrastructure developments and AI technologies provided by quantum computing and nanometre chips, increase transistor density and speed, while reducing power use, so that the AI response can be faster and automated, when compared to current response teams at the bank.

The data collection of Dark Web forum data, network traffic data in real-time or near real-time will be assisted by use of Anaconda Python ML libraries (pandas, Jupiter notebooks, TensorFlow). The steps begin with pre-processing of data, checking for missing data, data cleaning of data types and univariate data analysis. Data science methods are then used for exploratory observation of patterns and anomalies in parameter values that can raise an alert.

Machine Learning algorithms categorise the output data from each alert to further use classifiers for classification of each 'response experience' as part of the training of an ML model. This is where rapid training of a classifier model occurs automatically with a series of labelled real-time events, scaled from normal to anomalous. The outcome is rapid real-time or near real-time responses by monitoring teams with low latency. Furthermore, post-processing methods examine the historical content analysis of cases. Such observation of historical patterns then assists clustering and forecasting from the model.

As defined in the Cyber Security Applications book [19] it is important to build a Cyber Forensics Maturity Model as an added layer to the model. The Prevention-Detection-Response-Recovery (PDR^2) model was described in [20], as a Personal Cyber Security Model based on Self–Awareness and Intervention. The PARTD Model has Prevention, Detection, Response and Recovery as a series of iterative steps and can support the steps within this proposal model.

Prevention is the first important step. Companies and organisations prevent their systems by using firewalls and managed passwords. (Example: two-phased password protection of Commerzbank in Germany) Other issues of prevention are ethics and cyber security. The second iterative step is detection which always comes after prevention. It does not make sense to leave the system uncontrolled after the prevention process. It is important to decide how often the system should be controlled to detect input and output data. Prevention and Detection steps are performed by ML or AI techniques.

There are tools and teams which can support Response phase like CERT (Computer Emergency Response Team). It is possible for CERT to deliver active and up to dated responses on the network which also include system vulnerabilities. These responses can be sent as alerts. For example, if a system has Wireshark traffic and if CERT detects this traffic, it can alert this activity on time. Recovery is the next phase after response phase. If there are vulnerabilities in a system, it is important to recover the system from the vulnerabilities which are detected during the response phase. It is important to update the security and privacy level of the system.

4 Conclusion

It is obvious that there exists illegal forum activities inside the dark web every day. That is why, it is important to detect these activities faster with the best accuracy. Therefore, the purpose of this topic is to bring the results of the previous machine learning algorithms to the next level which are applied to detect illegal activities. Another issue is to get fingerprints of the illegal web sites which are visited by anonym users frequently. It is a common way to mix Machine Learning techniques to detect and train data quickly. The algorithms which have been included in this paper are the most updated and relevant ones to detect and extract data from dark web forums. Unfortunately, the hackers are also trying their best to not to be caught by the governments. That is why the research is not going to have an end. The technology evolves rapidly and that is why the types of illegal activities will vary during the evolution of the technology. Today it is a common way to use ML techniques to collect and examine the big data and this is also useful to monitor activities on the dark web.

Researchers have applied Machine Learning and Artificial Intelligence algorithms to detect the illegal forum activities in the dark web via training the data sets according to these patterns. On the other side, the users of Tor network were not idle against the outcomes of last research. They have also tried not to be caught. That is why it is always important to try new methods to detect them. Nowadays it became more important, because many people own IoT devices, and it is quite possible to hack those systems.

The algorithms which are included in this paper are the most updated and relevant ones to detect and extract data from dark web forums. Unfortunately, the hackers are also trying their best to not to be caught by the governments. That is why research is not going to have an end. The most challenging situation is to find the right algorithms to monitor the illegal activities on the dark web. That's why it is important to detect the gaps of previous research.

The technology evolves rapidly and that is why the types of illegal activities will vary during the evolution of the technology. It is very important to find new ways to build new algorithms to support the security of the evolving technology. That is why, this research project aims to help people to live in a more secure information superhighway. If the outcomes of this research can detect Dark Web threats faster, then this will help to protect all victims against future threats, through improved policies and procedures that enable quicker detection and response strategies and tactics by the IT professionals involved in frontline cyber security of their workplace.

This research will be informed by deep learning techniques from previous research which have found out as the most accurate method for web site fingerprinting attacks and other machine learning algorithms and open-source tools for the detection of illegal activities on the dark web. The cited papers in this research give inspiration and information of latest deep learning and machine learning algorithms which makes it possible to develop another accurate method.

References

1. Adewopo, V., Gönen, B., Varlioglu, S., Özer, M: Plunge into the underworld: a survey on emergence of darknet. In: International Conference on Computational Science and Computational Intelligence (CSCI), Las Vegas (2019)
2. Williams, K.: Untangling the dark web: taking on the human sex trafficking industry. IEEE Women Eng. Mag. **7**(2), 23–26 (2013)
3. Raaijmakers, S.: Artificial intelligence for law enforcement: challenges and opportunities. IEEE Secur. Priv. **17**(5), 74–77 (2019)
4. Harviainen, J.T., Haasio, A., Hämäläinen, L.: Drug traders on a local dark web marketplace. In: Proceedings of the 23rd International Conference on Academic Mindtrek, Tampere, Finland (2020)
5. Pantelis, G., Petrou, P., Karagiorgou, S., Alexandrou, D.: On strengthening SMEs and MEs threat intelligence and awareness by identifying data breaches, stolen credentials, and illegal activities on the dark web. In: ARES 2021: The 16th International Conference on Availability, Reliability and Security, Vienna Austria (2021)
6. Cimpanu, C.: Hackers breach FSB contractor, expose Tor deanonymization project and more, 20 July 2019. https://www.zdnet.com/article/hackers-breach-fsb-contractor-expose-tor-deanonymization-project/
7. The Guardian: Twitter launches privacy-protected site on dark web to bypass Russia's block, 09 March 2022. https://www.theguardian.com/technology/2022/mar/09/twitter-tor-version-russia-block?CMP=Share_iOSApp_Other
8. Tan, Q., Gao, Y., Shi, J., Wang, X., Fang, B.: A closer look at Eclipse attacks against TOR hidden services. In: IEEE International Conference on Communications (ICC), Paris, France (2017)

9. O'Cearbhaill, D.: Trawling TOR hidden service–mapping the DHT, 15 May 2013. https://donncha.is/2013/05/trawling-TOR-hidden-services/
10. Biryukov, A., Pustogarov, I., Weinmann, R.P.: Trawling for TOR hidden services: detection, measurement, deanonymization. In: IEEE Symposium on Security and Privacy, Berkeley, CA (2013)
11. Attarian, R, Hashemi, S.: Investigating the streaming algorithms usage in website fingerprinting attack against TOR privacy enhancing technology. In: 16th International ISC (Iranian Society of Cryptology) Conference on Information Security and Cryptology (ISCISC), Mashhad, Iran (2019)
12. Pfahringer, B., Holmes, G., Kirkby, R.: New options for hoeffding trees. In: Australasian Joint Conference on Artificial Intelligence, Goldcoast, QLD, Australia (2007)
13. Manapragada, C, Webb, G.I., Salehi, M.: Extremely fast decision tree. In: KDD 2018: Proceedings of the 24th ACM SIGKDD International Conference on Knowledge Discovery & Data Mining, London, United Kingdom (2018)
14. Hulten, G., Spencer, L., Domingos, P.: Mining time-changing data streams. In: KDD 2001: Proceedings of the seventh ACM SIGKDD International Conference on Knowledge Discovery and Data Mining, San Francisco California, US (2001)
15. Sun, Y., Edmundson, A., Feamster, N.: Chiang, M., Mittal, P.: Counter-RAPTOR: safeguarding TOR against active routing attacks. In: IEEE Symposium on Security and Privacy, San Jose, CA, USA (2017)
16. Nithyanand, R., Starov, O., Zair, A., Gill, P., Schapira, M.: Measuring and mitigating AS-level adversaries against TOR. In: NDSS 2016, San Diego, CA, USA (2015)
17. Kadoguchi, M., Hayashi, S., Hashimoto, M., Otsuka, A.: Exploring the dark web for cyber threat intelligence using machine learning. In: IEEE International Conference on Intelligence and Security Informatics (ISI), Shenzhen, China (2019)
18. Schäfer, M., Fuchs, M., Strohmeier, M., Engel, M., Liechti, M., Lenders, V.: BlackWidow: monitoring the dark web for cyber security information. In: 11th International Conference on Cyber Conflict (CyCon), Tallinn, Estonia (2019)
19. Türen, S. H., Islam, R., Eustace, K.: Analysing the threat landscape inside the Dark Web. Unpublished manuscript, submitted for publication (2022)
20. Eustace, K., Islam, R., Tsang, P., Fellows, G.: Human factors, self-awareness and intervention approaches in cyber security when using mobile devices and social networks. In: Lin, X., Ghorbani, A., Ren, K., Zhu, S., Zhang, A. (eds.) SecureComm 2017. LNICSSITE, vol. 239, pp. 166–181. Springer, Cham (2018). https://doi.org/10.1007/978-3-319-78816-6_13

Bitcoin as a New Payment Platform

Vivian Sultan(✉) and Garrett Tice

College of Business and Economics, California State University, Los Angeles, CA, USA
{vsultan3,gtice}@calstatela.edu

Abstract. Global e-commerce depends on mediums of exchange that allow users to make secure, quick, and easy transactions without the difficulties of traditional payment methods. We analyze cryptocurrency in general and inspect Bitcoin specifically as a digital-currency option for global e-commerce. Bitcoin can meet the needs of future e-commerce, but it suffers from several types of risks—including social, ethical, and economic—that can pose a threat to online users and must be addressed. Our goal with this research in progress is to review the literature on Bitcoin as a premier future online payment method, Bitcoin proponents must understand how it is being used in e-commerce now and then educate users about the value of digital currency as we move deeper into the digital age. In this work in progress, we define cryptocurrency, note the need for Bitcoin research, and discuss the pros and cons of Bitcoin as a payment platform.

Keywords: Cryptocurrency · Digital currency · Bitcoin · Blockchain · e-Commerce

1 Introduction

Traditional payment methods using cash are becoming antiquated. Why not opt for a futuristic payment like Bitcoin? Bitcoin is a digital currency without the oversight of financial institutions' governing policies. A digital currency "is a form of virtual currency that is electronically created and stored" [1]. Further, cryptocurrency is a "subset of digital currencies … [that] uses cryptography for security … [making] it extremely difficult to counterfeit" [1]. A user can control their Bitcoin in a virtual electronic wallet through a user-friendly platform, but users must be aware of several types of risks.

The anonymity afforded by Bitcoin gives rise to social risks as users can do business without revealing their identities. There is no centralized authority, so trust is a mutual gamble. For example, shadow figures can manipulate consumers into purchasing fake products. Bitcoin's ethical risks come from its potential to be used for such nefarious activities as human trafficking, the drug trade, and many others on the dark web. The economic risks of Bitcoin stem largely from its volatility and remain worrisome for potential investors. Despite the risks, Bitcoin does offer security and versatility as a payment platform for the future of e-commerce.

Bitcoin offers consumers and vendors the next level of flexibility and financial security. People like things at the click of a button and are inconvenienced by going to an ATM or carrying cash. Consumers are increasingly turning to ecommerce venues like

K. Daimi and A. Al Sadoon (Eds.): ICR 2022, AISC 1431, pp. 356–364, 2022.
https://doi.org/10.1007/978-3-031-14054-9_33

Amazon for their needs: food, household items, electronics, and more. Bitcoin has the potential to add the consumer's convenience in a preexisting digital marketplace. Already 6 years ago in 2016, Pew Research reported a survey of 4,787 U.S. adults and concluded that 24% of Americans make no cash transactions in their typical week and 39% are unconcerned about having access to cash [2]. "Nonwhites, low-income Americans and those 50 and older are especially likely to rely on cash as a payment method" [2]. Additionally, 12% have made purchases by tapping their mobile phone on a card processor. Also, "Awareness of the alternative currency Bitcoin is quite high, as 48% of Americans have heard of bitcoins" [2].

2 Discussion

Bitcoin is a useful medium of exchange for e-commerce. Without transaction fees when traveling abroad or sending money in a hurry, Bitcoin is fast and easy to use: One can order "beer in Berlin, order pizza in Amsterdam, … a taxi in Edinburgh, … a dental check-up in Ljubljana, [or] … Alpaca socks from Massachusetts" [1]. The convenience of using Bitcoin as a worldwide medium of exchange should be an obvious interest for new users [3].

Bitcoin should be attractive to younger and middle-aged users who often desire new products and services and ease of transactions. It can address many needs for e-commerce users that traditional payment methods cannot meet. The versatility of Bitcoin lies not only in where you can spend, but also in the fine grain increments available for any transactional situation [4]. A Bitcoin user can choose to charge 0.00000001BC for services rendered. This allows careful management of one's Bitcoin without a financial organization.

The use of Bitcoin in e-commerce can promote trust and financial security in countries with poor economies and fosters a sense of mutual trust because both parties are taking financial risks. The value of using Bitcoin on a global scale comes from the fact that transfers, once completed, cannot be reversed reducing merchants' risk of fraud [5].

A vendor selling specialized tea in China bogged down by foreign transaction fees could accept Bitcoin to sell globally and grow a profitable e-commerce business.

A country can have a poor economy for many reasons: political corruption and war, among others. The risk of losing your valuable objects like gold, cash, and physical belongings in these scenarios is very real. As a virtual currency, Bitcoin is intangibly stored in an electronic wallet. A digital currency like Bitcoin "would be physically safer than storing cash at home or buying gold jewelry. In addition, someone holding Bitcoin could exchange it for a more stable currency on one of the global Bitcoin exchanges" [6]. Despite the versatility of Bitcoin as a means of exchange, some social risks are important to Bitcoin users when entering the online market.

2.1 Social Risks

Bitcoin is an unregulated digital currency circumventing government agencies' manipulation, but this advantage is also a downside online. Bitcoin users trade in a digital world with no central authority to appeal to when transactions go wrong. Bitcoin is disruptive: It "disturbs governments and monetary authorities, consumers, and infrastructures. Government agencies will always try to play an important role in providing reliability in commercial transactions by imposing policies, laws and regulations" [3]. Without strict oversight, such activities as tax evasion are tempting.

Bitcoin allows users to make anonymous transactions. Social invisibility leaves an open door to numerous immoral behaviors. With no paper trail to confirm the identity of sellers and receivers aggressive and antisocial behaviors may ensue. Some users may even engage in criminal activities [3]. With no way to identify a user quickly and effectively, anonymity creates a significant problem when investigating cybercrime.

Anonymous vendors can easily swindle careless Bitcoin users in e-commerce with counterfeit products. Examples include the fake-handbag markets in Asia. The difficulty of determining a fraudulent vendor's profit at the misfortunate's expense creates social distrust. This situation also applies to a small vendor selling wine by accepting Bitcoin online. Potential customers take the risk of getting sick from a poorly produced product, and socially responsible companies conducting e-commerce with Bitcoin run the risk of tainting their reputation by association. Being transparent when using cryptocurrency and learning customers' or vendors' identities remains a challenge [6].

The lack of strict oversight by a central authority into the identities of online buyers and sellers leaves only mutual trust. In addition to its social risks, Bitcoin use also has ethical risks.

2.2 Ethical Risks

Bitcoin's anonymity characteristics help unethical users engage in illegal activities, leaving ethical users at risk of cybercrime. A look into the illegal activities shows that 26% of Bitcoin users and 46% of Bitcoin transactions are involved in some form of criminal endeavor as of April of 2017 [7].

These findings demonstrate the reality of Bitcoin: Anonymous users can conduct unethical activities to illicitly profit from a home computer. Bitcoin attracts cybercriminals because the risk of exposure to investigators is reduced, opening many options for unethical users.

The lack of a central governing authority to correct unethical Bitcoin transactions remains an issue. A central authority like a financial institution can help consumers with disputed transactions, Bitcoin offers no such feature to users [8].

Risking a purchase with anonymous users presents the issue of trust. Ethics remain in question because users cannot verify others' credibility. There are virtually no consequences for an offender even if a party could claim a "bad transaction." If a merchant is abroad without any intention of honoring a sale, the user has no appeal process to resolve the issue.

Because no regulations control Bitcoin, illegal activities can range widely. Copious opportunities remain for unethical users to prey on other users, including indirectly through tax evasion [9].

The dark web allows users to buy illegal merchandise such as drugs, human beings, and weapons with Bitcoin. Unethical activity remains prosperous and virtually consequence free for cybercriminals. The cryptocurrency protective layers of security prevent interested parties from unraveling the blockchain to reveal users' identities. Even with unethical behaviors, economic risks remain when getting into Bitcoin.

2.3 Financial Risks

Thinking of economic factors, skepticism about Bitcoin's future and its high volatility create another risk for users. Bitcoin can swing up and down in value. New users to cryptocurrency must monitor the market value of Bitcoin closely.

In May 2010 the first commercial transaction using Bitcoin was recorded where Laszlo Hanyecz, a Florida programmer, used 10,000 Bitcoin to purchase two pepperoni pizzas from Papa John's. Roughly valued at $60 at the time, Hanyecz figured that was enough Bitcoin for two pizzas and compensation for somebody's time but today that amount of Bitcoin would be worth about $5 million (Griswold, 2014) [1].

To illustrate Bitcoin's volatility, the 10,000 Bitcoins used by Laszlo was worth as much as $129,295,000 and as little as $33,590,000 in 2019. Its value ranged from $289,849,800 to $669,358,900 in 2021. That is a staggering change in the value of Bitcoin and proves the economic risk of cryptocurrency. This risk may be daunting for new users to the market.

With new competitors in the cryptocurrency market, Bitcoin might eventually be worthless altogether. Bitcoin will survive only if it remains popular among users and investment in the cryptocurrency remains strong. Bitcoin's competitors complicate the cryptocurrency's future stability as they offer more tools for developers. This is certainly the case with one top Bitcoin competitor, Ethereum, which offers to serve as a basis for new cryptocurrencies and other financial systems [10].

According to online source CoinRivet, there were "2,503 recognized cryptocurrencies as of November 21st, 2018" [11]. With so much cryptocurrency competition, developers must offer new features to interest users who desire versatility of application in online transactions.

Skepticism can hinder Bitcoin's economic growth as people are concerned about their financial futures. Thinking of tangible versus intangible value, a group of people would seem likely to invest in well-established currencies that provide such safeguards as those provided by the FDIC [1].

The point is that Bitcoin remains in its infancy and swings wildly in value. However, even with economic risks, the future of e-commerce using Bitcoin is still bright.

2.4 A Bright Future

Bitcoin can still be used as a platform for more secure transactions than traditional currencies. Bitcoin avoids the burden of counterfeit exchange [8]: "Fake Bitcoin" cannot exist whereas traditional currencies have been counterfeited throughout history.

The advantage of this characteristic is that it offers mutual trust between a seller and a customer. A digital currency like Bitcoin can teach users financial responsibility when making transactions without complicating merchants' situations.

Bitcoin is a fast and efficient medium of transaction for both users. According to Seaman, "Bitcoin also provides near instantaneous (within 10 to 30 min) undeniable confirmation that your money has been received or sent. No worrying about bounced checks" [8]. Traditional payments like cash on delivery, or credit card payment do not carry the same advantages. However, no central authority offers to issue a chargeback if a user is dissatisfied with the product. For e-commerce merchants, this is a solid win.

Despite the risks, users have many opportunities to quickly enter the Bitcoin market with ease while being aware of the risks and to engage in a futuristic medium of payment with benefits traditional currencies lack.

Financial security in transactions is a concern because consumers want to shop safely. Personal credit card information theft is a frequent news story. Bitcoin avoids those problems and offers this security around the world [1].

Foreign-transaction fees or concerns over losing a credit card while traveling are alleviated with Bitcoin. As a digital currency, Bitcoin is stored in an electronic wallet that can be accessed online. Both merchants and customers want to retain financial security and Bitcoin provides a modern approach on a virtual level to keep transactions safe and immediate.

Businesses can accept Bitcoin as payment with a few simple steps. The ease and convenience of using Bitcoin is similar to managing almost any other online financial client [8].

The benefit of Bitcoin e-commerce to business is the ease of operating a wallet and promoting a business to accept payment around the world, which can attract new clients.

Despite the skepticism about using Bitcoin as a means of payment, it should not be disregarded as an e-commerce option. We live in a fast-paced society where consumers want products and services without barriers. As a business, adapting to a wide-ranging customer base is essential for growth.

Bitcoin not only benefits businesses struggling to enter foreign markets, but also users who want security and convenience at the click of a button. It is important to understand why Bitcoin can affect the future of e-commerce growth and how it trumps traditional currencies as we move further into the digital age.

2.5 Advantages and Disadvantages

The economic benefits of poverty reduction, due to not having foreign-transaction fees when using Bitcoin, is a positive sign that can encourage a wide range of e-commerce businesses to participate. The cryptocurrency features help protect Bitcoin in comparison to storing hard currencies like gold and silver at home. Bitcoin should be attractive to a wide range of users from different socioeconomic backgrounds. Even with the potential for a positive future through Bitcoin e-commerce, it is important to tread cautiously as a user but to be flexible as a consumer and business when engaging with cryptocurrency. The advantages and disadvantages of Bitcoin can look both attractive and scary even after the COVID-19 pandemic.

Managing a digital currency like Bitcoin easier our devices than maintaining traditional currency and carrying cash. Online crypto markets are user friendly and require little personal info to maintain an digital wallet. Traditional currency requires much more information, and one must visit an ATM in person to withdraw cash or handle other types of transactions with an in-person banker. This physical-presence requirement and the sometimes-mandatory handwritten signatures can be inconvenient. Banks offer their customers numerous conveniences, including online money transfer, debit and credit cards, international money transfers, and ATM access. Yet, we must not ignore the power wielded by well-connected banks and the personnel required for bank operations. These factor into the energy requirements of fiat architectures [12].

A digital currency like Bitcoin has potential to become an ecofriendly option compared to the challenges of maintaining physical branches for banks and ATMs across the country. The convenience of managing digital currency from a device is more optimal than withdrawing cash during a potential crisis with long wait times. Bitcoin is attractive because it is also a time-saving option when handling transactions. The future of finance encompasses ecofriendly aspects and time-saving abilities along with less frustrating customer service experiences compared to personal banking. Bitcoin is a flexible tool from a software perspective versus the hardware required for physical bank branches with people [13]. "Bank queuing seems to be, or to have been at same times, in some places, a frequent problem. Conjectural bank queuing occurs in a economic crisis, when the government threatens to confiscate savings and accounts, or when there exists a risk of devaluation. Structural bank queuing is due to some systemic deficiency" (Pomsmeetings.org).

Bitcoin avoids tangible limitations compared to the current U.S. coin shortages due to the pandemic. A lack of circulating coins among cash-operated venues like laundromats, family-owned establishments, and brick-and-mortar businesses resulted in a lack of business [14].

Bitcoin can potentially benefit both consumers and businesses [15]. The lack of circulation and slow distribution of stimulus checks to Americans and increases in violent crimes across our nation should prompt consumers and businesses alike to ask, "Is converting to Bitcoin a better option?".

Bitcoin presents potential value, but the risk of external factors and resistance to change could prove problematic in becoming accepted as a mainstream U.S. currency.

External factors that could hinder Bitcoin's adoption are power outages or Internet failure. Access to physical cash and ATMs is a lifeline for consumers. ATMs are strategically placed by banking institutions to attract business and generate commerce. ATMs are operational even during emergencies. Even without the internet an ATM can still function and be serviced by a technician, while a power outage may only be limited to certain geographical areas.

Accessing a Bitcoin wallet through online market venues like Coinbase or Binance during natural disasters or cyberattacks is the difference between a digital platform and cash on hand. Transitioning to using Bitcoin for our daily needs should proceed with caution due to its security vulnerability [15].

The access to physical cash and ATMs that can generate cash during disaster situations will trump Bitcoin's use unless blockchains introduce ATMs for each cryptocurrency comparable to traditional currencies. However, if blockchains were able to introduce ATMs on a national scale, a country might consider the competition worth just creating a national cryptocurrency to rival Bitcoin and distribute to citizens. The very introduction of a cryptocurrency like Bitcoin has already been realized and the risks and rewards of such a massive change to a country's financial system must be analyzed further (Table 1).

Table 1. Bitcoin advantages and disadvantages.

Bitcoin advantages	Bitcoin disadvantages
Secured electronically as intangible currency	Cybercrime using Bitcoin is high risk in e-commerce
Vendors avoid high transactions fees	New high risks between vendors and consumers from anonymity
Multiple purchase options from products to services	No authority or institutional oversight to remedy bad transactions
Virtual exchange on numerous market platforms	Illegal activities are still rampant widely
No ATM requirements to withdraw funds physically during crisis and risk	Bitcoin use to purchase such illegal items as drugs, human beings, and weapons
More privacy for consumers	New competitors in the crypto market
Rapid distribution during a crisis like COVID-19	Inaccessible during service outages, electrical failure, and cyberattacks

Introducing Bitcoin on a national scale has been met with optimism and skepticism in El Salvador. Bitcoin can meet a developing country's needs even in the post-pandemic world. Travelers and migrants have been sending cash from the United States to El Salvador for decades, but the risks and timeliness remain antiquated as the potential for theft, and loss of cash is still significant. "El Salvador relies heavily on money sent back from workers abroad. World Bank data showed remittances to the country made up nearly $6 billion or around a fifth of GDP in 2019, one of the highest ratios in the world" [16]. Bitcoin can avoid the issues of remittances at least in a digital world. Greater timeliness and added convenience are what make Bitcoin a lucrative option. Reuters mentions the benefit of Bitcoin is that it's a "quick and cheap way to send money across borders without relying on remittance firms typically used for such transactions" [16]. The added convenience of using digital currency is not without potential pitfalls for a sensitive economy that historically relies on cash.

Another issue to consider is that Bitcoin on a national scale in El Salvador does pose significant issues to the fiat currency which has been reliant on a cash-based system historically. The convenience of use and speed of Bitcoin's transactions still face tradeoffs, though: older people who have relied on a cash system must adapt to a new digital currency. That can prove a greater risk if not managed correctly due to cybercrime. Although converting cash to Bitcoin should be easy and quick, "Converting local currencies to and from Bitcoin often relies on informal brokers, while trading often demands technical knowledge" [16]. Criminals and untrustworthy brokers could make an easy profit from unsuspecting clients, devastating an already fragile economy.

The ever-present risk of Bitcoin for everyday use is not just the general user's lack of knowledge, but also the risk of very talented cybercriminals looking to steal Bitcoin from accounts that are not properly secured. Cybertheft of cryptocurrencies is one of the biggest difficulties for a country switching to Bitcoin as the risk of theft increases exponentially with the size of the pool. Measures of protection, however, are available as markets like Binance offer two-factor authentication and strict identification periods requiring a photo ID and personal information. As the blockchain is developed and cryptocurrencies like Bitcoin evolve, so must the security and accountability among users if it is to be taken seriously.

3 Conclusion

Bitcoin is a versatile option as an exchange medium with economic advantages for e-commerce users. Bitcoin is still evolving as a cryptocurrency, and ethical, social, and economic risks remain, as well as advantages and disadvantages for e-commerce. Bitcoin is a versatile medium that can fit many e-commerce users' needs if they take precautionary steps when making e-commerce transactions.

A medium of exchange that is easy as sending a text message is invaluable in our modern age. Bitcoin is quick, fast, secure, and accepted on a global scale. In future e-commerce, Bitcoin can help poor economies and let new businesses reach wider markets for their products and services.

We need more Bitcoin research. Bitcoin proponents must understand how it is being used in e-commerce now and must educate users about the value of digital currency as we move deeper into the digital age.

Acknowledgements. In memory and acknowledgement of Professor Marshall Vallelunga whose inspiration and enthusiasm regarding cryptocurrency initiated this project.

References

1. Rose, C.: The evolution of digital currencies: Bitcoin, a cryptocurrency causing a monetary revolution. Int. Bus. Econ. Res. J. **14**(4), 617–621 (2015). https://doi.org/10.19030/iber.v14i4.9353
2. Smith, A., Anderson, M.: Online shopping and e-commerce: new technologies are impacting a wide range of Americans' commercial behaviors, from the way they evaluate products and services to the way they pay for the things they buy. Pew Research Center (2016). https://www.pewresearch.org/internet/2016/12/19/online-shopping-and-e-commerce/. Accessed 02 Apr 2022
3. Mendoza-Tello, J.C., Mora, H., Pujol-López, F.A., Lytras, M.D.: Disruptive innovation of cryptocurrencies in consumer acceptance and trust. IseB **17**, 195–222 (2019). https://doi.org/10.1007/s1025701900415w
4. Twesige, R.L.: Bitcoin. A simple explanation of Bitcoin and block chain technology. Scientific Essay (2015). https://www.grin.com/document/286736. Accessed 19 June 2021
5. Athey, S.: 5 ways digital currencies will change the world, 22 January 2015. https://www.weforum.org/agenda/2015/01/5-ways-digital-currencies-will-change-the-world/. Accessed 06 Nov 2019
6. Kbilashvili, D.: Influence of e-commerce and cryptocurrency on purchasing behavior of wine customers. Glob. J. Manag. Bus. Res.: E Mark. **18**(3), 2468 (2018). https://journalofbusiness.org/index.php/GJMBR/article/view/2468. Accessed 17 June 2021

7. Foley, S., Karlsen, J.R., Putniņš, T.J.: Sex, drugs, and Bitcoin: how much illegal activity is financed through cryptocurrencies? Rev. Financ. Stud. **32**(5), 1798–1853 (2019). https://doi.org/10.1093/rfs/hhz015
8. Seaman, D.: The Bitcoin primer: risks, opportunities, and possibilities. 123doc.net (2014). https://www.danodemano.com/Downloads/Bitcoin_Primer_Book.pdf. Accessed 19 June 2021
9. Dierksmeier, C., Seele, P.: Cryptocurrencies and business ethics. J. Bus. Ethics **152**(1), 1–14 (2016). https://doi.org/10.1007/s1055101632980
10. Laura, M.: Bitcoin Alternative: Best Altcoins & Top Bitcoin Competitors, 23 October 2019. https://www.bitdegree.org/tutorials/Bitcoin-alternative/. Accessed 04 Nov 2019
11. Bright, J.: How many cryptocurrencies are there? 28 November 2018. https://coinrivet.com/how-many-cryptocurrencies-are-there/. Accessed 05 Nov 2019
12. Usama, M.: Bitcoin and its energy usage: existing approaches, important opinions, current trends, and future challenges. KSII Trans. Internet Inf. Syst. **14**(8), 3243–3256 (2020). https://www.koreascience.or.kr/article/JAKO202026061057938.1ff8page. Accessed 02 Apr 2022
13. Machline, C., Serson, F.M.: A study of queues and customer service in retail bank agencies. Prod. Oper. Manag. Soc. (2014). https://www.pomsmeetings.org/confpapers/051/051-1233.pdf. Accessed 02 Apr 2022
14. Board of Governors of the Federal Reserve System: Are U.S. coins in short supply? https://www.federalreserve.gov/faqs/why-do-us-coins-seem-to-be-in-short-supply-coin-shortage.htm. Accessed 18 Dec 2021
15. Wadsworth, A.: The pros and cons of issuing a central bank digital currency. Bulletin of the Reserve Bank of New Zealand, 01 June 2018. https://www.rbnz.govt.nz/-/media/ReserveBank/Files/Publications/Bulletins/2018/2018jun81-07.pdf. Accessed 18 Dec 2021
16. Renteria, N., Wilson, T., Strohecker, K.: In a world first, El Salvador makes Bitcoin legal tender. Reuters, 09 June 2021. https://www.reuters.com/world/americas/el-salvador-approves-first-law-bitcoin-legal-tender. Accessed 18 Dec 2021

A Conceptual Model for Data-Driven Threat Analysis for Enhancing Cyber Security

Mohammed K. S. Alwaheidi[1], Shareeful Islam[2,4](✉), and Spyridon Papastergiou[3,4]

[1] School of Architecture Computing and Engineering, University of East London, London, UK
u1724270@uel.ac.uk

[2] School of Computing and Information Science, Anglia Ruskin University, Cambridge, UK
shareeful.islam@aru.ac.uk

[3] Department of Informatics, University of Piraeus, Piraeus, Greece
paps@unipi.gr

[4] Focal Point, Brussels, Belgium

Abstract. Technology has become increasingly adopted by businesses for achieving overall objectives. Systems within these technologies generate a huge amount of data. It is necessary to identify the data and undertake appropriate controls to protect the data from any potential threats. Data, in general, is different types, such as operational and business which have different costs and impact on the overall business continuity. Threat analysis needs to consider various data types and associated weaknesses related to an organisational context's systems and applications. There are numerous threat models available, but there is a lack of focus on analysing and prioritizing threats relating to the data. This paper presents a data-driven approach for threat analysis and a conceptual model. The model includes several concepts, i.e., actor, infrastructure, data and weakness, to analyse the data and threats from three phases management, control and business. Finally, a running example is used to demonstrate the applicability of the work.

Keywords: Threat modelling · Cyber attack · Management data · Data levels · Control data · Weakness

1 Introduction

Organizations are increasingly adopting new technologies to grow their businesses, where data is constantly generated from the systems and applications within these technologies relating to business and operational activities. It is essential to understand the data and associated dependencies on the overall organizational operational activities. For instance, data can reveal behaviour patterns, identify weaknesses in security controls, and predict future security events. Organizations need to analyse the data held, processed, or transmitted by the systems and applications. Hence, businesses are always looking for effective analysis techniques to help them understand the threat landscape and take appropriate action to safeguard this data. As a result, developing a threat model for an organization's systems and data will provide decision-makers with long-term strategies

K. Daimi and A. Al Sadoon (Eds.): ICR 2022, AISC 1431, pp. 365–374, 2022.
https://doi.org/10.1007/978-3-031-14054-9_34

and a more focused understanding of the overall security posture. There are a number of threat models focused on detecting attacks against popular technologies, i.e., IoT [1], Software-Defined Networks (SDN) [2], as well as 5G Core networks [3]. Moreover, threat models like STRIDE [4], PASTA [5], and Attack Tree [6] are also widely known, which aim to focus on attacks, threats, or threat actors. However, generally, there is a lack of focus on the data as a foundation for threat analysis throughout the life cycle of the data. Some models have contributed to analysing a specific type of data, such as control data or a particular system. The paper presents a data-driven threat model (d-TM) from all aspects of data generated from the systems and applications within an organization. Our research considers three types of data, i.e., management, control and business and identifies weaknesses and threats related with the data. d-TM identifies a number of concepts to identify and analyse the threats. Finally, a real-life use case scenario is used to demonstrate the applicability of the d-TM. The results show that d-TM identifies related data from the studied system context and analyse the data for possible threats and vulnerabilities.

2 Related Works

There are a number of widely used threat modelling approaches, including attack-tree, STRIDE, kill-chain, and PASTA. The attack tree is regarded as one of the oldest threat modelling approaches, which uses diagrams to depict potential attacks on a system. The model is designed in the form of a tree such that the root of the tree shows the goal of the attack, while its leaves are the methods through which the goal is to be realized [6]. The STRIDE model has undergone several evolutionary changes over time to include the use of threat-specific tables and other variants [6]. The cyber kill chain model involves using seven specific steps proposed by the Lockheed Martin defence company [8]. Each step is characterized by particular data types depending on the associated activities. PASTA is a risk-centric model of threat modelling developed in 2015 [5] that consists of seven distinct stages. Each stage harbours multiple activities intended to perform various purposes in the threat prediction, and counteraction processes/The National Institute of Standards and Technology (NIST) (SP 800–154) aims to provide a guide to data-centric system threat modelling. The proposed model focuses on data at a particular system and is based on Attack-side (as vulnerability, attack vector, threat, exploit and attack) and defence (risk, security controls and objectives) [7].

These works contribute to understanding and analysing the threats, but there is a lack of focus on data by these approaches. Current practice focuses on domains like assets, attacks, and software. NIST SP 800–154 provides a similar scope in the context of standards based on business data for a particular system or host that lacks a complete understanding of all types of data. Our work addresses these limitations by proposing a considering various types of data. The proposed model is superior to existing contributions in several ways. Firstly, it considers related concepts and meta-models for threat analysis. Secondly, the approach considers data from three different levels of abstraction, such that the threat vector is analysed for data relating to management, business, and control. This approach ensures that the model offers complete visibility and control over the data's location at any part of its lifecycle. Table 1 summarizes some features among common existing threat models and d-TM.

Table 1. Threat models comparison.

Factors\Models	Pasta	Stride	d-TM
Area of focus	Attacker/Risk-Centric	Threat-centric	Data-Centric
Mitigation support	Yes	Yes	Yes
Business impact alignment	Yes	No	Yes
Threat prioritisation	Yes	No	Yes
Threat/Weakness library	Dynamic	Static	Dynamic
Defined attack surface	No	No	Yes
Driven outcome	Application/System	Application/System	Data
Asset coverage	- Network - Compute - Application	- Compute - Application	- Data/user agent - Network/compute - Application
Data orientation	Single category, three phases	Single category	Management/Control/Business Three phases
Target audience	Senior Security Architect/analyst	Security Analysts	Security Architect/analyst
Analysis flow	- Business - Asset/application - Motivation/scenario - Vulnerability - Control	- Asset - Vulnerability - Threat - Control	- Business/Asset - Data/ Vulnerability - Threat - Control - Assurance
Technical implementation guidelines	High-level (fewer details)	Detailed	Detailed

3 Background – Data-Driven Threat Model

3.1 Data Levels

The model focuses on three abstraction levels of data, i.e., Management, Control and Business. Each data level is also could be in three data phases: rest, process, and transmit. Rest indicates that the data has not yet been processed and is simply sitting on storage devices such as hard drives or servers. The process occurs when data is read into the CPU. Transmit is the process by which data is sent to an external entity. The abstraction levels are equally important. An attack could directly or indirectly impact the business through any of these levels. The rationale behind d-TM abstraction levels is to secure any data regardless of its location in the digital infrastructure; hence, data could be anywhere and serve three contexts system management, control functionality and Business support (see Fig. 1).

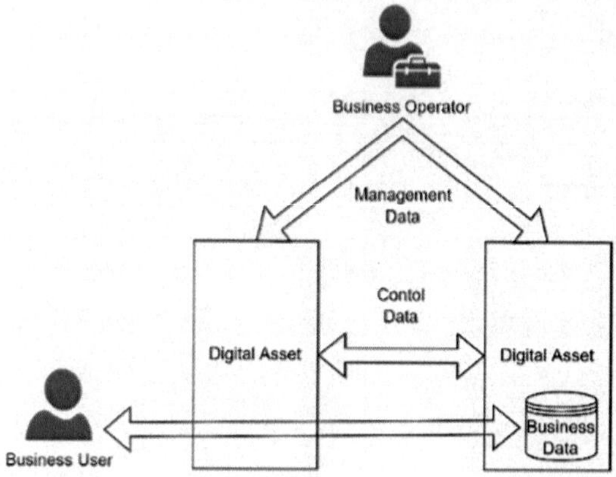

Fig. 1. Data-levels at digital systems.

- **Level 1 Management Data:** represents data linked to system administration, such as identity and access management, where admins initiate data to access systems for various administrative activities (Admin-to-System). The data could be authentication, authorization, or protocols to facilitate access to software, compute or network devices. The security assurance of infrastructure management access is an essential activity as compromising this layer is the ultimate goal of any attacker. For instance, stealing login credentials provides superior control over computing or network device. Therefore, the data generally consists of usernames or any other identifiable information, password, and associated privileges. Management data is used for authentication and authorization to access system functions (control data). The access can be user-based or system-based, systems using different mechanisms to interact with each other's, such as SSH, Telnet, FTP. It is vulnerable to some types of attacks such as brute force attack, privilege escalation, session hijacking, etc.
- **Level 2 Control Data:** represents data related to systems' functionalities, where data is exchanged between systems to support the business (System-to-System). Control data could be routing information, statistics update, application inquiries, or configuration updates. Control data could be used to share data between systems, such as business information. For instance, applications using Application Programmable Interface (*API*) for system-to-system information sharing; likewise, network routers provide packet routing functionality between networks using different protocols, such as Border Gateway Protocol (*BGP*), the routers using this protocol to exchange routing information among each other. Control data is vulnerable to many threats depending on its presentation in the environment, if locally or remotely. Insecure practices of the control data could lead to a major compromise in the network; for instance, the absence of a secure configuration to control information exchange between systems

could inject rouge information and manipulate or exfiltrate business-related data. Control data is subject to many threats, such as Man-in-The-Middle (MITM) attacks.

- **Level 3 Business Data:** represents data related to the organization's business services (User-to-System). Business Data is subject to compromise. It runs on software that could be taken over if an attacker compromises control or management data. For example, a network device uses the concept of a data plane where business data is presented; the data plane gets instructions from the control plane about actions that should be applied to particular traffic at a particular time. In this case, assuming the attacker exploited the control plane, business data could be redirected to his computer. Business Data is vulnerable to attacks that could interfere with business continuity, such as DDoS attacks.

4 Data-Driven Threat Model (d-TM)

This section presents an overview of the proposed d-TM. As mentioned previously, d-TM focuses on three different data types, i.e., management, control, and business and threat identification and analysis focus on these types. Therefore, d-TM investigates the data-level abstraction associated with the identified assets within an organizational current business context.

4.1 Conceptual View

This section presents the d-TM's conceptual view from holistic aspects of data and its surrounding environment. The model includes a number of relevant concepts for threat analysis. In addition, the model takes into account data from three different abstraction levels as management, business and control. Data abstraction gives a complete insight into the status of the data. It helps to identify the most common types of threats targeting specific data in any part of the organization's business ecosystem. Depending on the organization context, abstraction levels could help to define the priority of data threat assessment. d-TM model is founded on well-defined conceptual linkages and features.

- **Actor:** This is a general term referring to a person who intends to access an organization's data. The actor can be authorized or unauthorized and have benign or malicious intent. The model considers three purposes: "users", representing an actor accessing the service legitimately and looking for a particular service advantage with no harm intended. Moreover, "Operator" means an actor who accesses the service to maintain administration or operation tasks like troubleshooting. Lastly, the "threat-actor" represents a malicious user who looks after weakness in the service or abuses the system for non-legitimate gain.
- **Data**: It represents any data that an organization could run in infrastructure, including business or operational data. The model considers threats targeting data directly or indirectly, where data could be management, control and business. Also, data has different statuses, i.e., at rest, in process or transit.

- **Asset**: represents any hardware or software that an organization uses to run or access underlying business services. The model considers five infrastructure assets: Agent, Network, Compute, Application and Storage. Also, each asset act as a potential attack surface to data. The first is ***Agent***, which is considered a tool the actor uses to access an organization's data or resources. It is also the first point of interaction between organization infrastructure and external /internal actors; the Agent could be a web browser. While the ***network*** represents any intermediate devices that facilitate access to compute resources or applications. Switch and router are examples of network assets. Moreover, ***Compute*** refers to a machine that runs an operating system used to host business applications, i.e., hp servers (ubuntu OS). Lastly, The ***Application*** is software running the business service and hosted by a compute, and ***Storage*** refers to a local or remote data store.
- **Threat**: Cyberthreats refer to the potential of performing any malicious act to harm organization infrastructure data [9]. Moreover, threats could target any asset in the infrastructure, any level of data at any state. Threats also include attempts to access, infiltrate, or steal valuable information [9].
- **Control**: Control represents a set of policies, procedures or techniques to reduce or eliminate the impact of any cyber threats [9]. The controls could be technical, administrative or both. For instance, the firewall is a technical control, and the access policy is administrative control.
- **Weakness**: it refers to a weakness in the system that a threat actor could utilize to maintain the wrong action; the weakness could be a flow/gap in the running code, configuration or architecture of the system. However, defects could be identified at early stages compared to a vulnerability announced after system usage.

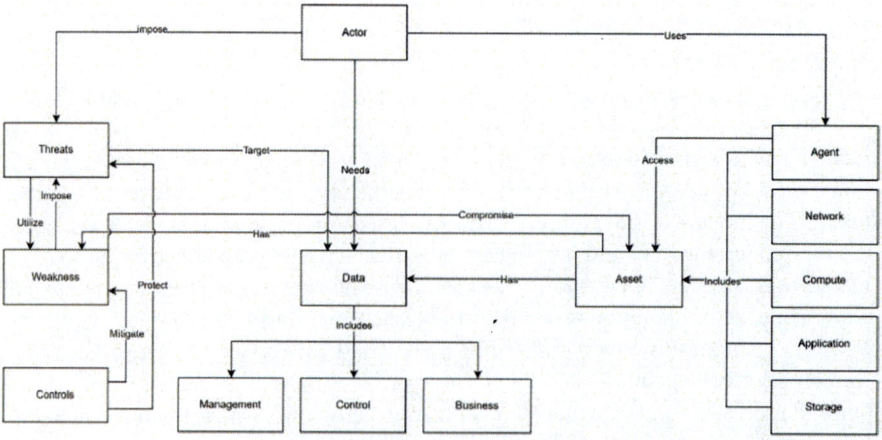

Fig. 2. d-TM conceptual model.

Figure 2 depicts the conceptual model of d-TM, which provides a complete analysis of any layer involved in the organization's data lifecycle. Additionally, it finds multiple attack surfaces aligned with today's organization operational layers, including Agent, Network, Compute, Application, and Storage, to analyse attacks.

5 Running Example

This section describes an industrial use case scenario that demonstrates the applicability of the proposed d-TM concept.

5.1 Industrial Context

The context is about a cybersecurity services provider located in the Middle East, providing services to others institutions, including banks, government agencies, and commercial. Due to confidentiality reasons, we cannot provide any identifying details of that service provider and use the anonymous name XTS. XTS provides cybersecurity services, including solutions, training, managed services, professional services and consultancy services in cybersecurity. However, XTS topology contains a set of network devices and computes facilitating its MSS platform (see Fig. 3). XTS is experiencing challenges in keeping its infrastructure and customer data safe. Due to the increasing demand for managed security services, XTS is experiencing a growth in the number of attacks targeting its services, especially services related to its Managed Security Services (MSS) platform. Recently, XTS got compromised by multiple attacks targeting its infrastructure that support the MSS platform. Due to the nature of the services XTS provides for their customers, these attacks keep happening when it extends its infrastructure to the internet. Mainly, the recent attacks focus on Denial of service and Account takeover.

5.2 Result

As a result of implementing the d-TM, XTS can identify a possible weakness that could be exploited to compromise data. Due to page restrictions, this section briefly presents the results. The infrastructure consists of several devices that serve MSS application; business customers access the application for monitoring their devices. Likewise, XTS analysts. The analysts are accessing the application along with its underlying assets for operation purposes. Figure 4 shows d-TM concepts, which are applied to one of MSS components, "Edge router-1". Whereas, "Juniper Networks" is the router's manufacturer, which has the model number MX104 and runs "JunOS" software. The router belongs to the network layer. The following outputs are produced by using d-TM.

- **Actor:** The model considers three types of actors dealing with data, business ***Users*** who use MSS services and are entitled to generate business data. ***Operator***, where XTS analysts deal with management data and define control data. ***Threat-actor*** is a source of threat that could interfere MSS management, control and business data.
- **Assets:** The MSS service is made up of several devices that, as shown below, map underlying infrastructure to d-TM asset layers. These layers serve as a potential attack surface. The table has information about assets, such as asset layer and name. While, to maintain the space restriction, detailed information about each asset is not provided.

- Agent: Web browser (google Chrome), SSH client software (Putty)
- Network: Edge-router-1, Edge-firewall-1, DMZ-switch-1, User-access-switch-1, User-access-switch-1, Core-switch-1, Core-firewall-1, Servers-access-switch-1
- Compute: MSS-console or customer, MSS-event-processor/collector
- Application: IBM Qradar application, Network-storage-1

- **Data:** MSS services components are identified, data is collected and ready to be classified to the d-TM three levels of data. Because of the confidentiality of using the router's specific configuration and the paper's space constraints, descriptive information is used to demonstrate data (see Table 2). In the end, the descriptive information will be used to identify flaws in each data level.
- **Weakness:** Figure 4 depicts the results of analysing "Edge-router-1" collected data. The assessment is security-driven, which necessitates that the analyst has a security background as well as knowledge of vendor-related security best practices. Also, Analysts can use any weaknesses database to enumerate the vulnerability on collected information such as MITRE CWE [10]. For instance, the router is configured to use basic username/password authentication mechanism, which is vulnerable to multiple types of attacks.

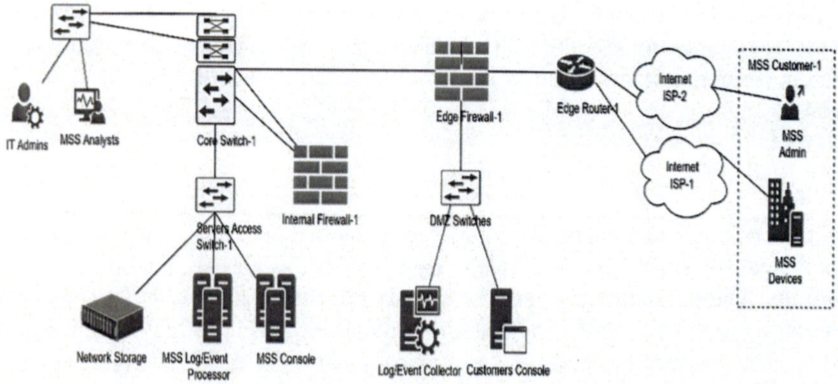

Fig. 3. XTS topology.

- **Threat:** Once weaknesses in MSS data are identified, the weaknesses have to be assigned to potential threats. The threats to weaknesses can be determined using several threat knowledge bases such as MITRE CAPEC [12] is considered to determine attacks for particular weaknesses. Hence, password brute-forcing is considered here as a potential threat to the asset Edge-router-1 under the management data level.
- **Control:** At this stage, Threats to MSS data have already been identified. Therefore, each threat must be mitigated. The mitigation strategy is determined by the threats and weaknesses that must be eliminated or reduced. Technical and administrative controls are required in relation to the MSS identified threat. Finally, to control the threat of

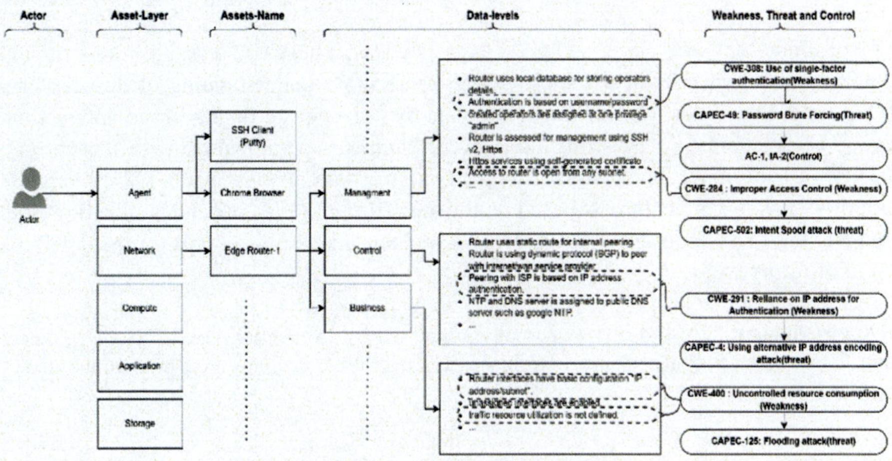

Fig. 4. d-TM to MSS application.

Table 2. MSS infrastructure to d-TM layers.

Asset layer/Name	Data-level
Network edge–router 1	Management • Router uses local database for storing users' details • Authentication is based on username/password • Created operators are assigned to single privilege "superuser" • Router is assessed for management using SSH v2, Https • Https services using self-generated certificate • Access to router is open from any subnet Control • Router uses a static route for internal peering and BGP to peer with internet/wan service provider • Peering with ISP considered with basic configuration (no authentication) • NTP and DNS server is assigned to public server such as google NTP Business • Router interfaces have a basic configuration "IP address/subnet" • Unassigned interfaces are enabled • Traffic resource utilization is not defined

"weak password requirements", with reference to the NIST control list, AC-1 and IA-2 [14] are considered as a part of the mitigating actions.

6 Conclusion

Organizations need to understand the data and possible threats targeting the data so that potential risks relating to the data can be tackled. In addition, it is essential to know what type of threat they are facing and what associated weakness could result in this threat. Data classification is critical for providing an accurate understanding of threats; The d-TM model provides a novel threat analysis by considering data at three abstraction levels. Understanding data from three-levels empower organization with the correct view of threat impact. The results from the example demonstrate that d-TM effectively supports to analyses the threats based on the data from the systems and application. We are planning to develop a systematic process and automate tool support for the d-TM as a part of future work.

Acknowledgment. This work was partially supported by the AI4HEALTHSEC EU project, funded from the European Union's Horizon 2020 research and innovation programme under grant agreement No 883273.

References

1. Casola, V., De Benedictis, A., Rak, M., Villano, U.: Toward the automation of threat modeling and risk assessment in IoT systems. Internet Things **7** (2019)
2. Tanyi, F.: Attack modeling and risk assessments in software defined networking (SDN) (2019)
3. Pell, R., Moschoyiannis, S., Panaousis, E., Heartfield, R.: Towards dynamic threat modelling in 5g core networks based on mitre att&ck a preprint (2021)
4. Kohnfelder, L., Garg, P.: The threats to our products, Microsoft Interface, Microsoft Corp., vol. 33 (1999)
5. UcedaVelez, T., Morana, M.M.: Risk Centric Threat Modeling: Process for Attack Simulation and Threat Analysis. John Wiley & Sons, Hoboken (2015)
6. Shevchenko, N.: Threat Modeling: 12 Available Methods (2018). https://insights.sei.cmu.edu/sei_blog/2018/12/threat-modeling-12-available-methods.html. Accessed 25 Feb 2020
7. Scarfone, K., Souppaya, M.: Draft NIST Special Publication 800–154 Guide to Data-Centric System Threat Modeling Draft NIST Special Publication 800–154 Guide to Data-Centric System Threat Modeling (2016)
8. Bharathi, B.B., Babu, E.S.: A novel approach to cyber hazard management intelligence system. Int. J. Eng. Technol. **7**, 473–479 (2018)
9. Bradshaw, S.: Chapter eight: combatting cyber threats: CSIRTS and fostering, Cyber Secur. a Volatile World, p. 105 (2016)
10. CWE–Common Weakness Enumeration (2022). https://cwe.mitre.org/index.html. Accessed 18 Jan 2022
11. CWE–CWE-521: Weak Password Requirements (4.6). https://cwe.mitre.org/data/definitions/521.html. Accessed 27 Jan 2022
12. CAPEC–Common Attack Pattern Enumeration and Classification (CAPEC^{TM}) (2022). https://capec.mitre.org/. Accessed 18 Jan 2022
13. CAPEC–CAPEC-49: Password Brute Forcing (Version 3.6). https://capec.mitre.org/data/definitions/49.html. Accessed 27 Jan 2022
14. Joint Task Force: National Institute of Standards and Technology Special Publication 800–53, Revision 5 : Security and Privacy Controls for Information Systems and Organizations, NIST Spec. Publ., p. 465 (2020)

Survey on Fake Accounts Detection Algorithms on Online Social Networks

Jad Shamseddine, Mohammad Malli, and Hussein Hazimeh(✉)

Arab Open University, Beirut, Lebanon
{jss008,mmalli,hhazimeh}@aou.edu.lb

Abstract. Online Social Networks (OSNs) are the most popular web services nowadays. They provide users with different kinds of services. Anyone can create his account on a certain OSN such as Facebook, using an email and password for registration. In addition, a single user can own one or more accounts. However, this feature has a lot of disadvantages and security drawbacks, such as creating fake accounts. A fake account is a profile that exists physically on OSN. Nonetheless, it is missing identity information such as names, last name, profile photo, and other profile attributes. Owners of fake accounts exploit them (accounts) for malicious internet activities like phishing, hacking, and more. Recently, this problem attracted considerably the research community. In this context, a lot of approaches have been emerged to solve fake account detection on OSNs. However, despite its importance, this field of research is still missing a systematic review. In this paper, we introduce a survey on sixteen kinds of research studies that have proposed solutions for solving the detection of fake accounts problem. We analyzed the following themes: Social networking platforms, evaluation metrics, machine learning algorithms, and models, data scale, features, and result accuracy were studied and analyzed in this survey.

Keywords: Fake account · Algorithms · Social media analysis · Survey · Machine learning

1 Introduction

Nowadays, the most used platforms on the web are social media services. According to statista.com ("Statista managed to establish itself as a leading provider of market and consumer data"), there are 13.37 billion active users on social networks as of October 2019. There are multiple types of users on these platforms and every type of them has its own reason to use these platforms. Some users use social media platforms to connect with friends, others to share media or opinion, and other users might be business owners or marketers that use social media platforms for marketing purposes.

Users might use one or more social media platforms. Some of them are interested in social connections only while others might be interested in business connections only or both, so no single social media platform for all. Facebook, Twitter, Instagram, LinkedIn, and Google+ are from the top social media platforms used worldwide. Facebook is a social networking site that is available for free; it allows users to chat with each other,

K. Daimi and A. Al Sadoon (Eds.): ICR 2022, AISC 1431, pp. 375–380, 2022.
https://doi.org/10.1007/978-3-031-14054-9_35

share media and text, post comments, and react, besides, business owners also can have their own pages and groups on this platform and can benefit from many features that are available on Facebook to help them market their products and services. For instance, lately ordering food became one of the available services on Facebook. Twitter is a social networking site that is available for free; it allows users to post and comment on posts in which is called tweet and retweet. Posts or tweets must be short no more than 140 characters to be specific. Furthermore, some users create accounts just to follow celebrities and receive their news. Instagram is a mobile application that is available for free on all mobile operating systems; it allows users to share photos and videos. Users can post, like, and comment on posts. Also, users can be business owners as well because Instagram has special features for businesses that help them in marketing their business, products, and services. LinkedIn is a social networking site that is made available for professionals, job seekers, recruiters, and anyone interesting in creating a professional network. Users can present their resumes, search for jobs, and get certificates while on the other hand business owners can recruit candidates, post jobs or seminar events, and more. LinkedIn is available for free with an optional subscription version for more features; however, the free version can be more than enough for regular users. Google+ is a social networking site that is also available for free. It was similar to Facebook and one of its first competitors, but in April 2019 Google+ was shut down due to disclosure of the design flaws of its software which allowed developers from outside to access the personal information of the users. The low engagement of users was also a reason behind shutting down the platform [20]. However, Google+ is still available for "G Suite" now called "Google Currents". In Table 1, we listed and compared 16 research paper in terms of social media platform(s) used, dataset size, ML algorithm, evaluation, and year of publication.

2 Social Media Platforms

As mentioned earlier in this analysis, five online social networks have been involved namely Facebook, Twitter, Instagram, LinkedIn, and Google+ that are ranked the top social media platforms worldwide. This section will discuss what platforms did the researchers use and what is the most used platform and why.

Multiple researchers have done studies on the mentioned platforms. Researchers in [1, 3, 5–8, 12, 17] have done studies and analysis on Facebook platform. On the other hand, researchers in [5, 8–10, 8–10, 18] have used Twitter in their analysis and studies. Furthermore, LinkedIn was studied and analyzed by researchers in [13], and [19]. Moreover, researchers in [5] used Google+ in their studies and analysis. Finally, Instagram was analyzed and studied by researchers in [11, 16].

Thus, Facebook is the most used platform in the studies and analysis. Researchers are using Facebook since it the most commonly used platform which is available on the web and also available as a mobile app. According to statista.com ("Statista managed to establish itself as a leading provider of market and consumer data"), the most popular social media platform as of October 2019 was Facebook with 2.41 billion active users. However, Multiple researches show that 20% to 40% of accounts on Facebook are fake profiles [1]. Fake profile detection techniques for Facebook accounts are very few

Table 1. Information about attributes used by researchers

Attribute \ Paper	[14]	[19]	[25]	[26]	[27]
Social Media Platforms	Facebook	Facebook Google+ Twitter	Facebook	Facebook	Facebook, Twitter
Data Size	N/A	Facebook: 4039 Accounts Twitter: 4000 Accounts Google+: 3045 Accounts	N/A	400 Accounts	2818 Accounts
Machine Learning Algorithm	Support Vector Machine, Decision tree, Artificial Neural Network, and Naïve Bayes'	Deterministic Finite Automaton (DFA), and Regular Expression techniques no ML used.	Support Vector Machine, and Naïve Bayes'	Support Vector Machine, Naïve Bayes', Decision tree, K-nearest Neighbors, and Random Forest	Neural Networks, Support Vector Machines, and Random Forest
ML Model	Supervised Machine Learning algorithms	N/A	supervised machine learning algorithms	supervised machine learning algorithms	supervised machine learning algorithms
Result Accuracy	93(%) -> 97(%)	89(%) → 90(%)	N/A	60(%) -> 80(%)	93(%)
Year Published	2016	2014	2018	2019	2019

Attribute \ Paper	[33]	[34]	[35]	[36]	[37]	[38]
Social Media Platforms	Twitter	Twitter	Instagram	Facebook	Twitter	LinkedIn
Data Size	4950 Accounts	13000 Accounts	696 Accounts	4,708 Accounts	6825 Accounts	74 Accounts
Machine Learning Algorithm	Decision Tree, Naïve Bayes', Neural Networks, Support Vector Machines, and Random Forest	Support Vector Machines, Simple Logistic, and k-Nearest Neighbors	Random Forest, and Logistic Regression	k-Nearest Neighbor, Naïve Bayes', Decision Tree, Decision Rule based, Support Vector Machines	Support Vector Machine, Artificial Neural Network, Random Forest, and k-Nearest Neighbors	Neural Network, and Support vector machine
ML Model	supervised machine learning algorithms	supervised machine learning algorithms	supervised machine learning algorithms	supervised machine learning algorithms	supervised machine learning algorithms	supervised machine learning algorithms
Result Accuracy	99.58(%)	98.74(%)	95(%)	80 (%)	99.2(%)	84(%)
Year Published	2016	2017	2019	2017	2019	2014

and limited. Facebook has its own security system for protecting users' credentials from scamming, phishing, etc. which is called Facebook Immune System (FIS) [2–4], however, it was not effective in detecting fake profiles on Facebook. Fake profiles can have a very bad impact on real users since they can use duplicate profiles of real users or create profiles for users that are not yet registered online, which can deceive real users as all the data of the profiles are real. The intruder can pretend to be an actual person and send friend requests to other existing users, then start collecting data from their profiles and that affects their privacy and security. Finding an alternative to Facebook Immune System (FIS) has become a must and that is how the story began.

3 Evaluation Metrics

In Fig. 1, we present multiple types of evaluation metrics that have been used by researchers namely accuracy, precision, recall, f1-score, AUC, and ROC. The accuracy results of a number of papers are presented in Fig. 2.

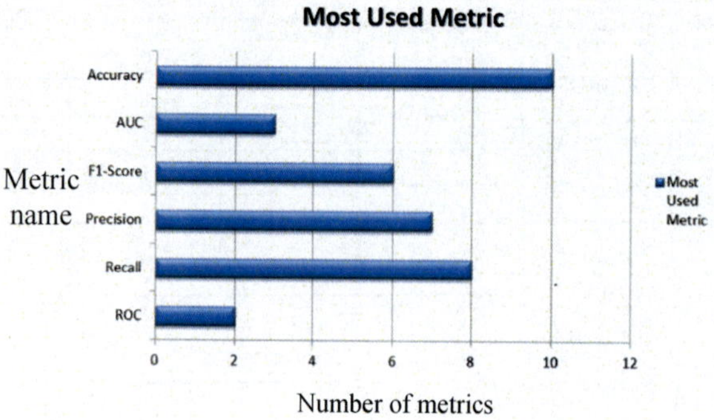

Fig. 1. The performance evaluation metrics.

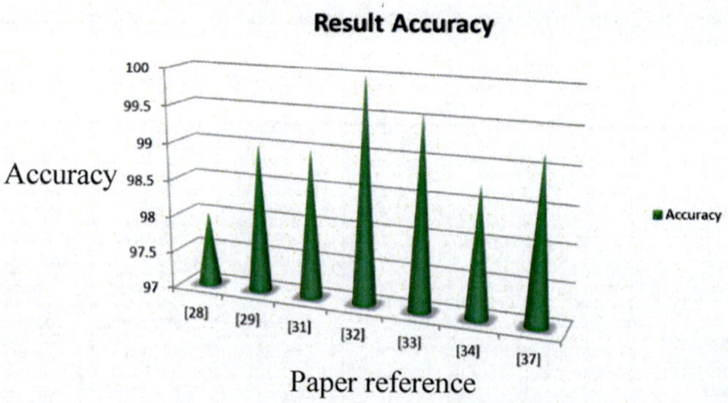

Fig. 2. The accuracy rates scores.

4 Machine Learning Algorithms

In this section, we will state what are the machine learning algorithms used by each study and what type of machine learning algorithms have been used by each of them as presented in Fig. 3. There are multiple types of machine learning models. The most commonly used are two which are supervised learning, unsupervised learning.

Supervised Learning: a group of training examples that are made up of correct answers that are given and based on this group of training; the algorithm works towards answering all the probable inputs appropriately. The same is referred to as learning from exemplars. There are several supervised learning algorithms, as stated: linear regression, Polynomial Regression, logistics Regression, artificial neural networks, Sequential Minimal Optimization (SMO), k-Nearest Neighbor, Decision Tree, Naive Bayes, Random Forest, and Support Vector Machines.

Unsupervised Learning: In this case, appropriate and correct answers are not offered; instead, the algorithm tries to recognize similarities among the inputs such that all the data that have a thing in common are placed together. The mathematical approach to unsupervised learning is defined as density estimation.

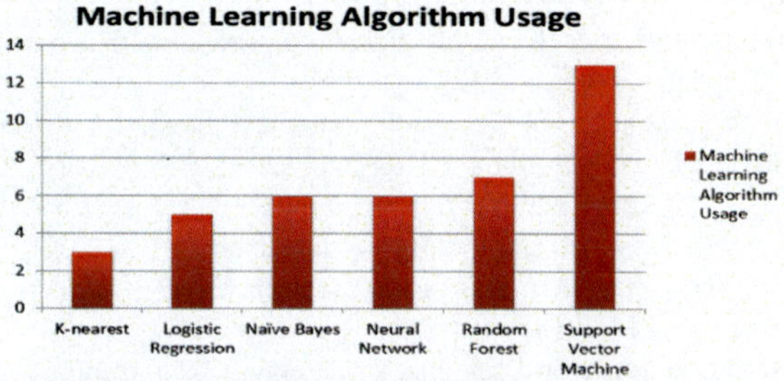

Fig. 3. Most used machine learning algorithms

Clearly, Support Vector Machine (SVM) is the most used machine learning algorithm by researchers as shown in Fig. 3 with 13 usages out of sixteen, almost every researcher use the SVM algorithm in his study. There is a huge difference between the number of usages of Support Vector Machines (SVM) and the other machine learning algorithms.

At the end of this section, we are able to tell that supervised learning is the most common if not the only machine learning type used by analysis. A wide range of machine learning algorithms was used by the authors of those papers. The most used algorithm was Support Vector Machines (SVM).

5 Conclusion

In this paper, we conducted a survey that compares and analyses sixteen research studies that tried solving the problem of detecting fake accounts on online social networks. Our comparison involved multiple aspects of research studies into consideration which are social network platform, evaluation metrics, machine learning algorithms, machine learning models, data scale, features, and result accuracy. At the end of the comparison, we were able to conclude that Facebook was the most used platform, Supervised learning was the most used machine learning model, Support Vector Machine (SVM) was the most used machine learning algorithm, and that accuracy was the most used metric. % and one result accuracy of 100% was detected. In the process of finding the best solution among the sixteen proposed solutions, we have developed our own benchmarking metrics that evaluated multiple factors, then we have applied them to the sixteen research studies. Benchmarking metrics result indicated that every single factor has an important role in detecting fake accounts on social networks.

References

1. Wani, S.Y., Kirmani, M., Ansarullah, S.: Prediction of fake profiles on Facebook using supervised machine learning techniques-a theoretical model. Int. J. Comput. Scie. Inf. Technol. **7**(4), 1735–1738 (2016)
2. DeBarr, D., Wechsler, H.: Using social network analysis for spam detection. In: Chai, S.-K., Salerno, J.J., Mabry, P.L. (eds.) SBP 2010. LNCS, vol. 6007, pp. 62–69. Springer, Heidelberg (2010). https://doi.org/10.1007/978-3-642-12079-4_10
3. Conti, M., Poovendran, R., Secchiero, M.: Fakebook: detecting fake profiles in online social networks, pp. 1071–1078, August 2012
4. Stein, T., Chen, E., Mangla, K.: Facebook immune system. In: Proceedings of the 4th Workshop on Social Network Systems - SNS 2011 (2011)
5. Meligy, A., Ibrahim, H., Torky, M.: Identity verification mechanism for detecting fake profiles in online social networks. Int. J. Comput. Netw. Inf. Secur. **9**, 31–39 (2017)
6. Rao, P., Gyani, J., Narsimha, D.G.: Fake profiles identification in online social networks using machine learning and NLP (2018)
7. Smruthi, M., Harini, N.: A hybrid scheme for detecting fake accounts in Facebook. Int. J. Recent Technol. Eng. (IJRTE) **7** (2019)
8. Shama, S., Nandini, K., Anjali, P., Manaswi, K.: Fake profile identification in online social networks. Int. J. Recent Technol. Eng. **8**, 11190–11194 (2019)
9. Khaled, S., El-Tazi, N., Mokhtar, H.M.O.: Detecting fake accounts on social media. In: 2018 IEEE International Conference on Big Data (BigData), pp. 3672–3681 (2018)
10. Mohammadrezaei, M., Shiri, M., Rahmani, A.: Identifying fake accounts on social networks based on graph analysis and classification algorithms. Secur. Commun. Netw. **2018**, 1–8 (2018)
11. Akyon, F., Kalfaoglu, E.: Instagram fake and automated account detection, September 2019
12. Singh, Y., Banerjee, S.: Fake (Sybil) account detection using machine learning. SSRN Electron. J. (2019)
13. Xiao, C., Freeman, D., Hwa, T.: Detecting clusters of fake accounts in online social networks, pp. 91–101, October 2015
14. Elazab, A., Mahmood, M., Hefny, H.: Fake account detection in Twitter based on minimum weighted feature set. Int. J. Comput. Electr. Autom. Control Inf. Eng. **10**(1), 2016 (2016)
15. Khalil, A., Hajjdiab, H., Al-Qirim, N.: Detecting fake followers in Twitter: a machine learning approach. Int. J. Mach. Learn. Comput. **7**, 198–202 (2017)
16. Dey, A., Reddy, H., Dey, M., Sinha, N., Joy, J.: Detection of fake accounts in Instagram using machine learning. Int. J. Comput. Sci. Inf. Technol. **11**, 83–90 (2019)
17. Gupta, A., Kaushal, R.: Towards detecting fake user accounts in Facebook. In: 2017 ISEA Asia Security and Privacy (ISEASP), pp. 1–6 (2017)
18. Rahman, M.D., Likhon, A.M., Rahman, A.S., Choudhury, M.H.: Detection of fake identities on Twitter using supervised machine learning, May 2019
19. Adikari, S., Dutta, K.: Identifying fake profiles in Linkedin. In: Proceedings - Pacific Asia Conference on Information Systems, PACIS 2014, January 2014
20. Mike, S.: Google sets April 2 closing date for Google+, download your photos and content before then. USA Today, 1 February 2019

Internet of Things

Sensor Networks with Edge Intelligence for Reliable Air Quality Monitoring in the Covid-19 Era

Eleftheria Katsiri(✉)

Department of Electrical and Computer Engineering,
Democritus University of Thrace, 67100 Xanthi, Greece
ekatsiri@gmail.com

Abstract. Rapid advancements in affordable, miniaturised air pollution sensor technologies offer the potential to capture the high variability of personal exposure to air pollution during daily life with unprecedented spatial and temporal resolution. However, concerns remain regarding the suitability of these novel technologies for scientific and policy purposes due to their lack of reliability.

The aim of this work is the development of three types of portable air quality devices that monitor particulate matter, differential pressure and outdoor emissions (CO, CO2, O3 and VOCs) with high reliability using low-cost sensors and communicating measurements to the cloud in real time. Reliability is strengthened in all three places: at the sensor level, the device/edge level and at the cloud, cashing data until network connectivity is restored. In order to evaluate their efficiency, two case studies were deployed: (a) in a modern industrial setting and (b) in an IT office space in Greece and the findings are reported.

Keywords: Low-cost sensors · Air quality monitoring · Internet of things · Raspberry pi · Arduino · Wireless sensor networks · Printed circuit boards · Delay tolerant networking · Middleware · Publish/subscribe

1 Introduction

In recent years the development of low-cost sensor technology has been a critical factor that changed the pollution detection paradigm allowing for the measurement of air pollution ad hoc and in great spatio-temporal resolution [9], which is required for advanced processing and analytics functions, such as the estimation of aggregated exposure of individuals and their children, especially in underdeveloped areas. The combination of great spatio-temporal resolution and real-time monitoring makes it possible to answer new questions about the underlying causes of poor air quality, ensure more accurate modelling and prediction at local scales, improve the ability to identify the links between air quality and human health or environmental degradation, identify potential air pollution "hot

K. Daimi and A. Al Sadoon (Eds.): ICR 2022, AISC 1431, pp. 383–396, 2022.
https://doi.org/10.1007/978-3-031-14054-9_36

spots", enhance the ability to quantify the impacts of pollutant mitigation techniques and promote savings through *on-demand ventilation* [20].

Furthermore, recent developments link covid-19 to poor air quality. The authors of [6] found that when the daily concentration of PM2.5 rises above $50\,\mathrm{ug/m}^3$, the number of cases doubles while [5] reports that during long term exposure, even $1\,\mathrm{ug/m}^3$ raise in daily concentration of PM10 leads to an 8% increase in mortality rate with 98% confidence level. According to Quéré et al. [8] the day-to-day global CO2 releases, was decreased by −17% (−11 to −25%) by April 2020, taking into account the emissions realised on 2019. On the other hand, indoor emissions such as VOCs were found to have grown by 30% during the first lockdown. The above issues make reliable measurement and control of air pollution a priority in the policy making agenda.

However, the plausibility of data from networks of low-cost measurement devices is a contentious point; although low cost sensors are commercially available for a large range of air pollutants they suffer in the field from temperature and humidity interference, and baseline drift, which is partly due to the deterioration of the sensing surface [11,12] while NO and NO_2 sensors exhibit cross-correlation towards O_3 [12]. To boot, he great degree of heterogeneity and lack of standardisation in air quality sensors and their electronics makes it hard to create a common architecture that will suit every single low-cost sensing technology. What is required for the successful exploitation of low-cost sensors is specialised knowledge about sensing principles, careful design of electronics, calibration in the laboratory and in the field, complex processing, monitoring and adaptive control, issues that hinder their adoption.

The aim of this work is the specification of three types of highly-reliable air quality measurement devices for ***particulate matter, differential pressure, indoor*** *gases* using a systematic approach. At the sensor level, the above devices integrate pre-calibrated, low-cost sensors that by means of low-noise electronics and good design of both the sensors and their electrodes, achieve *parts-per-billion* (ppb, 10^{-9}) level sensitivity in laboratory conditions [11]. The sensors that have been certified by their individual providers, thus allowing for the measurements produced by the device to be considered *certified.* At the device level novel embedded software components exploit sensor calibration sheets in order to eliminate noise while novel *store&forward* middleware components cache measurements for up to 24 h in case of network disruption. At the cloud level, raw data from different sources is integrated to provide high-level context such as indexes, using the interoperable Grafana visualisation platform.

2 Related Work

Previous research has successfully constructed some monitoring systems that provide real-time micro-level air pollution information, flexible data access, and user-friendly data visualization by utilizing the low-cost sensors and WSNs together with mobile web apps. Systems proposed in [26,36–38] were mainly focused on the system architecture and implementation. An urban scale wireless networking testbed was proposed and implemented in [37] based on 100 Wi-Fi enabled Linux PCs equipped with a set of low-cost sensors, mounted on the streetlight poles and powered by electrical grid. In [38], a real-time air monitoring system was proposed and implemented by utilizing the stationary low-cost sensors, powered by solar panels, and the General Packet Radio Service (GPRS) wireless link. In [26], a handheld sensor node with six environmental sensors was implemented. This sensor node was able to transmit data tagged with Global Positioning System (GPS) information to user's smartphone through Bluetooth or directly upload the data to a server through GPRS or 802.15.4 radio. In [36], a NoSQL database was chosen for the backend server considering the need for storing the time sensory data at any time from many sources. All of these systems are able to provide fine-grained air pollution information through mobile apps in real-time. However these approaches are not systematic and the monitoring reliability is not proven. On the other end of the spectrum of air quality monitors, the use of low-cost monitors (costing less than USD $3000) is increasing [26,32–35]. Most of the works reported in the literature have deployed low-cost-sensor devices outdoors, either as stationary networks (e.g., [21]) or mounted on buses or trucks. The latter [22,25] provide insufficient repetitive frequency to reveal long-term spatial air quality trends in a city [24,28,29]. Other works have focused on fusing low-cost sensors with satellite imaging [30], using neural networks [39] and using calibration [12,40,44]. Some works aimed to increase both reliability and energy consumption by substituting GPS components with energy-efficient localisation techniques [41,42], or by clustering nodes [43]. An air exchange rate based indoor air quality sensing method was proposed in [41] Privacy issues, user behavior, and data visualization were studied in [45–47].

Our focus is on a systematic approach, an overall architecture that encompasses multiple, heterogeneous sensors and interfaces, that is end-to-end reliable in the presense of sensor and network failure, and robust enough for the strict quality assurance requirements of the workspace domain.

3 System

Three types of reliable air quality measurement devices, *Particulate Matter (PM)*, ***Differential Pressure (DP)***, *Air quality Outdoor Gases (AQG)* were developed as shown in Table 1 where limits indoors are also mentioned where they exist. They can operate in either an *online* mode, sending measurements to the cloud or in an *autonomous* mode, storing data locally to a database where they can be retrieved through a USB interface. All devices are suitable for both indoor and outdoor use. They support wireless communication via WiFi and Bluetooth 4.0 as well as Ethernet. They are powered by mains and are also portable by integrating a power-bank which lasts for approximately 24 h before requiring recharging. They can be accessed and controlled remotely through an embedded TeamViewer micro-server.

A raspberry pi 4 (RPi4) was chosen as the microprocessor as it includes not only a high-performance 64-bit quad-core processor, dual-band 2.4/5.0 GHz wireless LAN, Bluetooth 5.0 and Gigabit Ethernet but also 4 GB persistent (flash)

Table 1. Device air quality sensor specification

Device name	Sensor	Range	Limits indoors
PM	PM1	0.38–1.0 ug/m^3	na
PM	PM2.5	0.38–2.5 ug/m^3	25 ug/m^3 [a]
PM	PM10	0.38–40 ug/m^3	40 ug/m^3 [b]
DP	diff. pressure	−125 to 125 Pa	n/a
AQG	CO	1 ppb to 50 ppm	na
AQG	CO_2	0 ppm to 5000 ppm	1000 ppm
AQG	O_3	0 ppb to 20 ppm	na
AQG	VOC	1 ppb to 50 ppm	na
AQG	NO_2	0 ppb to 20 ppm	na

[a] Average value aggregated over 24 h
[b] Average value aggregated over 24 h

local storage. An Arduino Uno (ARD), based on the ATmega328P, was chosen as the micro-controller featuring 14 digital input/output pins and 6 analog inputs. Furthermore, sensor boards were designed by the author to drive the PM and DP sensors while for the AQG sensors (CO, NO2, CO2, O3 and VOC), DFE and AFE boards that were initially procured by the sensor manufacturers were eventually replaced by custom sensor boards. Each sensing device is associated with a Grafana [50] dashboard that provides time-series graphs of all pollutants, temperature and relative humidity over a period of time defined by a widget on the top right of the screen. Visual analytics are possible by means of these dashboards.

4 Middleware

The software that underpins the reference architecture is structured as an infinite loop where at each iteration, four steps take place:

1. Sensors are polled.
2. Sensor data are calibrated, aggregated, combined and indices are calculated.
3. Pre-processed data are formatted and stored locally before transmission.
4. Data is visualised and analysed at the cloud; alerts are generated.

Typically, steps 1 and 2 take place at the micro-controller, step 3 takes place at the micro-processor and Step 4 takes place at the cloud. Each device runs either a store-and-forward or a publish-subscribe version of the middleware. The former provides delay and disruption tolerance by first cashing the data locally until an internet connection is available while the latter first stores a copy of each data tupple persistently in the local database; next it transmits it to the cloud using MQTT; The store-and-forward logic is shown schematically in Fig. 1. In terms of implementation, the publish-subscribe version is written entirely in Python and uses the AWS MQTT client for communication; whereas the store-and-forward version is

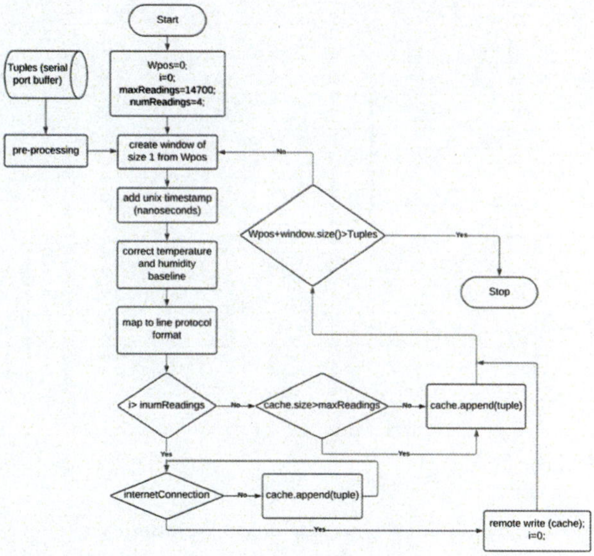

Fig. 1. Store-and-forward middleware functions

written both in Python and in Processing 3.0 [52] and the Telegraf open-source suite is used for deplay-tolerant communication.

5 Device Development

Core to the **PM measuring device** is the **PM sensor**: first, particles are classified according to their diameter in 24 bins that cover the range from 0.35 to 40 ug/m^3. Based on the histogram of the distribution of particle sizes, particle concentrations in ug/m^3 are calculated next, considering the particle density and the refraction index. Typical values are 1.65 g/ml for density and 1.5 for the refraction index. Particular matter load (mass) is calculated next for three typical classes $PM_{10}, PM_{2.5}$ and $PM_{1.0}$, respectively. The RPi4 controls the PM sensor via the *Serial Peripheral Interface (SPI)*: initialisation, sleep intervals, laser intensity and sampling rate are configurable via HEX commands while the specific threshold values depend on the level of ambient PM concentration.

As one of the PM sensor pins operates on 3.3 V while the ARD produces 5 V, a *voltage divider* circuit was constructed using two resistors (R_1, R_2) connected in series, with the input voltage applied across the resistor pair and the output voltage emerging from the connection between them according to Eq. 1.

$$V_{out} = R_2/(R_1 + R_2) * V_{in} \tag{1}$$

Both the SPI interface and the voltage divider were implemented as a *through-hole PCB sensor board* (Fig. 2(a)).

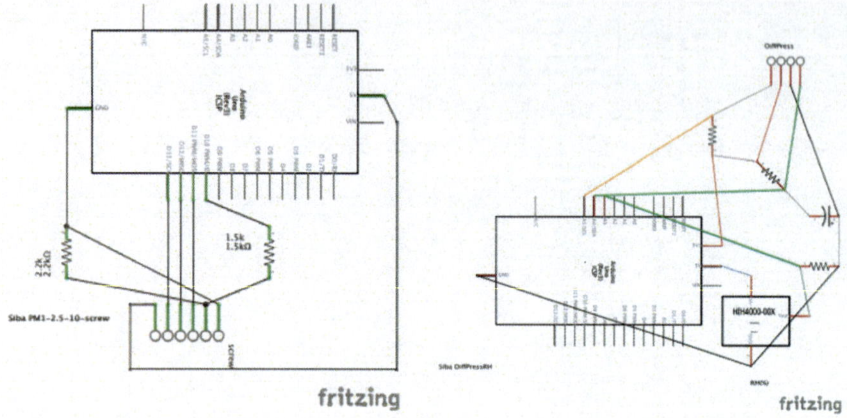

(a) PM sensor board (b) DP sensor board

Fig. 2. Device sensor board schematics

5.1 The DP Sensing Device

The DP sensing device comprises the *SDP800 CMOS* differential pressure sensor with measurement range in [−125 Pa, 125 Pa]. The sensor is fully calibrated and temperature compensated offering highest accuracy and resolution, especially at very low differential pressure. The sensor uses a thermal mass flow sensing element based on a calorimetric measurement principle and also includes an embedded thermistor. The board also comprises a Honeywell *HIH-4000* accurate analogue temperature and relative humidity sensor to provide a $RH\%$ measurement.

A through-hole printed circuit board was designed in order to connect the DP sensor to the micro-processor using I^2C (Fig. 2(b)). The RPi4 polls the sensor for both DP and temperature values (produced by the embedded thermistor). The DP sensor is configured to operate in an average till read mode with a sampling period of 10 ms. In this mode, all measurements since last read out or, when no read has occurred yet, since last start measurement command, are averaged. During the first 25 ms of averaging the averaged value is obtained as the arithmetic mean (Eq. 2).

$$\bar{x} = Sum_{i=1}^{N}(x_i/N)/for\ x < 25\,\mathrm{ms} \tag{2}$$

When the reading speed is even slower than 25 ms, the sensor will continue to average using an exponential smoothing algorithm with a smoothing factor $a = 0.05$ (Eq. 3)

$$S_k = a * x_i + (1 - a) * S_{k-1},\ S_0 = \bar{x}, for\ x > 25\,\mathrm{ms} \tag{3}$$

A medium flexible PVC tube of diameter 6 mm was procured from which pairs of two, three and five meter pieces, respectively, were cut and used as air hoses at different distances from the device. The particular diameter was chosen after testing with 2 mm, 8 mm and 10 mm diameters and different degrees of tube hardness; For the 3 m and 5 m long hoses, the pressure drop of the hose was compensated for an accurate differential pressure measurement using Eq. 4 (Hagen-Poiseuille law).

$$dp = 2 * dp_{hose} + dp_{sensor} \tag{4}$$

while the pressure drop Δp of non-turbulent air or gas in a long narrow hose with circular cross section, is:

1. proportional to the Length L and flow m
2. inversely proportional to the 4th power of the diameter D.

To test the compensation, first, all three devices were placed in the same location next to each other and the measurements were compared. All values were very close to one another, which indicated that the drop along the hose was negligible possibly due to the large diameter of the hose ($6\,mm$).

5.2 The AQG Sensing Device

The AQG Sensing Device integrates the following sensors: *CO A4 Carbon Monoxide 4-Electrode Sensor* (for concentrations in [*10ppb*, *2000ppm*]), O_x *A4 Ozone 4-Electrode Sensor* (for concentrations in [*10ppb*, *50ppm*]), *PID-AH2 VOC Sensor* (for concentrations in [*1ppb*, *50ppm*] (Isobutylene)) and an *IRC-A1 Carbon Dioxide Sensor* (for concentrations in [*0ppm*, *5000ppm*]). The CO, O_x and VOC sensors are mounted on a *810-0020-00 4-Way Analog Front End (AFE)*, which allows the power source and signal connections to be easily achieved. Furthermore, the AFE ensures low-noise electronics and achieves the temperature stability of the sensors - by means of a simple heater drive bridge circuit - whose performance is strongly dependent on the operating temperature.

The analogue signal is processed by the *SouthCoastScience DFE*, an electronic interface between the sensors and the RPi4 that converts it to digital so that it can be read by the RPi4. The CO_2 NDIR sensor is mounted on a separate transmission board that offers both a $4 - 20\,mA$ and USB outputs. The USB output is connected to the USB port of RPi4 that also powers the CO_2 sensor. The *Adafruit Pi Foundation 7" Touchscreen Display for Raspberry Pi* was mounted on the RPi4 to provide a GUI for the user.

5.3 Testing

A three stage testing plan was carried out. During development each custom sensor board was first tested thoroughly using a multi-meter (solder-joins in the base of headers, pico-molex receptors, screw terminals and the voltage drop over resistors and capacitors). Next, the assembled devices were tested in terms of sensing performance. The PM device was tested first in the proximity of a kitchen while a steak was being cooked. The result showed very quick response time in picking up the activity, very high concentrations of particulate matter while air quality remained poor for over an hour after cooking. The DP sensors were tested by placing a finger at one output port and measuring pressure at the other end. To test the CO sensor, a mosquito repellent coil was ignited that caused a peak in the CO concentration and a slight peak in the Ozone concentration. To test the CO_2 sensor response time, the tester breathed periodically very close to the sensor, which caused a significant narrow peak $> 1000ppm$ to the CO_2 concentration but also to the CO sensor showing correlation. Figure 3(a) shows comparison of differential pressure during staging. As can be seen from these figures, three devices, that are either without enclosure (DP1), or without lid (DP3) or without tubes (DP5) are closer in values through all experiments measurements. DP4, fitted with $1m$ long tubes shows lower DP values while DP2 fitted with even longer $5m$ tubes measures even lower values. However, the differences among devices are still very small around 0.3 Pa. Figure 3(b) shows that the number of samples per day for one of the devices is stable within one year period, indicating a stable performance of the device during rollout. The total samples amounts to 2291991.

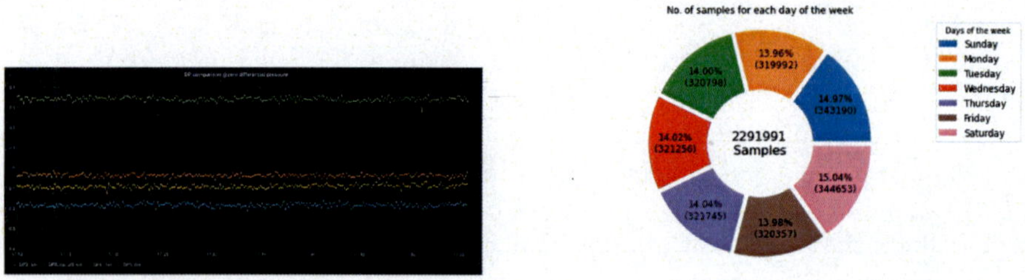

(a) DP timeseries comparison

(b) Number of samples per day

Fig. 3. Testing results

6 Results

Eighteen sensing devices were deployed at a dairy factory in the South of Greece. Three devices were deployed outdoors and twelve indoors, in three different production areas that range from *Critical Environment* (highly sensitive to contaminants) to *hygienic environment*. For the monitoring of air flow, 2 more DP sensing devices were deployed. The following aspects were monitored by means of the devices developed in this work.

1. Monitor in real-time the concentration of $PM_{10}, PM_{2.5}, PM_{1.0}$ in the fifteen device locations in the three production areas.
2. Monitor the real-time differential pressure between a ventilator in an existing production area and that of a new extension, in order to verify whether the extension was adequately ventilated from this ventilator.
3. Monitor in real-time the negative pressure in a critical environmental area in order to check conformance with the designated threshold value (5 Pa).

4. Monitor in real-time the change of differential pressure between two adjacent production areas that is caused by the opening of a door connecting the two.

A timeseries of DP measurements in the extension area over seven days, from the 6/2/2022 to 13/2/2022 is shown in Fig. 4. It can be observed that the average pressure is approximately at 7 Pa, which is a small difference indicating a small air flow. However, on 12/2/22 the average pressure increases to 10 Pa, which indicated a better air flow. Furthermore, several peaks, indicate changes in ventilation rate or some obstruction.

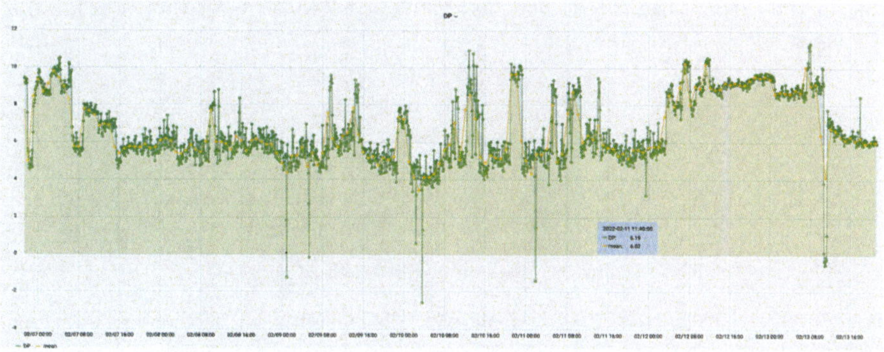

Fig. 4. Differential pressure in the extension area

6.1 Municipality Office Space

Two PM devices and one AQG device were deployed at a municipality office building to test the microclimate. To this extent, the following air pollutants were monitored: particulate matter, carbon monoxide, carbon dioxide, ozone, VOCs and humidity and temperature. Sensing devices were installed in separate areas of the office space where they operated for several hours up to two days. This process was supervised manually by an observer who noted all interesting events in the notebook and subsequently added the annotation on the graphs where they are shown in a light blue dotted vertical lines (e.g., Fig. 5). At the end of this period the devices were moved to the next room and the process was repeated until all areas of interested had been covered. The findings discussed below were reported to the health&safety officer and the ISO inspector.

The first area located at the back of the building overlooked a quiet alley and hosted offices with up to two people. Typically the windows were open and the air-conditioning was also on during the experiments. Although emission pollutant concentration indoors were negligent, particulate matter concentrations were slightly increased. Peaks crossed the threshold of 40 um/m^3 several times in an hour, although for very short duration. It was observed that they reached a peak during the spontaneous vacuum cleaning of the room by the cleaning contractors, as shown in Fig. 5(c) at 20 : $32pm$, indicating dust accumulation in the carpet.

The second area that is in the front of the building overlooking a busy road with significant traffic has an open-space configuration with some small offices. During the experiments an open window allowed slightly increased ozone concentrations to penetrate the space from outdoors; this dropped initially when the window was shut by two thirds and subsequently stabilised slightly higher (Fig. 5 (a)). Furthermore, it was observed that each person walking through this area caused a peak in particulate matter concentration, indicating accumulation of dust in the carpet (Fig. 5 (b)) and making it possible to count the total number of passers by counting the peaks.

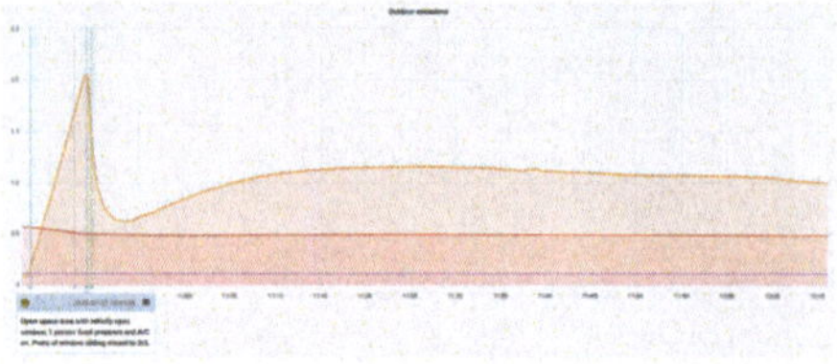

(a) CO, NO, O_3, VOC concentration in office over busy road

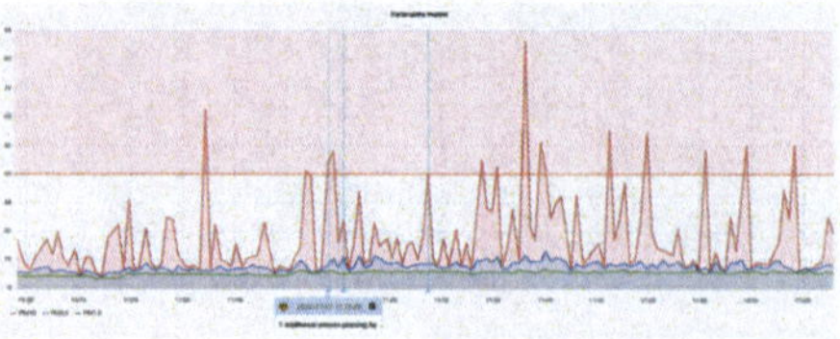

(b) PM concentration in office over busy road

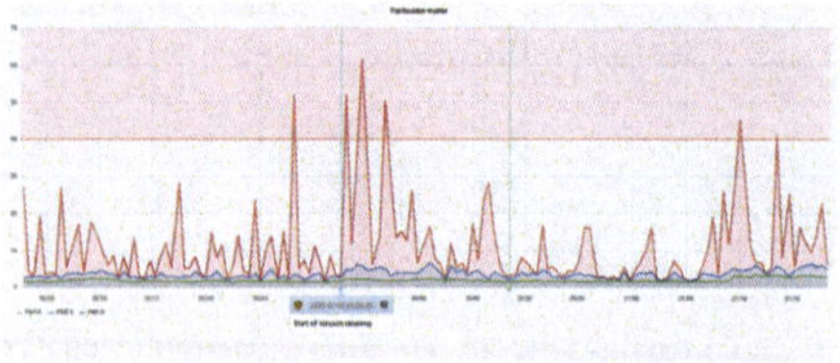

(c) PM concentration in office over quiet road

Fig. 5. Pollutant concentrations in office space

7 Conclusions

Low cost sensors make it possible to answer new questions about the underlying causes of poor air quality. Artificial intelligence in the broad sense appears to be a necessary companion to this work as it would provide insight and understanding in monitored patterns. For example, using a peak detection algorithm on the timeseries of Fig. 5(b) the number of passers-by could be detected in real-time, which could be useful in case of evacuation. Preventive maintenance is another area that could benefit from findings of this work, as the devices would indicate when is a good time for cleaning the carpets or perform cleaning tasks safely. Last, findings provide an insight on ventilation strategies seeming to suggest that in the front areas in proximity of heavy polluted roads, one should refrain from opening the window and should rather use the A/C retrofited with HEPA filters to purify the air.

References

1. Krzyzanowski, M., Martin, R.V., Van Dingenen, R., van Donkelaar, A., Thurston, G.D.: Exposure assessment for estimation of the global burden of disease attributable to outdoor air pollution. Environ. Sci. Technol. **46**, 652–660 (2012)
2. Samet, J.M., Dominici, F., Curriero, F.C., Coursac, I., Zeger, S.L.: fine particulate air pollution and mortality in 20 U.S. cities, 1987–1994. N. Engl. J. Med. **343**, 1742–1749 (2000)
3. Bano, N.: Assessment of indoor environmental impacts on human health (Case study: Glass city, Firozabad (India). Pollution **3**(2), 175–183 (2017)
4. **Setton, E., et al.: The impact of daily mobility on exposure to traffic-related air pollution and health effect estimates.** J. Expo. Sci. Environ. Epidemiol. **21**(1), 42–48 (2011)
5. Setti, L., et al.: Evaluation of the potential relationship between particulate matter (PM) pollution and COVID-19 infection spread in Italy:first observational study **based on initial epidemic diffusion.** BMJ Open 2020 **10**, e039338 (2020). https://doi.org/10.1136/bmjopen-2020-039338
6. Wu, X., Nethery, R.C., Sabath, M.B., Braun, D., Dominici, F.: Air pollution and COVID-19 mortality in the United States: strengths and limitations of an ecological regression analysis. Sci. Adv. **6**(45), eabd4049 (2020). https://doi.org/10.1126/sciadv.abd4049
7. Saadat, S., Rawtani, D., Hussain, C.M.: Environmental perspective of COVID-19. Sci. Total Environ. **728**, 138870 (2020). https://doi.org/10.1016/j.scitotenv.2020.138870
8. Le Quéré, C., et al.: Temporary reduction in daily global CO2 emissions during the COVID-19 forced confinement. Nat. Clim. Chang. **10**, 647–653 (2020). https://doi.org/10.1038/s41558-020-0797-x
9. Masiol, M., Squizzato, S., Chalupa, D., Rich, D.Q., Hopke, P.K.: Spatial-temporal variations of summertime ozone concentrations across a metropolitan area using a network of low-cost monitors to develop 24 hourly land-use regression models. Sci. Total Envirn. **2019**(654), 1167–1178 (2019)
10. Delgado-Saborit, J.M.: Use of real-time sensors to characterise human exposures to combustion related pollutants. J. Environ. Monit. **14**(7), 1824–37 (2012)
11. Mead, M.I., et al.: The use of electrochemical sensors for monitoring urban air quality in low-cost, high-density networks. Atmos. Environ. **70**, 186–203 (2013)
12. **Afzal, A., Cioffi, N., Sabbatini, L., Torsi, L.:** NO_x sensors based on semiconducting metal oxide nanostructures: progress and perspectives. Sens. Actuators B Chem. **171**, 25–42 (2012)
13. Hasenfratz, D., Saukh, O., Thiele, L.: On-the-fly calibration of low-cost Gas sensors. In: Picco, G.P., Heinzelman, W. (eds.) EWSN 2012. LNCS, vol. 7158, pp. 228–244. Springer, Heidelberg (2012). https://doi.org/10.1007/978-3-642-28169-3_15
14. Borrego, C., et al.: Assessment of air quality microsensors versus reference methods: the EuNetAir joint exercise - Part II. Atmos. Environ. **193**, 127–142 (2018)
15. Singhal, A., Cowie, M.R.: The role of wearables in heart failure. Curr. Heart Fail. Rep. **17**(4), 125–132 (2020). https://doi.org/10.1007/s11897-020-00467-x
16. Williams, D.E.: Low cost sensor networks: how do we know the data are reliable? ACS Sens. **4**(10), 2558–2565 (2019). https://doi.org/10.1021/acssensors.9b01455
17. Lightweight Machine to Machine Technical Specification, Open Mobile Alliance. http://www.openmobilealliance.org/release/LightweightM2M/V1_0-20170208-A/OMA-TS-LightweightM2M-V1_0-20170208-A.pdf

18. Katsiri, E., Bacon, J., Mycroft, A.: Linking sensor data to context-aware applications using abstract events. J. Pervasive Comput. Commun. (JPCC), Spec. Issue Managing Context Inf. Mobile Pervasive Environ. 4(3), 347–377 (2007)
19. Katsiri, E., Lopez-Ipina, D.: An ECA rule-matching service for simpler development of reactive applications. Published as a Supplement to the Proceedings of Middleware (2001)
20. Kumar, P., et al.: Indoor air quality and energy management through real-time sensing in commercial buildings. Energy Build. **111**, 145–153 (2016). https://doi.org/10.1016/j.enbuild.2015.11.037
21. Hagan, D.H., et al.: Inferring aerosol sources from low-cost air quality sensor measurements: a case study in Delhi. India. Environ. Sci. Technol. Lett. **6**, 467–472 (2019)
22. Nayeb Yazdi, M., Arhami, M., Delavarrafiee, M., Ketabchy, M.: Developing air exchange rate models by evaluating vehicle in-cabin air pollutant exposures in a highway and tunnel setting: case study of Tehran, Iran. Environ. Sci. Pollut. Res. **26**(1), 501–513 (2018). https://doi.org/10.1007/s11356-018-3611-9
23. deSouza, P., Lu, R., Kinney, P., Zheng, S.: Exposures to multiple air pollutants while commuting: evidence from Zhengzhou. China Atmos. Environ. **247**, 118168 (2020)
24. Bukowiecki, N., et al.: A mobile pollutant measurement laboratory–measuring gas phase and aerosol ambient concentrations with high spatial and temporal resolution. Atmos. Environ. **36**, 5569–5579 (2002). https://doi.org/10.1016/S1352-2310(02)00694-5
25. Apte, J.S., Messier, K.P., Gani, S., Brauer, M., Kirchstetter, T.W., Lunden, M.M., et al.: High-resolution air pollution mapping with google street view cars: exploiting big data. Environ. Sci. Technol. **51**, 6999–7008 (2017). https://doi.org/10.1021/acs.est.7b00891
26. Dutta, P., Aoki, P.M., Kumar, N., Mainwaring, A., Myers, C., Willett, W., et al.: Common sense: participatory urban sensing using a network of handheld air quality monitors. In: Proceedings of the 7th ACM Conference on Embedded Networked Sensor Systems, SenSys 2009, Association for Computing Machinery, Berkeley, California, pp. 349–350 (2009). https://doi.org/10.1145/1644038.1644095
27. Mahajan, S., Kumar, P.: Evaluation of low-cost sensors for quantitative personal exposure monitoring. Sustain. Cities Soc. **57**, 102076 (2020)
28. Anjomshoaa, A., Duarte, F., Rennings, D., Matarazzo, T.J., deSouza, P., Ratti, C.: City scanner: building and scheduling a mobile sensing platform for smart city services. IEEE Internet Things J. **5**, 4567–4579 (2018). https://doi.org/10.1109/JIOT.2018.2839058
29. DeSouza, P., Anjomshoaa, A., Duarte, F., Kahn, R., Kumar, P., Ratti, C.: Air quality monitoring using mobile low-cost sensors mounted on trash-trucks: methods development and lessons learned. Sustain. Urban Areas **60**, 102239 (2020)
30. deSouza, P., Kahn, A.R., Limbacher, A.J., Marais, A.E., Duarte, F., Ratti, C.: Combining low-cost, surface-based aerosol monitors with size-resolved satellite data for air quality applications. Atmos. Meas. Tech. **13**(10), 5319–5334 (2020). https://doi.org/10.5194/amt-13-5319-2020
31. Koukouli, M.E., et al.: Sudden changes in nitrogen dioxide emissions over Greece due to lockdown after the outbreak of COVID-19. Atmos. Chem. Phys. **21**(21), 1759–1774 (2020)
32. Kumar, P., Morawska, L., Martani, C., Biskos, G., Neophytou, M., Di Sabatino, S., et al.: The rise of low-cost sensing for managing air pollution in cities. Environ. Int. **75**, 199–205 (2015). https://doi.org/10.1016/j.envint.2014.11.019

33. Morawska, L., Thai, P.K., Liu, X., Asumadu-Sakyi, A., Ayoko, G., Bartonova, A., et al.: Applications of low-cost sensing technologies for air quality monitoring and exposure assessment: how far have they gone? Environ. Int. **116**, 286–299 (2018). https://doi.org/10.1016/j.envint.2018.04.018
34. Snyder, E.G., Watkins, T.H., Solomon, P.A., Thoma, E.D., Williams, R.W., Hagler, G.S.W., et al.: Applications of low-cost sensing technologies for air quality monitoring and exposure assessment: how far have they gone? Environ. Sci. Technol. **47**, 11369–11377 (2013). https://doi.org/10.1021/es4022602
35. Elen, B., Peters, J., Poppel, M.V., Bleux, N., Theunis, J., Reggente, M., et al.: The Aeroflex: a bicycle for mobile air quality measurements. Sensors **13**(2013), 221–240 (2013)
36. Capezzuto, L., et al.: A maker friendly mobile and social sensing approach to urban air quality monitoring. In: Proceedings of the 2014 IEEE on SENSORS, Valencia, Spain, pp. 12–16 (2014)
37. Murty, R.N., et al.: Citysense: an urban-scale wireless sensor network and testbed. In: Proceedings of the 2008 IEEE Conference on Technologies for Homeland Security, Waltham, MA, USA, 12–13 May, pp. 583–588 (2008)
38. Kadri, A., Yaacoub, E., Mushtaha, M., Abu-Dayya, A.: Wireless sensor network for real-time air pollution monitoring. In: Proceedings of the 2013 1st International Conference on Communications, Signal Processing, and their Applications (ICCSPA), Sharjah, United Arab Emirates, 12–14 February, pp. 1–5 (2013)
39. Postolache, O.A., Pereira, J.M.D., Girao, P.M.B.S.: Smart sensors network for air quality monitoring applications. IEEE Trans. Instrum. Meas. **58**, 3253–3262 (2009)
40. Hasenfratz, D., Saukh, O., Sturzenegger, S., Thiele, L.: Participatory air pollution monitoring using smartphones. Mobile Sensing **1**, 1–5 (2012)
41. Jiang, Y., et al.: MAQS: a personalized mobile sensing system for indoor air quality monitoring. In: Proceedings of the 13th International Conference on Ubiquitous Computing, Beijing, China, 17–21 September, ACM, New York, NY, pp. 271–280 (2011)
42. Jelicic, V., Magno, M., Brunelli, D., Paci, G., Benini, L.: Context-adaptive multimodal wireless sensor network for energy-efficient gas monitoring. IEEE Sens. J. **13**, 328–338 (2013)
43. Mansour, S., Nasser, N., Karim, L., Ali, A.: Wireless sensor network-based air quality monitoring system. In: Proceedings of the 2014 International Conference on Computing, Networking and Communications (ICNC), Honolulu, HI, USA, pp. 545–550 (2014)
44. Sun, L., et al.: Development and application of a next generation air sensor network for the Hong Kong marathon 2015 air quality monitoring. Sensors **16**, 211 (2016)
45. Honicky, R., Brewer, E.A., Paulos, E., White, R.: N-smarts: networked suite of mobile atmospheric real-time sensors. In: Proceedings of the Second ACM SIGCOMM Workshop on Networked Systems for Developing Regions. Seattle, WA, USA, 18 August, ACM, New York, NY, USA, pp. 25–30 (2008)
46. Lane, N.D., Miluzzo, E., Lu, H., Peebles, D., Choudhury, T., Campbell, A.T.: A survey of mobile phone sensing. IEEE Commun. Mag. **48**, 140–150 (2010)
47. Helbig, C., Bauer, H.-S., Rink, K., Wulfmeyer, V., Frank, M., Kolditz, O.: Concept and workflow for 3D visualization of atmospheric data in a virtual reality environment for analytical approaches. Environ. Earth Sci. **72**(10), 3767–3780 (2014). https://doi.org/10.1007/s12665-014-3136-6

48. Fadhel, M., Sekerinski, E., Yao, S.: A comparison of time series databases for storing water quality data. In: Auer, M.E., Tsiatsos, T. (eds.) IMCL 2018. AISC, vol. 909, pp. 302–313. Springer, Cham (2019). https://doi.org/10.1007/978-3-030-11434-3_33
49. Purpose-built, open-source time-series database: InfluxDB. https://www.influxdata.com
50. Grafana: The open observability platform. https://grafana.com
51. Elasticsearch. https://www.elastic.co/what-is/elasticsearch
52. Reas, C., Fry, B.: Processing: A Programming Handbook for Visual Designers MIT Press, Cambridge, Massachusetts, USA, p. 710 (2007). ISBN 978-0-262-18262-1

Information Quality Management for the Medical Wearable Devices: Validation Study

Rawhi Alrae[1](✉), Manar Abu Talib[2], and Qassim Nasir[3]

[1] Engineering Management Department, University of Sharjah, Sharjah, United Arab Emirates
alrae.rawhi@gmail.com
[2] Computer Science Department, University of Sharjah, Sharjah, United Arab Emirates
mtalib@sharjah.ac.ae
[3] Electrical Engineering Department, University of Sharjah, Sharjah, United Arab Emirates
nasir@sharjah.ac.ae

Abstract. Researchers have focused on wearable devices as viable Internet of Things (IoT) solutions in the recent decade. After the epidemic of COVID-19, they are receiving increasing attention. Wearable Internet of Things (IoT) systems must have high information quality (IQ) to be useful. In earlier publications, we developed a comprehensive framework for systematically managing the total information quality of IoT systems. By performing a comparative study, the framework was first shown to be accurate and reliable. In the last publication, medical wearable systems were selected as a single-case experiment to test the framework's usefulness by focusing on the assessment phase. This paper effectively uses the single case to test the rest of the framework phases: awareness and action. In addition, this work clearly illustrates the significance of the framework's three pillars: data quality, IoT, and IQ management procedures.

Keywords: Information quality · Internet of Things · Medical wearable devices · Quality management framework · Data quality dimensions · IoT elements

1 Introduction

In an earlier publication, we developed a framework to assist IoT managers and developers in maintaining their systems' information quality (IQ) [1]. Wieringa's [2] comparative study was used to validate the system. However, we agreed that a single case shows the context's applicability and stakeholders' responses. The COVID-19 crisis has boosted scholars' interest in wearable devices [3]. Therefore, we studied IQ management for the medical wearable IoT systems to discover current practices and develop future IQ methods for new trends and prospects. Moreover, this motivates us to use the medical wearable IoT devices as a single-case experiment.

This paper discusses the single-case validation structure in Sect. 2. Then Sect. 3 highlights the perspectives of our earlier developed framework. These are the data quality dimensions of IQ, the IoT technical elements, and the IQ management processes.

K. Daimi and A. Al Sadoon (Eds.): ICR 2022, AISC 1431, pp. 397–406, 2022.
https://doi.org/10.1007/978-3-031-14054-9_37

Section 4 focuses on the first stage of the case by testing the IQ assessment processes for medical wearable devices. Consequently, this stage defines the data dimensions of IQ for health systems and assigns relative importance to the dimensions. After that, the same section determines the IoT elements of wearable devices and identifies the activities per IoT element. Afterward, Sect. 5 defines IQ awareness processes, while Sect. 6 defines IQ action processes. Finally, Sect. 7 summarizes the results, concludes the work, and discusses how future works can benefit from the developed framework to manage IQ for IoT systems.

2 Methodology

The single-case goal is to oversee the complete quality of medical wearables using the developed framework. Moreover, it creates a macro quality system as general quality advocacy, rather than focusing on a particular application. Accordingly, our framework is based on the HoQ approach for managing information quality. Therefore, Fig. 1 summarizes how we implemented the IQ processes for the single-case [1]. These processes start with defining the data quality and IoT elements for medical wearables, then structure the quality relationships matrix and the technical interrelationships. The last processes are for building the planning and technical improvement plans. Figure 1 shows that the IQ assessment results in the ability to structure the quality relationships matrix and the technical interrelationships.

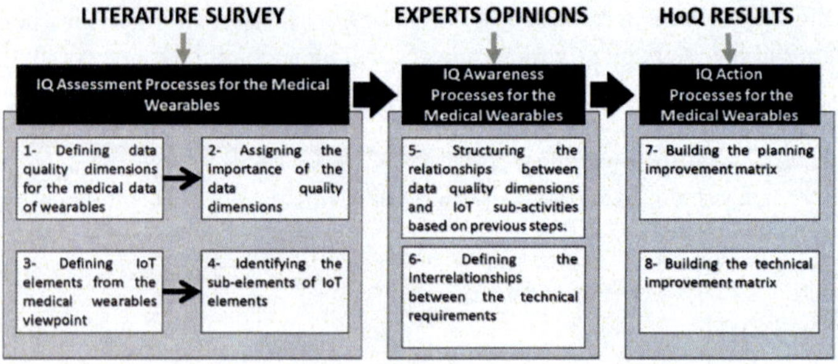

Fig. 1. IQ processes implementation for the single-case.

2.1 Expert Opinion Mythology

When the literature survey was conducted for the single-case to accomplish the IQ assessment, the first round of the Delphi represents building IQ awareness and IQ action through the experts' opinion. Therefore, the framework divided IQ management for wearables into eight stages, as shown in Fig. 1. This study uses the Delphi technique to get input from a group of experts. The Delphi method brings together the viewpoints of a diverse set of specialists based on the subject at hand [4–6]. Preparing questionnaires for improved data gathering is also recommended. This process allows the facilitator to gather, display, and evaluate the information. In order to reach a broad agreement and assure continual improvement, the questionnaire cycles may be repeated as many times as necessary. The first step in adopting the system is to get IQ assessment results. Based on these findings, a 15-question survey was built. To answer these questions, the expert must fill in a correlation matrix. The correlation definition determines each cell's response in multiple-choice selection. "No connection", "weak", "moderate", and "strong" are the four correlation definitions. According to the definitions, the scales are 0, 1, 3, and 9. This correlation scaling is adopted from many publications that discuss HoQ design, such as [7–11]. These publications suggested to have a significant variation between the moderate and strong correlation, and we agree that it ensures remarkable weight for the strong correlation.

Based on Delphi standards that match our case, we agreed with the University of Sharjah's Research Ethics Committee that the sample size should be roughly ten experts. Furthermore, we decided to choose the experts based on their academic qualifications or technological accomplishments in the field of IoT, Data Science, and information quality. After collecting data from experts, analyzing data, and presenting results, build the total IQ roadmap using the HoQ technique. Part of the case study can be addressed in the future for continuous improvements. Publications that discuss the "house of quality" agree that using the methodology can continuously build a circular quality management framework that keeps the quality cycle rolling [7–19].

3 Background and Related Work

The assumption of information as a product of IT systems can be seen in several publications such as [7, 20]. To this end, we devised an innovative and systematic approach to overseeing the IoT systems' overall information quality. Information quality is ensured by using the framework's defined methods and techniques. The framework's viewpoints are the IQ data quality dimensions, the IoT technical elements, and the IQ management processes [1].

This section discusses the developed framework published in [1], highlighting the IQ assessment process published in [3].

3.1 The Developed Framework

Having a framework for managing information quality in the IoT system was outlined in an earlier publication. In order to fulfill customer expectations, the suggested framework employs TQM methodologies to implement technological procedures. We indicated that IQ might be maintained by a matrix of product quality qualities and needed technical processes. Thus, information product quality is determined by its data quality dimensions. However, the IoT elements show the technical procedures of product quality [1].

IoT systems' IQ matrix should be carefully prepared and structured. To aid the IoT developer in controlling the system's IQ, each part of the matrix should be subsegmented. Assessment, awareness, and action are the three basic IQ management procedures shown in Fig. 2.

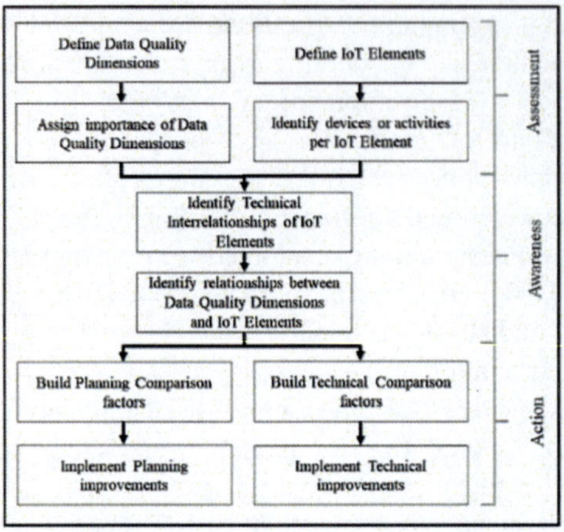

Fig. 2. IQ framework for IoT systems [1].

Our research found that awareness and action are more trend or application-focused. Specialist groups can help IoT developers identify and resolve trade-off issues. As shown in Fig. 2, awareness processes detect technical relationships between IoT elements and IQ data dimensions. The continuous improvement structure is defined by action processes portrayed by components that are assessed qualitatively. In other words, action processes can help marketing research and expert feedback.

4 IQ Assessment for Medical Wearables

Figure 2 depicts the proposed IQ framework for IoT system evaluation. These steps have been split into two groups to assist IoT developers. The first group determines the IQ data quality dimensions and their relative weights for IoT systems, and the second group defines IoT elements and their devices or activities. To analyze this case, one must determine the IQ aspects of data quality for health systems, prioritize them, and specify sub-elements per IoT element.

4.1 Defining and Prioritizing the Data Quality Dimensions for Health System

According to recent studies, based on our earlier observations in [1], clinical practice and healthcare research are the primary uses of wearables. Data quality dimensions are defined by focusing on these two characteristics. These dimensions are Security, Accessibility, Concise Representation, Representational Consistency, Ease of Understanding, Interpretability, Amount of Data, Completeness, Timeliness, Relevancy, Value-Added, Reputation, Believability, Objectivity, and Accuracy. Nevertheless, we showed in [3] that clinical practice and healthcare research publications tended to concentrate on the dimensions in diverse ways.

We were able to have better understand the significance of these dimensions in the literature because of these variances. These variations were used to calculate the importance weights by sorting the value of the data that represent the publications. The sorting values indicate the weight suggested by studying the recent literature studies on wearables for clinical practice and healthcare research work. The sorting takes the ascending order for the importance weight, so the higher the value, the higher the weight. These results are placed on the left side of the HoQ of Fig. 3.

4.2 Determining the IoT Elements of Wearable Devices and Identifying Their Technical Sub-elements

In [1], we proposed a comprehensive 7-elements view of the IoT elements. The implementation and existence of the IoT elements differ by the type of use of the wearable. Therefore, we validate the IoT elements structure by conducting a literature survey on wearable IoT systems. In this subsection, the survey determines the IoT elements by studying their definitions from the wearables' perspectives. Moreover, the survey identified the activities per IoT elements of wearables.

In [3], we conducted a literature search to ascertain the IoT elements of medical wearable systems. Additionally, the literature review was utilized to determine the technical tasks associated with each IoT element. We concentrated on sub-elements that had been endorsed by more than 90% of the chosen publications. The 90% threshold was assumed to favor the sub-elements with the most significant influence on the information quality of wearables based on the publication's focus. As a second part of the assessment, the results define the health wearables' IoT elements and the sub-elements' identification. These results are placed on the top side of the HoQ of Fig. 3. It is just below the roof.

5 IQ Awareness for Medical Wearables

5.1 Relating Data Quality Dimensions to IoT Sub-elements of Medical Wearables

The first part of the awareness is the relationship matrix between data quality dimensions to IoT sub-elements of medical wearables. This stage's findings are shown in the center of Fig. 3's HoQ. The matrix values are complex, and they pertain to three metrics. The first metric is indicated by the meanings of the symbols, which are "weak", "moderate", and "strong" relationships represented by a triangle, circle, or bullet, respectively [7, 12–17].

These relationships were established using the experts' most often expressed preferences. The symbols, which are based on the HoQ approach, have a numerical scale for each objective criterion. The numerical scale is the second dimension in which the matrix values are expressed. The scales used in the definitions are 1, 3, and 9. However, cells devoid of symbols indicate "no relationship" and hence have a value of zero [8–10, 19].

The third metric is shown by the percentages beside the symbols, representing the ratio of the most often selected expert opinion. For instance, the matrix's first cell represents the link between "dynamic identification" and "accuracy". Given that it takes the form of a circle with 58%, this number indicates that 58% of experts agree on the existence of a "moderate" link between the two variables.

5.2 Defining the Interrelationships Between the Technical Requirements

The interrelationships between IoT sub-elements of medical wearables comprise the second portion of the awareness outcomes. When the difference between scales is zero, then the two technical sub-elements are closely connected in the data quality dimension of the particular scale. Furthermore, zero-valued differences were counted to reflect the links between technical sub-elements. Since the number of DQ dimensions is 15, the intensity of interrelationships is represented by its proximity to the number 15. As a result, we created categories by splitting the range 0 to 15 into four quadrants as follows:

- The no-correlation for the values of 0 to 3.
- The weak correlation for the values of 4 to 7.
- The moderate positive correlation for the values of 8 to 11 denoted by the 'x'.
- The strong positive correlation for the values of 12 to 15 denoted by double 'x'.

Typically, operational teams and technical stakeholders have distinct roles for IoT elements and sub-elements. The roof of HoQ enables groups with a variety of responsibilities to choose who they can learn from or exchange experiences in terms of IQ management.

6 IQ Action for Medical Wearables

6.1 Building the Quality Improvement Plan

The quality improvement plan is the first portion of the action section. The five columns on the HoQ's left side illustrate this idea. These columns show how the data quality dimensions' present stage may be used to enhance the quality. They are as follows: DQ importance, the DQ weighted importance, the DQ relative percentage of importance, the DQ review urgency, and the DQ relative percentage of review urgency.

The DQ importance is calculated by adding the values of the symbols in each row of the relationship matrix. Additionally, the DQ-weighted importance results from multiplying DQ importance with the DQ importance weight. The outcome of the multiplication reflects both the ranking criteria provided in the literature review and the expert opinions. As a result, DQ relative importance quantifies the proportion of significance assigned to data quality attributes. The greater the DQ relative importance, the greater the dimension's effect on the information quality of the medical wearable system. As a result, Fig. 3 demonstrates that "accuracy" has the most significant influence on the medical wearable's IQ, while "ease of understanding" and "representational consistency" have the least.

On the other hand, the "DQ review urgency" of the findings by counting the symbols whose percentages are less than 50% for each row in the connection matrix. The urgency counters tell precisely what needs to be changed and where compromises are required. As a result, "DQ relative review urgency" quantifies the degree of urgency with which experts' comments should be reviewed concerning data quality aspects. The greater the urgency of the "DQ relative review", the more critical it is to verify the definition or classification of the DQ dimension for the information quality of the medical wearable

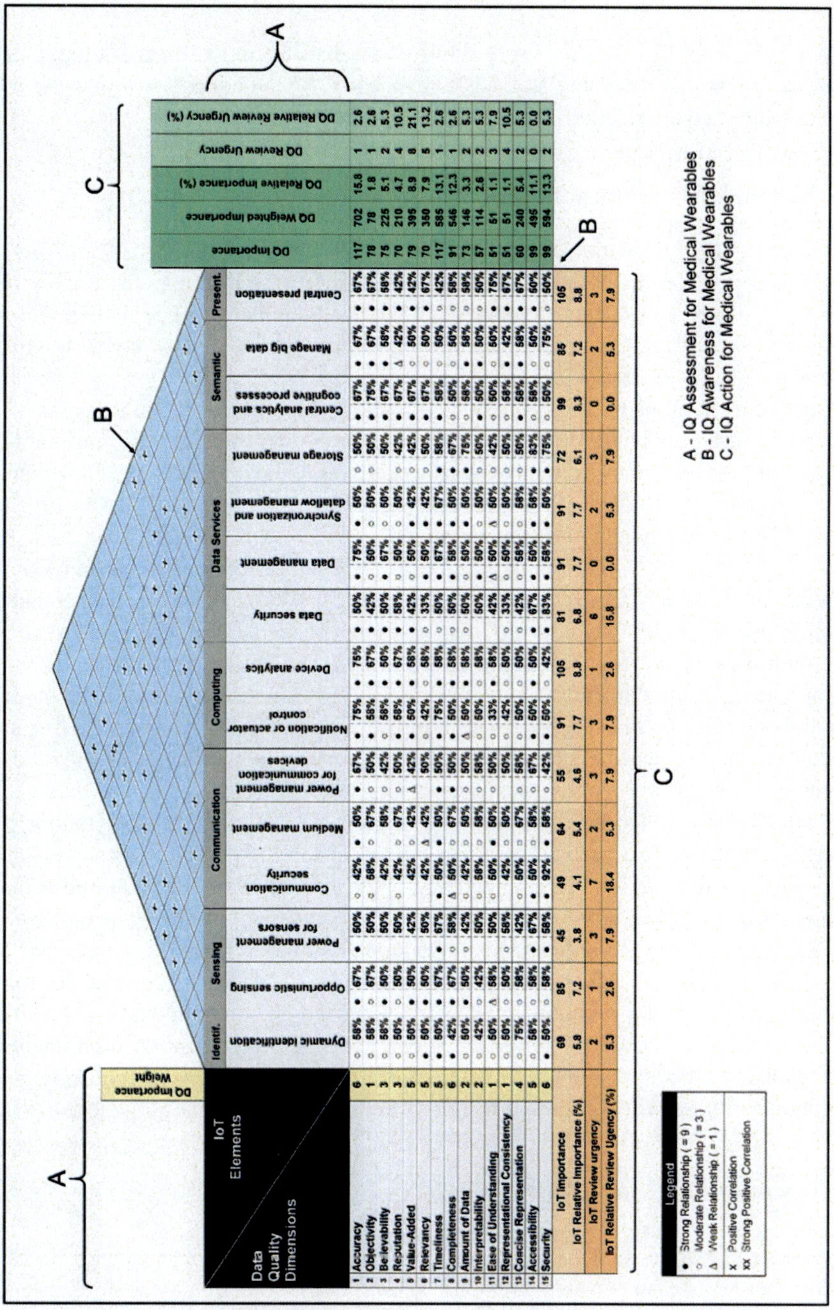

Fig. 3. HoQ as a result for the IQ management for the medical wearables.

system. As seen in Fig. 3, when "accessibility" receives the most consistent input, there is a high urgency in assessing and sub-categorizing "Value-added," as it has the most considerable urgency relative percentage.

6.2 Building the Technical Improvement Plan

The second part of the action section is the technical improvement plan. The four rows present this plan on the base of the HoQ. These rows describe how the quality may improve by studying the current stage of the IoT sub-elements. They include the IoT importance, the IoT relative percentage of importance, the IoT review urgency, and the relative percentage of review urgency.

The technical improvement plan is the second portion of the action processes. The four rows on the base of the HoQ show this plan. These rows illustrate how the quality of the IoT sub-elements may be improved by examining their present state. They include the IoT importance, the IoT relative percentage of importance, the IoT review urgency, and the relative percentage of review urgency.

The IoT importance represents the sum of the symbols' values of each column in the relationship matrix. Consequently, "IoT relative importance" defines the percentage of importance relatively linked to IoT sub-elements of the system. The greater the relative relevance of IoT, the greater the effect of technical activities associated with the appropriate IoT sub-element on implementing the information quality of the medical wearable system. As a result, Fig. 3 demonstrates that the sub-elements "notification or actuator control" and "central presentation" have the most influence on the medical wearable, while "power management for sensors" has the least.

On the contrary, "IoT review urgency" represents the counting of the symbols' percentages below 50% for each column in the relationship matrix. The urgency counters tell precisely what needs to be changed and where compromises are required. Consequently, "IoT relative review urgency" defines the percentage of urgency to review the experts' feedback that is comparatively linked to IoT sub-elements. The greater the "IoT relative review urgency", the more critical it is to revise the definition or classification of IoT sub-elements as the technological structure for the information quality of medical wearable systems. Therefore, since Fig. 6 can accurately represent "central analytics and cognitive processes", there is a high level of urgency to evaluate and sub-categorize "communication security", as it has the largest relative proportion of urgency.

7 Results and Conclusion

The case demonstrates how to use the framework developed to create a comprehensive structure for IQ assessment, awareness, and action. The first section of the IQ assessment specifies and prioritizes data quality characteristics for the IoT system. Additionally, the IQ assessment outlines the elements and sub-elements of the Internet of Things.

The awareness stage establishes linkages between data quality dimensions and IoT sub-elements in order to instruct the technical team on their degree of awareness for each data quality dimension during each technical activity. Furthermore, information stakeholders may leverage the links between data quality dimensions and IoT sub-elements to identify the IoT elements that contribute to each DQ dimension. Although the relationships matrix is at the core of the awareness stage and framework, it is helpful to define interrelationships between technical elements in IQ awareness. The technical interrelationships matrix defines the links between the IoT elements and sub-elements. These interrelationships refer to a technical group about the awareness correlation with other groups. Teams with good correlations may benefit from one another's experiences and knowledge.

The single-case study explored and demonstrated that the action stage adequately reflects the present cumulative influence of each DQ dimension and IoT element. Additionally, the action stage establishes qualitative and technical goals for ongoing progress.

In summary, the single case demonstrates to practitioners how the created framework maintains the IQ of medical wearable systems. Practitioners must be aware that this framework is not a tool to technical measure the quality of a specific unit.

However, practitioners must understand that this is a framework for continuous quality management. Publications discussing the "house of quality" concur that using the technique enables the development of continuous and circular quality management frameworks that keep the quality cycle rolling. As a result, the single-case study demonstrates the dynamic behavior of the developed framework when used in conjunction with the HoQ. The number of implementation cycles controls the behavior and the assumptions used for each cycle.

References

1. Alrae, R., Nasir, Q., Abu Talib, M.: Developing house of information quality framework for IoT systems. Int. J. Syst. Assur. Eng. Manag. **11**(6), 1294–1313 (2020). https://doi.org/10.1007/s13198-020-00989-6
2. Wieringa, R.J.: Single-case mechanism experiments. In: Wieringa, R.J. (ed.) Design Science Methodology for Information Systems and Software Engineering, pp. 247–267. Springer, Heidelberg (2014). https://doi.org/10.1007/978-3-662-43839-8_18
3. Alrae, R., Abutalib, M., Nasir, Q.: Information quality assessment for the medical wearable devices: validation study. In: Proceedings of the 2020 14th International Conference on Innovations in Information Technology, IIT 2020 (2020)
4. Linstone, H.A., Turoff, M.: The Delphi Method. Addison-Wesley, Reading (1975)
5. Skulmoski, G.J., Hartman, F.T., Krahn, J.: The Delphi method for graduate research. J. Inf. Technol. Educ. Res. **6**, 1–21 (2007)
6. Okoli, C., Pawlowski, S.D.: The Delphi method as a research tool: an example, design considerations and applications. Inf. Manag. **42**, 15–29 (2004)
7. Al-Hakim, L.: Information quality function deployment. In: Challenges of Managing Information Quality in Service Organizations, pp. 26–51. IGI Global (2007)
8. Temponi, C., Yen, J., Tiao, W.A.: House of quality: A fuzzy logic-based requirements analysis. Eur. J. Oper. Res. **117**, 340–354 (1999)
9. Hauser, J.: How Puritan-Bennett used the house of quality. Sloan Manage. Rev. **34**, 61 (1993)
10. Shen, X.X., Tan, K.C., Xie, M.: The implementation of quality function deployment based on linguistic data. J. Intell. Manuf. **12**, 65–75 (2001)
11. Hauser, J.R., Clausing, D.: The House of Quality (1988)
12. Ramalingam, T., Christophe, B., Samuel, F.: How to find a minimum viable product in IoTA. In: ERTS 2018 (2018)

13. Alptekyn, S.E., Alptekin, G.I.: A framework for customer-oriented IoT product design. In: Proceedings - 2018 2nd European Conference on Electrical Engineering and Computer Science, EECS 2018 (2018)
14. Ramalingam, T., Christophe, B., Samuel, F.W., et al.: Assessing the potential of IoT in aerospace. In: Kar, A.K., et al. (eds.) I3E 2017. LNCS, vol. 10595, pp. 107–121. Springer, Cham (2017). https://doi.org/10.1007/978-3-319-68557-1_11
15. Sharma, M., Chandna, S.: House of quality for complex software development decisions in mobile, wearables and IoT (2015)
16. Martí Bigorra, A., Isaksson, O.: Combining customer needs and the customer's way of using the product to set customer-focused targets in the House of Quality. Int. J. Prod. Res. **55**, 2320–2335 (2017)
17. Lee, S.H., Haider, A.: A framework for information quality assessment using six sigma approach. Commun. IBIMA (2011)
18. Lin, G., Jing, G., Fang-fang, D.: Evaluation method of enterprise information quality based on QFD. In: 2011 International Conference on Consumer Electronics, Communications and Networks (CECNet), pp. 325–328 (2011)
19. Haider, A., Lee, S.H.: A critical to quality factors choice: an integrated AHP-QFD model for information quality. In: Abramowicz, W., Domingue, J., Węcel, K. (eds.) BIS 2012. LNBIP, pp. 127–138. Springer, Heidelberg (2012). https://doi.org/10.1007/978-3-642-34228-8_13
20. Eppler, M.J., Wittig, D.: Conceptualizing Information quality: a review of information quality frameworks from the last ten years. IQ **20** (2000)

RFID Based Remote Monitoring Techniques for IoT Smart Parking System

Pujan Pradhananga[1], Javad Rezazadeh[2](✉), AB Emran Salahuddin[2], and Anchal Shrestha[2]

[1] Study Group Australia, Sydney, Australia
[2] Kent Institute Australia, Sydney, Australia
{javad.rezazadeh,emran.salahuddin,anchal.shrestha}@kent.edu.au

Abstract. The RFID based techniques help overcome the problem of parking system by using smart technology which is based on IoT (Internet of Things). The paper focuses on improving the issues occurring at the parking which affects the area due to the gathering of the crowd at their nearby places. The aim of doing this research is to create an RFID based parking system for improvement of proper transportation facilities at the public places. In this paper we compare and evaluate highlighted methods based on the three important components, Data receiving, Monitoring and Displaying information (DMD). These components are very helpful in the smart parking techniques, such as the data about the parking area is received with the help of sensors or video camera and the information is displayed on the monitor screen or on the smartphones, the detection system is based on RFID, with the help from this system. Information can be shared and displayed to the server from where it can be monitored easily. The system has proposed results in monitoring the parking with the help of smart methods, such as monitoring with the help of smart sensors based on IoT.

Keywords: RFID · IoT · VANET · Cloud computing · Smart City

1 Introduction

The Internet of Things (IoT) is one of the leading technologies in ubiquitous computing and the key solution for providing the smart environments [1]. The technology used is unconstrained optimization method which is very useful in the Smart parking system which uses RFID (Radio Frequency Identification) [2]. The purpose of this project is to reduce the crowd level at the public places due to which any kind of problems can occur such as security, parking issues, traffic congestion, etc. [3]. The issues can be resolved with the help of proposed taxonomy i.e. Data receiving, monitoring, and displaying information (DMD) [4]. With the help of these components, the information can be shared, displayed and improved for the future purpose [5]. The technology used for this project is RFID which helps in monitoring the vehicles in the parking area with the help of smart sensors [6]. As the project is based on monitoring of the vehicles coming to the parking area and it helps collect information about the vehicle. The limitation of this project is that it is only able to monitor the objects but sometimes due to bad

K. Daimi and A. Al Sadoon (Eds.): ICR 2022, AISC 1431, pp. 407–416, 2022.
https://doi.org/10.1007/978-3-031-14054-9_38

weather conditions the images [7] becomes blur due to which the exact information is not monitored, so as the images become blur and the information is not processed correctly [8]. The main objective of this project is to create safe and secure parking which do not affect the nearby places [9]. By classifying the data receiving, monitoring, and displaying information components for parking system it becomes easy to distinguish what kind of approach can be taken for the betterment of the project [10]. This project is based on RFID which performs the monitoring process with the help of sensors and can be used in the smart parking system [11]. The work steps followed in this is as follows: step2 includes literature review through which all the collected papers can be used for research [12] Step 3 includes state of the art solution. Step 4 includes the proposed model [13] Step 5 includes validation and evaluation [14] Step 6 includes verification technique [15] Step 7 includes a discussion of the project. Step 8 includes the conclusion of comprehensive research [16]. DMD taxonomy is a technique which is used as a component for classification of the smart parking system which includes remote monitoring techniques [17]. It is used for the improvement of security and parking facilities [18].

2 Literature Review

Previously the parking area was monitored manually which was not that efficient as efficiency was not up to the mark and was less than 40%, but smart parking systems which includes RFID gives more efficient results and gives the efficiency rate up to 80% [19]. The proposed system in [20] is used for reducing the influence of position and accuracy on the performance of AVG (Automated Guided Vehicle). The solutions for improving monitoring of parking system are implemented with RFID.

The input is taken in the form of radio signals which is processed using the probabilistic technique, and the output is given in the form of data [21]. This process is used to study the LPDA (Log-Periodic Dipole Array) antenna which provides radiation efficiency of 80% but the major issues occur on positioning system is the time delay that it was due to the less efficiency of the system. If the positioning systems do not function properly, then the productivity of the whole system will be affected as given by, the iBeacon algorithm is used to improve the positioning mechanism of the car parking system [22]. It also aims at minimizing the use of human resources in this system so that the needed accuracy is achieved for Smart Parking System. The main focus of the research is on smart parking system with the help of mobile applications, that is the details of the vacant space, or occupied space available in the parking area can be tracked by the mobile application so that the ticketing system can be improvised. Some limitations such as low penetrating power of the system, low range of Bluetooth device needed to be improved in the system [23].

The model based on IoT is applied to provide the empirical path loss model to be implemented in WSN for outdoor and indoor parking for the use of a Smart Car Parking System. It has a Comparison between proposed mode and theoretical model which is for smart car parking [24]. The Cloud-based SVPS (Smart Vehicle parking systems) model is used for a smart vehicle parking system by using cloud-based Vehicular Ad Hoc Network (VANET) for the use of Smart vehicle parking [25]. It has been proposed that the number of vehicles has increased over time and the parking space is limited. Due to this on an average about 7.5 min are wasted by the users in searching available parking space [26]. Although the author has proposed that the research provides an effective solution for the parking system by implementing cloud based SVPS. It also uses the novel algorithm to provide available parking space [27]. In [28] the IoT is a technique which is used for the security of the system which is based on IoT for the betterment of Security of Smart parking system. It has been observed that the signaling overheads are reduced to 52.5% to 87.3%. The research provided the security of the parking management system using Lora WAN technique; but some issues are occurring on it that the technique has few features for security due to the high-power consumption of the more secure system [29]. In [30], the model based on IoT is to develop a framework to be implemented in the smart parking and smart city that contains features such as storage for big data, processing in real time and IoT for the Smart Environments. The Ultrasonic distance measurement technique is used for providing such a system which is used to transmit the data with ranging accuracy of RFID tags. Mobile wireless sensor networks [31] should be used to cover all space of the parking and use blockchain [32] to provide appropriate security and also apply accurate localization methods [33, 34] to find location of vehicles in an intelligent VANET systems [35].

3 System Components

This system is proposed for smart parking system such as Data receiving, Monitoring, and displaying information (DMD), which is originated from ritual criteria. It is selected based on RFID based remote monitoring for smart parking system which is used for both parking and security purposes. This development is doing on considering the issues like Check-ins and Check-outs of vehicles involved in parking and controlling of the crowd in public areas. Furthermore, DMD Taxonomy will be applied on premises owned by management and their area of coverage to facilitate their work.

In this paper all important components of smart parking are evaluated. These are required for the domain and help complete the project of smart parking system for security and management purpose. Thus, important steps have to be followed below:

- What are the techniques and equipment required for the monitoring of the parking system with RFID technology?
- For completion of this research work what type of information is required?
- How can the problems of parking be improved with the help of RFID technology?

Hence, contact of remote sensing technique is implemented to give correct monitoring for security and parking purpose with explained three all-inclusive factors as Data receiving, Monitoring, and Displaying information.

The first part of the DMD taxonomy is Data receiving. It contains data about the parking lot of vehicles. By containing the data of the parking lot, it becomes easy for remote sensor-based controlling. Highly sensitive sensors will cover parking lot area which facilitates monitoring and security for parking purposes. Data receiving component receives and records vehicle data that are entering the premises. Monitoring, the second step of the proposed taxonomy, which helps to monitor the vehicles that are coming for parking, currently inside or leaving the premises. The third component of the proposed taxonomy is displaying information. This component will depend on first two component i.e., Data receiving and Monitoring. Information received from the sensors are stored, processed, and managed by the server and displayed at different display points and report.

With combination of these three steps, all vehicles in parking lot remains secure and managed. Therefore, remote sensing technology with RFID tool is very helpful for the maintenance and security of the vehicles. We have design Fig. 1 that shows all the three components Data receiving, Monitoring and Displaying information Sensing, with given instances.

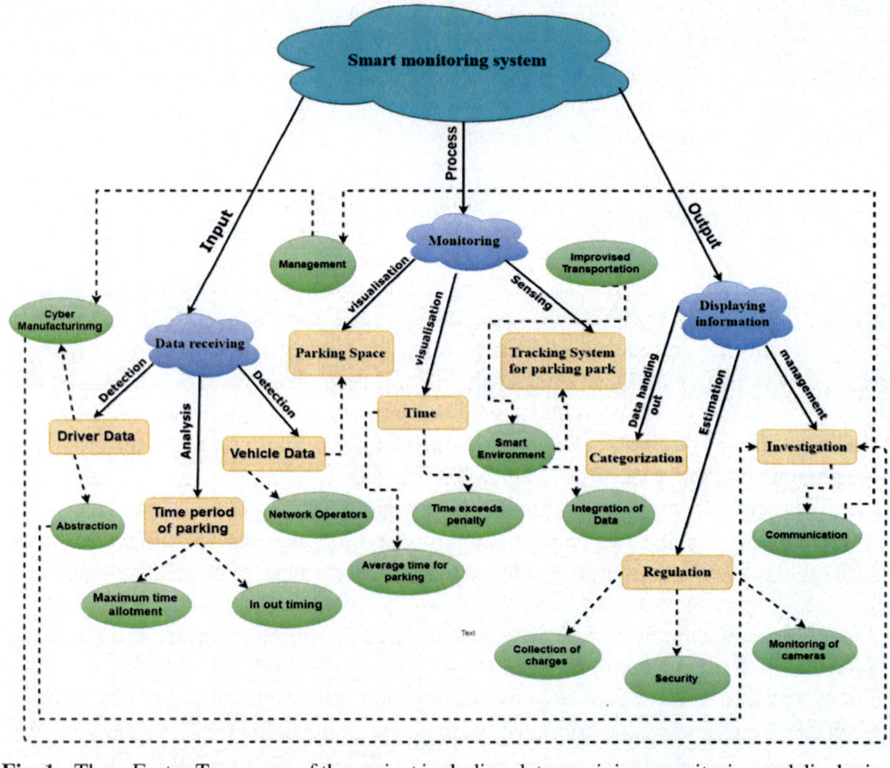

Fig. 1. Three Factor Taxonomy of the project including data receiving, monitoring and displaying information and their interrelationship.

Data Receiving. The main purpose of this step is about the collection of the data which is installed in the sensors. To do the complete processing of the stored information data integration method is used for the fulfilment of the parking and security. Virtual sensors are used for extracting the information about the vehicles and types of vehicles are coming in a parking lot. The whole process is completed with the help of data synchronization technique.

Monitoring. The purpose of monitoring is to monitor the surroundings and the vehicle park in the lot with the help of wireless acoustic sensors. There are several tools and devices such as sensors and wearable devices used in this procedure. Moreover, the security process involved the software and hardware approach.

Displaying Information. It is used to display the output of the input given to the system. It is used to give the output of the system in the tactile form; the output is given in the electronic form. The result is extracted from the system in the digital form with the help of sensors and wearable devices. The input information is given in the system in the form of an electrical signal form.

The Table 1 describes the main components of the Taxonomy with Data receiving, monitoring and Displaying Information.

Table 1. Classifies the research work according to the primary components

References	Used technology	Domain	Data receiving		Monitoring		Displaying information	
			Driver data	Vehicle data	Parking space	Tracking system	Investigation	Categorization
Lu et al. 2017	Unconstrained optimization	Smart factories	Cyber manufacturing	Proper management	Coordination technology	Communication system	Available parking space	GPS
Olasupo et al. 2018	IoT (Internet of Things)	Smart car parking	Smart parking meters	Geographic area	Occupancy per areas	Smart mobile devices	Real-time monitoring	Vehicle real time
Celesti & Fazio 2018	Internet of things	Smart environments	Spout	Bolt	Allyn	Environment AJSC	Remote monitoring	Improvised transportation
Ahmed et al. 2018	Optimization techniques	Smart street	Speed protocol	Node deployment	complex devices	Interaction	Database	Gateway
Carotenuto et al. 2018	Ranging RFID tags	RFID,Remote Sensor	ranging accuracy	Energy harvesting	RF transmitter	RFID Relay	RFID Sensor	Peak detection time
Tang et al. 2018	Genetic algorithm	Highly populated	DGP algorithm	IoT	Micro controller	Distance based	Signal amplitude	RFID-remote sensor
Rizvi et al. 2018	Computer simulation	Populated urban areas	ASPIRE	Visualization tool	IOT nodes	Vehicle monitor	Accurate parking	ASPIRE
Habibzadeh et al. 2018	Machine intelligence	Soft sensing tool	Flexible	The sensor node is wired	Monitoring	Linear network	KNN Optimize	Accuracy
Sobral et al. 2018	Fuzzy Q-algorithm	RFID enabled parking	Spaces management	Multiple transmissions	RFID anti collision	Google -map	Process time	Ant colony opt
Karpenko et al. 2018	Semantic data model	Enabling smart parking	Data sharing	Self–parking	API Data model	Hybrid sensor	Sending data over IPv6	Data format

4 System Verification

The method for evaluating ontology (taxonomy) recommended as a very important factor. In this quantitative and qualitative approaches have been used for the evaluation of ontologies. It includes domain which has expertise in the given taxonomy which full fills the criteria for the given task.eg. Monitoring, reviewing, data extraction and uniformity. There were other approaches like the optimization techniques which were used for solving the issues of ontology. Since the approach is statistical so to differentiate between the different ontologies' corpus method is used for making the comparison between the different ontologies.

System Acceptance. To calculate the DMD taxonomy, it has been checked about the overlap of terms among literature and taxonomy. Basically, it has been examined about the overlap of terms between the instances that class or components in a given taxonomy can be used or not. It was exactly not conceivable to completely automate the method because the used terms in the taxonomy are fully dependent on context. For example, the parking of vehicle involving smart techniques includes a sensor, so the parking is dependent on sensors and it depends on the tracking system of the vehicle. We provide the criteria of validation and evaluation of highlighted related papers in the Table 2. Most papers improved the performance and accuracy of smart parking with RFID.

Table 2. Validation and evaluation table

Author	Study criteria	Validation		Component validate	Evolution	Result
		Input	Output			
Lu et al. 2017	Smart Factories	Evaluation on the services provided	Evaluation index is different	Smart cells	Communication technology	7% for smart cities, 9% for administration
Olasupo et al. 2018	Smart car parking	Embedded system is applied	Big data analysis	Data analytics	Cloud & remote monitoring	Enhances performance
Celesti et al. 2018	Smart environments	Theoretical model	WSN for accuracy	Path loss models	Propagation model	Deviation is 10% to 46%
Ahmed et al. 2018	Smart street	The number of vehicles	Dynamic allocation	Using PSU	Infrastructure high computing	On an average, about 7.5 min
Carotenuto et al. 2018	Remote sensor	Ranging code runs on machine	Achieve ranging rate of 1 Hz	Prototype Design	Chirp frequency bandwidth	Distance based
Tang et al. 2018	Populated area	Localization technique	Fog computing and VANET	Fog Computing	Fog node for the parking time	Parking distance
Rizvi et al. 2018	Highly populated urban areas	RFID based sensor detects the IOT chip	Efficient in solving parking	Transmitting information	Transmitting information	Parking slot allotted to the vehicle
Habibzadeh et al. 2018	Soft sensing for smart parking	Dynamic demand response (D2R)	Easily sharing of data	Intelligence data processing	Driver's decision support framework	Sensor fusion (τ) set at 0.8 & threshold 0.65
Sobral et al. 2018	RFID enabled parking	Ant colony optimization	EPC C1–G2 anti-collision	RFID & WSN Integration	RFID & WSN enable ranging	Electronic Product Code
Karpenko et al. 2018	Enabling smart parking	Error rate with traffic load	Interoperability is functionless	Open API Data model	Initiate Low-level network	1% for users & 7% traffic

The percentage of research papers shown that represents the class of the factor within the taxonomy. Figure 2 shows percentage of component used different technologies.

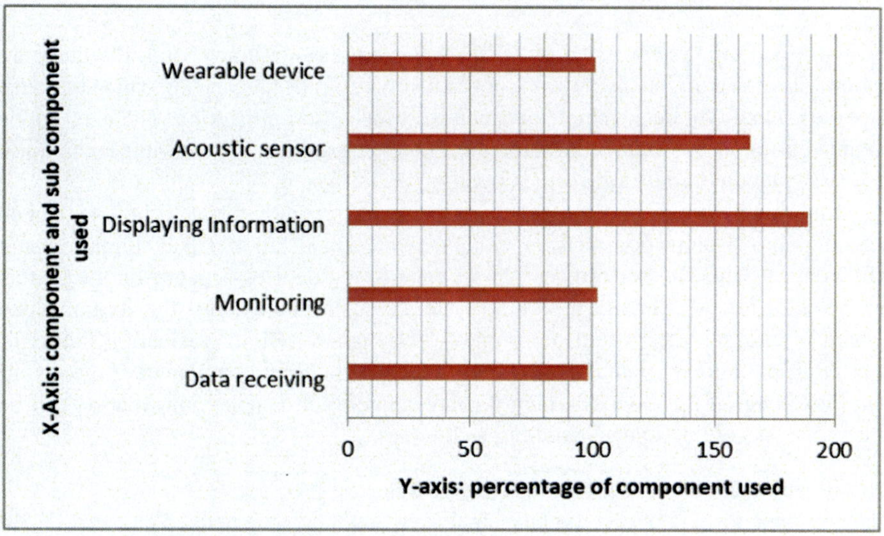

Fig. 2. Occurrence of system components and their subcomponents

Completeness. According to [3], the criteria due to which failure can occur the proposed system area hybrid approach of the simulation model. The reason for the failure is that the simulation model needs different condition according to the environment. Due to the different model, there occurs the problem of security of server of IoT. Table 3 shows the frequency used for different Technologies.

Table 3. Frequency table

Term	Frequency	Term	Frequency
RFID	90	Detection	70
Internet of Things	80	Information	75
Acoustic sensor	60	Sensors	90
Display devices	90	Tracking System	65
Monitoring	95	Identification	85
Smart parking	85	Optimization	80
Vehicles	95	Acquisition	60
Mobility	55	Interfacing	50

5 System Discussion

As per the research, in the discussion section, it is necessary to discuss the components of taxonomy in this research DMD. To show the importance of DMD taxonomy in the smart parking system based on RFID, the examples are drawn from the literature review. The first component of the proposed taxonomy is Data receiving which has been classified into driver data, vehicle data and the time period of parking. The data can be obtained from various extraction, detection techniques and machine learning techniques. The large amount of data affects the operation of the system.

Monitoring is the second component of the taxonomy, monitoring techniques can be classified into visualization, sensors, cloud network, localization, cloud computing and RFID devices etc. The performance of the monitoring devices depends on the performance of the internet. Smart car parking system uses the cloud computing as embedded system to enhance the system performance. Use smart cells in evaluation index for smart transportation system. Display Information is the third component of the taxonomy including all the devices which displays the output. Display information can be categorized according to data handling techniques.

Data Receiving: Driver Data and Vehicle Data

The very specific data of raw has been analyzed, and they were defined and share in all the respected publications and just some papers were up to the mark and fulfilling the conditions and giving accurate information. The data which has been derived supports the data of driver to be recognized for the safe parking, and the vehicle data has also been stored with the help of sensors for secure parking of the vehicles. So, for the secure parking vehicle data and driver data has been stored with the help of sensors.

Monitoring: Parking System and Tracking System

Monitoring plays a vital role in smart parking based on RFID. In monitoring parking space as well as a tracking system is important which is based on remote monitoring techniques for smart parking system. Sensors are used for the remote monitoring of the vehicles. Some of the papers require the optimization techniques for the smart parking system which is different from other techniques, and it is very useful. It is time dependent technique. With the help of monitoring indoor and outdoor navigation are provided for the welfare of the parking system.

Displaying Information: Categorization and Investigation

From above all publications selected, many of the research papers are not up to the required domain and technique. Only a few of the papers fulfil the required conditions of the research. Displaying information is a part of the output for the parking system. LED indicators and LED display are used for the output with the help of sensors. Information is collected from satellite networks for the radio frequency propagation.

6 Conclusion

The research has the aim of focusing on proposed DMD taxonomy for smart parking system based on RFID technology. With the proper monitoring and systematic approach to the parking method, problems related to parking can be solved easily. This research has the limitations that such as problems that occur previously when vehicles were parked on the roads which result in long traffic jams and were very common, but with the help of this smart parking system, the frequency of traffic jams is reduced abruptly, as the Ultra High RFID network is built to approach the parking rage to get the easy source.

References

1. Rezazadeh, J., Sandrasegaran, K., Kong, X.: A location-based smart shopping system with IoT technology. In: 2018 IEEE 4th World Forum on Internet of Things (WF-IoT), Singapore, pp. 748–753 (2018)
2. Sobral, J.V.V., Rodrigues, J.J.P.C., Rabelo, R.A.L.: A framework for enhancing the performance of internet of things applications based on RFID and WSNs. J. Netw. Comput. Appl. **107**(11), 56–68 (2018)
3. Chen, C., Liu, X., Qiu, T., Liu, L., Sangaiah, A.K.: Latency estimation based on traffic density for video streaming on the internet of vehicles. Comput. Commun. **111**(1), 176–186 (2017)
4. Chen, J., et al.: Service-oriented dynamic connection management for software-defined internet of vehicles. IEEE Trans. Intell. Transp. Syst. **18**(10), 2826–2837 (2017)
5. Choudhary, A., Gopal, K., Sood, D., Tripathi, C.C.: Development of compact inductive coupled meander line RFID tag for near-field applications. Int. J. Microw. Wirel. Technol. **9**(4), 757–764 (2017)
6. Colella, R., Tarricone, L., Catarinucci, L.: SPARTACUS: self-powered augmented RFID tag for autonomous computing and ubiquitous sensing. IEEE Trans. Antennas Propag. **63**(5), 2272–2281 (2015)
7. Karpenko, A., et al.:: Data exchange interoperability in IoT ecosystem for smart parking and EV charging. Sensors **18**(6) (2018)
8. Diro, A.A., Chilamkurti, N., Kumar, N.: Lightweight cybersecurity schemes using elliptic curve cryptography in publish-subscribe fog computing. Mob. Netw. Appl. **22**(5), 848–858 (2017). https://doi.org/10.1007/s11036-017-0851-8
9. Ding, K., Jiang, P., Su, S.: RFID-enabled social manufacturing system for inter-enterprise monitoring and dispatching of integrated production and transportation tasks. Robot. Comput.-Integr. Manuf. **49**(4), 120–133 (2018)
10. Abdelnour, A., Lazaro, A., Villarino, R., Kaddour, D., Tedjini, S., Girbau, D.: Passive harmonic RFID system for buried assets localization. Sensors **18**(11), 3635 (2018)
11. Feng, S., Setoodeh, P., Haykin, S.: Smart home: cognitive interactive people-centric internet of things. IEEE Commun. Mag. **55**(2), 34–39 (2017)
12. Habibzadeh, H., Qin, Z., Soyata, T., Kantarci, B.: Large-scale distributed dedicated- and non-dedicated smart city sensing systems. IEEE Sens. J. **17**(23), 7649–7658 (2017)
13. Hilmani, A., Maizate, A., Hassouni, L.: Designing and managing a smart parking system using wireless sensor networks. J. Sens. Actuat. Netw. **7**, 24 (2018)
14. Zhang, K., Ni, J., Yang, K., Shen, X.S.: Security and privacy in smart city applications: challenges and solutions. IEEE Commun. Mag. **55**(1), 122–129 (2017)
15. Ivanov, D., Dolgui, A., Sokolov, B., Werner, F., Ivanova, M.: A dynamic model and an algorithm for short-term supply chain scheduling in the smart factory industry 4.0. Int. J. Prod. Res. **54**(2), 386–402 (2016)
16. Javed, M.A., Hamida, E.B.: On the interrelation of security, QoS, and safety in cooperative ITS. IEEE Trans. Intell. Transp. Syst. **18**(7), 1943–1957 (2017)
17. Javed, M.A., Zeadally, S., Usman, M., Sidhu, G.A.S.: FASPM: fuzzy logic-based adaptive security protocol for multihop data dissemination in intelligent transport systems. Trans. Emerg. Telecommun. Technol. **28**, 3190 (2017)
18. Javed, M.A., Zeadally, S., Hamida, E.: Data analytics for cooperative intelligent transport systems. Veh. Commun. **15**(1), 63–72 (2019)
19. Tang, C., Wei, X., Zhu, C., Chen, W., Rodrigues, J.J.P.C.: Towards smart parking based on fog computing. IEEE Access **6**(19), 70172–70185 (2018)
20. Tsai, M.-F., Kiong, Y.C., Sinn, A.: Smart service relying on internet of things technology in parking systems. J. Supercomput. **74**, 4315–4338 (2018)

21. Kotb, A.O., Shen, Y., Huang, Y.: Smart parking guidance, monitoring, and reservations: a review. IEEE Intell. Transp. Syst. Mag. **9**(2), 6–16 (2017)
22. Rezazadeh, J., Subramanian, R., Sandrasegaran, K., Kong, X., Moradi, M., Khodamoradi, F.: Novel iBeacon placement for indoor positioning in IoT. IEEE Sens. J. **18**(24), 10240–10247 (2018)
23. Celesti, A., Fazio, M., Galletta, A., Carnevale, L., Wan, J., Villari, M.: An approach for the secure management of hybrid cloud–edge environments. Futur. Gener. Comput. Syst. **90**(4), 1–19 (2019)
24. Alelaiwi, A.: A collaborative resource management for big IoT data processing in Cloud. Clust. Comput. **20**(2), 1791–1799 (2017). https://doi.org/10.1007/s10586-017-0839-y
25. Lin, J., Yu, W., Yang, X., Yang, Q., Fu, X., Zhao, W.: A real-time en-route route guidance decision scheme for transportation-based cyberphysical systems. IEEE Trans. Veh. Technol. **66**(3), 2551–2566 (2017)
26. Alqazzaz, A., Alrashdi, L., Aloufi, E., Zohdy, M., Ming, H.: SecSPS: a secure and privacy-preserving framework for smart parking systems. J. Inf. Secur. **9**(4), 299–314 (2018)
27. Lin, T., Rivano, H., Mouël, F.L.: A survey of smart parking solutions. IEEE Trans. Intell. Transp. Syst. **18**(12), 3229–3253 (2017)
28. Lu, S., Xu, C., Zhong, R.Y., Wang, L.: An RFID-enabled positioning system in an automated guided vehicle for smart factories. J. Manuf. Syst. **44**(15), 179–190 (2017)
29. Ahmed, S., Rani, S.: hybrid approach, Smart Street use case and future aspects for IoT in smart cities. Futur. Gener. Comput. Syst. **79**(3), 941–951 (2018)
30. Rizvi, S.R., Zehra, S.: ASPIRE an agent-oriented smart parking recommendation system for smart cities. IEEE Intell. Transp. Syst. Mag. **1** (2018)
31. Rezazadeh, J., Moradi, M., Ismail, A.S.: Mobile wireless sensor networks overview. Int. J. Comput. Commun. Netw. **2**(1), 17–22 (2012)
32. Sharifinejad, M., Dorri, A., Rezazadeh, J.: BIS-A blockchain-based solution for the insurance industry in smart cities. arXiv:2001.05273 (2020)
33. Rezazadeh, J., Moradi, M., Ismail, A.S.: Message-efficient localization in mobile wireless sensor networks. J. Commun. Comput. **9**(3), 340–344 (2012)
34. Rezazadeh, J., Moradi, M., Sandrasegaran, K., Farahbakhsh, R.: Transmission power adjustment scheme for mobile beacon-assisted sensor localization. IEEE Trans. Ind. Inform. **15**(5), 2859–2869 (2019)
35. Fotros, M., Riahi Kashani, M. M., Rezazadeh, J., Ayoade, J.: A timely VANET multi-hop routing method in IoT. In: 2019 20th International Conference on Parallel and Distributed Computing, Applications and Technologies (PDCAT), pp. 19–24 (2019)

DOA Based Identification for Devices and Applications of IoT in Heterogeneous Networks

Mahmood Al-Bahri[1](✉) and Wasan Al Kishri[2]

[1] Faculty of Computing and IT, Sohar University, Sohar, Oman
mbahri@su.edu.om
[2] Faculty of Computer Studies, Arab Open University–Oman, Muscat, Oman
wasan.k@aou.edu.om

Abstract. This paper proposes a method for recognizing Internet of Things devices and applications in heterogeneous networks based on the Digital Objects Architecture (DOA). Also, the work discusses techniques for integrating a DOA identifier into IoT devices that support various wireless data transfer technologies and presents a metadata structure. A description of the structure of a typical IoT device and the resolution process based on the DOA is presented. Typical examples of implementing the represented methods and the interaction of the IoT device with the components of the DOA are considered. The potential for implementing the DOA-based identification of Internet of Things devices and applications in heterogeneous communication networks are examined. It is shown that the proposed integration should contribute to a more open exchange of data between different IoT devices and applications. The proposed method allows for identifying IoT devices and applications on a global scale.

Keywords: DOA · GHR · LHR · IoT · Devises · Identification · Network · Handle system

1 Introduction

Access to the Internet, both directly and through gateways, is one of the most important responsibilities for IT specialists. This is required for each object (IoT) to be represented electronically or physically, to have an address, and to be accessible via the Internet at any time and from any location. The Industrial Internet of Things is currently working on developing identifying techniques for a variety of device classes and types. It is also part of research in International Standards Organizations, both public and commercial.

The existing identification mechanisms used in various data transmission technologies were invented at the turn of the century. Despite this, there was no mention of the estimated number of connected IoT devices. Only a small number of IoT devices can benefit from an efficient system for assigning unique identifiers [1]. In addition, the existing identification methods, for the most part, do not support IoT devices that are briefly connected to the Internet, moving between various public and private communication

K. Daimi and A. Al Sadoon (Eds.): ICR 2022, AISC 1431, pp. 417–428, 2022.
https://doi.org/10.1007/978-3-031-14054-9_39

networks. The fact that IDs can contain information connected to a specific location of IoT devices in communication networks is also a disadvantage of these methods. IoT objects should have identifiers that do not depend on which network they are in or which users they belong to [2].

The conceptual gap between an item identification and its network address is another point to examine. The object identification and its address serve different purposes in the most general scenario. The former assigns a distinct identifier to the object. Nonetheless, the network address may differ depending on the object's physical location, logical membership in one or more networks, or role. When the object identifier and the address are different, the identifier is usually constructed using one of several different identification systems. Figure 1 shows the interaction between an object identifier and its network address.

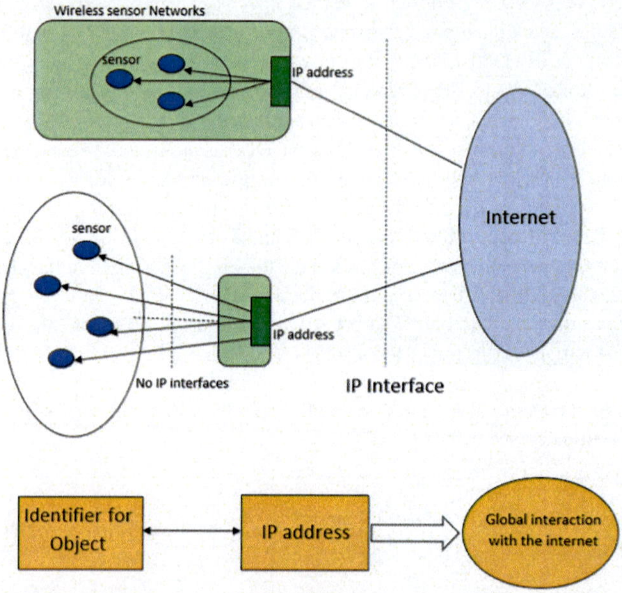

Fig. 1. Interaction between object identifier and its network address.

One of the most well-known entity identification techniques that may uniquely identify entities connected with an RFID tag is the Electronic Product Code (EPC). Another identification scheme, called the ubiquitous code (uCode), introduced by the uID centre in Japan, is a different coding system that is exclusively supported in Japan and Asia. Similarly, other addressing schemes may be various [3]. Objects that are currently connected to the Internet use the global IP addressing scheme (IPv4 or IPv6). In turn, some IoT devices cannot use global IP addressing because they connect to the Internet through a so-called gateway. The gateway, for example, can be a smartphone that communicates with a smartwatch using Bluetooth Low Energy technology [4].

2 Digital Object Architecture

The present information management systems on the network, as illustrated in work [9], are based on the classic client-server design. In such a system, the server is represented as a location for storing data and processing requests from clients to deal with it. DOA, on the other hand, takes a different approach, focusing on the context of a digital object rather than localization.

In this architecture, a digital object is defined by more than just its physical position. In addition, other information about the object itself can be obtained, such as access constraints, authentication, author information, and so on [8]. All of this information is entered by the digital object's creator. The DOA architecture incorporates a unique infrastructure that delivers the essential encryption and access verification.

The digital object, the identification resolution system (Handle System), and the repository and registration of digital objects are the three fundamental structural parts of DOA. Let's take a closer look at the resolution system's principles.

A unique identification - DOI - is assigned to each digital object in the defined architecture (Digital Object Identifier). This identification is similar to the URL, which is the foundation of the current Internet. In contrast to the latter, the allocated identifiers are constant and independent of the digital object's state. It's the resolution mechanism that connects the identification to information about a digital object's present state (location, access, and authenticity information) [11].

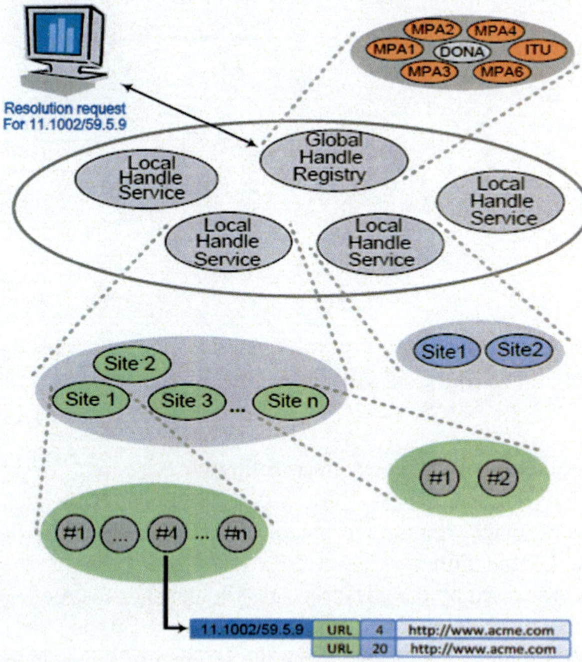

Fig. 2. Structure of the resolution system (Handle system)

The resolution system is two-level in the classical DOA architecture [10]. The first level of resolution is the global registry (GHR, from the English Global Handle Registry); the second level is a set of LHR (Local Handle Registry) or LHS (Local Handle Service).

In order to resolve the identifier in this subsystem, the global GHR registry is first queried, which reports information about the local LHR registry, which has the essential digital object information. Figure 2 depicts this procedure schematically.

The DOA identifier's structure also correlates to a two-level system [11]. Consider the following identifier: 10.1000/123abc. The prefix, which comes before the "/," is called a prefix, and the suffix, which comes after the "/," is called a suffix. It can be used the prefix to set information about the LHR digital object's local registry. The global GHR registry stores this prefix and administrator information mapping. The suffix already uniquely identifies a certain object, and this information is saved in the local LHR registry [13].

3 Laboratory Stand for Full-Scale Experiment

Figure 3 shows the laboratory structure stands for testing the application of methods for identifying IoT devices based on the DOA. During the experiment, it was necessary to test the possibility of using methods for identifying Internet of things devices. The experiment was carried out based on the model network of the laboratory of the Internet of Things of Sohar University.

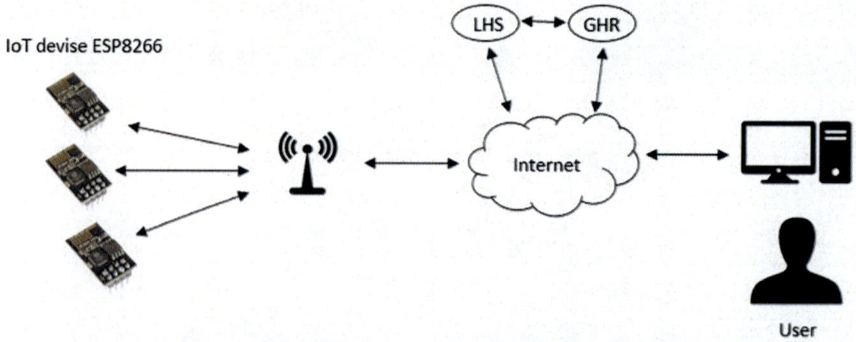

Fig. 3. Structure of laboratory stands

Identification of a digital object occurs as follows:

- The user (or user device) requests to obtain information about the object using the available public DOI identifier.
- This request is processed by the GHR service, which sends the request to the system of registries, then to the repository, where information about the LHS responsible for the requested digital object is located using the Internet of things technology (in our case, Wi-Fi technology was used).
- This information is sent to the user device, which establishes a secure connection with the LHS service using asymmetric encryption algorithms.

– After processing this request, the LHR sends data about the object to the user device.

The ID of a digital object is used to define information about the object's state, including the object's location, authentication methods, public keys, and other relevant data. Since a digital object is essentially a string of bits that can be uniquely identified, a part of the object can also be identifiable. Thus, when an IoT device is used as an object, it can be identified. The structure of metadata that can be used in digital object architecture for IoT devices to validate originality.

4 Identifying IoT Devices in Heterogeneous Networks Based on DOA

Based on the approaches presented in ITU-T Rec. Y.4459 Architecture for IoT Interoperability, the proposed schema defines a minimum set of required architectural components, protocols and services that together form a framework that implements standard information functions and service interoperability. The core of the structure is the architecture of digital objects. Any digitally presented information can be organized into a digital object with a globally unique identity [12].

This identifier returns the ancillary information of the digital object that exists in the resolution system regardless of any changes made to the digital object by any entity. Data such as location, metadata, checksums, digital signatures, certificates, public keys, and other ancillary information may be included. Attributes of a digital thing are the components of accompanying information linked with the digital entity. Regardless of data transmission protocols, a digital object can be used to represent IoT entities, for example, on top of the TCP/IP protocol stack.

Any digital information previously structured as a digital object can be securely identified using the described architecture, regardless of the system, service, or application where the data was created or stored. As you may be aware, DOA is made up of three main components that work together to provide the following services: global identification, digital object storage, and digital object registration. The process of constructing a digital object and assigning attributes is depicted in Fig. 4.

The global identity service will allow any digital object to be assigned a global identifier. This service offers a resolution and management methodology for determining the auxiliary data associated with a digital object:

- The storage location.
- The origin of information.
- The possibility of retrieval and management in compliance with the necessary security measures.

The identification service should be a distributed system with built-in protection mechanisms to guarantee the service's integrity, non-repudiation, and data integrity.

The availability of selective access control for any metadata linked with the identification, as well as authentication and confidentiality of actions with stored data, are also required. The secure storage, access, and transfer of things using identifiers is made

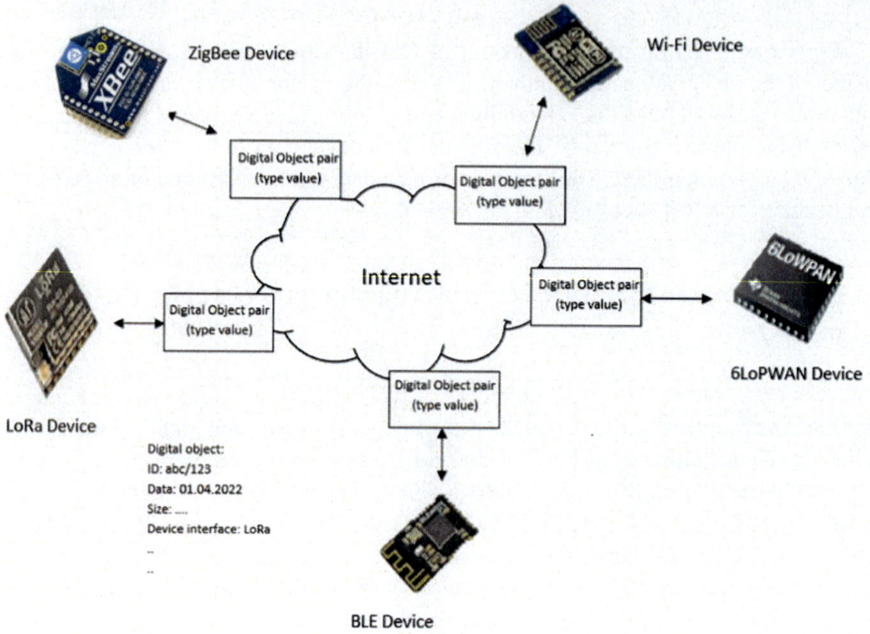

Fig. 4. The process of creating a digital object and assigning attributes.

easier using a set of distributed digital object storage services. The vault is a digital item that can contain other digital objects [7]. A digital object can do a variety of things, such as interact with other digital objects, create new digital objects, and so on. A digital object store can be a collection of Internet of Things (IoT) devices that are also digital objects.

Many qualities associated with a real object can be found in a digital object. Part of the properties could be used to characterize the IoT device's nature. The object may contain control properties connected with the program, allowing direct interaction with the IoT device's functionality, such as turning the system on or off and collecting readings from the device's temperature sensor. Furthermore, a digital object may include attributes that define the accessibility of basic device properties, so determining who can interact with the IoT device using the interface provided in the object's attributes. Figure 5 shows the interaction diagram of IoT devices connected to a communication network using various data transfer technologies and digital architecture components.

A digital representation of a physical IoT device can be used to create the structure of a digital object.

The component system, namely the registry, can define how such entities can be found and accessed. In terms of the Internet of Things, the interoperability criterion indicates the presence of an API that allows digital objects to interact with the devices to which they are connected. This method can be used to achieve specific access controls for each repository's convenience. On the other hand, the storage may provide access to data generated by a particular IoT device. The architecture of digital objects does not limit the number of possible storages [5, 6].

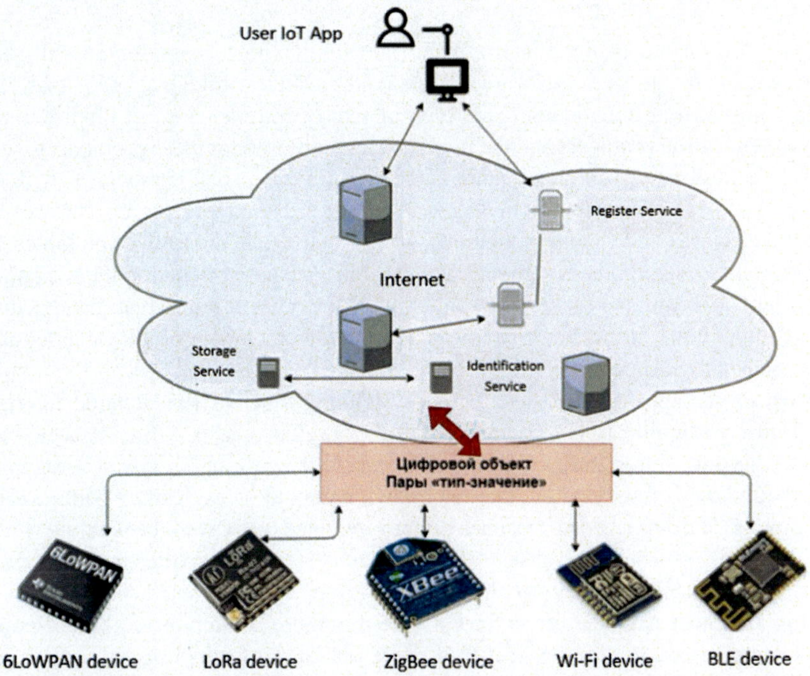

Fig. 5. Scheme of IoT devices interaction with digital architecture components.

A set of digital object registry services within one area (which is part of the MPA) allows the discovery of any digital object. A digital object registry may also allow users to search metadata or simple data contained within a digital object [1, 14]. It can be used the registry to find digital things based on a variety of characteristics, such as:

1) Search for different types of metadata records of digital objects within various registry services.
2) Search by different levels of network interaction within different services-registries.
3) Search for different types of data management services.
4) Search by different types of security and access control systems.

The access policy must be explicitly defined, including authentication and authorization of client requests applied to a set of MPAs.

Currently, products, approaches and initiatives related to the issue of IoT interoperability are still under development. The proprietary nature of the release of IoT devices was observed until 2017, which created the prerequisites and the need to develop requirements for device compatibility both for mutual interaction tasks and for collaborative identification tasks. So that one IoT device understands another IoT device. An example is systems built on a standard service layer and implementations of familiar service entities, service-oriented architectures, digital object architectures, and the domain name system [15].

There are various types of interoperability: technical interoperability, usually associated with software and hardware components, systems, and platforms that allow machine-to-machine interaction. This type of interoperability is most often based on the communication protocols and the infrastructure required for these protocols to work. Another kind of compatibility, syntactic compatibility, is usually associated with data formats. There is no doubt that all messages transmitted using protocols must have explicitly defined syntax and encoding methods, even if they are in the form of bit tables. The third kind of compatibility is semantic compatibility, usually related to the meaning of the content, affecting the human interpretation of the content rather than the machines. Thus, compatibility at this level means a common understanding of the meaning of the exchanged content (information).

Most of the approaches listed focus on defining a set of fundamental interfaces within different applications. The architecture of digital objects defines a basic set of services that allow information to be encapsulated, registered, and discovered, regardless of the boundaries of application, thereby allowing data to be exchanged within various applications. The described approaches can be integrated into any of the previously listed interoperability aspects (typical service level, service-oriented architecture, etc.), which will allow the exchange of information within various applications.

Digital Object Architecture defines a bare minimum of architectural requirements components, protocols, and services to provide standard information and service interoperability. The description here is technologically neutral and can also be implemented with existing technologies for global IoT identification tasks. This will facilitate the interoperability of IoT devices' identification, description, presentation, access, storage, and security. The implementation of DOA for Internet of Things devices implies the assignment of its identifier (handle) to each IoT device [16].

5 Structure of a Typical IoT Device and the Resolution Process Based on DOA

The presence of an identification service, including the resolution process, is a key requirement for IoT systems and, at the same time, the basic principle of DOA. However, the architecture of digital objects has a special requirement for identifiers within the architecture, namely the ability to resolve the identifier into metadata about the object whose resolution is taking place, or, in our case, about the object of the IoT. The access control system implemented on the servers provides access only to metadata-specific values.

One of the primary goals that can be implemented based on the DOA in IoT is the fight against counterfeiting in IoT products and services. The user gets the opportunity to check the characteristics of the IoT device using the Handle system. The end-user can extract the identifier prefix using special technology by requesting the GHR server to determine the location of the LHS service, which has direct information about the IoT device. The GHR responds to such a request with a message containing the address of the requested LHS. The device makes a new request to the received address. In response, it gets a message with data on a specific identifier, including all the necessary information controlled and modified only by the device manufacturer. Figure 6 shows the processes and structure for checking by an IoT device for counterfeit detection based on the architecture of digital objects.

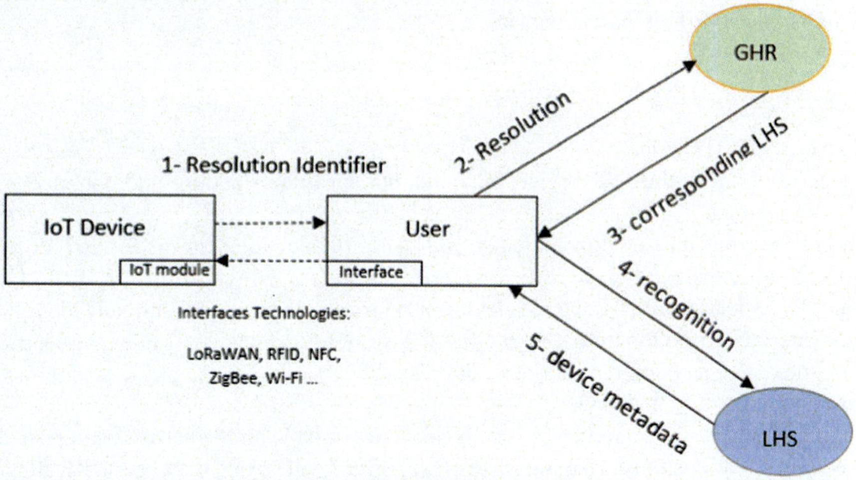

Fig. 6. Structure and procedures for checking the IoT device for counterfeit detection.

The resolution result must be in the form of a type-value pair.

In the DOA data structure, a digital object is a file, service, database, device, or combination [17].

The following is a list of characteristics that describe DOA identification systems that can be used in the context of IoT:

1. Ability to integrate with existing identification systems, such as OID (X.6660) or any other current identification systems currently used by IoT device manufacturers to ensure universal compatibility in resolving identifiers [18].
2. Verification of existence and uniqueness. A registry and a resolution system are needed to confirm the existence of a particular identifier and its uniqueness. This characteristic is key in confirming the global identity of any new IoT device.
3. The identity service is structured to provide valid, fail-safe functionality that the origin of a particular resolution service can verify. The most important is the presence of a mechanism that allows access methods by services or clients to authenticate the IoT device with which they interact. Reliability is achieved by having values signed by a digital object, using the object's key, on behalf of the IoT device.
4. Ability to use encryption. An IoT device may need to have certain levels of encryption to eliminate the risk of risks from attacks like "Man in the middle" attacks.
5. Access control. IoT devices may need access control capability to manage entities that can access information about the device or itself.
6. Means for the association of auxiliary information with the identifier of each digital object/device of the IoT. This information will be returned by a subsequent permission request as a set of type-value pairs. "Type" is directly a DOA identifier, which

produces a set of type descriptions. The flexibility of this process allows manufacturers in the IoT industries to use their proprietary systems to describe their own IoT devices while allowing the entire IoT community to have the information needed to process a specific type-value pair.

Examples of types and attributes are:

- the type of IoT device.
- a description of the IoT device, both for human understanding and for machine understanding.
- accompanying information includes information about the state of the IoT device (location, status, etc.).
- interface specifications. Each IoT device provides an identifier that uniquely identifies the interfaces used to interact with other IoT systems and devices. For example, such an interface specification provides a low-level description of the physical interfaces used to interact with a device.
- access to the service interface. Each IoT device available on the network can provide recommendations to service interfaces. For some devices, this may be a URI. It may be a simple IP address and any other options for others. A particular IoT device may have different service interfaces.
- relationship with the archive storage of the IoT device. Many IoT devices can generate data during operation. DOA can link the device to a store of similar data.

6 Access to IoT Devices with Identity Support Based on DOA

To ensure the availability of IoT devices, they need a standard interface for reading and writing data, setting parameters, and diagnosing specific operations for a particular device. These parameters necessarily vary from device to device. The variety of IoT devices is very wide.

Through the fundamental components of the Global Identity System, the Digital Object Store and the Digital Object Registry Service, the Digital Object Architecture can provide supported access to an IoT device. This functionality can be implemented using any standard lightweight protocol that uses the notion of globally derived types to refine the available operations. The result is the ability to directly access data or services using a special type of control or access request. It is equally important that this access method is discoverable, and the functionality is understandable to any interacting client within the digital object architecture.

A set of simple, type-based actions is designed to support all devices. The advantage of this approach is that DOA provides a flexible digital object-based data model that provides a basic, fully customizable, and extensible system for accessing data from any IoT device. DOA supports access to the IoT device using any protocol, which allows you to perform any device-dependent operations. For example, a IoT device provides the ability to perform specific actions to set accurate calibration parameters, configure the device, or add an entry to an internal proprietary database. A manufacturer can define such steps by creating a new digital object to represent device information, with a unique identifier and an associated description of the action in the accompanying information. When a client makes a request to an IoT device using the underlying protocol to get a list of possible activities performed by the IoT device, the IoT device returns that action specific to that manufacturer. Using the type of system that is native to the architecture of digital objects, the client can determine the type of operations and find out if these actions are helpful for use. Any IoT device vendor can use this intrinsic extensibility of protocols to develop new action types while still supporting old ones.

7 Conclusion

This research described a mechanism for identifying Internet of Things devices and applications in heterogeneous communication networks based on DOA, which enables for global identification of IoT devices and applications.

Also, methods for integrating a DOA identifier into IoT devices that support various wireless data transmission technologies are considered. A metadata structure can be used in the architecture of digital objects for IoT devices to confirm originality in conjunction with standard identifiers. The work suggested aspects of network interaction and compatibility of IoT devices and applications with integrated DOA identifiers in heterogeneous communication networks.

In the end, we described the structure of a typical IoT device and the resolution process based on DOA. Specific examples of implementing the described methods and the interaction of the Internet of things device with the components of the architecture of digital objects were mentioned.

References

1. Recommendation ITU-T T.181203: an architecture for IoT interoperability, p. 25. ITU-T, Geneva 2018
2. Danilov, K., Kulik, V., Kirichek, R.: Review and analysis of methods of identification and authentication of the internet of things devices. Sci. J. Inf. Technol. Telecommun. **1**(3), 49–57 (2016)
3. ISO, ISO 6709: Standard representation of geographic point location by coordinates (2008)
4. ISO 26324: 2012 Information and Documentation-Digital Object Identifier System. BSI British Standards (2012)
5. Recommendation ITU-T E.164: the international public telecommunication numbering plan, November 2010. https://www.itu.int/rec/T-REC-E.164-201011-I
6. Recommendation ITU-T P.10: vocabulary for performance and quality of service, p. 12. ITU-T (2006)
7. Vladimirov, S.S., Pirmagomedov, R., Kirichek, R., Koucheryavy, A.: Unique degradation of flash memory as an identifier of ICT device. IEEE Access **7**, 107626–107634 (2019)
8. Al-Bahri, M.: Combating counterfeit for IoT system based on DOA. In: Al-Bahri, M., Ateya, A.A., Muthanna, A., et al. (eds.) Proceedings of the 2018 10th International Congress on Ultra-Modern Telecommunications and Control Systems and Workshops (ICUMT) 2018, St. Petersburg, Russia, 5–9 November 2018, pp. 338–342. IEEE (2018)
9. Al-Bahri, M.: Smart system based on DOA and IoT for products monitoring and anti-counterfeiting. In: Al-Bahri, M., Yankovsky, A., Borodin, A., Kirichek, R. (eds.) 2019 4th MEC International Conference on Big Data and Smart City (ICBDSC), pp. 25–31. IEEE (2019)

10. Al-Bahri, M., Yankovsky, A., Borodin, A., Kirichek, R.: Testbed for identify IoT-devices based on digital object architecture. In: Galinina, O., Andreev, S., Balandin, S., Koucheryavy, Y. (eds.) NEW2AN ruSMART 2018. LNCS, vol. 11118, pp. 129–137. Springer, Cham (2018). https://doi.org/10.1007/978-3-030-01168-0_12
11. Digital object architecture for IoT. http://www.wileyconnect.com/home/2016/11/8/what-governmentsdecided-on-digital-object-architecture-foriot
12. Kahn, R.E.: The organization of computer resources into a packet radio network. In: Managing Requirements Knowledge, International Workshop (1975). https://www.computer.org/csdl/proceedings/afips/1975/5083/00/50830177.pdf
13. Kahn, R., Wilensky, R.: A framework for distributed digital object services. Int. J. Digit. Libr. **6**(2), 115–123 (2006)
14. Lam, K.Y., Chi, C.H.: Identity in the internet-of-things (IoT): new challenges and opportunities. In: Lam, K.Y., Chi, C.H., Qing, S. (eds.) ICICS 2016. LNCS, vol. 9977, pp. 18–26. Springer, Cham (2016). https://doi.org/10.1007/978-3-319-50011-9_2
15. Recommendation ITU-T Y.2066: Common requirements of the Internet of things, p. 12. ITU-T, Geneva (2014)
16. Al-Bahri, M., Alkishri, W.: DOA-A new approach to identify IoT devices. Appl. Comput. J. 66–76 (2021)
17. Kahn, R.: The role of architecture in internet defense: America's cyber future: security and prosperity in the information age. Center for a New American Security (CNAS), vol. II, Chap. XII, May 2011
18. Recommendation ITU-T X.1255: framework for discovery of identity management information. ITU-R, Geneva, April 2013. http://handle.itu.int/11.1002/1000/1195

Smart City and Smart Energy

A Blockchain Based Methodology for Power Grid Control Systems

Rouwaida Abdallah[1(✉)] and Rim Abdallah[2,3]

[1] CEA, LIST, 91120 Palaiseau, France
rouwaida.abdallah@cea.fr
[2] Normandie Univ., UNILEHAVRE, LITIS, SFlog, 76600 Le Havre, France
rim.abdallah@etu.univ-lehavre.fr
[3] HAROPA PORT, 71 Quai Colbert, 76600 Le Havre, France

Abstract. The increasing shift towards renewable energy has increased the complexity of power grid systems. Generally, power management is done through a centralized control architecture where a single entity governs the entire network. Centralized architecture is simple to manage but is not fault tolerant. If the centralized entity fails, the entire system will be impaired. Despite decentralized architecture's tolerance to the single point of failure, it highly affects the system's efficiency. A fragmented decentralized power grid lacks sufficient knowledge for optimal load distribution. In this study, we suggest the use of a distributed blockchain-based approach for power grid management. This novel approach overcomes both centralized and decentralized architectures' vulnerabilities. It offers a solution to the centralized dependent single point of failure while maintaining a secure data flow across the grid for optimal performance.

Keywords: Blockchain · Distributed power grid · Control architectures · Renewable energy · Smart grid

1 Introduction

In the last decade, institutions have invested in re-thinking and reforming traditional methods of energy supplies driven by worriment about global warming, energetic security, and price moderation [1]. Nowadays, electric power grids are becoming increasingly complex due to the widespread integration of intermittent renewable energy sources. Smart grids, which is an electrical grid that uses information and communication technology, promise to facilitate the integration of renewable energy [2, 3]. As integrating these sustainable resources into power grids originally built for traditional resources has not been without its challenges [4]. Therefore, to ensure the power system's stability and prevent its collapse or degradation as we attempt to sustain business and societal goals, novel approaches that overcome the complexity of energy networks should be considered for grid control systems.

In the literature, we distinguish between several types of control architectures. The main types are centralized, distributed and decentralized.

K. Daimi and A. Al Sadoon (Eds.): ICR 2022, AISC 1431, pp. 431–443, 2022.
https://doi.org/10.1007/978-3-031-14054-9_40

The centralized architecture (see Fig. 1-a) is easier to understand and operate than other types of architecture. This architecture revolves around a single central entity. A central controller (CC) governs the entire power grid and is responsible for decision-making amongst multiple connected local controllers (LCs). The LCs feed their data to the CC, which subsequently analyze the received data and control changes in the system. The main advantage of a centralized architecture is that the central controller CC responsible for the grid's control intelligence has global visibility over the entire network. This type of control is achieved through a simple architecture aiming for thorough visibility, that gives the CC the ability to make optimal decisions. [5].

However, the main drawback of centralized architecture is the weakness against Single Point Of Failure (SPOF) in communication, which can lead to a complete collapse, while only an occasional and transient loss of performance in distributed architectures [5, 6].

In a decentralized control architecture (see Fig. 1-b), independent controllers govern separate subsystems, that do not exchange any information between them. In the literature, the terms "decentralized" and "distributed controls", are sometimes used interchangeably [7]. Nevertheless, if there is an exchange of information between independent controllers, the control architecture is considered "distributed".

Unlike centralized strategies, in decentralized control, each entity is considered autonomous and independent using its local controller (Local Controller LC). We can also have groups of entities that are controlled separately by a leader (DC in Fig. 1-b). This leader could be elected by the LCs or could be a controller outside the LCs. A subsystem is a zone consisting of several LCs.

This overcomes the single point of failure vulnerability. When a decentralized controller DC is compromised, it will only cause partial system impairment, as opposed to a total failure in centralized architectures. Although this architecture overcomes the SPOF, it introduced new performance issues. The decentralized independent architecture does not require information exchange between its entities, neither locally nor globally. Thus, unlike the centralized system where the controller makes its decision based on the entire network's data, the lack of communication and the fragmented visibility has a direct impact on the system's operational optimality and stability.

This is why the application of a pure decentralized architecture in an electrical network without complete network visibility is not realistic. Communication between the different controllers is a crucial point for the overall stability of the network. Any fragmented control results in performance deterioration. A typical example of the consequences of the drawbacks of such a control strategy is the widespread blackout of August 2003 in North America [8]. In this incident, each subsystem only focused on maintaining its own subsystem stability and transferred the additional load to other subsystems. The lack of communication and global visibility deprived the network intelligence controllers of their ability to make adequate decisions and optimally distribute loads increasing overload severity and ultimately causing a cascading collapse of the whole system [9, 10].

Any new suggested architecture targeting electrical networks should consider the broad number of participants, the diversity of energy sources and should maintain informational exchanges between entities. And it is where we can clearly distinguish between decentralized and distributed control architecture. Distributed control (see Fig. 1-c), can be considered as decentralized control in which controllers are allowed to share information with neighbors. Thus, the distributed method can achieve stability, just like centralized architecture. Therefore, highly integrated distributed architectures can provide an optimal solution for grid management.

This architecture overcomes its previous architecture SPOF issue while maintaining global visibility. Any SPOF will not cause a cascading failure in the microgrid [10] and entities connectivity and information exchange will guarantee decisions optimality [11].

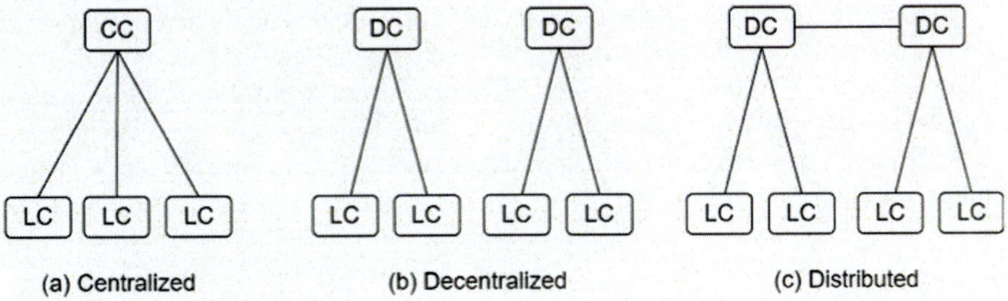

Fig. 1. Main types of control architecture: (a) Centralized, (b) Decentralized and (c) Distributed

The distributed technology called blockchain has been increasingly gaining interest, especially after its great success in the financial sector. The most prominent use of blockchain technology is cryptocurrencies such as Bitcoin, Ethereum, and others, whereas the technology has a broad spectrum of possible applications. The distributed and trusted nature of the technology can be applicable in power grid management. Decision-making in power grid control largely relies on a reliable data flow and communication in the environment. Theoretically, decentralized power grid control management lacks collaboration and communication to ensure decision optimality.

And the success of collaboration in a distributed environment relies largely on building a trusted environment for information exchange. Hence, the elimination of single points of failure while providing reliable verifiable information determines the eventual success of a distributed approach. This can be achieved using blockchain technology. Blockchain allows the storage of information across multiple nodes in a peer-to-peer network while anchoring cryptographic algorithms to ensure ledger immutability and security. And because of the distributed nature of the technology, single point of failure is eliminated. Each node possessed a cryptographically protected copy of the ledger making it impossible to alter data while maintaining data availability. Moreover, data appended to the ledger is verifiable and agreed upon through a consensus algorithm ensuring collaborative decision-making removing control from centralized single entities while maintaining accountability.

Our study builds on literature and application analysis of current power grid control studies along with theoretical framework studies of blockchain application in other sectors. And proposes the integration of blockchain features into a conceptual framework to allow efficient and distributed power grid control management enhancing renewable energy integration while maintaining reliable data exchanges.

2 Current Power Grid Control Architecture

2.1 Definition

The power grid control system is based on a reliable supply and demand system. It involves power generators and consumer loads. Loads are generally at liberty to consume as needed however, the power supply must be monitored and dispatched appropriately. Supply utilities became adept at power dispatching to preserve continuous stability between load demands and power supplies.

Generally, this balance is done using a centralized architecture where a unique CC is granted visibility over the entire power grid and takes its decisions accordingly.

The standard IEC 60050–351–55–09 [12] defines it as a "control structure with interconnected subprocesses, in which each partial control equipment considers the information of all subprocesses to form its output information" (International Electrotechnical Commission IEC).

2.2 Architecture

Power grid networks are an ecosystem whose foundations are based on the acquisition of information, monitoring, evaluation, and decision-making as well as control management. In this ecosystem, one of the most important properties is the real-time aspect.

In fact, if certain actions executed within the system can wait or can be delayed in time, others should be executed almost instantly, especially to respond to certain changes that could strongly affect the system. This criterion based on response time has mainly led to "hierarchical control functions".

In the literature, we mainly find three levels of control functions: primary, secondary, and tertiary [13]. System status information flows from the primary level to the tertiary level, and decision signals (commands and recommendations) flow from the tertiary level to the primary level to achieve overall operating goals. The primary controller has the smallest decision time step to regulate the voltage and frequency to the desired values. On the other hand, the tertiary controller collects system status information using the communication infrastructure and makes decisions to improve the overall performance of the grid; its decision time step is longer.

Depending on the architecture chosen, these functions can be mapped to the different types of controllers. In a centralized architecture, we distinguish between two types of Controllers: A unique central controller (CC), and local controllers (LCs).

Primary level functions are often mapped to LCs as they are closest to physical resources like substations and therefore can act faster than other types of controllers. Also in the same logic, the tertiary level is often mapped on the CC when it is present in the architecture. The secondary level functions will be mapped on the CC or LCs.

The central controller is implemented to send control commands and recommendations to Local controllers and receive status data from them. The main objective of the central controller is to predict the load demand and renewable power generation, so a set of operation plans of commands and recommendations is developed accordingly. The central controller mainly sends to each Local controller the threshold of productivity that it might respect. The local controller should try its best to attend to this threshold without exceeding it. The CC's commands and recommendations are not based solely on LCs' data (voltage, current, power, etc.) but also on other diverse data sources such as meteorology, marketplace, and others. The local controller should act in almost real-time to adjust the power output and this is to ensure the stability of voltage and frequency.

2.3 Effects of Centralization on Power Grid Control Systems

The load's use of electric power across the network can be inconsistent and intermittent. And until now, the use of the combination of a unique CC and LC's have proved adept to maintaining stable reliable grids. And some of the loads' inconsistent consumption create certain patterns, which allows the CC, after a full data analysis to make informed intelligent decisions.

Hence, the centralized architecture has proven effective. However, this type of architecture is often susceptible to SPOF. In a centralized system control, if the main CC fails for any software or hardware defect, it halts all network's processes. Upon failures, the network's architecture will convert from centralized into decentralized. And the disrupted communication on the network will eventually lead to a total blackout as aforementioned. Without the correct threshold to maintain the network's stability, LCs might exceed productivity possibly causing line congestions that may eventually lead to cascading failures resulting in a widespread network blackout.

Therefore, the availability of the entire system is heavily dependent on a single entity. And usually, to overcome this dependency, the use of decentralized architecture is suggested. But, in power grid management the use of a decentralized architecture will impact the operational optimality and network's performance. Despite that it solves the SPOF vulnerability, the lack of communication between controllers affects global monitoring of the grid and prevent the correct resources dispatching to balance between supply and demand since none of the controller have a complete overview of the entire grid. Thus, the search for alternative solutions has not yet presented any revolutionizing solutions despite theoretical grounds for distribution effectiveness in grid control overcoming centralized architecture's problem without compromising effectiveness [8, 9].

On that account, we propose in the next sections a distributed approach. A blockchain-based approach can achieve the desired distribution that overcomes centralized architecture's SPOF vulnerability and guarantee operational optimality since communication is maintained across the network in a distributed and trusted environment. The introduction of a new blockchain approach will necessitate a detailed plan of action. The approach, despite being innovative, may proffer advancements for the challenging and costly implementation of traditional energy grids without impairing our systems.

3 Blockchain

3.1 Structure and Categories

Blockchain can be dated back to 2008 when an entity by the name of Satoshi Nakamoto proposed stacking pre-existing technologies in an innovative approach [14]. This technological stacking was the origin of the later known technology as Blockchain. The paper proposed a solution called Bitcoin to the double-spend problem of electronic cash systems. It relied on notions such as timestamp, hashing, cryptographic signatures, and chaining to induce trust in the system's environment. Parties can transact digital currencies without unnecessary third parties. These digital currencies were later known as cryptocurrencies for their reliance on cryptography. Bitcoin was the first widespread cryptocurrency, but others shortly emerged evolving the technological infrastructure to include other features such as Smart contract in Ethereum [15]. Also, the infrastructural technology of these cryptocurrencies started being implemented in diverse applications such as gambling [16], escrow [17], proof of identity [18], and others [19, 20, 18, 21, 22].

3.2 Blockchain Structure

Blockchain is a distributed ledger technology [23, 24, 25]. It is a peer-2-peer network where participants are called nodes and have their own copy of the database. The database includes communications and transactions executed over the network. These data are grouped in the form of blocks. Blocks in the ledger are chained together using timestamps and cryptographical hashes. Each block contains the hash of its previous in addition to its data. Hash-chained blocks allow locating where data is stored on the network. The ledger is also replicated over nodes adding an additional trust layer to the network that renders the ledger had to alter. And since no single entity is responsible for maintaining the ledger, any network member can access, verify, and confirm data.

The transaction between network members is unmediated. Unnecessary third parties are eliminated since all transactions executed within the network are replicated and stored across nodes. The decentralization and replication allow all these members to vouch for the validity of stored transactions.

When a transaction is executed on the network, it is broadcasted across the network. When a node receives a transaction, it will try to construct a block to be appended to the ledger. Block characteristics are known across the network. The method that nodes use to append the block to the ledger is called consensus. There are several types of consensuses. For example, in a proof of work consensus, the block will contain the encryption of current data, a timestamp, a nonce, and the hash of its previous. Each node, upon receiving transactions will produce its own block that it will try to append to the ledger. The nonce in the block expresses the network difficulty level. And each node will try to calculate its block's corresponding nonce. When a node succeeds, it will broadcast its block on the network. Upon receipt, nodes will verify the block and append it to their own ledgers. Hence, we have replication across all network nodes that combined with the cryptographic chaining renders the network immutable.

Smart contracts are codes that can be automatically executed over the network. They are called contracts because they are agreed upon by all network nodes which makes them legally binding hence the automatic execution when all its conditions are fulfilled.

3.3 Blockchain Types

Literature has classified blockchain networks into distinct categories based on different attributes [26]. One common attribute is network management and accessibility. We distinguish between three categories of networks: public, private, and permissioned.

In all types of blockchain networks database decentralization and replication amongst network, participants remained.

In private and permissioned blockchain networks participants are identified before being granted access to the network. The network is thus maintained by known entities that agree amongst each others on operational conditions such as blocks attributes, length, frequency, and consensus. Therefore, private blockchains have a higher operational efficiency since transactions are processed, executed, and appended faster with fewer authorized members. The small number of members in private and permissioned blockchains makes reaching consensus and appending data to the ledger faster since fewer members have to agree. Moreover, the limited access scope to data by only authorized members limits risks related to privacy and data leakage. While private blockchains are completely isolated networks, permissioned blockchain can allow certain members to participate in its network using different access levels.

In a public blockchain, anyone can be a part of the network. Members' identities are concealed behind blockchain addresses for anonymity. Any member can write, verify and access data in the replicated decentralized ledger. Thus, the consensus in public blockchain is much more complex to achieve network immutability and maintain network security which requires immense amounts of computational power to run such networks and decrease operational efficiency since more time is needed to reach consensus and process transactions.

The use of this technology for power grid control can enhance scalability and improve operational efficiency. Information distribution across the grid can eliminate SPOF vulnerabilities while maintaining decisions optimality. And since traditional power grids are usually private where data is shared across private networks of authorized participants, we suggest maintaining this type of network for optimal operational efficiency.

4 Blockchain-Based Solution

Blockchain was first suggested as an electronic currency double spend solution. But over the past few years, the technology has been successfully implemented in application in different sectors. This allowed us to reflect on its use in power grid control management to benefit from its features.

4.1 New System Architecture

In our approach, the central controller is replaced by a set of d distributed controllers (DC). The local controllers are grouped into d zones based on their geographical location. A zone is a set of n_d neighboring local controllers and one distributed controller.

Each local controller communicates with the DC of its corresponding zone. Each DC communicates with all the other DCs (a peer-to-peer network) (Fig. 2).

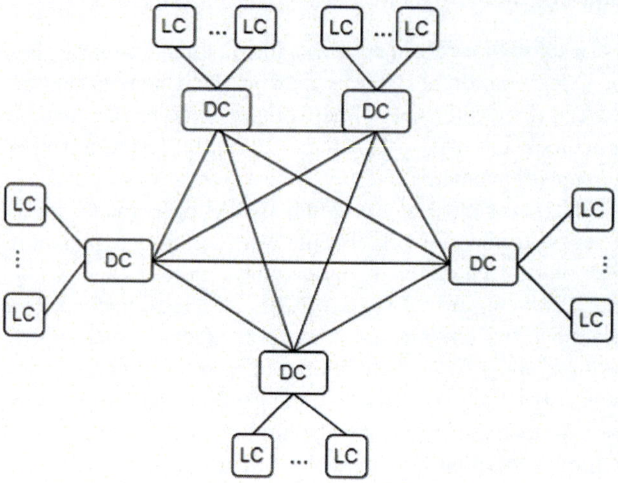

Fig. 2. The proposed distributed architecture

4.2 Methodology

We suggest the use of a private blockchain network as our system's infrastructure. The private peer-to-peer blockchain network setup requires common rules to establish synchronization between participants. A trusted entity will be chosen to assume the role of a network admin responsible for configuring the network, creating accounts, and adding authorized nodes to the network (for this trusted identity we might use the general concept of "decentralized identity" as defined in the standard UNE 71307–1:2020 [27]. In the network configuration, the admin will specify epochs upon which peers in the network will take action. This allows a more coherent network synchronization.

Peers in our network are DC nodes that are receiving data continuously from LCs. In our network, we distinguish between three types of DC nodes:

The first type is the "normal DC": The normal DC has similar tasks to the traditional CC; it receives and sends data to attached LCs. However, unlike the traditional CC, a normal DC is not responsible for computing commands and recommendations. It locally stores data that it receives periodically from LCs. When the agreed-upon time period T (T is specified in the network configuration) is up, the normal DC forwards the relevant LCs' data to the current "principal DC" and all the "validator DCs".

The second type is the "principal DC": The principal DC receives data from all other DCs periodically each T. It is characterized by its visibility over the totality of the network, which allows it to make an informed optimal decision (the set of commands and recommendations). Its role is to store all received data from normal DCs, hashes them, and incorporate them in a block. It then calculates the optimal commands and recommendations and appends them to the block as well. Commands and recommendations are added in clear to the block. Once the block is built, it is sent to be validated by the currently designated validator DC nodes. After the block is validated, the principal DC appends the block to the ledger. When a principal DC appends a new block to the ledger, each normal DC detects its corresponding LCs' recommendations and control from the new decision in the block's body and sends the needed data to the LCs to adjust accordingly.

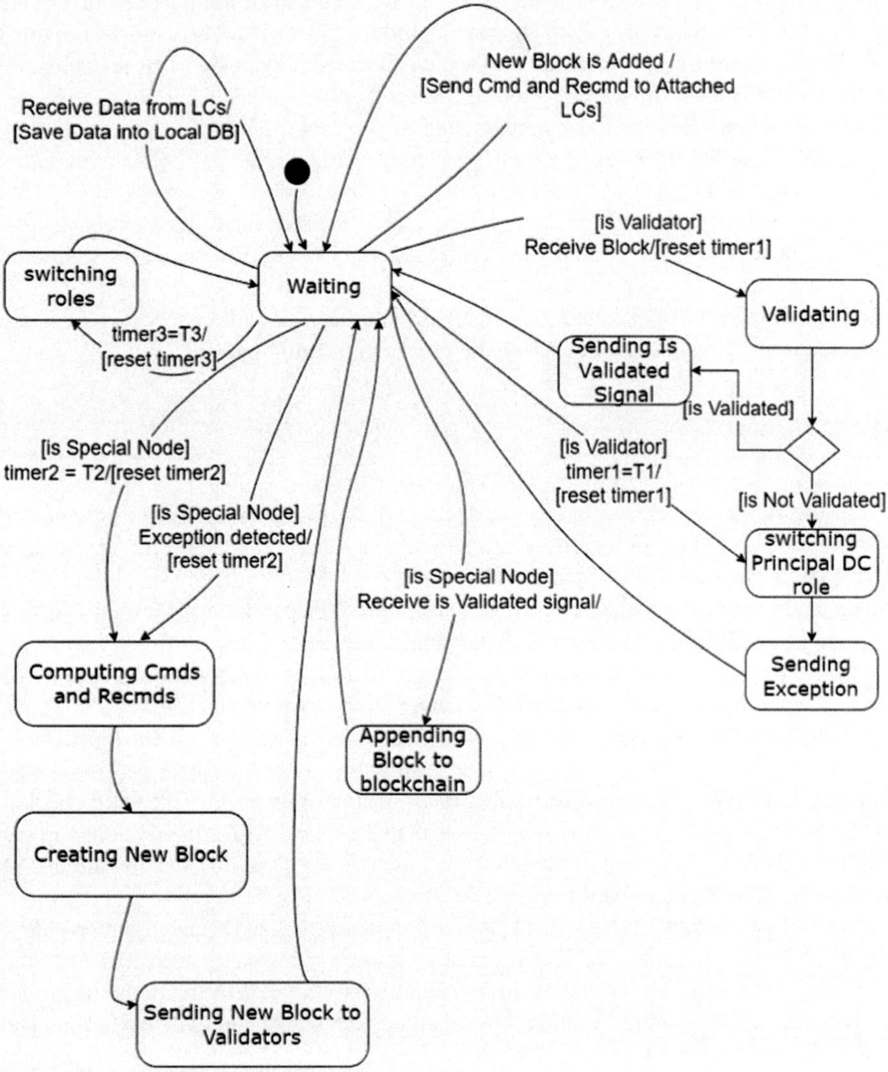

Fig. 3. This state machine diagram describes the behaviors of each DC node in the new architecture.

The third type is the "validator DC": The validator DC allows for distributed computation of commands and recommendations. It receives the same data received by the principal DC so it can do verify if the commands and recommendations are valid or not based on the received data. Just like a principal DC the validator DC stores the received data from other DCs then wait for an epoch T1 to receive a block from the principal DC. Once received, it double-checks the optimality of commands and recommendations, and if it agrees, it signs a confirmation response that it sends back to the principal DC. This step is called block validation. If the block is not validated or not received in T1, the principal DC will switch its role to normal DC and another DC will become the principal DC. The manner how new roles are attributed is decided previously in the specification of the blockchain (in the genesis block). If after T1, the validator did not receive any block, the switch role function is applied, and a new principal node is chosen.

Each T3 period, the roles of the DCs change, and new principal DC and validators will be designated.

Figure 3 presents a state machine diagram that describes the different behaviors of each DC node. Every DC node is by default a normal DC but can assume an additional role as a Principal DC or a Validator.

The values of T, T1, T2, and T3 as well as the process according to which roles are assigned in the network, are defined in the blockchain configuration.

4.3 Data Structure

In our approach, a block consists of a header and a body.

In the block header, we have: The hash of its previous block, a timestamp, the Merkle root, an index, an identity array. The identity array contains: First the identity of the decision-maker that appended the block. Second, the identity of the currently designated validators and their confirmation response. The confirmation response allows verifying the validators' approval of the appended block.

As for the block body, it contains the commands and recommendations in clear, and the hash of data the decision-maker DC received in the current epoch T.

So as we mentioned before the hash of the data only can be found in the blockchain, so if the data itself is needed (for example, using the data at the same period of time from the last year to help in some prediction or analysis process), we can still check it in the local database of the node that was principal DC and which is mentioned in the header of the block. Or even in the local databases of any validator node mentioned in the header of the block as well.

Each block contains the clear decisions made by the principal DC in its corresponding epoch T. Once appended to the ledger the block can be accessed by normal DCs on the network. Each normal DC can take into consideration its targeted instructions and ignore the rest. This allows adding additional transparency on the network where a normal DC node can have access to all other DCs' commands and recommendations. This might be particularly helpful in exceptional situations where DCs need to be aware of each other's statuses to take urgent decisions and avoid line congestions.

5 Related Works and Conclusion

Many works address the use of blockchain technology within the energy sector. For a good brief review, the reader is referred to [28]. In general, the applications in energy systems can be divided into two main categories of problems: (i) electrical energy and services trading in power markets; and (ii) renewable energy certification and active user tracing.

Our approach can be located in a new separate category, as it considers the management and the control at the power grid level not at the prosumers end level as it is proposed in some approaches.

In this paper, we present a preliminary road map for evolving power grid control. The conceptual framework is based on a distributed approach that addresses current power grid challenges. Current power grid control is mostly centralized unqualified to manage the network's increasing complexity due to the integration of distributed intermittent sustainable energy sources. Moreover, centralized architectures are most susceptible to SPOF failures. While decentralized architecture solves SPOF vulnerabilities, they fragment the network. This fragmentation can cause cascading failure that consequently imped the whole system. The adoption of distributed control approach, in theory, has the potential to overcome both approaches' challenges. It eliminates SPOF while maintaining communications responsible for network stability.

One important distributed technology is Blockchain. We propose a blockchain implementation that integrates power grids to allow a secure and distributed management of the network.

Our conceptual framework relates in its consensus to a pbft consensus [29, 30]. But lacks additional refinement and customization to address the power grids needs. Which requires the implementation of the framework and additional studies for a better-adjusted framework.

Additionally, the use of blockchain can allow the use of smart contracts to further automate power grid control. A smart contract is a software code stored on the blockchain that has a set of requirements. Its execution can be triggered by an event that satisfies the contract's requirements.

Furthermore, renewable resources supply is not always stable but can be sometimes predictable. For example, solar energy is at its lowest during the night but is widely available during the day when it's sunny. Currently, most implementations of renewable sources in power grids use storage to turn them into stable sources. We can store power generated from the sun during the summer to provide for the winter. Nevertheless, with the technological advancement in batteries and renewable energy price drops, prolonged energy storage can become costly. The current centralized architecture allows only balancing one side of the network. Any changes to balance loads consumption while maintaining high-efficiency levels that align with the grid's capabilities is not feasible since it's the main CC that holds the control intelligence across the grid. Controlled loads with local storage such as electric water heaters and EV chargers combined with grid visibility can theoretically balance both sides of our system. But this requires systems where loads, power generation, and storage are distributed while keeping the ability to control the entire grid for maximum operational efficiency. And the implementation of a distributed control system brings us one step closer towards such highly distributed systems that can manage both sides of our architecture for an optimal sustainable power grid.

We hope that this paper set the foundational stone for blockchain-based power grids for more reliable infrastructure. And in spite of the technology's promising utilization, it is also important in the future to study its feasibility in-depth. An example of a feasibility study is its regulatory aspects where innovation always tends to predate legislation. Data collected from power grids are liable to regulatory laws and methods to eliminate personal information such as aggregation, encryption, and steganography. Therefore, this should be taken into consideration well before storing information on the immutable ledger. Hence, this study offers a starting point for an extensive but very profitable new approach.

References

1. Rhodes, A., Skea, J., Hannon, M.: The global surge in energy innovation. Energies **7**, 5601–5623 (2014)
2. Camacho, E.F., Samad, T., Garcia-Sanz, M., Hiskens, I.: Control for renewable energy and smart grids. Impact Control Technol. Control Syst. Soc. **4**, 69–88 (2011)
3. Dib, M., Abdallah, R., Dib, O.: Optimization approach for the aggregation of flexible consumers. Electronics **11**(4), 628 (2022)
4. Taft, J., De Martini, P., Geiger, R.: Ultra large-scale power system control and coordination architecture. Pacific Northwest National Laboratory (PNNL) (2014)
5. Yamashita, D.Y., Vechiu, I., Gaubert, J.-P.: A review of hierarchical control for building microgrids. Renew. Sustain. Energy Rev. **118**, 109523 (2020)
6. Baghaee, H.R., Mirsalim, M., Gharehpetian, G.B., Talebi, H.A.: Unbalanced harmonic power sharing and voltage compensation of microgrids using radial basis function neural network-based harmonic power-flow calculations for distributed and decentralised control structures. IET Gener. Transm. Distrib. **12**(7), 1518–1530 (2018)
7. Kermani, M., Carnì, D.L., Rotondo, S., Paolillo, A., Manzo, F., Martirano, L.: A nearly zero-energy microgrid testbed laboratory: centralized control strategy based on scada system. Energies **13**(8), 2106 (2020)
8. Elbez, G., Keller, H.B., Hagenmeyer, V.: A new classification of attacks against the cyber-physical security of smart grids. In: Proceedings of the 13th International Conference on Availability, Reliability and Security, pp. 1–6 (2018)
9. Sabri, Y., El Kamoun, N., Lakrami, F.: A survey: centralized, decentralized, and distributed control scheme in smart grid systems. In: 2019 7th Mediterranean Congress of Telecommunications (CMT), pp. 1–11 (2019)
10. Feng, X., Shekhar, A., Yang, F., Hebner, R.E., Bauer, P.: Comparison of hierarchical control and distributed control for microgrid. Electr. Power Compon. Syst. **45**(10), 1043–1056 (2017)
11. Elmouatamid, A., Ouladsine, R., Bakhouya, M., El Kamoun, N., Khaidar, M., Zine-Dine, K.: Review of control and energy management approaches in micro-grid systems. Energies **14**(1), 168 (2021)
12. https://www.electropedia.org/iev/iev.nsf/display?openform&ievref=351-55-09
13. Elmouatamid, A., Naitmalek, Y., Ouladsine, R., Bakhouya, M., Khaidar, M., Zine-Dine, K.: A microgrid system infrastructure implementing IoT/Big-Data technologies for efficient energy management in buildings. In: Advanced Technologies for Solar Photovoltaics Energy Systems, pp. 571–600 (2021). https://doi.org/10.1007/978-3-030-64565-6_20
14. Nakamoto, S.: Bitcoin: a peer-to-peer electronic cash system. Decentralized Bus. Rev. 21260 (2008)

15. Wood, G.: Ethereum: a secure decentralised generalised transaction ledger. Ethereum Proj. Yellow Pap. **151**, 1–32 (2014)
16. Gainsbury, S., Blaszczynski, A.: How blockchain and cryptocurrency technology could revolutionize online gambling. Gaming Law Rev. **21**, 482–492 (2017)
17. Cha, S., Baek, S., Kim, S.: Blockchain based sensitive data management by using key escrow encryption system from the perspective of supply chain. IEEE Access **8**, 154269–154280 (2020)
18. Foroglou, G., Tsilidou, A.-L.: Further applications of the blockchain. In: 12th Student Conference on Managerial Science And Technology, vol. 9, (2015)
19. Swan, M.: Blockchain: Blueprint for a New Economy. O'Reilly Media Inc, Sebastopol (2015)
20. Tasatanattakool, P., Techapanupreeda, C.: Blockchain: challenges and applications. In: 2018 International Conference on Information Networking (ICOIN), pp. 473–475 (2018)
21. Gürcan, Ö., Agenis-Nevers, M., Batany, Y.-M., Elmtiri, M., Fevre, F.L., Tucci-Piergiovanni, S.: An industrial prototype of trusted energy performance contracts using blockchain technologies. In: 2018 IEEE 20th International Conference on High Performance Computing and Communications; IEEE 16th International Conference on Smart City; IEEE 4th International Conference on Data Science and Systems (HPCC/SmartCity/DSS), IEEE, pp. 1336–1343 (2018)
22. Brousmichc, K.-L., Anoaica, A., Dib, O., Abdellatif, T., Deleuze, G.: Blockchain energy market place evaluation: an agent-based approach. In: 2018 IEEE 9th Annual Information Technology, Electronics and Mobile Communication Conference (IEMCON), pp. 321–327. IEEE (2018)
23. Haring, T.W., Mathieu, J.L., Andersson, G.: Comparing centralized and decentralized contract design enabling direct load control for reserves. IEEE Trans. Power Syst. **31**, 2044–2054 (2015)
24. Aştefanoaei, L., Chambart, P., Del Pozzo, A., Rieutord, T., Tucci, S., Zălinescu, E.: Tenderbake – a solution to dynamic repeated consensus for blockchains, In: International Symposium on Foundations and Applications of Blockchain (FAB) (2021)
25. Amoussou-Guenou, Y., Del Pozzo, A., Potop-Butucaru, M., Tucci-Piergiovanni, S.: Correctness of tendermint-core blockchains. In: 22nd International Conference on Principles of Distributed Systems (OPODIS 2018). Schloss Dagstuhl-Leibniz-Zentrum fuer Informatik (2018)
26. Butterin, V.: On public and private blockchains (2015). https://blog.ethereum.org/2015/08/07/on-public-and-private-blockchains/. Accessed 28 Feb 2022
27. https://www.en.une.org/encuentra-tu-norma/busca-tu-norma/norma?c=N0064986
28. Foti, M., Vavalis, M.: What blockchain can do for power grids? Blockchain: Res. Appl. **2**(1), 100008 (2021)
29. Castro, M., Liskov, B.: Practical byzantine fault tolerance. In: OsDI, vol. 99, no (99), pp. 173–186 (1999)
30. Dib, O., Brousmiche, K.-L., Durand, A., Thea, E., Hamida, E.B.: Consortium blockchains: overview, applications and challenges. Int. J. Adv. Telecommun. **11**(1&2), 51–64 (2018)

Data Visualization Tool for Smart Buildings HVAC Systems

Iva Matetić, Ivan Štajduhar, Igor Wolf, Darko Palaić, and Sandi Ljubic(✉)

Faculty of Engineering, University of Rijeka, Vukovarska 58, 51000 Rijeka, Croatia
{iva.matetic,ivan.stajduhar,igor.wolf,darko.palaic,sandi.ljubic}@riteh.hr

Abstract. With the expected increase in world population and economic growth, the demand for energy is steadily increasing worldwide. To support the growing exploitation of energy resources, buildings must be made smart enough to use energy efficiently without wasting it. Heating, ventilation, and air conditioning (HVAC) systems consume a lot of energy and hence require effective control and analysis capabilities, which is one of the most important aspects of current smart buildings. If HVAC systems are not properly controlled, this can lead to poor user comfort, high utility bills due to excessive energy consumption, and a negative impact on the environment. This problem is aggravated in the context of hotel buildings. To support the overall energy consumption tracking, we propose a system integration with an analytical web application for data visualization that allows the user to perform an in-depth analysis of the sensory data measured. The motivation for developing the application is primarily to monitor the regulation of the HVAC system by providing an interactive analytical dashboard needed for future smart buildings. The data visualization tool provides a quick and easy way to visualize and compare time-series data. The visualizations provide insight into how different hotel rooms compare, deviations of room temperature from set-point temperature, data distribution, correlations between sensory data parameters, and the degree of correlation of room temperature compared to other parameters. The application is aimed at a wide range of users, from lay people and hotel staff to data analysts and scientists conducting research in this area.

Keywords: HVAC systems · Smart buildings · Data analytics · Monitoring tool

1 Introduction

With the rise of big data and technology advancements, it is possible to collect, visualize, and analyze data with the goal of making important decisions. As a result, it is often necessary to develop highly interactive and easy-to-use visualization tools for specific problems that need to be addressed in a given context.

K. Daimi and A. Al Sadoon (Eds.): ICR 2022, AISC 1431, pp. 444–453, 2022.
https://doi.org/10.1007/978-3-031-14054-9_41

For example, problems related to buildings' HVAC systems have been reported to be directly connected to the contribution of 30% CO_2 emissions and 40% towards total energy consumption in the European Union [1]. Furthermore, the majority of energy comes from non-renewable resources like fossil fuels, which contribute to environmental pollution and are not a sustainable resource of energy. To change this vicious cycle, problems of HVAC systems should be solved by making buildings smarter with the integration of sensory infrastructure, data acquisition protocols, proper visualization tools, and, ultimately, machine learning support.

As a contribution to the process of solving the mentioned problems, we propose a web application visualization tool specifically designed for HVAC systems deployed in smart buildings. We aimed for a solution with high usability in order to make the application user-friendly for both the professional analysts and non-experts, since it is important for hotel staff to have access to their analytics as well. The application can, in our case, serve as a monitoring and diagnostic tool for smart hotel rooms, with multiple goals that include anomaly detection, energy savings, and improvement of thermal comfort.

Following the literature review presented in the next section, we introduce the smart room concept and its software logic for controlling HVAC systems, as well as guest benefits and hotel employee HVAC control capabilities. Next, we describe the used dataset, development of the application, its tool categorization and visualization modules with the corresponding interpretations. The conclusion and directions for future work are outlined at the end of the paper.

2 Related Work

There are many research efforts related to smart rooms, smart buildings, and HVAC systems control; however, a considerably smaller number of papers specifically investigate the diagnostic and visualization tools for HVAC systems in such environments.

For example, some recent studies focused only on visualizations of HVAC systems can be found in [2–5]. The authors have shown a comparison between line chart visualization, RadViz, and matrix-based visualization of HVAC data to find the most efficient and insightful visualization method that can give an overview of the HVAC system operation in buildings. It has been concluded that RadViz is useful for familiarization with data behavior, line charts are beneficial for getting detailed information on data dependencies, and matrix-based visualizations are good for presenting detailed information and patterns. Based on RadViz visualizations, a specific visualization-driven approach for detecting anomalies in HVAC systems has been developed. However, this approach assumes that a user has beforehand knowledge about the RadViz visualizations.

Results on work concerning the use of Sankey diagrams to visualize HVAC performance has also been reported [6]. The proposed method can help in better understanding of HVAC components, but lacks in visualization and identification of anomalies.

Focused on data anomaly visualization, authors in [7] reported on pixel-based time-series and anomaly detection of energy consumption data. They experimented with the most common time-series visualization techniques (line charts, spiral visualizations, and recursive patterns). In summary, their method gave fine-grained results and an overview of data. They also concluded that spiral visualizations are a good way for quick detection and analysis of periodic patterns.

Next, a solution introduced in [8] represents an interactive web application tool for visualization and exploration of multivariate time-series data. With this tool, the authors plan to simplify the visualizations so that users with different expertise can explore data more easily. This tool can identify and map data-specific concepts, find high-level and long-term behavior, and traverse scales for later phenomenon detection. However, it has not been used specifically on HVAC systems but has been applied to three different use cases, meaning it is a multipurpose visualization tool. The related solution can be adjusted to support HVAC systems, but this involves the implementation of additional features because it is important to monitor the system as a whole rather than detecting anomalies only.

A review of all feasible visualizations of data related to energy consumption, along with the corresponding categorization and grouping, is provided in [9]. The authors concluded that traditional, two-dimensional visualizations are the most used and easy to interpret by non-expert users in this field. On the other hand, visualizations that specifically tackle time-series data are presented in [10].

Concerning exploratory data analysis of HVAC systems, the work presented in [11] mostly utilized line graphs, histograms, and joint relation plots for visualizing data. Room temperature parameter was the most important one for visualization because it was utilized within the machine learning model built for temperature prediction. The mentioned visualizations have proven to be helpful in interpreting seasonality, trends and data anomalies.

In general, existing HVAC-based data visualization solutions often lack online availability and a rich and user-friendly graphical user interface (GUI). Furthermore, some visualization tools are not suitable for non-expert users, and existing web applications do not offer an analytic dashboard for HVAC systems. By developing a visualization tool web application for HVAC systems, data monitoring would be more accessible to a wider range of users and could be available at any given time of the day, irrespective of the user's whereabouts, because it could be utilized from a mobile device as well.

Our solution is not designed to compete with commercially available diagnostic tools that provide various operational tracking capabilities for building operators (as discussed in [10,12], and [13]), but rather to support detailed data exploration. Such an exploratory approach can help improve the quality of HVAC monitoring process and, ultimately, contribute to the development of a machine learning system that can improve user comfort while saving energy.

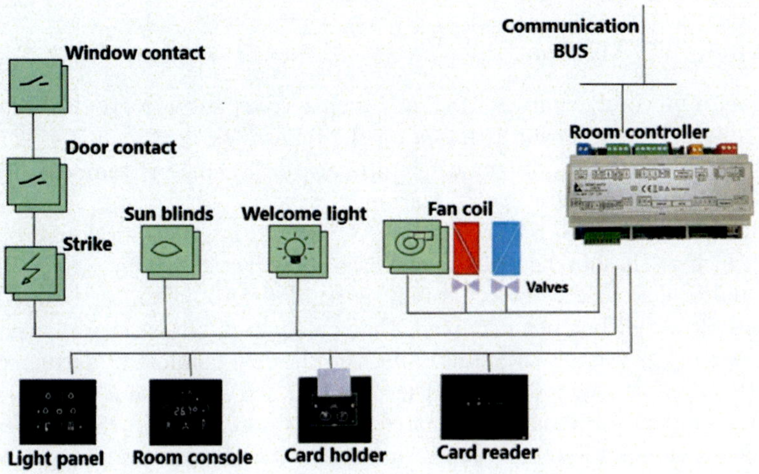

Fig. 1. A diagram of a typical smart room system.

3 Smart Room Concept

The smart room concept involves a microprocessor-controlled station that monitors all key parameters for a hotel room's proper functioning. Such stations are connected to the computer in order to increase efficiency, and the total control is centralized. In summary, it is a system for better energy management that may save money, provide better service to customers, boost the overall system's security, and allow hotel employees to be more efficient by having continual access to up-to-date information. This concept may assist hotels in having more structured administrative activities as well as improved management and supervision of the complete system. Figure 1 illustrates a room controller which gathers inputs from a user control panel and sensors.

3.1 System Functions

A smart room system typically utilized in hotels allows authorized staff to look up information about customers and rooms. It can show the current state of all sensory data, such as room temperature, open or closed doors and windows, fan speed, air conditioning status, and key card status. Furthermore, it can notify staff about electrical cabinet overheating, drops or rises of room temperature outside of predefined limits, power consumption, and flooding. Most importantly, authorized employees (operators) can manipulate HVAC systems by controlling room temperature settings. Other functions typically include monitoring of room cleanings, SOS alarms, unauthorized entries into rooms, etc.

On the other hand, guests can use the room control panel to set the proper temperature, control the air conditioning, activate the "Do Not Disturb" signal, notify the maid, and operate the room lights, valve, blinds, door, and windows.

3.2 Smart HVAC Control

The most important component of any smart room software is the control of HVAC system. Its operation is based on the following four parameters: (1) economic temperature, (2) pre-comfort temperature, (3) comfort temperature, and (4) scope of hotel temperature regulation.

When a room is not issued, the HVAC system is set to economic temperature, which is the hotel's established base temperature. Whenever a room is issued and occupied, the HVAC system is regulated to a comfort temperature. If a room is issued but not occupied, the pre-comfort temperature is set. This way, no energy is wasted on maintaining the thermal comfort of an unoccupied room. Pre-comfort temperature further helps in achieving the comfort temperature more quickly when a guest is present in a room. Finally, the temperature regulation scope of a hotel is a limitation for how much a guest may modify the comfort temperature on his/her own.

If the difference between room temperature and set temperature is higher than the input for economic or pre-comfort temperature value, then the system notifies the operators. In such a situation, operators correct the set parameters for the temperatures. This prevents prolonged exposure of the room to outside temperature, which would make it difficult to return to comfort temperature.

Other smart features include automatic valve shutdown when water temperature exceeds the set limit or when a window is left open for an extended length of time. Fan operating speed can increase or decrease automatically as well, based on the range of the difference between set temperature and room temperature.

4 Dataset and Data Visualization Tool

4.1 Dataset

To develop a custom visualization tool for smart buildings HVAC system, data were collected from a hotel in the Croatian capital of Zagreb. The related data includes indoor measurements collected from 2013 to 2021 for 166 hotel rooms. It is important to note that the obtained dataset was collected by an industrial log system with a sampling rate of one record in five minutes. Therefore, the available historical data cannot represent every event that may have occurred within the system, but they adequately demonstrate its operation in accordance with such discretized states. Furthermore, we also collected the related environmental measurements from the Croatian Meteorological and Hydrological Service [14]. Table 1 lists all parameters included in the dataset thus obtained.

4.2 Framework Technologies

We developed our web application using Dash framework – which combines Flask, React.js and Plotly.js – to create powerful interactive analytical online dashboards. Using the Dash framework and packages such as Plotly, we were able to construct our visualization tool entirely using Python programming language.

Table 1. Sensory measurements recorded in the dataset used in our research. While the upper part of the table refers to indoor (smart room) data, the lower part corresponds to measurements in the outdoor environment.

Parameter	Description	Data type
Timestamp.	Time-line of data being measured every 5 min	Date and time
Set temp	Desired temperature set by users	Continuous
Room temp	Current achieved temperature in the room	Continuous
HVAC speed	Fan speed with range from 0 to 3	Categorical
HVAC valve	Current status of the valve (open/closed)	Binary
Room occup.	Gives insight if a room is occupied or not	Binary
Window	Current status of the window (open/closed)	Binary
Irradiation	Solar radiation that falls upon a surface	Continuous
Humidity	The amount of vapor present in the atmosphere	Continuous
Outside temp	Current climate in the outside atmosphere	Continuous

On top of that, we utilized MongoDB as a NoSQL database to manipulate large amounts of data. It is worth noting that the Dash framework is both scalable and easily adaptable to the specific needs of the target application, hence a Dash-based solution can be effortlessly integrated into any smart building system.

4.3 Tool Categorization

HVAC system diagnostic tools have been researched and compared in [12]. The authors have noted that the most popular diagnostic objectives are energy waste, comfort control, and equipment operation. Accordingly, the main objective of our application is visual analysis of the temperature in hotel rooms, which forms the basis for comfort control.

There has been a distinction between available diagnostic tools by their level of automatization. Namely, they can roughly be divided into manual and automated tools. Automatization can be furthermore represented through four important functions of the diagnostic tools: (1) data acquisition, (2) data management and pre-processing, (3) anomaly detection, and (4) system diagnosis. In our application, data acquisition is automated since the system does not require manual import of new data. Data management and pre-processing is automated as well, because of integrated MongoDB database and interactive user interface which allows users to filter data. On the other hand, anomaly detection and system diagnosis are considered to be manual operations since users' reasoning for further identifications and conclusions is required.

In summary, the proposed visualization tool comes in the form of a responsive web application which can visualize different types of 2D interactive charts that can be filtered by target parameters and/or time periods. It also includes an interactive data table with sorting and filtering capabilities. Finally, it can display and compare basic indicators of descriptive statistics.

4.4 Visualization Dashboards

Application dashboards are divided into two web pages: (1) detailed analysis of one hotel room, and (2) comparison of two selected hotel rooms. The corresponding pages are shown in Fig. 2 and Fig. 3, respectively.

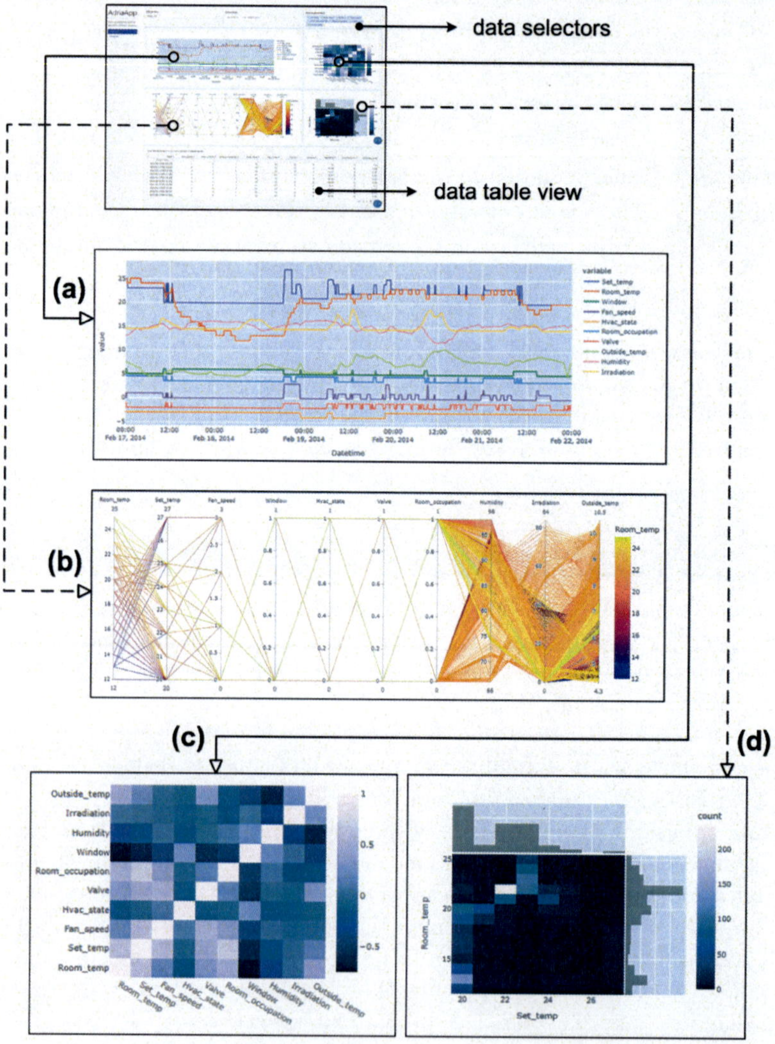

Fig. 2. First page visualizations: (a) Line graph – shows a drop in room temp. caused by a window that has been left open. (b) Parallel coordinates chart – shows degree of correlation of room temperature with other parameters. (c) Matrix chart – shows that set temp., room temp. and room occupation have the highest correlation between the observed parameters. (d) 2D histogram chart – further visualizes the relationship between set temp. and room temp. data; overall temperature density was at 22°C.

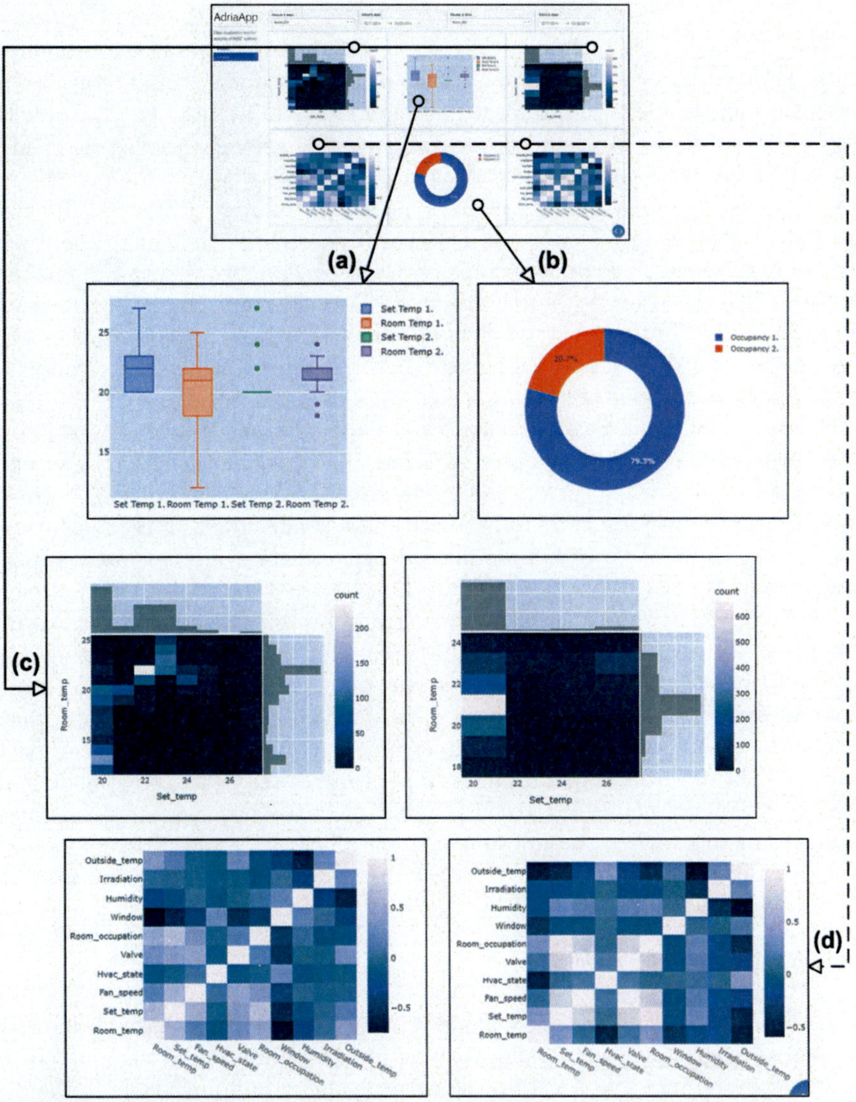

Fig. 3. Second page visualizations: (a) Box plot chart – Both rooms have similar temp. medians, indicating that the HVAC system is working well. Outliers and data skewness can signal anomalies that in turn can be attributed to sensor errors or human factor. (b) Pie chart – The first room was more occupied, so anomalies are more likely to be detected there. (c) 2D histogram charts – The set temp. of the first room varies more (because it is more occupied). Consequently, the temperature of the second room is more consistent and follows a normal distribution. (d) Matrix chart – The second room, with more static data, has stronger correlations between observed parameters, which indicates more HVAC functioning in the default mode.

The first web page, schematically explained in Fig. 2, provides an analysis for the selected hotel room in a given time period. It contains an interactive line graph that allows users to filter out parameters, zoom in and out, pan over the graph, hide or show lines, and hover over lines for getting detailed data information. The matrix chart depicts the correlations between all the parameters, providing insight into which parameters have the strongest or weakest influence on others. We also provided a parallel coordinates chart that might help with better interpretations of relationships between parameters by using room temperature as a base metric. Furthermore, a 2D histogram chart illustrates the density and distribution of set and room temperatures. It helps to further visualize the relationship between set and measured temperatures in the observed room. All visualizations are accompanied by a data table view.

On the second web page, schematically explained in Fig. 3, it is possible to select two different (in most cases adjacent) hotel rooms in order to visually explore and compare the corresponding data side-by-side. This page is both relevant and useful because hotel rooms with shared walls might affect each other's temperature value. As a result, we may identify whether a particular temperature anomaly is caused by nearby rooms. On the other hand, if HVAC system is functioning properly, data visualizations should produce similar uniform results throughout the observed hotel rooms. Box plot chart is used to visualize descriptive statistics of both set temperature and room temperature. We can assume temperature anomalies by looking at data similarities, outliers, and skewness. Box plots are accompanied by a simple pie chart which compares the occupancy of the two selected rooms, and temperature density plots to provide more detailed insights. Finally, matrix charts are included because they can reveal anomalies in cases when the low and high correlations between parameters are more diverse.

5 Conclusion

To briefly conclude, we have developed and presented a web-based data visualization tool that offers an exploratory approach to data analysis and can be easily scaled and integrated within the existing smart building system. The tool offers a simple and intuitive user interface and includes visualization dashboards for a better understanding of HVAC system data. Users can discover irregularities, monitor HVAC systems, analyze thermal comfort and make decisions on how to manage the hotel's energy consumption based on the application feedback. Furthermore, the tool does not exclude non-experts since it is designed to be used by a wide range of users, here including hotel's operators.

To make the tool more efficient and informative, it would require automated anomaly detection and diagnosis, as well as an updated dataset involving statistics on energy use and air quality. Further investigation on how to enhance the web application by integrating machine learning algorithms, with the goal to make useful predictions and support automated control, will be the focus of our future research.

Acknowledgment. This work was supported in part by European Regional Development Fund (ERDF) under grant agreement number KK.01.2.1.02.0303, project *Adria Smart Room*.

References

1. Ahmad, M.W., Mourshed, M., Yuce, B., Rezgui, Y.: Computational intelligence techniques for HVAC systems: a review. Build. Simul. **9**(4), 359–398 (2016). https://doi.org/10.1007/s12273-016-0285-4
2. Novikova, E., Bestuzhev, M., Shorov, A.: The visualization-driven approach to the analysis of the HVAC data. In: Kotenko, I., Badica, C., Desnitsky, V., El Baz, D., Ivanovic, M. (eds.) IDC 2019. SCI, vol. 868, pp. 547–552. Springer, Cham (2020). https://doi.org/10.1007/978-3-030-32258-8_64
3. Novikova, E., Bestuzhev, M., Kotenko, I.: Anomaly detection in the HVAC system operation by a RadViz based visualization-driven approach. In: Katsikas, S., et al. (eds.) CyberICPS/SECPRE/SPOSE/ADIoT -2019. LNCS, vol. 11980, pp. 402–418. Springer, Cham (2020). https://doi.org/10.1007/978-3-030-42048-2_26
4. Novikova, E., et al.: Usability assessment of the visualization-driven approaches to the HVAC data exploration. In: Proceedings of the 30th International Conference on Computer Graphics and Machine Vision (GraphiCon 2020), pp. 1–12. CEUR-WS (2020)
5. Novikova, E., Bestuzhev, M.: Exploration of the anomalies in HVAC data using image similarity assessment. In: 9th Mediterranean Conference on Embedded Computing (MECO 2020), pp. 1–4. IEEE (2020)
6. Abdelalim, A., O'Brien, W., Shi, Z.: Development of Sankey diagrams to visualize real HVAC performance. Energy Build. **149**, 282–297 (2017)
7. Janetzko, H., Stoffel, F., Mittelstädt, S., Keim, D.A.: Anomaly detection for visual analytics of power consumption data. Comput. Graph. **38**, 27–37 (2014)
8. Stopar, L., Skraba, P., Grobelnik, M., Mladenic, D.: Streamstory: exploring multivariate time series on multiple scales. IEEE Trans. Visual Comput. Graph. **25**(4), 1788–1802 (2018)
9. Murugesan, L.K., Hoda, R., Salcic, Z.: Design criteria for visualization of energy consumption: a systematic literature review. Sustain. Cities Soc. **18**, 1–12 (2015)
10. Fang, Y., Xu, H., Jiang, J.: A survey of time series data visualization research. IOP Conf. Ser. Mater. Sci. Eng. **782**(2), 022013 (2020)
11. Mao, J., Ryan, G.: Interpreting machine learning models for room temperature prediction in non-domestic buildings. arXiv:2111.13760 (2021)
12. Friedman, H., Piette, M.A.: Comparison of emerging diagnostic tools for large commercial HVAC systems. Technical report, Lawrence Berkeley National Lab. (LBNL), Berkeley, CA, USA (2001)
13. Balaji, B., Weibel, N., Agarwal, Y.: Managing commercial HVAC systems: what do building operators really need? arXiv:1612.06025 (2016)
14. Croatian Meteorological and Hydrological Service. https://meteo.hr/index_en.php. Accessed 08 Mar 2022

Solar Car Parking for Maximum Power Utilization at the United Arab Emirates University: Case Study

Prinu C. Philip[1], Faris Subaihi[2], Simon Musgun[1], Solomon Ghebretatios[1], and Fady Alnajjar[2](✉)

[1] Department of Electrical Engineering, UAE University, Al Ain 15551, UAE
{201990050,201640079,201850221}@uaeu.ac.ae
[2] Department of Computer Science and Software Engineering, UAE University, Al Ain 15551, UAE
{faris_subaihi,fady.alnajjar}@uaeu.ac.ae

Abstract. The demand for electricity and power from fossil fuels has been increasing in recent decades. The Greenhouse gases generated by such processes significantly impact the atmosphere. In addition, the cost of electricity production from these sources is very high; therefore, it is not affordable in the long run. Such a situation can be solved by utilizing renewable energy sources. This article presents a case study that is implementing a solar parking lot to generate energy by using existing car parking roofs at United Arab Emirates University. The generated power shall be fed to a grid. We have used PVSyst software to simulate various factors, including the shadow effect, and select proper solar parking that guarantees maximum solar power generation. Two cases with the fixed and the tracked PV panels were analyzed, considering power generation and the corresponding economic evaluation. The results suggested that the tracking PV panel produced more power and had less payback time energy than the fixed one.

Keywords: Solar energy · Parking lot solar system · Shading · Fixed and Dynamic PV panels · PVsyst

1 Introduction

The energy demand around the world is growing with population growth and urbanization. UAE population in 2020 is estimated to be around 9.28 million [1]. With the increasing population comes more electricity consumption. The UAE relies on natural gas for 98% of its electrical output to meet its demand [2]. The UAE has taken various measures to strengthen its energy security and diversify its energy profile through renewables and nuclear power. According to the UAE National Energy Strategy 2050, the plan will increase the contribution of clean energy from 25–50% by 2050. With the increase in energy production and the dependency on fossil fuels, the risk of increased GHG (Global Warming and Green House Gas) emissions also exists. UAE has been striving to improve its dependence on clean energy. The UAE National Energy Strategy

K. Daimi and A. Al Sadoon (Eds.): ICR 2022, AISC 1431, pp. 454–464, 2022.
https://doi.org/10.1007/978-3-031-14054-9_42

2050 emphasizes reducing carbon emissions from the power generating process by 70% [2]. Renewable energy sources such as geothermal, tidal, wind, and solar are abundant in nature and can quickly meet the growing demand for electrical energy. Solar energy is the primary source of producing clean energy in the UAE. Solar irradiance is the measure of solar power over a particular area. Solar irradiance at the surface of the earth is 1000 Wm^{-2}. Solar radiation with a photovoltaic (PV) system can be used to generate clean electricity. Urban area lands are often too costly for setting up PV systems [3]. Building-integrated photovoltaics technology has gained popularity due to its cost-effectiveness in urban areas [4]. But the PV deployment on building rooftops created uncertainties regarding building geometrics, urban layouts, orientation, and architectural configuration. Therefore, car parking roofs in urban areas were suggested for PV system installation [5]. Commercial buildings, educational institutions, residential complexes, and shopping malls car parking are good hotspots for PV system installation. The UAE receives over 10 h of sunlight on average – highly significant considering that the country has roughly 350 sunny days per year on average. Total solar energy received is about 6.5 kWh/m^2/day, and direct average solar radiation is 4–6 kWh/m^2/day, depending on location and time of the year [4]. In this research work, we have proposed implementing a solar car parking system at the United Arab Emirates University, Al Ain. The purpose of installing this system is to offset the grid electrical energy by using the photovoltaic system. The proposed car parking area is the Male Sidecar parking of the UAE University in Al Ain, UAE. Figure 1 shows the geographical coordinates of the site, which is located at 24.1967 latitudes, 55.6843 longitudes, and 249 m above sea level.

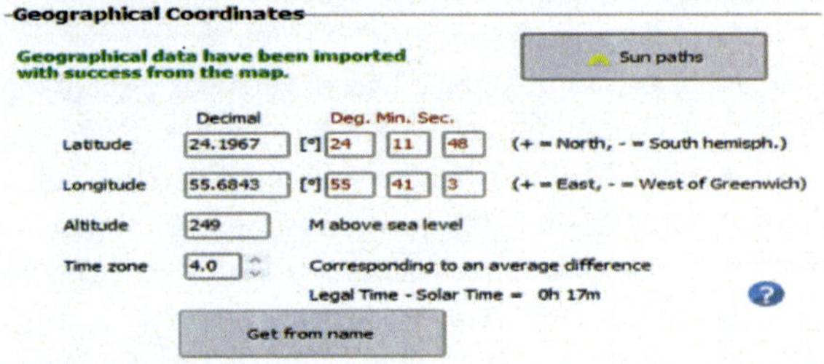

Fig. 1. Geographical coordinates of the UAE university male side F3 car parking.

2 Review of Literature

In [5], a case study was carried out on the King Fahd University of Petroleum and Minerals (KFUPM) campus in the Kingdom of Saudi Arabia to find out the forecasts for installing PV modules on building rooftops. Modeling approaches for solar radiation simulation and PV system energy generation were made using ArcGIS and PVsyst software. Considering all the obstructions in the available roof area like HVAC systems, skylights, water tanks, etc., the net general roof area for PV installation was 25–41% of the total building roof area. PV modeling was performed with the help of PVsyst software for both slanted and horizontal installations to optimize system efficiency and space use. PV panels set at a 24° tilt angle was found to be 9% more efficient than those installed horizontally. The modeling results suggested a net yearly output of 37,750 and 46,050 MWh from 21.44 and 28.51 MW of tilted and horizontal PV panels, respectively. This could compensate for 16% and 20% of campus electricity. In this study, only the building rooftops were considered for PV installation, whereas the car parking roofs were left out.

In [6], a capstone project was conducted at the University of Illinois at Urbana-Champaign. This project aimed to assess the possibility of using the open parking as solar car parks for power generation. 65.75 acres of parking spaces were allotted for this project. 967 parking strips were identified over this area and considered for this analysis. Annual solar power generated was estimated using ArcMap. For year-round solar radiation, the estimated potential energy from the parking strips was 257.25 GWh. After examination, it was found that solar carports could generate power ranging from 28.94 GWh to 46.3 GWh, contributing to clean energy ranging from 6.2% to 10% of the overall power needed by campus as of 2016. The efficiency of the solar panels was 15%, with a performance ratio of 0.75.

In [7], a project was conducted to evaluate the solar cell utilization and yield potential at the De Uithof campus in Utrecht, Netherlands. This project used solar energy to develop building-attached photovoltaic, solar parking lots and charging electric cars. The estimated yield production (MWh/year) through this work for two cases, VC0 and VC1, was 27.229 and 35.285, respectively. The performance ratio for the cases were 0.775 and 0.757, respectively. The project was economically feasible as the payback period was 7.69 years and the lifetime of the project was 25 years.

In [8], the project power generation idea was implemented at the King Abdulaziz University (KAU), Jeddah, in Saudi Arabia. The project was carried out as a trial phase to implement solar power generation across KSA, utilizing the car parking spaces to generate power. Cars require shading when parked in KSA due to the year-round high temperatures and direct irradiation. This provides a cooler climate and protects the vehicles. The project will also offer site owners a plan for utilizing PV technology in a dual role of power generation and vehicle shading. The PV installation capacity of the unshaded areas of the case study was found to be 16.1 MWp, generating energy of 29.3 GWh/year. Furthermore, the PV installation capacity for existing shaded canopies was anticipated to be around 20.3 MWp, with a potential electricity generation of 36.9 GWh/year. Overall, the campus car parks can install approximately 36.4 MWp of PV capacity, generating around 66.2 GWh of power per year.

In [9], a solar car parking system was installed at the Islamia University of Bahawalpur in Pakistan to balance the cost of grid electricity by employing a solar PV system. Using Folsom Labs' HelioScope software, a complete analysis of solar car parking site selection, maximum solar electric power output, and capacity implications with neighboring trees and buildings were completed. The monopitch canopy seemed to be the optimum to be installed at solar-powered parking areas at an inclination angle of 10°, according to the rigorous optimization and choosing of parking space canopies at a different set of standards tilt degrees to produce optimum sun photovoltaic energy. The analysis also conducted thorough economic research, revealing that installing a solar car parking lot at the proposed site would save 14% on power costs while reducing annual grid energy use by 17%. The parking facility and photovoltaic system's entire investment cost could be repaid in 6–7 years.

Parking lots covered 2647 hectares, or 0.06% of the national territory, according to Swiss land use statistics from 1994. Using images captured from the cameras, in Frauenfeld, a city in Switzerland, forty-eight large parking lots were spotted to install solar carports. These parking lots span a total area of 125140 m^2 and range in size from 112 to 6080 m^2. Individually, the orientation of the Photovoltaic panel towards the south, as well as the incline of 15 of the PV generators, were considered. PV syst was used for the simulation. The yield, efficiency, and effectiveness of the PV carport for the particular parking spot were calculated using different horizons. These parking spaces were then classified into one of three categories based on their simulated yield [10]. The purpose of the research done in [11] was to analyze and evaluate the energy provided by a PV system built on the university's parking lot, as well as the energy required for charging an electric vehicle. This was carried out at the Federal University of Technology in Curitiba, Paraná, Brazil. During its 24 months of operation, the solar carport system had produced an average of 465.37 kWh [12].

3 Methodology

In our study, a series of experiments were carried out. These included measurement of annual solar irradiation at the parking location, identifying if there is any shadow from the nearby buildings or trees at the proposed site, simulation using the proposed area in square meters, and economic analysis. These experiments were performed using PVSyst version 7.2.9. PVsyst is designed to be used by architects, engineers, and researchers. It is worldwide used for photovoltaic system installation. It is a PC software package for the study, sizing, and data analysis of complete PV systems. It deals with grid-connected, stand-alone, pumping, and DC-grid PV systems and includes extensive meteonorm and PV systems components databases [13]. The proposed site car parking for PV installation in our work did not have any shadows from the nearby trees or buildings. Therefore, we performed the PV car parking analysis without the shading effect of trees and buildings.

3.1 Car Parking Structure

Case 1 (Fixed Structure): The proposed site is the car parking area of the male side of the UAE University. The location is situated at a latitude of 24.20ºN and a longitude of 55.68ºE. The car parking site has an area of $44.25 \times 12.7 = 561.975$ m^2. For simulation accuracy, we approximate it to 562 m^2. The proposed site has several other similar area parking sites. The total available area for car parking is 26,200 m^2. For the PV analysis, we are considering one parking area. The albedo at the site is found to be 0.20. We have considered the Meteonorm 8.0 data for the analysis. By using PVsyst version 7.2.9, it is found that the total nominal power of 89.1 kWp is available at this site. We have considered a grid-connected system while performing the simulation. The PV field orientation for the fixed system is placed at an angle of 25º for maximum power which is shown in Fig. 2.

The number of PV modules required for this setup is 330 units, and the number of necessary inverters is 22 units. The total produced energy obtained for this setup is 158.3 MWh/year, with a performance ratio of 81.42. The Performance Ratio is the ratio of the energy effectively produced (used) concerning the energy produced if the system was continuously working at its nominal STC efficiency. PV modules used in this analysis are the globally available LG Electronics LG 270 S1C-B3 model with a unit nom. power of 270 Wp. Inverters used in this case are Mitsubishi PV-PNS04ATL – GER model with a unit norm. Power of 3.30 kW. Table 1 shows the detailed configuration of the PV module and the matching inverter selected for the simulation using PVSyst 7.2.9.

Table 1. PV Array Characteristics

PV module		Inverter	
Manufacturer	LG Electronics	Manufacturer	Mitsubishi
Model	LG 270 S1C-B3	Model	PV-PNS04ATL – GER
Unit norm. power	270 Wp	Unit norm. power	3.30 kWac
Nominal (STC)	89.1 kWp	Total power	72.6 kWac
Modules	22 strings × 15 in series	Pnom ratio	1.23

Case 2 (Tracking/Dynamic): Figure 3 shows that the tracking system's PV field orientation is placed at a tilt axis of 10° with an axis azimuth angle of –30°, and a rotating angle around the axis is placed between –60° to 60°. The number of PV modules required for this setup is similar to case 1 at 330 units, and the number of necessary inverters is 22 units. The produced energy for this tilted axis system is 185 MWh/year with a performance ratio of 81.52. The PV module and inverter make model are the same as that of case 1.

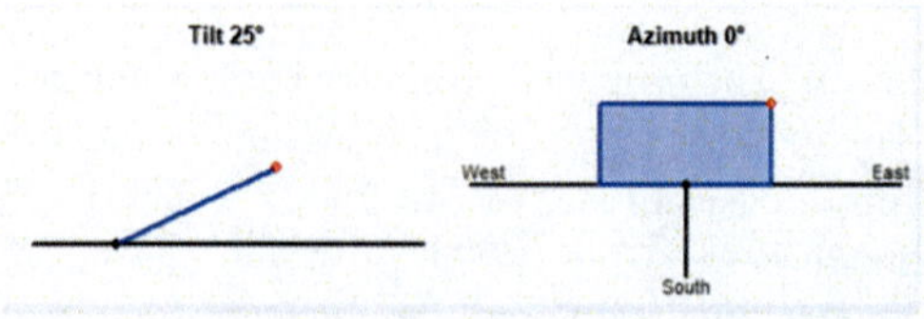

Fig. 2. Fixed tilt angle of the PV module for maximum solar power generation

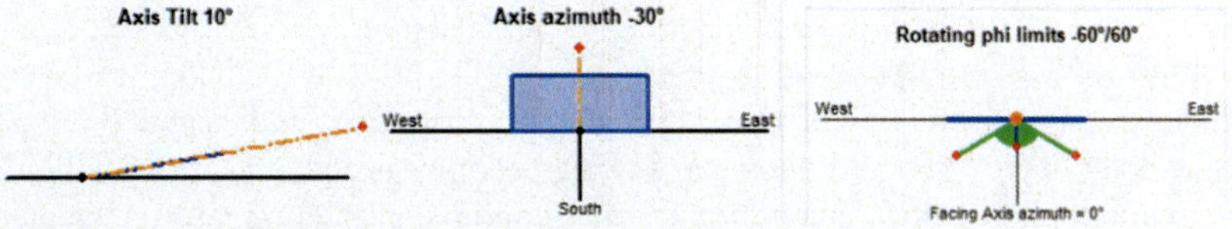

Fig. 3. Axis tilt, Axis Azimuth and rotating phi limits of the tracking PV module for maximum solar power generation

4 Results

Case 1

Normalized Energy: These indicators are related to the incident energy GlobInc in the collector plane and are normalized by the Pnom = Array nominal installed power at STC, as given by the PV-module manufacturer [kWp] [14]. The following results were obtained for Case 1:

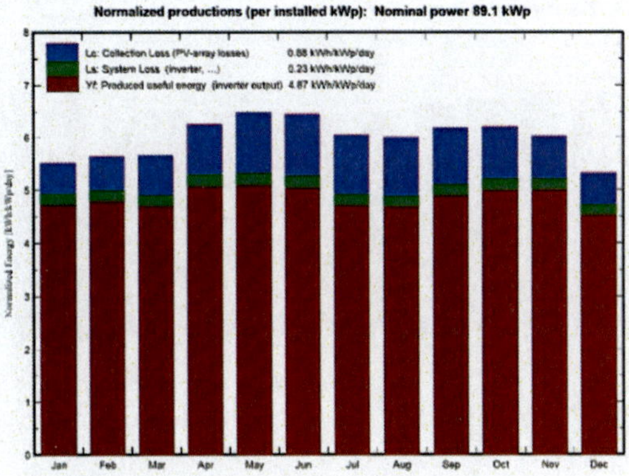

Fig. 4. The normalized energy production per installed kWp for each month in a year

Figure 4 shows the yearly normalized energy production, explicitly showing each month's production. The violet bar represents the PV array losses, called collection loss, which is 0.88 kWh/kWp/day. The green bar represents the system loss. System loss is 0.23 kWh/kWp/day. The maroon-colored bar indicates the produced useful energy, which is 4.87 kWh/kWp/day.

Performance Ratio: The Performance Ratio is the ratio of the energy effectively produced (used) concerning the energy produced if the system continuously worked at its nominal STC efficiency [14]. Figure 5 shows the performance ratio for each month in a year. The average for the year was found to be 0.814.

Economic Evaluation: Previous studies and their findings suggest that solar energy generation on car parking canopies is feasible with their optimal maximum photovoltaic generation [15]. Every operation is determined by the amount of money invested, the advantages received, and the time it takes to pay off. Prior case studies and findings suggest that solar energy generation on car parking canopies is conceivable with their optimal maximum photovoltaic generation [5–9]. Economic evaluation tells us the invested amount and the payback period estimate. For case 1, the amount invested was found to be payback in 7.4 years. Table 2 shows the detailed costs and the payback period for case 1.

Case 2

Normalized Energy: Figure 6 shows the yearly normalized energy production, explicitly showing each month's production. The violet bar represents the PV array losses, called collection loss, which is 1.03 kWh/kWp/day. The green bar represents the system loss. System loss is 0.26 kWh/kWp/day. The maroon-colored bar indicates the produced useful energy of 5.69 kWh/kWp/day.

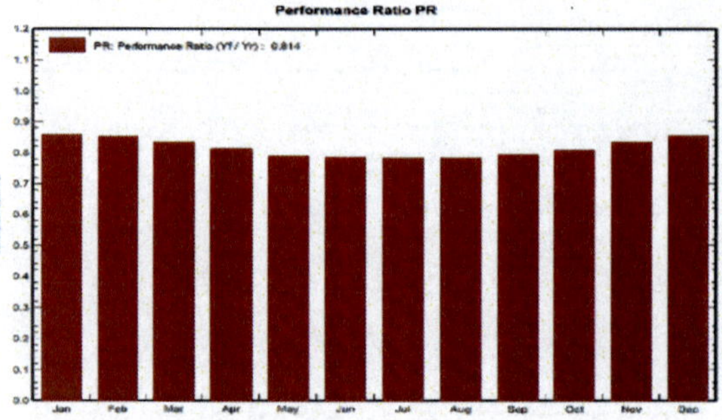

Fig. 5. Performance ratio for each month in a year

Table 2. Investment and payback period

Components	Cost (USD)
Cost of PV modules + support for modules	66825.00
Cost of inverter	53460
Installation + other components	60588
Total	180873.00
Produced energy	158 MWh/year
Payback period (years)	7.4

Performance Ratio: The Performance Ratio is the ratio of the energy effectively produced (used), with respect to the energy which would be produced if the system was continuously working at its nominal STC efficiency. Figure 7 shows the performance ratio for each month in a year. The average for the year was found to be 0.815.

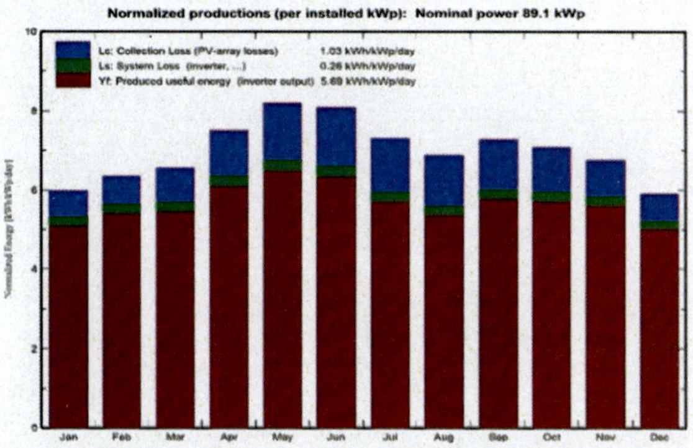

Fig. 6. The normalized energy production per installed kWp for each month in a year

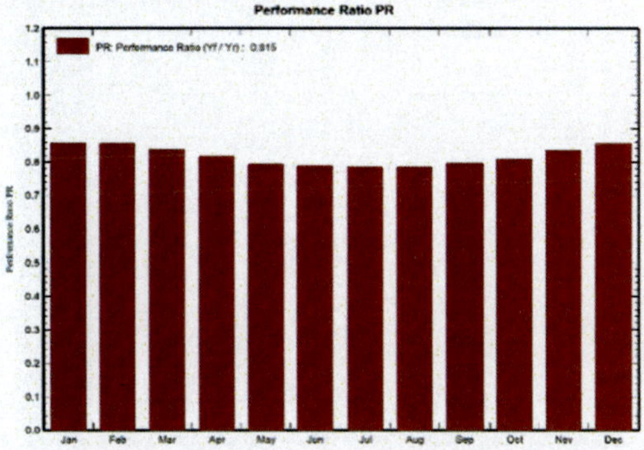

Fig. 7. The normalized energy production per installed kWp for each month in a year

Economic Evaluation: Every operation is determined by the amount of money invested, the advantages received, and the time it takes to pay off. Prior case studies and findings suggest that solar energy generation on car parking canopies is conceivable with their optimal maximum photovoltaic generation. Economic evaluation tells us the invested amount and the payback period estimate. For case 2 the amount invested was found to be payback in 6.2 years. Table 3 shows the detailed costs and the payback period for case 2.

Performance Analysis of the Fixed and the Tracking PV Panels Throughout the Year: The climate of the UAE consists of four **season's** summer, autumn, winter, and spring [16]. Summer season begins from May and lasts till September. Autumn season is from September to December. Winter begins from late December to mid-March. Spring season lasts from mid-March to May. The performance of the fixed and the tracking panels has been shown in Fig. 8.

Table 3. Investment and payback period

Components	Cost (USD)
Cost of PV modules + support for modules	66825.00
Cost of inverter	53460
Installation + other components	69498
Total	189783.00
Produced energy	185 MWh/year
Payback period (years)	6.2

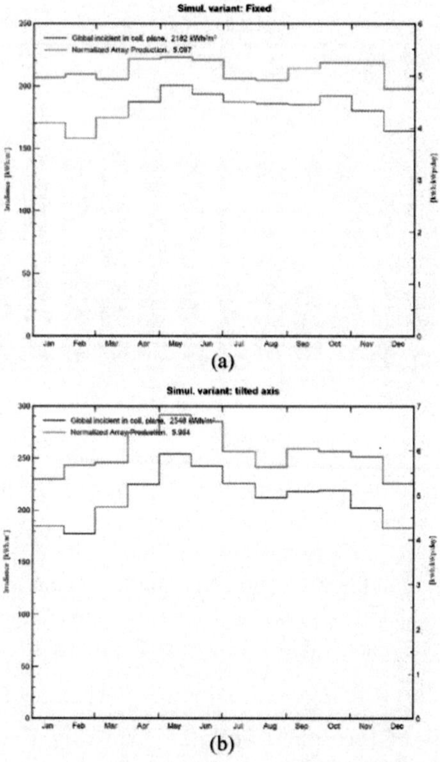

Fig. 8. The normalized energy production vs Irradiance for each month in a year for fixed (above) and Dynamic PV panels (.

5 Conclusion

University campuses have car parks that cover large areas. Such places have a lot of potential for integrating solar PV systems and contributing to electrical power services for local loads or grid export.In this work, we have utilized the existing car parking of UAE university to generate solar power and contribute to the power requirement of the university. This provides a dual advantage of power production and solar shading. Also, it will offset the university's monthly energy demand and reduce the campus's carbon footprint. This helps to develop a sustainable community within the university campus. In this research work, the available car parking area was simulated using PVsyst software to generate power fed to a grid. This analysis considers two cases with fixed and tracking/dynamic PV panels. The results revealed that tracking PV panels could generate more power than fixed panels. The economic analysis showed that the payback period for the tracking panels was less as compared to the fixed PV panel setup.

Acknowledgement. The authors would like to acknowledge the Research Office of the United Arab Emirates University for the financial support extended for the project.

Conflicts of Interest. The authors declare no conflicts of interest.

References

1. United Arab Emirates: Article IV Consultation—Press Release and Staff Report. International Monetary Fund, February 2022 (2021)
2. UAE State of Energy Report 2050: Ministry of Energy, United Arab Emirates (2017). ISBN-10: 1542953324
3. Salim, A.M., Dabous, S.A.: SWOT analysis of solar photovoltaic systems in public housing projects in the United Arab Emirates. In: 2022 Advances in Science and Engineering Technology International Conferences (ASET). IEEE (2022)
4. Alnaser, W.E., Alnaser, N.W.: The status of renewable energy in the GCC countries. Renew. Sustain. Energy Rev. **15**(6), 3074–3098 (2011)
5. Asif, M., Hassanain, M.A., Nahiduzzaman, K.M.: Techno-economic assessment of application of solar PV in building. Smart Sustain. Built Environ. **8**(1), 34–52 (2019)
6. Badami, P.: Assessment of open parking lots to locate potential solar carport installations for power generation at the university of illinois at urbana-champaign. http://hdl.handle.net/2142/111666
7. de Oliveira, T. D.: Facades and Solar Parking Yield Estimation at Ultrecht University, Diss. Universidade de Evora (Portugal) (2020)
8. Alghamdi, A.S., Bahaj, A.S., Yue, W.: Assessment of large-scale photovoltaic power generation from carport canopies. Energies **10**(5), 686 (2017)
9. Umer, F., et al.: Design and optimization of solar carport canopies for maximum power generation and efficiency at Bahawalpur. Int. J. Photoenergy **2019** (2019)
10. Neumann, H.-M., Schär, D., Baumgartner, F.: The potential of photovoltaic carports to cover the energy demand of road passenger transport. Prog. Photovoltaics Res. Appl. **20**(6), 639–649 (2012)
11. Kulik, A.C., et al.: Analysis of scenarios for the insertion of electric vehicles in conjunction with a solar carport in the city of Curitiba, Paraná—Brazil. Energies **14**(16), 5027 (2021). https://doi.org/10.3390/en14165027
12. Miceli, R., Viola, F.: Designing a sustainable university recharge area for electric vehicles: technical and economic analysis. Energies **10**(10), 1604 (2017). https://doi.org/10.3390/en10101604
13. Bremer, P., Kunz, S., Voltz, R.: METEONORM . vol 1 (Théorie), vol 2 (Données), vol 3 (Procédures de calcul), vol 4 (Sources de données). Office Fédéral de l'Energie, Berne (1986)

14. Kumar, N.M., Kumar, M.R., Rejoice, P.R., Mathew, M.: Performance analysis of 100 kWp grid connected Si-poly photovoltaic system using PVsyst simulation tool. Energy Procedia, **117**, 180–189 (2017). ISSN 1876-6102. https://doi.org/10.1016/j.egypro.2017.05.121
15. Erickson, L.E., Robinson, J., Brase, G., Cutsor, J.: Solar Powered Charging Infrastructure for Electric Vehicles: A Sustainable Development. CRC Press, Boca Raton (2016)
16. Abuelgasim, A., Farahat, A.: Effect of dust loadings, meteorological conditions, and local emissions on aerosol mixing and loading variability over highly urbanized semiarid countries: United Arab Emirates case study. J. Atmos. Solar Terr. Phys. **199**, 105215 (2020)

Learning and Education

Learner Performance-Based Behavior Optimization Algorithm: A Functional Case Study

Shahad A. Salih[1,2] and Tarik A. Rashid[3](✉)

[1] Computer Science Department, University of Duhok, Duhok, Iraq
[2] Da Vinci Studio School, Duhok, Iraq
[3] Computer Science and Engineering Department, University of Kurdistan Hewler, Erbil, Iraq
tarik.ahmed@ukh.edu.krd

Abstract. A novel algorithm called learner performance-based behavior algorithm (LPB) was proposed for single and multi-objective by Chnoor M. Rahman and Tarik A. Rashid in 2021. LPB proved its ability to deal with complex optimization problems compared to the dragonfly algorithm *(DA),* genetic algorithm *(GA),* and particle swarm optimization (*PSO*). This paper presents and explains the implementation of the LPB algorithm, and it applies it as a model in a case study to maximize a fitness function. As a result, the LPB algorithm is successfully improved the initial population and achieved the optimal solution.

Keywords: Metaheuristic · Learner performance-based behavior · Optimization algorithm

1 Introduction

Metaheuristic refers to higher-level heuristics, which have been developed for solving a variety of optimization problems. Various metaheuristic algorithms have recently been successful in tackling intractable situations. The advantage of employing these algorithms to solve complicated problems is that they produce the approximate solutions in a short amount of time, even for very complex problems [1]. Optimization is used in almost all areas of our lives, such as engineering, medicine, business planning, control, energy, etc. These algorithms intelligently select the best solutions from a wide range of choices [2]. Some widely used optimization algorithms are extracted from natural systems, such as Genetic Algorithm (GA), Particle Swarm Optimization (PSO), Ant Colony Optimization (ACO) [3].

Recently, a learner performance-based behavior algorithm (LPB) has been proposed by Chnoor M. Rahman and Tarik A. Rashid in 2021 [4, 5] to mainly tackle single and multi-objective problems. The main contribution of the paper is to apply LPB to a case study to maximize and obtain optimal solutions. A simple step-by-step guide is demonstrated for this purpose. The paper also serves as a guide for researchers to develop, enhance or hybridize the algorithm.

K. Daimi and A. Al Sadoon (Eds.): ICR 2022, AISC 1431, pp. 467–482, 2022.
https://doi.org/10.1007/978-3-031-14054-9_43

The rest of the paper is organized into sections, where section two explains LPB in brief. In section three, a case study has been designed to evaluate LPB. Finally, in section four, the main points are concluded.

2 Learner Performance-Based Behavior Algorithm

LPB algorithm is inspired by the idea of accepting graduates from high school to university. Through the steps that are applied during the admission of Learners, which are the methods used to divide learners and group them according to their cumulative rate. Also, these methods are used to improve the behavior and level of performance of the individuals after admission to the departments. Learners need to use new study habits because the methods they used to study in junior high do not work properly in college [6–8]. In this algorithm as a first step, a group of individuals is selected from the population. These individuals are then divided into sub-groups, and the best individuals are then selected from the subgroups depending on their fitness. Their behavior and performance are then improved by having them work as groups. Where teamwork will provide information sharing among themselves when they study (crossover), this method will affect their behavior randomly (mutation). LPB uses crossover and mutation techniques of the genetic algorithm. LPB algorithm works as shown in Fig. 1.

```
1.  Randomly Initial a main population: M
2.  Calculate fitness of all M individuals
3.  Initial the parameters: the number of required individuals N, Crossover rate and mutation rate
4.  Use dp parameter to randomly create sub population O from M
5.  Sort the individuals in O (descending order) depending on their fitness
6.  Divide O to two populations, good (Highest fitness) and bad (Lowest fitness)
7.  while termination condition is not met
8.  Find the highest fitness in good and bad populations
        if      an individual from M has fitness ≤ highest fitness in the bad population
                Move M individual to the bad population (BP)
        else if an individual from M has fitness ≤ highest fitness in the good population
                Move M individual to the good population (GP)
        else
                Move M individual to the perfect population (PF)
        end if
        while k ≤ N
            if      PF is not empty
                    Select an individual from PF
                    Apply Crossover between PF individual and individual from O Good
            else if GP is not empty
                    Select an individual from GP
                    Apply Crossover between GP individual and individual from O Good
            else
                    Select an individual from BP
                    Apply Crossover between BP individual and individual from O Good
            end if
            k = k+1;
        end while
9.  Mutation
10. Termination
11. Repeat the procedure from step 4 until the termination condition is met.
12. end while
13. Optimal Solution: Select the best solution from the perfect population
```

Fig. 1. LPB pseudocode

Figure 2 show the flowchart of LPB.

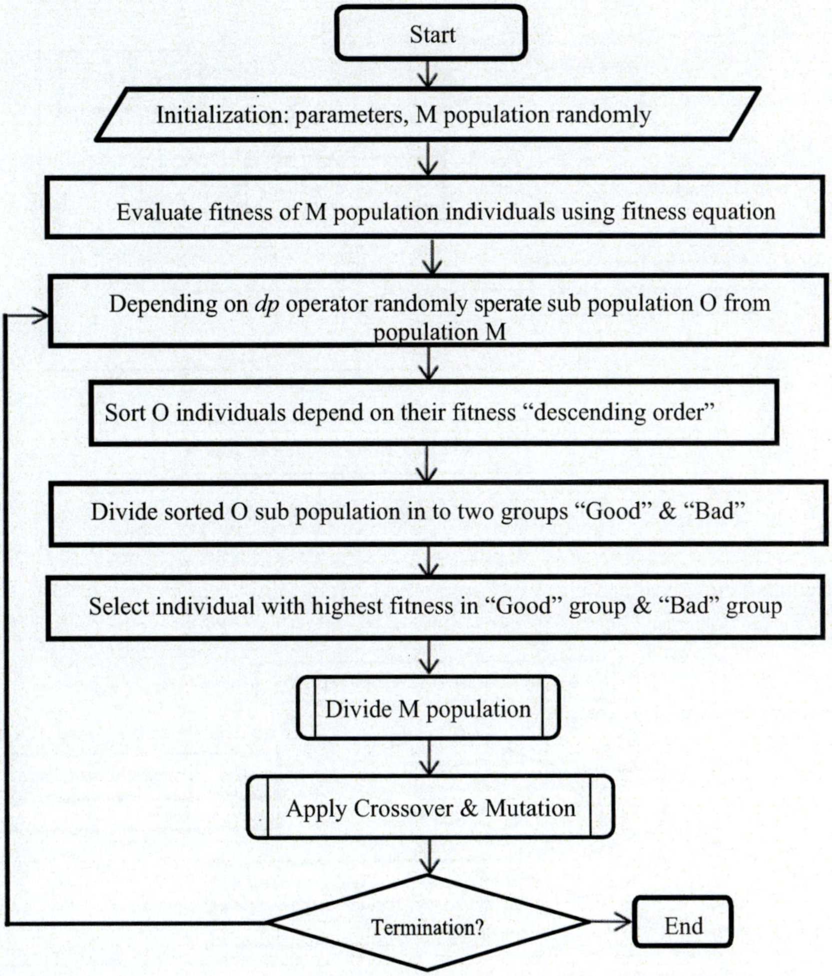

Fig. 2. LPB algorithm flowchart

Figure 3 shows how to divide *M* population flowchart.

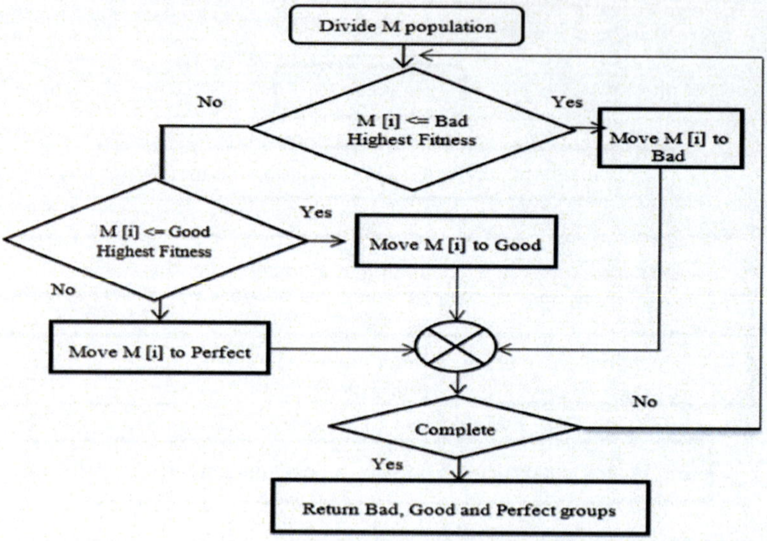

Fig. 3. Divide M population flowchart

Figuer 4 shows the processes of Crossover & Mutation.

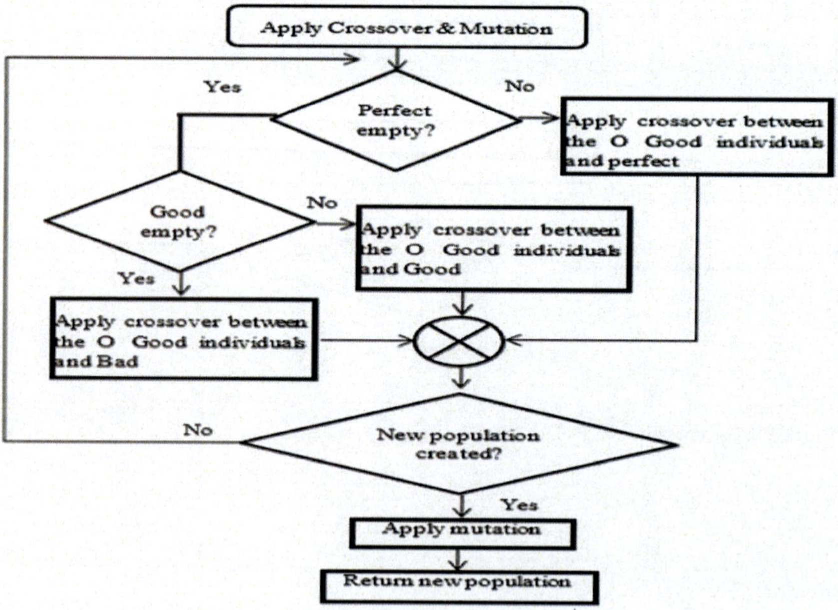

Fig. 4. Apply Crossover & Mutation

3 A Case Study

For a maximizatnion type of optimization as oppoosed to a minimization type; consider the following function: *f(x)*, where $f(x) = x_1^2 + x_2^2$; for integer *x*, $0 \le x_1 \le 5000$ *and* $0 \le x_2 \le 5000$.

Itreation 0

Step 1: Let *M* consists of 16 individuals. Then evaluate the fitness of all *M* individuals by the fitness equation. Let $N = 4$ where *N* is the number of required individuals. Calculate the summation, average and find maximum fitness form *M* as shown in Table 1:

Table 1. Randomly create an *M* population and evaluate the fitness of all individuals.

Mi	X_1	X_2	X_1^2	X_2^2	$Fitness\ (Mi) = X_1^2 + X_2^2$
M1	3770	3362	14,212,900	11,303,044	25,515,944
M2	703	1264	494,209	1,597,696	2,091,905
M3	3235	2191	10,465,225	4,800,481	15,265,706
M4	3989	3940	15,912,121	15,523,600	31,435,721
M5	1716	1065	2,944,656	1,134,225	4,078,881
M6	2394	4020	5,731,236	16,160,400	21,891,636
M7	1600	2559	2,560,000	6,548,481	9,108,481
M8	3639	2013	13,242,321	4,052,169	17,294,490
M9	3500	3275	12,250,000	10,725,625	22,975,625
M10	1890	1105	3,572,100	1,221,025	4,793,125
M11	4044	4038	16,353,936	16,305,444	32,659,380
M12	4065	1122	16,524,225	1,258,884	17,783,109
M13	2673	3580	7,144,929	12,816,400	19,961,329
M14	3829	1473	14,661,241	2,169,729	16,830,970
M15	245	2484	60,025	6,170,256	6,230,281
M16	2212	3382	4,892,944	11,437,924	16,330,868

Sum fit. (Mi) = 264,247,451
Average fit. (Mi) = 16,515,466
Max fit. (Mi) = 32,659,380.

Iteration 1

Step 2: Randomly create a subpopulation; let *O* consists of 8 individuals. Then Sort *O* descending order. Divide *O* into two groups; Good and Bad. Select that individual with the highest fitness from good and bad as shown in Table 2.

Table 2. *O* population, finding the highest fitness from Good and Bad groups.

Mi	Oi	Fitness (Oi)	Groups
M11	O1	32,659,380	Good
M9	O2	22,975,625	
M8	O3	17,294,490	
M14	O4	16,830,970	
M16	O5	16,330,868	Bad
M7	O6	9,108,481	
M10	O7	4,793,125	
M5	O8	4,078,881	

Good High Fitness is O1 = 32,659,380
Bad High Fitness is O5 = 16,330,868.

Step 3: Compare *M* individuals with *O* Good and Bad highest fitness to divide *M* (Table 3).

Table 3. Comparing *M* individuals with *O* Good and Bad highest fitness to divide *M*, Fitness (Fit.).

Mi	Fitness (Mi)	Fit. (Mi) ≤ Fit. (O5)	Fit. (Mi) ≤ Fit. (O1)	Perfect group
M1	25,515,944		Good	
M2	2,019,905	Bad		
M3	15,265,706	Bad		
M4	31,435,721		Good	
M5	4,078,881	Bad		
M6	21,891,636		Good	
M7	9,108,481	Bad		
M8	17,294,490		Good	
M9	22,975,625		Good	
M10	4,793,125	Bad		
M11	32,659,380		Good	
M12	17,783,109		Good	
M13	19,961,329		Good	
M14	16,830,970		Good	
M15	6,230,281	Bad		
M16	16,330,868	Bad		

Step 4: Check if the Perfect population is not empty, select individuals from PF. If the PF is empty select individuals from the Good population (GP) when it's not empty, if the GP is empty, then select individuals from the Bad population (BP). The selected individuals will be used in the crossover operator. Note that the number of selected individuals equals the number of required individuals N, which we specify in the first step.

Table 4. Selected individuals.

Selected Individuals to Crossover with O_Good Individua's		
M1	25,515,944	Good
M4	31,435,721	Good
M6	21,891,636	Good
M12	17,783,109	Good

Step 5: Apply crossover between selected individuals from Table 4 and good individuals from Table 2.

Table 5. Apply crossover.

P, Ch	Ind.	X_1	X_2	X1 (Binary)	X2 (Binary)
P1	M1	3770	3362	**1110 10**11 1010	**1101 00**10 0010
P2	O1	4044	4038	1111 11**00 1100**	1111 11**00 0110**
Ch1	New	3724	3334	1110 1000 1100	1101 0000 0110
Ch2	New	4090	4066	1111 1111 1010	1111 1110 0010
P3	M4	3989	3940	**1111 10**01 0101	**1111 01**10 0100
P4	O2	3500	3275	1101 10**10 1100**	1100 11**00 1011**
Ch3	New	4012	3915	1111 1010 1100	1111 0100 1011
Ch4	New	3477	3300	1101 1001 0101	1100 1110 0100
P5	M6	2394	4020	**1001 01**01 1010	**1111 10**11 0100
P6	O3	3639	2013	1110 00**11 0111**	0111 11**01 1101**
Ch5	New	2423	3997	1001 0111 0111	1111 1001 1101
Ch6	New	3610	2036	1110 0001 1010	0111 1111 0100
P7	M12	4065	1122	**1111 11**10 0001	**0100 01**10 0010
P8	O4	3829	1473	1110 11**11 0101**	0101 11**00 0001**
Ch7	New	4085	1089	1111 1111 0101	0100 0100 0001
Ch8	New	3809	1506	1110 1110 0001	0101 1110 0010

Step 6: Apply mutation on new individuals (Child), to maximize the function (randomly convert 0 --> 1) 1bit for each individual (Table 6).

Table 6. Apply mutation.

Child	X_1	X_2	X_1 Binary	X_2 Binary
Ch1	3724	3334	1110 1000 1100	1101 0000 0110
Ch2	4090	4066	1111 1111 1010	1111 1110 0010
Ch3	4012	3915	1111 1010 1100	1111 0100 1011
Ch4	3477	3300	1101 1001 0101	1100 1110 0100
Ch5	2423	3997	1001 0111 0111	1111 1001 1101
Ch6	3610	2036	1110 0001 1010	0111 1111 0100
Ch7	4085	1089	1111 1111 0101	0100 0100 0001
Ch8	3809	1506	1110 1110 0001	0101 1110 0010

New individuals are shown in Table 7:

Table 7. New individuals after mutation.

X_1new (Binary)	X_2 new (Binary)	X_1	X_2
1110 1100 1100	1111 0000 0110	3788	3846
1111 1111 1011	1111 1111 0010	4091	4082
1111 1110 1100	1111 1100 1011	4076	4043
1101 1001 0111	1110 1110 0100	3479	3812
1001 1111 0111	1111 1001 1111	2551	3999
1110 0101 1010	1111 1111 0100	3674	4084
1111 1111 1101	0100 1100 0001	4093	1217
1111 1110 0001	0101 1111 0010	4065	1522

Step 7: Calculate the fitness of new individuals as shown in Table 8.

Table 8. Calculate fitness for new individuals.

Child	X_1	X_2	X_1^2	X_2^2	Fitness(Chi) $= X_1^2 + X_2^2$
Ch1	3788	3846	14,348,944	14,791,716	29,140,660
Ch2	4091	4082	16,736,281	16,662,724	33,399,005
Ch3	4076	4043	16,613,776	16,345,849	32,959,625
Ch4	3479	3812	12,103,441	14,531,344	26,634,785
Ch5	2551	3999	6,507,601	15,992,001	22,499,602
Ch6	3674	4084	13,498,276	16,679,056	30,177,332
Ch7	4093	1217	16,752,649	1,481,089	18,233,738
Ch8	4065	1522	16,524,225	2,316,484	18,840,709

Step 8: Find the sum, average, and max between new individuals from Table 8 and the parents (Pi) from Table 5.

Table 9. Find sum, average, and max.

Ind.	X_1	X_2	X_1^2	X_2^2	Fitness (Ind.) $= X_1^2 + X_2^2$
M1	3770	3362	14,212,900	11,303,044	25,515,944
O1	4044	4038	16,353,936	16,305,444	32,659,380
M4	3989	3940	15,912,121	15,523,600	31,435,721
O2	3500	3275	12,250,000	10,725,625	22,975,625
M6	2394	4020	5,731,236	16,160,400	21,891,636
O3	3639	2013	13,242,321	4,052,169	17,294,490
M12	4065	1122	16,524,225	1,258,884	17,783,109
O4	3829	1473	14,661,241	2,169,729	16,830,970
Ch1	3788	3846	14,348,944	14,791,716	29,140,660
Ch2	4091	4082	16,736,281	16,662,724	33,399,005
Ch3	4076	4043	16,613,776	16,345,849	32,959,625
Ch4	3479	3812	12,103,441	14,531,344	26,634,785
Ch5	2551	3999	6,507,601	15,992,001	22,499,602
Ch6	3674	4084	13,498,276	16,679,056	30,177,332
Ch7	4093	1217	16,752,649	1,481,089	18,233,738
Ch8	4065	1522	16,524,225	2,316,484	18,840,709

Sum fitness = 398,272,331
Average fitness = 24,892,021
Max fitness = 33,399,005.

The new population is shown in Table 9. Table 10 just rename the (Ind.) column to (Mi) to show that it's the New *M* Population. That should generate *O* subpopulation from it.

Table 10. The new *M* population.

Mi	X_1	X_2	X_1^2	X_2^2	Fitness (Ind.) = $X_1^2 + X_2^2$
M1	3770	3362	14,212,900	11,303,044	25,515,944
M2	4044	4038	16,353,936	16,305,444	32,659,380
M3	3989	3940	15,912,121	15,523,600	31,435,721
M4	3500	3275	12,250,000	10,725,625	22,975,625
M5	2394	4020	5,731,236	16,160,400	21,891,636
M6	3639	2013	13,242,321	4,052,169	17,294,490
M7	4065	1122	16,524,225	1,258,884	17,783,109
M8	3829	1473	14,661,241	2,169,729	16,830,970
M9	3788	3846	14,348,944	14,791,716	29,140,660
M10	4091	4082	16,736,281	16,662,724	33,399,005
M11	4076	4043	16,613,776	16,345,849	32,959,625
M12	3479	3812	12,103,441	14,531,344	26,634,785
M13	2551	3999	6,507,601	15,992,001	22,499,602
M14	3674	4084	13,498,276	16,679,056	30,177,332
M15	4093	1217	16,752,649	1,481,089	18,233,738
M16	4065	1522	16,524,225	2,316,484	18,840,709

Sum fitness = 398,272,331
Average fitness = 24,892,021
Max fitness = 33,399,005.

Iteration 2
The previous steps (2 to 8) will be repeated till the required number of iterations or the stop condition is met, then the optimal solution is returned.

Repeat **steps 2 to 8**, to do the second iteration.

Step 2: Create a new *O* sub-population from new *M* population Table 10.

Table 11. Randomly create *O* population and select the highest fitness from Good and Bad.

Mi	Oi	Fitness (Oi)	Groups
M11	O1	32,959,625	Good
M3	O2	31,435,721	
M9	O3	29,140,660	
M12	O4	26,634,785	
M1	O5	25,515,944	Bad
M16	O6	18,840,709	
M15	O7	18,233,738	
M7	O8	17,783,109	

Good High Fitness is O1 = 32,959,625
Bad High Fitness is O5 = 25,515,944.

Step 3: Compare the new *M* individuals Table 10 with *O* Good and Bad highest fitness (Table 12).

Table 12. Comparing *M* individuals with *O* Good and Bad highest fitness.

Mi	Fitness (Mi)	Fit. (Mi) ≤ Fit. (O5)	Fit. (Mi) ≤ Fit. (O1)	Perfect group
M1	25,515,944	Bad		
M2	32,659,380		Good	
M3	31,435,721		Good	
M4	22,975,625	Bad		
M5	21,891,636	Bad		
M6	17,294,490	Bad		
M7	17,783,109	Bad		
M8	16,830,970	Bad		
M9	29,140,660		Good	
M10	33,399,005			Perfect
M11	32,959,625		Good	
M12	26,634,785		Good	
M13	22,499,602	Bad		
M14	30,177,332		Good	
M15	18,233,738	Bad		
M16	18,840,709	Bad		

Step 4: Check if the Perfect population is not empty select individuals from PF, if the PF is empty, select individuals from the good population when it's not empty, if the GP is empty, select individuals from the BP. The selected individuals will be used in the crossover operator.

Note: The number of selected individuals will equal the number of required individuals *N*, which we specify in the first step.

Table 13. Selected individuals.

Selected Individuals to Crossover with O_Good Individua's		
M10	33,399,005	Perfect
M2	32,659,380	Good
M14	30,177,332	Good
M4	22,975,625	Bad

Step 5: Apply crossover between selected individuals from Table 13 and good individuals from Table 11.

Table 14. Apply crossover.

P, Ch	Ind.	X_1	X_2	X1 (Binary)	X2 (Binary)
P1	M10	4091	4082	**1111 1111** 1011	**1111 1111** 0010
P2	O1	4076	4043	1111 11**10 1100**	1111 11**00 1011**
Ch1	New	4076	4043	1111 1110 1100	1111 1100 1011
Ch2	New	4091	4082	1111 1111 1011	1111 1111 0010
P3	M2	4044	4038	**1111 1100** 1100	**1111 1100** 0110
P4	O2	3989	3940	1111 10**01 0101**	1111 01**10 0100**
Ch3	New	4053	4068	1111 1101 0101	1111 1110 0100
Ch4	New	3980	3910	1111 1000 1100	1111 0100 0110
P5	M14	3674	4084	**1110 0101** 1010	**1111 1111** 0100
P6	O3	3788	3846	1110 11**00 1100**	1111 00**00 0110**
Ch5	New	3660	4038	1110 0100 1100	1111 1100 0110
Ch6	New	3802	3892	1110 1101 1010	1111 0011 0100
P7	M4	3500	3275	**1101 1010** 1100	**1100 1100** 1011
P8	O4	3479	3812	1101 10**01 0111**	1110 11**10 0100**
Ch7	New	3479	3300	1101 1001 0111	1100 1110 0100
Ch8	New	3500	3787	1101 1010 1100	1110 1100 1011

Step 6: Apply mutation on new individuals (Child) to maximize the function (randomly convert 0 bit to 1 bit) 1bit for each individual (Table 15).

Table 15. Apply mutation process on the new child.

Child	X_1	X_2	$X_{1\ Binary}$	$X_{2\ Binary}$
Ch1	4076	4043	1111 1110 1100	1111 1100 1011
Ch2	4091	4082	1111 1111 1011	1111 1111 0010
Ch3	4053	4068	1111 1101 0101	1111 1110 0100
Ch4	3980	3910	1111 1000 1100	1111 0100 0110
Ch5	3660	4038	1110 0100 1100	1111 1100 0110
Ch6	3802	3892	1110 1101 1010	1111 0011 0100
Ch7	3479	3300	1101 1001 0111	1100 1110 0100
Ch8	3500	3787	1101 1010 1100	1110 1100 1011

New individuals are shown in Table 16.

Table 16. New individuals after mutation.

X_1new (Binary)	X_2 new (Binary)	X_1	X_2
1111 1111 1100	1111 1100 1111	4092	4047
1111 1111 1111	1111 1111 1010	4095	4090
1111 1101 1101	1111 1110 0101	4061	4069
1111 1100 1100	1111 0110 0110	4044	3942
1110 0100 1110	1111 1101 0110	3662	4054
1111 1101 1010	1111 0111 0100	4058	3956
1111 1001 0111	1100 1111 0100	3991	3316
1101 1110 1100	1110 1110 1011	3564	3819

Step 7: Calculate the fitness of new individuals by fitness equation, as shown in Table 17.

Table 17. Calculate fitness for new individuals.

Child	X_1	X_2	X_1^2	X_2^2	Fitness (Chi) $= X_1^2 + X_2^2$
Ch1	4092	4047	16,744,464	16,378,209	33,122,673
Ch2	4095	4090	16,769,025	16,728,100	33,497,125
Ch3	4061	4069	16,491,721	16,556,761	33,048,482
Ch4	4044	3942	16,353,936	15,539,364	31,893,300
Ch5	3662	4054	13,410,244	16,434,916	29,845,160
Ch6	4058	3956	16,467,364	15,649,936	32,117,300
Ch7	3991	3316	15,928,081	10,995,856	26,923,937
Ch8	3564	3819	12,702,096	14,584,761	27,286,857

Step 8: Find the sum, average, and max between new individuals from Table 17 and the parents (Pi) from Table 14.

Table 18. Find sum, average, and max.

Ind.	X_1	X_2	X_1^2	X_2^2	Fitness (Ind.) $= X_1^2 + X_2^2$
M10	4091	4082	16,736,281	16,662,724	33,399,005
O1	4076	4043	16,613,776	16,345,849	32,959,625
M2	4044	4038	16,353,936	16,305,444	32,659,380
O2	3989	3940	15,912,121	15,523,600	31,435,721
M14	3674	4084	13,498,276	16,679,056	30,177,332
O3	3788	3846	14,348,944	14,791,716	29,140,660
M1	3770	3362	14,212,900	11,303,044	25,515,944
O4	3479	3812	12,103,441	14,531,344	26,634,785
Ch1	4092	4047	16,744,464	16,378,209	33,122,673
Ch2	4095	4090	16,769,025	16,728,100	33,497,125
Ch3	4061	4069	16,491,721	16,556,761	33,048,482
Ch4	4044	3942	16,353,936	15,539,364	31,893,300
Ch5	3662	4054	13,410,244	16,434,916	29,845,160
Ch6	4058	3956	16,467,364	15,649,936	32,117,300
Ch7	3991	3316	15,928,081	10,995,856	26,923,937
Ch8	3564	3819	12,702,096	14,584,761	27,286,857

Sum fitness = 489,657,286
Average fitness = 30,603,580
Max fitness = 33,497,125.

The new population is shown in Table 18. Table 19 just rename the (Ind.) column to (Mi) to show that it's the New *M* Population. That should generate *O* subpopulation from it.

Table 19. The new *M* population.

Ind.	X_1	X_2	X_1^2	X_2^2	Fitness (Ind.) = $X_1^2 + X_2^2$
M1	4091	4082	16,736,281	16,662,724	33,399,005
M2	4076	4043	16,613,776	16,345,849	32,959,625
M3	4044	4038	16,353,936	16,305,444	32,659,380
M4	3989	3940	15,912,121	15,523,600	31,435,721
M5	3674	4084	13,498,276	16,679,056	30,177,332
M6	3788	3846	14,348,944	14,791,716	29,140,660
M7	3770	3362	14,212,900	11,303,044	25,515,944
M8	3479	3812	12,103,441	14,531,344	26,634,785
M9	4092	4047	16,744,464	16,378,209	33,122,673
M10	4095	4090	16,769,025	16,728,100	33,497,125
M11	4061	4069	16,491,721	16,556,761	33,048,482
M12	4044	3942	16,353,936	15,539,364	31,893,300
M13	3662	4054	13,410,244	16,434,916	29,845,160
M14	4058	3956	16,467,364	15,649,936	32,117,300
M15	3991	3316	15,928,081	10,995,856	26,923,937
M16	3564	3819	12,702,096	14,584,761	27,286,857

Sum fitness = 489,657,286
Average fitness = 30,603,580
Max fitness = 33,497,125.

Thus, it can be noted from the results that the population has been improved and the efficiency of individuals is increased. Table 20 shows a comparison between the summation and the average and the optimal value for each iteration.

Table 20. Comparison between the results of 3 iterations.

Iteration N	Sum	Average	Max
Iteration 0	264,247,451	16,515,466	32,659,380
Iteration 1	398,272,331	24,892,021	33,399,005
Iteration 2	489,657,286	30,603,580	33,497,125

4 Conclusion

This study presents Learner based Performance algorithm. A case study is designed to describe the crossover and mutation processes that may confuse readers of this algorithm. In the experimental results, LBP proved its potential in improving and developing qualities and likewise finding the optimal solution. LPB improves and obtains better solutions iteratively. The authors recommend that this algorithm can be enhanced to reduce the processing time. In addition, changing the GA's crossover and mutation operations with other operations or mathematical equations from other competitive optimization algoirhtms might lead to a better performance of LBP.

References

1. Dokeroglu, T., Sevinc, E., Kucukyilmaz, T., Cosar, A.: A survey on new generation metaheuristic algorithms. Comput. Ind. Eng. **137**, 106040 (2019)
2. Hussain, K., Mohd Salleh, M.N., Cheng, S., Shi, Y.: Metaheuristic research: a comprehensive survey. Artif. Intell. Rev. **52**(4), 2191–2233 (2018). https://doi.org/10.1007/s10462-017-9605-z
3. Wong, W.K., Ming, C.I.: A review on metaheuristic algorithms: recent trends, benchmarking and applications. In: 2019 7th International Conference on Smart Computing & Communications (ICSCC), pp. 1–5. IEEE, June 2019
4. Rahman, C.M., Rashid, T.A.: A new evolutionary algorithm: learner performance based behavior algorithm. Egypt. Inform. J. **22**(2), 213–223 (2021)
5. Rahman, C.M., Rashid, T.A., Ahmed, A.M., Mirjalili, S.: Multi-objective learner performance-based behavior algorithm with five multi-objective real-world engineering problems. Neural Comput. Appl. **34**, 6307–6329 (2021). https://doi.org/10.1007/s00521-021-06811-z
6. Qayyum, A.: Student help-seeking attitudes and behaviors in a digital era. Int. J. Educ. Technol. High. Educ. **15**(1), 1–16 (2018). https://doi.org/10.1186/s41239-018-0100-7
7. Chew, S.L.: Improving classroom performance by challenging student misconceptions about learning. Association for Psychological Science - APS (2010). https://www.psychologicalscience.org/observer/improving-classroom-performance-by-challenging-student-misconceptions-about-learning. Accessed 10 Feb 2022
8. Cao, L., Nietfeld, J.L.: College students' metacognitive awareness of difficulties in learning the class content does not automatically lead to adjustment of study strategies. Aust. J. Educ. Dev. Psychol. (2006). https://eric.ed.gov/?id=EJ815620. Accessed 10 Feb 2022

Hybrid Model for Predicting Educational Use of Mobile Cloud Computing Services in Higher Education

Muhammad Burhan[1], Razwan Mohmed Salah[2], Sruja l Patel[3], Syed Altaf[3], Ali A. Alwan[4(✉)], and Shayma Ismail Ali[5]

[1] Study Group Australia, Sydney, Australia
[2] The University of Duhok, Duhok, KRG, Iraq
razwan.mayi@uod.au
[3] Kent Institute Australia, Sydney, Australia
{srujal.patel,syed.altaf}@kent.edu.au
[4] Ramapo College of New Jersey, Mahwah, NJ, USA
aaljuboo@ramapo.edu
[5] Cihan University, Duhok, KRG, Iraq
shayma.ali@duhokcihan.edu.krd

Abstract. In the recent decade, there has been growing interest towards exploring research opportunities in the higher education sector of technology. This interest comes from the immense amount of information related to education that can be exploited using IT. Adopting technology in higher education has been proved very beneficial and resulted in many successes. However, it is yet to investigate the negative impact of technology adoption in higher education. This paper attempts to discuss the works related to the predictive modelling problem that deals with the technology adoption factors. This paper also strives to examine and evaluate the current issues with technology adoption in higher education. The paper shows that there is a major gap in the previous research studies and most of the studies carried out only investigated some of the components of mobile cloud computing services in higher education, which make it inefficient for current researchers.

Keywords: Mobile cloud computing · Behavioural intentions · Technology adoption · Higher education · Prediction analysis

1 Introduction

Mobile Cloud Computing (MCC) is the subclass of cloud computing technology that exploits the distributed cloud computing paradigm to process and share data among the infrastructure, domain, and applications. The usage of MCC facilitates the process of data management such as data storage, and data transmission using mobile devices. In most situations, MCC provides solutions to both organizations and individuals. Adopting MCC introduces a lot of benefits to cloud computing. Due to its importance, technology integration in higher education is a must in most societies. It is also necessary to examine the negative challenges of technology adoption in higher education. However, that

K. Daimi and A. Al Sadoon (Eds.): ICR 2022, AISC 1431, pp. 483–489, 2022.
https://doi.org/10.1007/978-3-031-14054-9_44

requires a reliable prediction model which leads to producing an accurate assessment of the user intentions towards technology adoption in higher education. The proposed model encompasses three main components, namely: prediction, adoption motivators and future intention of technology adoption based on the adoption effects.

This research paper emphasizes on discussing numerous cloud models such as software and infrastructure as service models to be used for various purposes [1]. MCC has been considered a practical solution, offering its services at the higher education level. Despite the numerous benefits of mobile cloud computing, however, it has several limitations as well, such as energy efficiency and large computational strength. However, it is issues of data privacy and security that stop many from choosing to adopt the cloud as a platform to run their businesses [2]. These limitations impose serious challenges when deciding on the adoption of MCC. This research paper aims at analysing a group of well-known prediction modelling techniques, using machine learning or classical SEM-based to predict both the positive and negative aspects of adopting mobile cloud computing services from the user perspective in higher education.

2 Literature Review

Numerous aspects affecting technology adoption such as information storage, sharing and application were analysed in the previous papers. This section concentrates on studying and examining these previous studies. The paper identifies numerous variables and factors that affect the adoption of technology in education which are directly linked with the prediction analysis.

The work in [3] proposed a model which uses a comparative analysis based on proposed models of research competing models to learn the adoption of cloud computing effects. The proposed models help to understand the factors that affect the aspects of cloud computing adoption [3]. The work contributed by [4] investigates the relationship between perceived usefulness and expectation for knowledge management. The study also argued that education and training and innovativeness are highly correlated with ease-of-use perceptions [4]. The work contributed in [5] developed and tested a model that predicts the impact of mobile cloud computing adoption determinants [5].

The work contributed in [6] concentrates on the validation of a proposed model which is for the prediction of technology continuation. The proposed model has been tested in a limited environment which was the only limitation in its validation of it [6, 7]. Lastly, the work contributed in [8] proposed a unified model by combining six theoretical models and presenting the combination of the factors from all six theories.

2.1 Key Factors in the Adoption of Technology

Mobile cloud computing is used at both individual and organization levels. For example, the work introduced in [9] applied the UTATU (unified theory of Acceptance and Use of Technology). Results of their work suggested that key predictors are effort expectancy, social influence, performance expectancy and social adoption for the determination of behavioural intentions [9].

2.2 Prediction Theories, Frameworks

Numerous works extended or used the existing theories such as TAM through surveys but these theories are limited because they can't be generalized specifically. To solve this issue numerous researchers have used the extended version of these theories, [10].

2.3 Modelling Adoption Intention

Various studies have worked on the relationship of information sharing service models. These researches show the significance of information and system quality [9]. The work reported in [11] focuses on the services provided by the technology. Results suggested that irrespective of the lower cost of the technology, information sharing hardware requires continuous maintenance [11].

2.4 Continue Intention of Technology

Substantial theoretical works had included continuance intention such as information sharing continuance [12] and after adoption usage of technology. Researchers have used prior theories such as the theory of planned behaviour (TPB), which explains the user's behaviours and intentions to use IT services [7].

3 Proposed MMC Taxonomy

The prediction techniques are based on the variables affecting the adoption of MCC in education. This enhances our knowledge related to different variables' effects on adoption and user's intuitions.

3.1 Hybrid Model Prediction

Numerous techniques were analysed in this research. Prediction techniques considered in this study are of two types, namely machine learning techniques and classical SEM-based approach. These models include data mining and learning techniques as well as a comparative analysis of previous research.

3.2 Technology Adoption and Continued Intention of Technology Use in Education

The second component of the suggested taxonomy is technology adoption. In this research, technology adoption was based on three main features. Behavioural Intentions, Business Performance and Cloud Usefulness.

The aim of the continued intention of the technology component is to provide enough evidence to support the technology adoption. This is based on adoption intentions, usage intentions and demographic effects (Fig. 1).

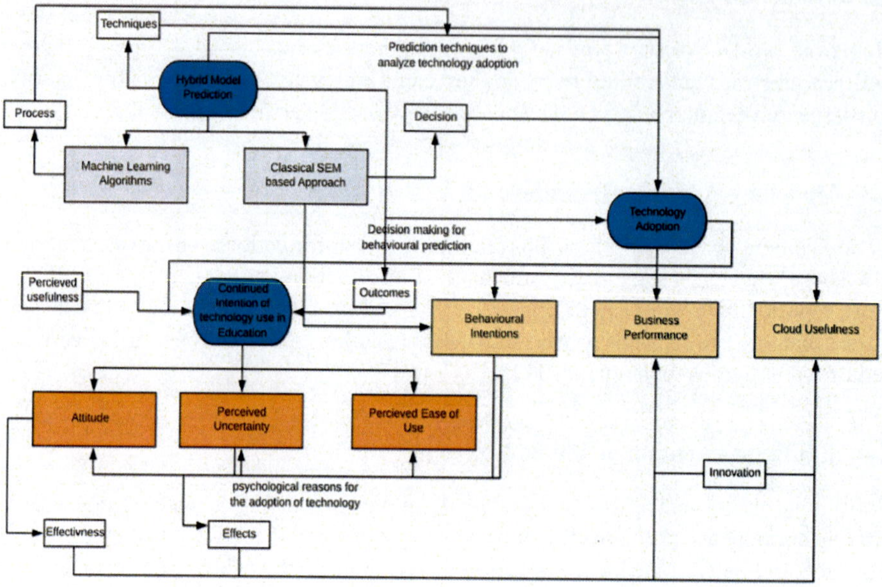

Fig. 1. Proposed MMC taxonomy components and their relationships

4 System Classification

Publications included in this study described an adoption technique for the use of MCC technology in education, even if they focused on only one aspect. Table 1 presents the details of the evaluation of the system components to understand the previous works

Table 1. Evaluation of system components

Ref.	Prediction		Technology Adoption			Continued Intention of Technology use in Education		
	Machine Learning	Classical SEM	Behavioural Intentions	Business Performance	Cloud Usefulness	Attitude	Perceived Uncertainty	Ease of Use
[11]	✗	✗	✗	Useful business solutions	Enhanced computing resources	✗	✗	Better resource management.
[2]	Kaiser-Meyer-Olkin (KMO)	Factor Analysis and Cronbach's alpha	Monitoring	Information	Social Network Services	Privacy and security concerns	Uncertainty Risk	Information symmetry
[9]	✗	✓	Facilitation conditions	Behavioural intentions	Effort Expectancy	Social Influence	Performance Expectancy	Facilitation conditions
[5]	Neural Network modelling (Multilayer perception)	✓	Social Influence	Resource sharing	Perceived usefulness	Collaboration	Demographic variables	Perceived Enjoyment
[6]	Control Theory and QN Model	Statistical analysis techniques	✗	Working environment		Enjoyment/ Perception	Computer self-efficacy	Perceived effectiveness
[8]	T-Test, Reliability	✓	Behavioural control	Ease of use	Application service quality	Relative Advantages	Voluntariness compatibility	PEOU, PU, PP

carried out. From the table, it is obvious that no attention has been paid to analysing the prediction of the user intentions to use MCC.

5 System Components Validation and Evaluation

Table 2. Validation of system components

Ref.	Application Area	Component Validation	Components Evaluation	Study Criteria	Considered Parameters	Adopted Methodology
[11]	Mobile cloud computing issues and challenges	Cloud architecture	Cloud applications	Adoption techniques	MCC effecetivness and efficency	Survey
[2]	Mobile cloud computing implications	Adoption of MCC	Computation offloading	comparative analysis using tables and graphs	Data and Computation Offloading	Machine Learning and Classical SEM Theory
[9]	MCC education adoption at tertiary level	Use Behaviours	Model Evaluation	Seven Point Likert scale	PE, EE, SI, FC, PBC, BI	SEM
[5]	Education	Adoption Intention	Model Evaluation	Hypothesis testing using Hybrid modelling	SI, PU, PE, RS, C, UI, BI,	Hybrid Modeling
[6]	E-Learning	Technology Acceptance in Education	Research Hypothesis evaluation	Survey Analysis using SPSS	Continue intention	Hybrid Modeling
[8]	Classroom	Students BI	United Model of Behavioural Intentions	Chi-squared statistics	ATT, CP, CSE, OSE, CSQ, PBC, PEOU, PP, PU, RD, SN, ASQ, TRI, VIS, VOL	Hybrid Modeling

ATT: attitude; CP: compatibility; CSE: computer self-efficacy; BI: behavioural intention; OSE: cloud self-efficacy; CSQ: cloud service quality; PBC: perceived behaviour control; PEOU: perceived ease of use; PP: perceived playfulness; PU: perceived usefulness; RD: result demonstration; SN: subjective norm; ASQ: application service quality; TRI: trialability; VIS: visibility; VOL: voluntariness, UB: User behaviour.

In determining the most relevant factors of an MCC system, we found the components that needed to be evaluated and validated to see if there is any added value in using the system. Table 2 summarizes these validations and evaluations of the system components for the previous approaches considered in this work.

6 Discussion

This section discusses the components of the proposed taxonomy. From the literature review, we have reviewed a few components and subcomponents which were considered by some researchers in MCC adoption in education. These components are related to the proposed taxonomy.

A. **Prediction (Pre-analysis validation of Input)**

In this research paper, selected journals have discussed at least one of two prediction techniques of hybrid modelling. Pre-analysis validation of data inputs was considered by a few researchers but not all. Pre-analysis validation is an important aspect of prediction because it provides the support for accurate data analysis and validation. Normally this is done using Cronbach's Alpha which describes the validity of selected data samples.

B. **Adoption (Psychological Factors)**

Adoption of MCC in education is dependent upon numerous such as self-efficacy, perceived network externalities and subjective norms. Subjective norms include the social influence which is a salient social referent. Adoption intention requires these psychological factors in the prediction to provide strong results. The work contributed in [13] has included these factors in its modelling due to which the prediction modelling shows a strong result for adoption intentions.

C. **Continue Intentions (Perceived usefulness)**

Technology adoption is only valid if it is used continuously after the adoption. This is dependent upon sub-components of knowledge sharing, storage and discovery or creation. These sub-components were not discussed by many researchers. As discussed by the work introduced in [4], the proposed model that perceived usefulness is linked with PEOU and Attitude which led to continued use of intentions.

D. **Limitation for the adoption of MCC:** Conducted surveys, tested hypotheses and proposed models were mostly tested on the professionals, not on the generic audience which could thus raise numerous problems such as the audience was aware of technology so limitations were ignored.

E. **Hybrid Modelling** minimizes the error chances with the best prediction results but is not adopted by numerous publications because complex mathematical calculations and error chances are high.

F. **Prediction Motivators** are not just limited to a few factors. Every selected study has included a few as it is not realistically possible to consider every factor. The work contributed by [12] discusses the delay and financial cost factors that were not adopted by most of the researchers but have a strong impact on the adoption of mobile cloud computing.

G. **Continued Intentions** are linked with the technology risk and adoption motivators. These risk factors should be adopted by every researcher but only [2] and [13] discussed security, IT and perceived adoption risk in their research. This factor wasn't included in the sub-components of the continued intention but is important for the validation of the adoption of MCC in education. Prediction of adoption leads to continued intentions of MCC adoption, but this requires a real-time modelling implementation, and this requires more study as a separate component.

Lack of sampling size and feeding of non-validated data to prediction models were the factors not considered by numerous researchers. However, we believe this poses a strong impact on the validation of the system and enhances the validation of the results. Similarly, in adoption factors, psychological factors were not a choice of numerous researchers in their proposed models but adoption intentions and motivators are somehow dependent on these as it provides a helpful understanding of the user's intentions and supports the behavioural intentions. Technology is only validated after its continued use and usefulness require real-time implementation results. Prediction of adoption leads to continue intention of MCC adoption, but this requires a real-time modelling implementation, and this requires more study as a separate component.

7 Conclusion

This study discusses the prediction modelling used to predict the factors that affect MCC adoption in higher education. Machine learning algorithms were analysed with existing structural equation modelling theories and then used for the prediction of adoption effects of MCC adoption. This study analysed the existing study, proposed a taxonomy based on the literature review, and defined the components of this study for classification, verification and validation. The findings share the factors required for the adoption of mobile cloud computing and its continued intention of usage in the discussed domain. Lastly, the proposed taxonomy provides an effective classification of mobile cloud computing services applications in the higher education domain to develop efficient and reliable platforms for higher education services.

References

1. Abdo, J.B., Demerjian, J.: Evaluation of mobile cloud architectures. Pervasive Mob. Comput. **39**, 284–303 (2017)
2. Akherfi, K., Gerndt, M., Harroud, H.: Mobile cloud computing for computation offloading: Issues and challenges. Appl. Comput. Inf. **14**, 1–16 (2018)
3. Shaukat, K., Hassan, M. U.: Cloud security through encryption techniques. Transylvanian Rev. **1** (2017)
4. Arpaci, I.: Antecedents and consequences of cloud computing adoption in education to achieve knowledge management. Comput. Hum. Behav. **70**, 382–390 (2017)
5. Sharma, S.K., Al-Badi, A.H., Govindaluri, S.M., Al-Kharusi, M.H.: Predicting motivators of cloud computing adoption: a developing country perspective. Comput. Hum. Behav. **62**, 61–69 (2016)
6. Lew, S.-L., Lau, S.-H., Leow, M.-C.: Usability factors predicting continuance of intention to use cloud e-learning application. Heliyon **5**, e01788 (2019)
7. Gan, C.L., Balakrishnan, V.: Mobile technology in the classroom: what drives student-lecturer interactions? Int. J. Hum.-Comput. Interact. **34**, 666–679 (2018)
8. Shiau, W.-L., Chau, P.Y.: Understanding behavioral intention to use a cloud computing classroom: a multiple model comparison approach. Inf. Manag. **53**, 355–365 (2016)
9. Amin, M.K., Rahman, M.A., Khan, T., Karim, M.T.: Investigating students' adoption and usage behavior of educational technology (EduTech) at tertiary level (PLS-SEM Approach). AIUB J. Sci. Eng. (AJSE) **17**, 25–30 (2018)
10. Khalilzadeh, J., Ozturk, A.B., Bilgihan, A.: Security-related factors in extended UTAUT model for NFC based mobile payment in the restaurant industry. Comput. Hum. Behav. **70**, 460–474 (2017)
11. Noor, T.H., Zeadally, S., Alfazi, A., Sheng, Q.Z.: Mobile cloud computing: Challenges and future research directions. J. Netw. Comput. Appl. **115**, 70–85 (2018)
12. Haghighi, V., Moayedian, N.S.: An offloading strategy in mobile cloud computing considering energy and delay constraints. IEEE Access **6**, 11849–11861 (2018)
13. Priyadarshinee, P., Raut, R.D., Jha, M.K., Gardas, B.B.: Understanding and predicting the determinants of cloud computing adoption: a two staged hybrid SEM-Neural networks approach. Comput. Hum. Behav. **76**, 341–362 (2017)

Data Analytics on eXtended Reality (XR) for Pedagogy Education: Educators' Awareness for the Future of Education in Smart Cities

Eleni Mangina[1(✉)], Georgia Psyrra[1], Thomas Phelan[1], and Michael Schwaiger[2]

[1] School of Computer Science, University College Dublin, Dublin, Ireland
{eleni.mangina,thomas.phelan}@ucd.ie,
georgia.psyrra@ucdconnect.ie

[2] European Network for Transfer and Exploitation of EU Project Results–E.N.T.E.R., Graz, Austria
michael.schwaiger@enter-network.eu

Abstract. The future of education in smart cities is connected with the metaverse and eXtended Reality (XR) applications. Educators know so little or nothing about helpful digital learning opportunities because they never heard about them during their pedagogic studies. To rapidly change this, European educational institutions join forces in the Erasmus + XR4Ped project to provide answers to questions and help foster digitisation in higher education in general and promote XR-based Virtual Reality (VR), Augmented Reality (AR) and the combination and further extension of both to Extended Reality (XR) immersive learning in particular. This poster will present the results of the anonymous data provided through a qualitative online questionnaire, highlighting the differences of XR technologies' awareness in Europe.

Keywords: eXtended Reality · Smart cities · Education · Augmented Reality · Pedagogy

1 Introduction to XRforPED EU Project

XRforPed [1] European project fosters digitization in education in general and the promotion of XR-based immersive learning. One of the main objectives of this project has been the implementation of a quantitative online questionnaire survey within 200 European educators at all levels to obtain a clear picture about their awareness, experiences, demands and needs with regard to digital and immersive learning as well as their experiences and lessons learnt during the Covid-19 lockdowns.

The data set used for this analysis consist of responses given by European teachers/trainers to an XR-related questionnaire for Pedagogical Education. The questionnaire was translated into English, German and Slovenian, since these were representative of the consortium partners. The survey consisted of 23 questions regarding three main domains:

K. Daimi and A. Al Sadoon (Eds.): ICR 2022, AISC 1431, pp. 490–493, 2022.
https://doi.org/10.1007/978-3-031-14054-9_45

1. General characteristics like (gender, years of experience, country, and training)
2. Technology equipment of institutes during the pandemic
3. AR and VR technology awareness and interest.

Each question that is included in the questionnaire includes a set of sub questions, which will be the characteristics to be analyzed in this survey. Free response submissions and personally identifiable information have been removed from the results to protect the privacy of respondents. The survey involved **324 respondents from 26 different countries** in total: 80 Slovene speakers; 100 German speakers; and 144 English speakers. The participants completed the questionnaire between 26/10/2021 and 2022/02/10.

Based on Eurostat statistics [2], 5.8 million people worked as school teachers in European Union in 2017. These are teachers who work at primary through to upper secondary level. Considering these statistics, we assume that the sample of educators (school and higher education) in EU would not be higher that 10 million people. Using the SurveyMonkey Sample size calculator [3], a sample of 273 participants in a population of 10 million people would be capable for conclusions based on 90% Confidence Level and 5% Margin Error. In conclusion the sample of 324 respondents who participated in the survey can be considered enough for accurate results on a statistical analysis based on 90% Confidence Level and 5% Margin Error. The results' findings provide the specific level of educators' awareness on XR applications, which is crucial for the future applications [4].

2 Participants' Profile

Most of participants were female (60.80%). Male participants were 36.11% of the sample while the percentages of non-binary/genderqueer are low. Additionally, most of participants range from 31 to 60 years old. Regarding the level/area of participants' main teaching activity, the 5 most common are: Higher education (42.28%), High school (18.52%), Secondary school (16.36%), Primary school (13.89%) and Vocational education and training (VET) (12.35%). Fewer respondents teach on Preschool, General adult education, Social pedagogy or other areas/levels of education.

3 Discussion

Within this poster the following results will be presented in graphs:

- Most of participants (87.7%) agree with the statement: "Remote learning increases loneliness". Only some teachers (8.6%) disagree with this statement, while less respondents (3.7%) did not answer the question.
- Participants tend to agree that: "Learners also want to be taught digitally/remote to a certain extent in the future". However, a significant number of participants tend to disagree.
- The level of AR awareness was found somewhere in between of VR and XR technologies and participants did not reveal a significant difference in the levels of AR awareness.

- In terms of the number of times that respondents have tested AR/VR/XR technologies in the past, the percentages revealed that they have not used such technologies a lot. In more detail: Half of respondents (50.92%) have never used AR/VR/XR technologies and 1/4 have used such technologies up to 3 times.
- Most of participants (90.43%) have not used VR/AR/XR technologies in their own teaching (Fig. 1).

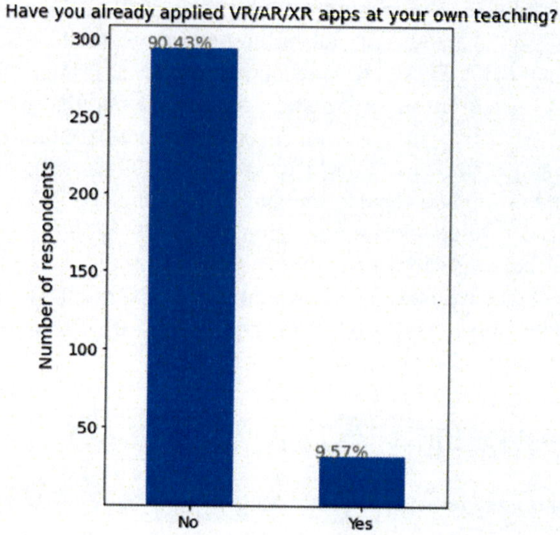

Fig. 1. How many educators have applied AR/VR/XR in their own teaching?

4 Conclusions

In October 2021, to mark World Teachers Day, the EU has launched a new online tool for teachers in the EU and beyond to reflect on how they use digital technologies in their teaching activities [5]. Within the Digital Education Action Plan (2021–2027) the challenges and opportunities of the COVID-19 pandemic, which has led to the unprecedented use of technology for education, had led to the increased need for immersive education. The data analysis of the survey described in this poster, focused on the readiness of the educators for XR applications in education, which revealed the lack of expertise and training for the teachers at all levels, given the urgent need for availability of an XR marketplace and open-source authoring toolkits. It is absolutely necessary to tackle teachers' XR digital skills for our future smart cities' educational systems.

Acknowledgement. The publication has been supported by the European Union's Horizon 2020 Research and Innovation program under grant agreement No 856533, project ARETE and data collected through the project XRforPED: 2020–1-SI01-KA226-HE-093633.

References

1. XRforPED project homepage. https://www.xr4ped.eu/. Accessed 17 Apr 2022
2. Eurostat homepage. https://ec.europa.eu/eurostat/web/products-eurostat-news/-/edn-20191004-1. Accessed 01 Apr 2022
3. SurveyMonkey homepage. https://www.surveymonkey.com/mp/sample-size-calculator/. Accessed 01 Apr 2022
4. Roizin, E., Wang, M.: X-Reality (XR) and immersive learning: theories, use cases, and future development. In: 2021 IEEE International Conference on Engineering, Technology & Education (TALE), pp. 751–754 (2021). https://doi.org/10.1109/TALE52509.2021.9678595
5. SelfieForTeachers. https://ec.europa.eu/commission/presscorner/detail/en/IP_21_4964. Accessed 25 Apr 2022

Author Index

K. Daimi and A. Al Sadoon (Eds.): ICR 2022, AISC 1431, pp. 495–497, 2022.
https://doi.org/10.1007/978-3-031-14054-9